Carbohydrate Chemistry

Proven Synthetic Methods

Volume 1

Carbohydrate Chemistry: Proven Synthetic Methods

Series Editor: Pavol Kováč

National Institutes of Health, Bethesda, Maryland, USA

Carbohydrate Chemistry: Proven Synthetic Methods, Volume 1, by Pavol Kováč

Carbohydrate Chemistry | Proven Synthetic Methods Series

Carbohydrate Chemistry

Proven Synthetic Methods

Volume 1

Edited by
Pavol Kováč

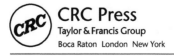

CRC Press
Taylor & Francis Group
Boca Raton London New York

CRC Press is an imprint of the
Taylor & Francis Group, an **informa** business

CRC Press
Taylor & Francis Group
6000 Broken Sound Parkway NW, Suite 300
Boca Raton, FL 33487-2742

First issued in paperback 2019

© 2012 by Taylor and Francis Group, LLC
CRC Press is an imprint of Taylor & Francis Group, an Informa business

No claim to original U.S. Government works

ISBN-13: 978-1-4398-6689-4 (hbk)
ISBN-13: 978-0-367-24680-8 (pbk)

Library of Congress Cataloging-in-Publication Data

Carbohydrate chemistry : proven synthetic methods / edited by Pavol Kovac.
      p. cm.
    ISBN 978-1-4398-6689-4 (hardcover : alk. paper)
    1. Carbohydrates--Synthesis. I. Kovác, Pavol, 1938- II. Title.

QD322.S95C37 2011
547'.27--dc22   2011010495

**Visit the Taylor & Francis Web site at
http://www.taylorandfrancis.com**

**and the CRC Press Web site at
http://www.crcpress.com**

This series is dedicated to Sir John W. Cornforth, the 1975 Nobel Prize winner in chemistry, who was the first to publicly criticize the unfortunate trend in chemical synthesis, which he described as "pouring a large volume of unpurified sewage into the chemical literature."[1]

1. Cornforth, J. W. *Austr. J. Chem.* 1993, *46*, 157–170.

Contents

Foreword by Derek Horton xiii
Foreword by Paul Kosma xv
Foreword by Bert Fraser-Reid xvii
Introduction xix
Contributors xxiii

PART I   Synthetic Methods

Chapter 1   Acetolysis of 6-Deoxysugars Controlled by
Armed–Disarmed Effect 3

*Emiliano Bedini, Luigi Cirillo, Ian Cumpstey, and
Michelangelo Parrilli*

Chapter 2   NaH/Im₂SO₂-Mediated Preparation of Hex-2- and
Hex-3-Enopyranoside Enol Ethers 11

*Emanuele Attolino, Giorgio Catelani, Felicia D'Andrea,
Lorenzo Guazzelli, and Marie-Christine Scherrmann*

Chapter 3   Enhancement of the Rate of Purdie Methylation by
Me₂S Catalysis 27

Shujie Hou, Thomas Ziegler, and Pavol Kováč

Chapter 4   Synthesis of Oligosaccharides by Preactivation-Based
Chemoselective Glycosylation of Thioglycosyl Donors 43

*Zhen Wang, Gilbert Wasonga, Benjamin M. Swarts,
and Xuefei Huang*

Chapter 5   The Use of Hypophosphorous Acid in Radical Chain
Deoxygenation of Carbohydrates 53

Karsten Krohn, Ivan Shuklov, Ishtiaq Ahmed, and Alice Voss

Chapter 6   Diphenylsulfoxide-Trifluoromethanesulfonic Anhydride: A
Potent Activator for Thioglycosides 67

*Jeroen D.C. Codée, Thomas J. Boltje,
and Gijsbert A. van der Marel*

Chapter 7 Preparation of Glycosyl Chlorides from Glycopyranoses/
Glycofuranoses under Mild Conditions 73

*Chih-Wei Chang, Chin-Sheng Chao, Chang-Ching Lin, and
Kwok-Kong T. Mong*

Chapter 8 *C*-Glycosylation Starting from Unprotected *O*-Glycosides 83

*Barbara La Ferla, Laura Cipolla, Wouter Hogendorf, and
Francesco Nicotra*

Chapter 9 Palladium-Catalyzed Sonogashira Coupling on *p*-Iodophenyl
α-D-Mannopyranoside 91

Tze Chieh Shiao, Jacques Rodrigue, and Mohamed Touaibia

Chapter 10 Synthesis by "Click Chemistry" of an α-D-Mannopyranoside
Having a 1,4-Disubstituted Triazole as Aglycone 95

Tze Chieh Shiao, Denis Giguère, and Mohamed Touaibia

Chapter 11 Synthesis of Methyl Glycuronates by Chemo- and
Regioselective TEMPO/BAIB-Oxidation 99

*Marthe T.C. Walvoort, Deepak Sail, Gijsbert A. van der Marel,
and Jeroen D.C. Codée*

Chapter 12 Synthesis of Sugar Nucleotides: A Phosphoramidite Approach 107

*Henrik Gold, Karine Descroix, Jeroen D.C. Codée, and
Gijsbert A. van der Marel*

Chapter 13 Conversion of *N*-2,2,2-Trichloroethoxycarbonyl-Protected
2-Aminoglycosides into *N*-Alkylated 2,3-*N,O*-Carbonyl
Glycosides 113

Thomas Honer, Siegfried Förster, and Thomas Ziegler

Chapter 14 TIBAL-Induced Rearrangement: Synthesis of *gem*-
Difluorocarbagalactose.. 129

*João Sardinha, Amélia Pilar Rauter, Matthieu Sollogoub, and
Yves Bleriot*

Chapter 15 Pyranose-Fused Butenolides: An Expedient Preparation from
Furanose Synthons 137

Nuno M. Xavier, Sebastian Kopitzki, and Amélia Pilar Rauter

Chapter 16 Glycal Dimerization with High Diastereoselectivity 159

Andreas H. Franz, Paul H. Gross, and Katja Michael

Chapter 17 Regioselective Debenzylation of *C*-Glycosylpropene 167

Laura Cipolla, Barbara La Ferla, Amélia Pilar Rauter, and Francesco Nicotra

Chapter 18 Synthesis of Azido-Functionalized Carbohydrates for the
Design of Glycoconjugates 175

Samy Cecioni, Mehdi Almant, Jean-Pierre Praly, and Sébastien Vidal

Chapter 19 Synthesis of Thioglycosides and Thioimidates from Glycosyl
Halides 181

Archana R. Parameswar, Daniel Mueller, Lin Liu, Cristina De Meo, and Alexei V. Demchenko

Chapter 20 Synthesis of Thioglycosides and Thioimidates from Peracetates 187

Archana R. Parameswar, Akihiro Imamura, and Alexei V. Demchenko

PART II   Synthetic Intermediates

Chapter 21 2-Acetamido-4,6-*O*-Benzylidene-2-Deoxy-D-Glucopyranose 199

Sergey S. Pertel, Sergey A. Gunchak, Elena S. Kakayan, Vasily Ya. Chirva, and Sébastien Vidal

Chapter 22 Synthesis of 1,3,4,6-Tetra-*O*-Acetyl-2-Azido-2-Deoxy-
α,β-D-Glucopyranose and 2-Azido-4,6-*O*-Benzylidene-2-
Deoxy-α,β-D-Glucopyranose 205

Rafael Ojeda, José Luis de Paz, Ricardo Lucas, Niels Reichardt, Lin Liu, and Manuel Martín-Lomas

Chapter 23 An Easy Access to 2,3,4,6-Tetra-*O*-Benzyl-D-Galactopyranose
and 2,3,6-Tri-*O*-Benzyl-D-Glucopyranose 213

Ian Cumpstey, Riccardo Cribiu, and Lorenzo Guazzelli

Chapter 24 Benzyl 2,3,6,2′,3′,6′-Hexa-*O*-Benzyl-β-Cellobioside 221

Deepak Sail, Paula Correia da Silva, and Pavol Kováč

Chapter 25 One-Step Syntheses of 1,2,3,5,6-Penta-*O*-Benzoyl-α,β-
D-Galactofuranose and 1,2,3,5-Tetra-*O*-Benzoyl-α,β-D-
Arabinofuranose.. 231

Carla Marino, Lucía Gandolfi-Donadío, Carola Gallo
Rodriguez, Yu Bai, and Rosa M. de Lederkremer

Chapter 26 Stereoselective Synthesis of α-*C*-Sialyl Compounds 239

Jin-Hwan Kim, Fei Huang, Sayaka Masuko, Deepak Sail,
and Robert J. Linhardt

Chapter 27 Synthesis of *O*-Acetylated *N*-Acetylneuraminic Acid Glycal 245

Nadezhda Y. Kulikova, Anna M. Shpirt, A. Chinarev, and
Leonid O. Kononov

Chapter 28 Substituted Benzyl Glycosides of *N*-Acetylneuraminic Acid 251

A. Chinarev, A.B. Tuzikov, A.I. Zinin, and N.V. Bovin

Chapter 29 Synthesis of 1,5-Di-*C*-Alkyl 1,5-Iminoxylitols Related to
1-Deoxynojirimycin.. 259

Vincent Chagnault, Philippe Compain, Olivier R. Martin, and
Jean-Bernard Behr

Chapter 30 Synthesis of 1,6-Anhydro-2,3,5-Tri-*O*-Benzoyl-α-D-
Galactofuranose 269

Sujit K. Sarkar, Ambar K. Choudhury, Ján Hirsch,
and Nirmolendu Roy

Chapter 31 Synthesis of Prop-2-Ynyl 2,3,4,6-Tetra-*O*-Acetyl-α-D-
Mannopyranoside 275

Yoann M. Chabre, Tze Chieh Shiao, Sébastien Vidal,
and René Roy

Chapter 32 Synthesis of 3-*C*-(2,3,4,6-Tetra-*O*-Acetyl-β-D-
Galactopyranosyl)prop-1-Ene... 279

Subhash Rauthu, Tze Chieh Shiao, Dominique Lafont,
and René Roy

Chapter 33 Synthesis of (*E*)-Methyl 4-(2,3,4,6-Tetra-*O*-Acetyl-β-D-
Galactopyranosyl)but-2-Enoate by Cross-Metathesis Reaction 285

Denis Giguère, Jacques Rodrigue, David Goyard, and René Roy

Chapter 34 Preparation of *O*-β-D-Galactopyranosylhydroxylamine 289

*Tze Chieh Shiao, Alex Papadopoulos, Olivier Renaudet, and
René Roy*

Chapter 35 Synthesis of 2,3,4,6-Tetra-*O*-Acetyl-1,5-Anhydro-D-*Lyxo*-Hex-
1-Enitol and Its Conversion into a Hex-3-Enopyranosid-2-Ulose
Analogue of Levoglucosenone 295

*Verónica E. Manzano, Evangelina Repetto, María Laura Uhrig,
Marek Baráth, and Oscar Varela*

Chapter 36 Efficient Synthesis of Methyl(Allyl 4-*O*-Acyl-2,3-Di-*O*-Benzyl-
β-D-Galactopyranosid)uronates from D-Galacturonic Acid 303

*Alice Voss, Navid Nemati, Hmayak Poghosyan,
Hans-Ulrich Endress, Andreas Krause, and Christian Vogel*

Chapter 37 Methyl(Ethyl 2,3,5-Tri-*O*-Benzoyl-1-Thio-α,β-D-
Galactofuranosid)uronate 327

*Ambar K. Choudhury, Dirk Michalik, Andreas Gottwald, and
Nirmolendu Roy*

Chapter 38 *p*-Tolyl 2,3,5-Tri-*O*-Benzoyl-1-Thio-α-D-Arabinofuranoside:
A Useful Thioglycoside Building Block in the Synthesis of
Oligoarabinofuranosides 341

Maju Joe, Yu Bai, Lucía Gandolfi-Donadío, and Todd L. Lowary

Chapter 39 Ethylene Dithioacetals of Common Hexoses 349

*Rui C. Pinto, Marta M. Andrade, Cécile Ouairy,
and Maria Teresa Barros*

Chapter 40 Preparation of 2,6-Anhydro-Aldose Tosylhydrazones 355

Marietta Tóth, László Somsák, and David Goyard

Chapter 41 Preparation of *Exo*-Glycals from (*C*-Glycopyranosyl)
formaldehyde Tosylhydrazones 367

Marietta Tóth, Sándor Kun, László Somsák, and David Goyard

Chapter 42   Synthesis of *O*-(6-Deoxy-α- and β-ʟ-Galactopyranosyl)
Hydroxylamines (α- and β-ʟ-Fucopyranosylhydroxylamines)......... 377

*Isabelle Bossu, Barbara Richichi, Pascal Dumy,
and Olivier Renaudet*

Chapter 43   Functionalization of Terminal Positions
of Sucrose—Part I: Synthesis of 2,3,3′,4,4′-Penta-*O*-
Benzylsucrose and Differentiation of the Terminal Positions
(1,6,6′)... 387

Mateusz Mach, A. Zawisza, B. Lewandowski, and S. Jarosz

Chapter 44   Functionalization of Terminal Positions of Sucrose—Part II:
Preparation of 1′,2,3,3′,4,4′-Hexa-*O*-Benzylsucrose and 6,6′-*Bis*-
O-(2-Hydroxyethyl)-1′,2,3,3′,4,4′-Hexa-*O*-Benzylsucrose............... 413

B. Lewandowski, A. Listkowski, K. Petrova, and S. Jarosz

Index... 431

Foreword

In long-established carbohydrate laboratories around the world there are to be found dog-eared and tattered, but precious, copies of early volumes of the "Methods in Carbohydrate Chemistry" series dating from the 1960s, which were edited by Whistler and Wolfrom. These volumes constitute a trove of valuable proven procedures for the synthesis of sugars and their derivatives and methods for their analysis. Most of the articles were written by the original investigators and include enough practical detail to enable a competent technician, rather than an experienced researcher, to repeat them.

Unfortunately the "Methods" series has long been out of print and is not accessible online. Consequently, investigators in the numerous new laboratories now focusing on carbohydrates can thank Paul Kováč for his initiative in launching a new series—*Carbohydrate Chemistry: Proven Synthetic Methods*. This promises to revive the concept of the "Methods" series and make it accessible to today's greatly expanded community of researchers working in the field of carbohydrate chemistry. Selecting from a broad international pool of respected contributors, this first volume features a wide range of general synthetic methods, together with procedures for particular useful intermediates, written with careful attention to reproducible experimental detail.

Research on carbohydrates was once the province of a handful of determined investigators bold enough to work in a "difficult" field of multifunctional compounds that often gave unpredictable results and afforded complex mixtures presenting formidable challenges in separation. The eventual characterization of pure products employed the classical criteria of combustion analysis, recrystallization to constant melting point, specific optical rotation, and later the revolutionary tool of NMR spectroscopy.

Nowadays, recognition of the great significance of carbohydrates in a multitude of important applications has led to a veritable explosion of research effort throughout the world, and with it a vast increase in the number of research reports in the literature. Target structures of great complexity have been attained by improved synthetic methods, coupled with advanced separation methodology and powerful spectroscopic tools.

However, along with this augmentation of the literature record there has been a regrettable trend toward the suppression of much experimental detail and a decrease in the quality of characterization of new compounds. Authors frequently resort to "preliminary communications" to stake a claim, but fail to follow up with publication of satisfactory experimental detail. Even when experimental procedures are recorded, many authors fail to provide sufficient information to permit another investigator to repeat the procedure, and frequently omit such traditional criteria of identity as elemental analysis, crystallinity, chiroptical data, and proof of homogeneity, to the point that the veracity of many claimed new structures may be called into question.

Such periodicals as *Organic Syntheses* and *Biochemical Preparations* have earned high respect because of their policy of inviting volunteer "checkers" to repeat submitted procedures in the laboratory and subsequently share coauthorship of the article. This practice, although difficult in today's grant-driven and targeted research, has nevertheless been adopted by Dr. Kováč in this series. Users of this and subsequent volumes can therefore take confidence in the reliability of the selected procedures. Authors of stature in the field attest to the validity of their contributions. The efforts of the independent checkers serve to verify that the methods are reproducible and that sufficient detail is given to the procedures and the thorough characterization of the products and intermediates described.

It is to be hoped that this series will provide a significant contribution to ongoing research with its trustworthy collection of procedures. It should help in preventing much wasteful hit-or-miss experimentation aimed at repeating the synthesis of compounds claimed in the literature, but offered with unjustifiably inflated yields and woefully inadequate characterization or procedural detail.

Dr. Kováč is to be commended upon his initiative to help today's researchers with reliable experimental access to key structures and synthetic methodology, and it is to be hoped that other investigators will be encouraged to submit new procedures and to serve as independent checkers.

Derek Horton
Emeritus Professor of Chemistry
Ohio State University

Foreword

The rapid and dynamic growth in the area of glycosciences has been based on modern techniques provided by genetics, enzymology, and advanced analytic instrumentation as well as on the key expertise and methodology developed by carbohydrate chemists, thereby linking organic chemistry with medicinal chemistry and glycobiology. The experience that has accumulated over the past years, however, has not always been fully transmitted to younger glycoscientists, and the general annotation of the field is seen as a rather challenging part of natural product chemistry. The inherent difficulties of carbohydrate chemistry, which are related to the presence of many stereogenic centers, multiple conformations, the need for stereoselective and high-yielding transformations of the anomeric center, a well-conceived choice of protecting groups, and elaborated analytical techniques, have further labeled the field for "dedicated experts only."

The novel series, *Carbohydrate Chemistry: Proven Synthetic Methods*, edited by Paul Kováč, aims at bridging this gap between potential newcomers and experienced glycochemists by providing a compendium of preparatively useful procedures that have been checked by independent research groups elsewhere. Thus, the main concept of this series follows other successful precedents in the field of general organic synthesis. The compilation of protocols covers both common and important analytical and synthetic methods as well as illustrates the synthesis of selected carbohydrate intermediates with general utility. The major focus is devoted to the proper practice of state-of-the-art preparative procedures, including the detailed description of the starting materials used, reaction setup, and work-up and isolation of products followed by identification and proof of purity of the final material (nota bene: regrettably, this requirement is not always fulfilled in many of the papers published nowadays). In addition, general information regarding convenience of operation and comments on safety issues have been addressed, where appropriate. Versatile and practically useful methods that have not received long-lasting recognition or that are difficult to access from their primary sources have also been revitalized and brought forward to the attention of the reader.

The reliability and reproducibility of the methods contained in this collection have been carefully established and will thus be highly valued and appreciated by the scientific community, in particular by postdoctoral staff as well as PhD students with less "hands-on" experience.

A series of this type has long been overdue, and Volume 1 should be followed by many future volumes in due course of time. One can safely expect that this series will receive a warm reception from organic chemists, biochemists, and glycoscientists and will be consulted many times during daily experimental benchwork.

Paul Kosma

Foreword

In setting up my initial research group at the University of Waterloo, one of my first purchases was Volumes I and II of "Methods in Carbohydrate Chemistry." Unsaturated sugars were central to our research plans, and triacetyl glucal was to be our starting material. The compound was either not commercially available or was beyond our economic means, so it had to be prepared. The literature procedure was brief and somewhat dense, but fortunately, the authors' version in "Methods" was highly detailed and user-friendly. Indeed, the "Methods" procedure was so reliable that Mark Yunker, our undergraduate intern, was able to mass-produce triacetyl glucal by using a plastic garbage pail as his reaction vessel. In order to efficiently stir the large amount of zinc required, he borrowed a stirrer from the university's swimming pool, facilitated by the fact that he was on the water polo team.

Today's carbohydrate literature with its myriad experiments in organic synthesis biology, biochemistry, etc., presents even more formidable obstacles. For this reason, the advent of the first volume of *Carbohydrate Chemistry: Proven Synthetic Methods* is timely, and these volumes will be seen as equivalent to *Organic Syntheses*. Now that glycoscience is attaining well-deserved prominence, a ready compilation that gives easy access to user-friendly methods not only for synthesis but also for biochemistry and biology will be welcome.

Dr. Kováč is to be warmly congratulated for his vision in championing this new series.

Bert Fraser-Reid

Introduction

The idea to start the *Carbohydrate Chemistry: Proven Synthetic Methods* series was conceived after many discussions with colleagues at conferences, symposia, and also privately, when the conversation almost invariably ended with joint complaints about "a lot of junk in the synthetic literature." What we primarily meant was that results of many papers on synthetic methods published recently could not be reproduced because of lack of data presented or inflated yields. In some publications, inclusion of data had been so carefully avoided that one could easily write such papers even without doing any work in the laboratory. Another pile of "junk" in the chemical literature is formed by a large number of new synthetic compounds that have not been properly characterized. The 1975 Nobel Prize winner in chemistry, Sir John Cornforth, obviously had not much regard for such substances when he referred to them very appropriately as "unpurified sewage."[1] Encouraged by Sir John, I had first written my commentaries[2,3] and later tried to find a sponsor for the publication of a series in preparative carbohydrate chemistry that would be similar to what already existed in general organic chemistry, and where the reproducibility of every protocol would be ensured by results of an independent "checker." My thanks are due to CRC Press/Taylor & Francis and, in particular, to Hilary Rowe (acquisition editor) and Jennifer Ahringer (project coordinator), who were instrumental in launching this series.

Reproducibility of synthetic work has always been of concern to chemists, and irreproducibility, which was recently eloquently criticized,[4] has become a serious problem. The days are long gone when authors included in their publications parallel preparative experiments to document reproducibility of their work (e.g., Ref. [5]) and when journals would publish such papers. Fierce competition for priority and funding often leads to hasty publication of synthetic work without optimizing reaction conditions and/or without proper characterization of products. It also often results in including in papers on synthesis unproven, unreliable experimental protocols. Responsibility for publishing manuscripts that describe such work lies mainly with editors of journals because it is the editors who have the final say as to what does and what does not get published. This state of affairs with publishing synthetic chemistry is alarming knowing that Guidelines for Authors, which most journals make available to authors, state clearly the strict requirements for acceptance of papers for publication. Among those, many journals that publish synthetic chemistry require that proof of purity be provided by correct analytical figures obtained by combustion analysis. That notwithstanding, editors often do not adhere to those requirements and routinely accept manuscripts that would not pass criteria of what once used to be considered acceptable standards. Those criteria are not something that may be arbitrarily changed. What is pure is pure, and what is not is not. Sadly, the current norm seems to be HRMS figures, which provide no clues about the purity and which even the clumsiest chemist can readily obtain. Authors and editors alike seem to have forgotten that it used to go without saying that reports of syntheses of new, simple, stable compounds had to either include combustion analysis figures as the criterion of purity or, in preliminary communications, a statement to that effect. With the ever-increasing number of individuals involved in organic synthesis, as well as with the exploding number of journals available for publication of synthetic work, it is virtually impossible to sort out laboratories or individuals whose work is reliable. With that in mind, I have ventured to start a series for publication of selected preparative procedures whose reliability has been verified by independent checkers. I have done so in the hope that a compilation of methods that have been checked would be of great value to the present and future generations of carbohydrate chemists, as has been the case with a revered, independent, now apparently defunct previous series in the field of carbohydrate chemistry.

I realize that by what I said above and what follows I may be stepping on some toes. If this sounds like I am trying to shake up the establishment a little, then this writing fulfilled its purpose, and I am doing this in the hope that the field of synthetic organic chemistry will benefit from it. The good work of contributors to the first volume of *Proven Synthetic Methods* and this Introduction is supposed to be a wake-up call to the community of synthetic organic chemists, which will have to police itself, lest the misguided, prevailing trend of executing and publishing organic chemistry might continue.

Now, when a group of dedicated carbohydrate chemists had put extra effort into making a volume of reliable synthetic protocols available to their peers, I was disturbed to see that the editor in chief of a major organic chemistry journal, which has been referred to as a "high-impact journal," has informed the potential contributors that his journal has softened its requirements for accepting papers for publication. One can surmise from the tone of the announcement that the editor was actually proud to make it known that as part of "ongoing efforts to streamline the publication process for authors," the journal has "made a significant change to the purity requirements for manuscripts submitted in 2009." While in the past the journal "required that the purity of all tested compounds should be not less than 98% and that documentation be provided as evidence of purity," the journal's revised policy requires that "tested compounds, whether synthesized or purchased, should possess a purity of not less than 95%." And as if the above were not shocking enough, the information continued as follows: "No documentation for purity is required in the manuscript." It is incredible that this can come from a journal that is highly relevant to the life sciences, where purity and proper characterization of chemicals is particularly important when such substances are used as probes or as drugs, lest the effect of more potent minor impurity might be misinterpreted as that of the major component.

Even in the prevailing "publish or perish" atmosphere, it is hard to understand the obsession of authors with the desire to have their work published in the so-called high-impact journals when, judging by any standard, *what* is published is more important than *where*. The flaws of the system that grants the impact status to journals are obvious and well documented, as a simple Google search can quickly reveal. To all those examples found on Google of how the impact factor can be manipulated to go up without a valid reason, one could readily suggest another one: Soften the requirements for quality of work to be acceptable for publication. The impact factor is, essentially, calculated as a ratio of the number of citations over the number of papers published during a two-year period. It can be reasonably assumed that when the number of papers published—good or bad—increases, so does the number of citations. Taking that into consideration, lowering the stick that some journals use to categorize submissions as acceptable or not acceptable for publication becomes now quite understandable, although not condonable. The best proof of inadequacy of the concept of high-impact journals is the high impact of journals that publish review articles. The value of review articles is indisputable, but it is the *authors* who deserve the credit, since it is their work that made the high impact on science and not the *journals* that publish such articles. Journals that publish review articles get a disproportional number of citations and, consequently, readily win the status of high-impact factor journals mainly because readers take shortcuts and seek information in review articles instead of searching for it primarily in the original publications. It is actually the authors of valuable work and not the journals who should be given the high-impact factors. Should we respect Emil Fisher and Albert Einstein for their accomplishments and ideas that changed the world or glorify journals that published their work? The answer to this question should be a no-brainer. However, it is neither possible nor necessary to assign a numerical impact factor to authors. We cannot objectively rank authors either by number of papers or citations. Doing the former would encourage fragmentation of results, and if we were to do the latter, anybody could collect a lot of citations by publishing an idea that would be later proven wrong. The only objective method of evaluating the quality of any scientist's work would be the one based on discussions his or her peers have during coffee breaks at scientific meetings. It is there that conferees freely voice among themselves appreciations, or lack thereof, of the work of their colleagues. In this context, I cannot but express sadness over the nothing but profit-driven mushrooming of scientific journals. Just look how many more "Letters," "Natures," "Trends," and the like have been created during the last decade or two. Or should we, perhaps, cheer because that is supposed to reflect the ever-increasing volume of good science produced by the new generation of scientists? Hardly. Instead of contributing to the advancement of science, publishers of these offshoot journals have, in fact, done a great service to Parkinson, by confirming the validity of his law of scientific publishing: "The progress of science varies inversely with the number of scientific journals published," which is no longer funny.

In this high-impact-journal mania, it should not, perhaps, be surprising to see some unscrupulous editors prey on potentially gullible contributors for their new journals, which came into existence for no other than economical reasons. I can only guess how it resonated with hundreds of colleagues who received the same invitation to contribute as I did, but the following e-mail from the editor of a new journal came to me as a shock (I shall be kind here, and not name the editor or the journal): "WX Publishing recently announced the online publication of the first issue of YZ Publication, a new high-impact, peer-reviewed journal for the rapid publication of research in the XY Field." Reading this highly misleading, pathetic advertising is analogous to a "We are #1"-type desperate sales pitch by a used-car dealer. I could not resist and responded to the sender with a query: "Could you please explain how has it been determined that YZ Publication is a new *high-impact* journal when only one issue has been published?" I did not expect any answer because if I had been the sender of that note, I would have felt embarrassed and rather not responded.

However, there came a reply, and it addressed the issue in the following way: "At WZ Publishing, our aim when launching new journals is for them to be amongst the leading and highest-impact publications in the field. Our inclusion of the term 'high-impact' reflects our belief that amongst the articles published in the first issue and beyond will be work which the MN community will see as high-quality and thought-provoking." Well, I wish the new journal the impact they hope for. Nevertheless, as long as the scientific community requires that the content of a paper published in a respectable journal be based on solid scientific evidence supported by data and not *belief*, the same standards should be required of and maintained by the publishers and the editors. Just because one *believes* that one is a bird does not mean one actually can fly, and one should be careful or one may get hurt. Examples of the same go back to ancient mythology.

Volume 1 of *Carbohydrate Chemistry: Proven Synthetic Methods* is organized a little differently than similar, existing series. The most important part of each topic is, of course, the experimental protocol. In *Proven Synthetic Methods*, it often contains more experimental details and data than is normally found in full papers or communications on synthesis. In addition to numerical data, copies of 1D NMR spectra of compounds prepared are also included. These are presented at the end of each contribution to give readers an idea about the purity they can expect of the products described.

In addition to those I mentioned above, I should like to thank all authors who contributed to this volume, which made it possible to get this series started. My undiminished thanks are also due to all those who have acted as checkers, accepting thereby a great part of the responsibility for the reproducibility of protocols contained in this volume. The work of Dr. Amélia Pilar Rauter, who has proofread the carbohydrate nomenclature with the aid of Bernardo Herold and Gerry Moss, is hereby gratefully acknowledged.

It is commendable, and I highly appreciate it, that many contributors to this volume belong to the new generation of young carbohydrate chemists. This volume could have been even more valuable if many more laboratories known for producing credible work had participated, and I trust that they will do so when the future volumes of *Proven Synthetic Methods* will be in preparation.

Pavol Kováč
National Institutes of Health
Bethesda, Maryland

REFERENCES

1. Cornforth, J. W. *Austr. J. Chem.* 1993, *46*, 157–170.
2. Kováč, P. *Chem. Biodivers.* 2004, *1*, 606–608.
3. Kováč, P. *An Open Letter to the Community of Organic Chemists*; Colombo, G. P. and Ricci, S., Eds.; Nova Science Publishers, Hauppauge, NY, 2009, pp. 1–5.
4. Hudlický, T.; Wernerová, M. *Synlett* 2010, *18*, 2701–2707.
5. Zemplén, G.; Gerécs, A.; I, H. *Chem. Ber.* 1936, *69*, 1827–1829.

Contributors

Ishtiaq Ahmed
Department of Chemistry
University of Paderborn
Paderborn, Germany

Mehdi Almant
Laboratoire des Glucides
Institut de Chimie de Picardie
Université de Picardie Jules Verne
Amiens, France

Marta M. Andrade
Faculdade de Ciências e Tecnologia
Departamento de Química
Centro de Química Fina e Biotecnologia
Rede de Química e Tecnologia
Universidade Nova de Lisboa
Lisbon, Portugal

Emanuele Attolino
Dipartimento di Scienze Farmaceutiche
Università di Pisa
Pisa, Italy

Yu Bai
Alberta Ingenuity Centre for
    Carbohydrate Science

and

Department of Chemistry
Gunning-Lemieux Chemistry Centre
University of Alberta
Edmonton, Alberta, Canada

Marek Baráth
Slovak Academy of Sciences
Institute of Chemistry
Bratislava, Slovakia

Maria Teresa Barros
Faculdade de Ciências e Tecnologia
Departamento de Química
Centro de Química Fina e Biotecnologia
Rede de Química e Tecnologia
Universidade Nova de Lisboa
Lisbon, Portugal

Emiliano Bedini
Dipartimento di Chimica Organica e
    Biochimica
Università degli Studi di Napoli
Naples, Italy

Jean-Bernard Behr
Institut de Chimie Moléculaire de Reims
Center for Natural Resource Studies
Université de Reims-Champagne
    Ardennes
Reims, France

Yves Bleriot
Laboratoire de Synthèse et Réactivité
    des Substances Naturelles
Université de Poitiers
Poitiers, France

Thomas J. Boltje
Leiden Institute of Chemistry
Leiden University
Leiden, the Netherlands

Isabelle Bossu
Département de Chimie Moléculaire
Université Joseph Fourier
Grenoble, France

N.V. Bovin
Laboratory of Carbohydrates
Shemyakin and Ovchinnikov Institute
  of Bioorganic Chemistry
Russian Academy of Sciences
Moscow, Russia

Giorgio Catelani
Dipartimento di Scienze Farmaceutiche
Università di Pisa
Pisa, Italy

Samy Cecioni
Laboratoire de Chimie Organique
Institut de Chimie et Biochimie
  Moléculaires et Supramoléculaires
Villeurbanne, France

Yoann M. Chabre
Department of Chemistry
Université du Québec à Montréal
Montréal, Québec, Canada

Vincent Chagnault
Institut de Chimie Organique et
  Analytique
Center for Natural Resource Studies
Université d'Orléans
Orléans, France

Chih-Wei Chang
Department of Applied Chemistry
National Chiao Tung University
Hsinchu, Taiwan

Chin-Sheng Chao
Department of Applied Chemistry
National Chiao Tung University
Hsinchu, Taiwan

A. Chinarev
Laboratory of Carbohydrates
Shemyakin and Ovchinnikov Institute
  of Bioorganic Chemistry
Russian Academy of Sciences
Moscow, Russia

Vasily Ya. Chirva
Department of Organic and Biological
  Chemistry
Tavrida National V.I. Vernadsky
  University
Simferopol, Ukraine

Ambar K. Choudhury
Sami Laboratories Limited
Bangalore, India

Laura Cipolla
Department of Biotechnology and
  Biosciences
University of Milano-Bicocca
Milano, Italy

Luigi Cirillo
Dipartimento di Chimica Organica e
  Biochimica
Università degli Studi di Napoli
Naples, Italy

Jeroen D.C. Codée
Leiden Institute of Chemistry
Leiden University
Leiden, the Netherlands

Philippe Compain
Laboratoire de Synthèse Organique et
  Molécules Bioactives
European Center of Pharmaceutical
  Medicine
Université de Strasbourg
Strasbourg, France

Riccardo Cribiu
Arrhenius Laboratory
Department of Organic Chemistry
Stockholm University
Stockholm, Sweden

Ian Cumpstey
Arrhenius Laboratory
Department of Organic Chemistry
Stockholm University
Stockholm, Sweden

Felicia D'Andrea
Dipartimento di Scienze
  Farmaceutiche
Università di Pisa
Pisa, Italy

Alexei V. Demchenko
Department of Chemistry and
  Biochemistry
University of Missouri
Columbia, Missouri

Karine Descroix
School of Pharmacy
University of East Anglia
Norwich, United Kingdom

Pascal Dumy
Département de Chimie Moléculaire
Université Joseph Fourier
Grenoble, France

Hans-Ulrich Endress
Herbstreith & Fox KG Pectin-Fabriken
Neuenbuerg, Germany

Barbara La Ferla
Department of Biotechnology and
  Biosciences
University of Milano-Bicocca
Milano, Italy

Siegfried Förster
Institute of Organic Chemistry
University of Stuttgart
Stuttgart, Germany

Andreas H. Franz
Department of Chemistry
University of the Pacific
Stockton, California

Lucía Gandolfi-Donadío
Facultad de Ciencias Exactas y
  Naturales
Departamento de Química Orgánica
Centro de Investigaciones en Hidratos
  de Carbono
Universidad de Buenos Aires
Buenos Aires, Argentina

Denis Giguère
Department of Chemistry
Université du Québec à Montréal
Montréal, Quebec, Canada

Henrik Gold
Leiden Institute of Chemistry
Leiden University
Leiden, the Netherlands

Andreas Gottwald
Department of Chemistry
University of Rostock
Rostock, Germany

David Goyard
Laboratoire de Chimie Organique
Institut de Chimie et Biochimie
  Moléculaires et Supramoléculaires
Université Lyon
Villeurbanne, France

Paul H. Gross
Department of Chemistry
University of the Pacific
Stockton, California

Lorenzo Guazzelli
Dipartimento di Scienze Farmaceutiche
Università di Pisa
Pisa, Italy

Sergey A. Gunchak
Department of Organic and Biological
  Chemistry
Tavrida National V.I. Vernadsky
  University
Simferopol, Ukraine

Ján Hirsch
Institute of Chemistry
Slovak Academy of Sciences
Bratislava, Slovakia

Wouter Hogendorf
Faculty of Science
Leiden University
Leiden, the Netherlands

Thomas Honer
Institute of Organic Chemistry
University of Tuebingen
Tuebingen, Germany

Shujie Hou
National Institute of Diabetes and
    Digestive and Kidney Diseases
National Institutes of Health
Bethesda, Maryland

Fei Huang
Department of Chemistry and Chemical
    Biology
Center for Biotechnology and
    Interdisciplinary Studies
Rensselaer Polytechnic Institute
Troy, New York

Xuefei Huang
Department of Chemistry
Michigan State University
East Lansing, Michigan

Akihiro Imamura
Department of Chemistry and
    Biochemistry
University of Missouri
Columbia, Missouri

S. Jarosz
Polish Academy of Sciences
Institute of Organic Chemistry
Warsaw, Poland

Maju Joe
Alberta Ingenuity Centre for
    Carbohydrate Science

and

Department of Chemistry
Gunning-Lemieux Chemistry Centre
University of Alberta
Edmonton, Alberta, Canada

Elena S. Kakayan
Department of Organic and Biological
    Chemistry
Tavrida National V.I. Vernadsky
    University
Simferopol, Ukraine

Jin-Hwan Kim
Department of Chemistry and Chemical
    Biology
Center for Biotechnology and
    Interdisciplinary Studies
Rensselaer Polytechnic Institute
Troy, New York

Leonid O. Kononov
N.D. Zelinsky Institute of Organic
    Chemistry of the Russian Academy
    of Sciences
Moscow, Russia

Sebastian Kopitzki
Faculty of Sciences
Department of Chemistry
University of Hamburg
Hamburg, Germany

Pavol Kováč
National Institute of Diabetes and
    Digestive and Kidney Diseases
National Institutes of Health
Bethesda, Maryland

Andreas Krause
Institute of Organic Chemistry
Leibniz University Hannover
Hannover, Germany

Karsten Krohn
Department of Chemistry
University of Paderborn
Paderborn, Germany

Nadezhda Y. Kulikova
N.D. Zelinsky Institute of Organic
Chemistry of the Russian Academy
of Sciences
Moscow, Russia

Sándor Kun
Department of Organic Chemistry
University of Debrecen
Debrecen, Hungary

Dominique Lafont
Laboratoire de Chimie Organique
Institut de Chimie et Biochimie
Moléculaires et Supramoléculaires
Université Lyon
Villeurbanne, France

Rosa M. de Lederkremer
Facultad de Ciencias Exactas y
Naturales
Departamento de Química Orgánica
Centro de Investigaciones en Hidratos
de Carbono
Consejo Nacional de Investigaciones
Científicas y Técnicas
Universidad de Buenos Aires
Buenos Aires, Argentina

B. Lewandowski
Polish Academy of Sciences
Institute of Organic Chemistry
Warsaw, Poland

Chang-Ching Lin
Department of Chemistry
National Tsing Hua University
Hsinchu, Taiwan

Robert J. Linhardt
Department of Chemistry and Chemical
Biology
Center for Biotechnology and
Interdisciplinary Studies
Rensselaer Polytechnic Institute
Troy, New York

A. Listkowski
Polish Academy of Sciences
Institute of Organic Chemistry
Warsaw, Poland

Lin Liu
Department of Chemistry
Iowa State University
Ames, Iowa

Todd L. Lowary
Alberta Ingenuity Centre for
Carbohydrate Science

and

Department of Chemistry
Gunning-Lemieux Chemistry Centre
University of Alberta
Edmonton, Alberta, Canada

Ricardo Lucas
Instituto de Investigaciones Químicas
Centro de Investigaciones
Científicas "Isla de la Cartuja"
Seville, Spain

Mateusz Mach
Polish Academy of Sciences
Institute of Organic Chemistry
Warsaw, Poland

Verónica E. Manzano
Facultad de Ciencias Exactas y
  Naturales
Departamento de Química Orgánica
Centro de Investigaciones en Hidratos
  de Carbono
Consejo Nacional de Investigaciones
  Científicas y Técnicas
Universidad de Buenos Aires
Buenos Aires, Argentina

Gijsbert A. van der Marel
Leiden Institute of Chemistry
Leiden University
Leiden, the Netherlands

Carla Marino
Facultad de Ciencias Exactas y
  Naturales
Departamento de Química Orgánica
Centro de Investigaciones en Hidratos
  de Carbono
Consejo Nacional de Investigaciones
  Científicas y Técnicas
Universidad de Buenos Aires
Buenos Aires, Argentina

Olivier R. Martin
Institut de Chimie Organique et
  Analytique
Centre National de la Recherche
  Scientifique
Université d'Orléans
Orléans, France

Manuel Martín-Lomas
Department of Functional
  Nanomaterials
Centro de Investigacion Cooperativa en
  Biomateriales BiomaGUNE
Donostia-San Sebastian, Spain

Sayaka Masuko
Department of Chemistry and Chemical
  Biology
Rensselaer Polytechnic Institute
Center for Biotechnology and
  Interdisciplinary Studies
Troy, New York

Cristina De Meo
Department of Chemistry
Southern Illinois University
Edwardsville, Illinois

Katja Michael
Department of Chemistry
University of Texas
El Paso, Texas

Dirk Michalik
Leibniz Institute for Catalysis
University of Rostock
Rostock, Germany

Kwok-Kong T. Mong
Department of Applied Chemistry
National Chiao Tung University
Hsinchu, Taiwan

Daniel Mueller
Department of Chemistry
Southern Illinois University
Edwardsville, Illinois

Navid Nemati
Institute of Chemistry
University of Rostock
Rostock, Germany

and

Leibniz Institute for Catalysis at
  University Rostock
Berlin, Germany

Francesco Nicotra
Department of Biotechnology and
Biosciences
University of Milan Bicocca
Milan, Italy

Rafael Ojeda
Carbohydrate Group
Instituto de Investigaciones Químicas
Centro de Investigaciones
Científicas "Isla de la Cartuja"
Seville, Spain

Cécile Ouairy
Institut de Chimie des Substances
Naturelles
Centre de Recherche de Gif
Gif-sur-Yvette, France

Alex Papadopoulos
Department of Chemistry
Université du Québec à Montréal
Montréal, Québec, Canada

Archana R. Parameswar
Department of Chemistry and
Biochemistry
University of Missouri
St. Louis, Missouri

Michelangelo Parrilli
Dipartimento di Chimica Organica e
Biochimica
Università degli Studi di Napoli
Naples, Italy

José Luis de Paz
Instituto de Investigaciones Químicas
Centro de Investigaciones
Científicas "Isla de la Cartuja"
Seville, Spain

Sergey S. Pertel
Department of Organic and Biological
Chemistry
Taurida National V.I. Vernadsky
University
Simferopol, Ukraine

K. Petrova
Faculdade de Ciências e Tecnologia
Departamento de Química
Centro de Química Fina e Biotecnologia
Rede de Química e Tecnologia
Universidade Nova de Lisboa
Lisbon, Portugal

Rui C. Pinto
Faculdade de Ciências e Tecnologia
Departamento de Química
Centro de Química Fina e Biotecnologia
Rede de Química e Tecnologia
Universidade Nova de Lisboa
Lisbon, Portugal

Hmayak Poghosyan
Institute of Chemistry
University of Rostock
Rostock, Germany

Jean-Pierre Praly
Laboratoire de Chimie Organique
Institut de Chimie et Biochimie
Moléculaires et Supramoléculaires
Villeurbanne, France

Amélia Pilar Rauter
Faculdade de Ciências
Departamento de Química e
Bioquímica
Centro de Química e Bioquímica
Universidade de Lisboa
Lisbon, Portugal

Subhash Rauthu
Department of Chemistry
Université du Québec à Montréal
Montréal, Québec, Canada

Niels Reichardt
Department of Functional
  Nanomaterials
Centro de Investigacion Cooperativa en
  Biomateriales BiomaGUNE
Donostia-San Sebastian, Spain

Olivier Renaudet
Département de Chimie Moléculaire
Université Joseph Fourier
Grenoble, France

Evangelina Repetto
Facultad de Ciencias Exactas y
  Naturales
Departamento de Química Orgánica
Centro de Investigaciones en Hidratos
  de Carbono
Consejo Nacional de Investigaciones
  Científicas y Técnicas
Universidad de Buenos Aires
Buenos Aires, Argentina

Barbara Richichi
Dipartimento di Chimica Organica
Polo Scientifico e Tecnologico
Universita' degli Studi di Firenze
Florence, Italy

Jacques Rodrigue
Department of Chemistry
Université du Québec à Montréal
Montréal, Québec, Canada

Carola Gallo Rodriguez
Facultad de Ciencias Exactasy Naturales
Departamento de Química Orgánica
Centro de Investigaciones en Hidratos
  de Carbono
Consejo Nacional de Investigaciones
  Científicas y Técnicas
Universidad de Buenos Aires
Buenos Aires, Argentina

Nirmolendu Roy
Department of Biological Chemistry
Indian Association for the Cultivation
  of Science
Kolkata, India

René Roy
Department of Chemistry
Université du Québec à Montréal
Montréal, Québec, Canada

Deepak Sail
National Institute of Diabetes and
  Digestive and Kidney Diseases
National Institutes of Health
Bethesda, Maryland

João Sardinha
Faculdade de Ciências
Departamento de Química e
  Bioquímica
Centro de Química e Bioquímica
Universidade de Lisboa
Lisbon, Portugal

and

Glycochimie Organique Biologique et
  Supramoléculaire
Institut Parisien de Chimie
  Moléculaire
Université Pierre et Marie Curie
Université de Paris
Paris, France

Sujit K. Sarkar
Syngene International Limited
Bangalore, India

Marie-Christine Scherrmann
Institut de Chimie Moléculaire et des
  Matériaux d'Orsay
Laboratoire de Chimie des Procédes et
  des Substances Naturelles
Université Paris-Sud
Orsay, France

Tze Chieh Shiao
Department of Chemistry
Université du Québec à Montréal
Montréal, Québec, Canada

and

Department of Chemistry and
  Biochemistry
Université de Moncton
Moncton, New Brunswick, Canada

Anna M. Shpirt
N.D. Zelinsky Institute of Organic
  Chemistry of the Russian Academy
  of Sciences
Moscow, Russia

Ivan Shuklov
Leibnitz Institute for Catalysis
University of Rostock
Rostock, Germany

Paula Correia da Silva
Instituto Superior de Ciências da Saúde
  Egas Moniz
Universidade Nova de Lisboa
Lisbon, Portugal

Matthieu Sollogoub
Glycochimie Organique Biologique et
  Supramoléculaire
Institut Parisien de Chimie Moléculaire
Université Pierre et Marie Curie
Université de Paris
Paris, France

László Somsák
Department of Organic Chemistry
University of Debrecen
Debrecen, Hungary

Benjamin M. Swarts
Department of Chemistry
Wayne State University
Detroit, Michigan

Marietta Tóth
Department of Organic Chemistry
University of Debrecen
Debrecen, Hungary

Mohamed Touaibia
Department of Chemistry and
  Biochemistry
Université de Moncton
Moncton, New Brunswick, Canada

A.B. Tuzikov
Laboratory of Carbohydrates
Shemyakin and Ovchinnikov Institute
  of Bioorganic Chemistry
Russian Academy of Sciences
Moscow, Russia

María Laura Uhrig
Facultad de Ciencias Exactas y
  Naturales
Departamento de Química Orgánica
Centro de Investigaciones en Hidratos
  de Carbono
Consejo Nacional de Investigaciones
  Científicas y Técnicas
Universidad de Buenos Aires
Buenos Aires, Argentina

Oscar Varela
Facultad de Ciencias Exactas y
  Naturales
Departamento de Química Orgánica
Centro de Investigaciones en Hidratos
  de Carbono
Consejo Nacional de Investigaciones
  Científicas y Técnicas
Universidad de Buenos Aires
Buenos Aires, Argentina

Sébastien Vidal
Laboratoire de Chimie Organique
Institut de Chimie et Biochimie
  Moléculaires et Supramoléculaires
Université de Lyon
Villeurbanne, France

Christian Vogel
Institute of Chemistry
University of Rostock
Rostock, Germany

Alice Voss
Institute of Chemistry
University of Rostock
Rostock, Germany

Marthe T.C. Walvoort
Leiden Institute of Chemistry
Leiden University
Leiden, the Netherlands

Zhen Wang
Department of Chemistry
Michigan State University
Detroit, Michigan

Gilbert Wasonga
Department of Chemistry
Michigan State University
Detroit, Michigan

Nuno M. Xavier
Faculdade de Ciências
Departamento de Química e
    Bioquímica
Centro de Química e Bioquímica
Universidade de Lisboa
Lisbon, Portugal

A. Zawisza
Department of Organic and Applied
    Chemistry
University of Łódź
Łódź, Poland

Thomas Ziegler
Institute of Organic Chemistry
University of Tübingen
Tübingen, Germany

A.I. Zinin
N.D. Zelinsky Institute of Organic
    Chemistry of the Russian Academy
    of Sciences
Moscow, Russia

Part I

Synthetic Methods

1 Acetolysis of 6-Deoxysugars Controlled by Armed–Disarmed Effect

Emiliano Bedini,* Luigi Cirillo, Ian Cumpstey,[†] and Michelangelo Parrilli

CONTENTS

Experimental Methods 4
General Methods 4
Acetolysis Procedure 6
Acknowledgments 7
References 10

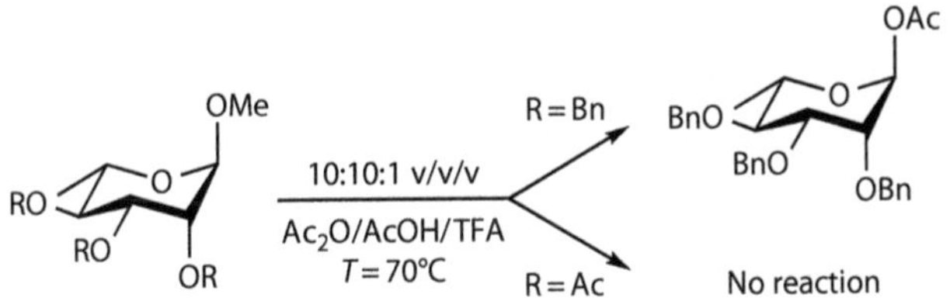

Acetolysis is a widely used reaction in both synthetic and analytical carbohydrate chemistry.[1] Its main synthetic application is to convert alkyl or aryl glycosides into 1-*O*-acetylated derivatives, which are useful building blocks easily transformable into other derivatives. Owing to the importance of acetolysis of carbohydrates in synthetic glycochemistry, several studies on the mechanism of this reaction exist in the literature.[2] There are no general protocols for acetolysis, and the conditions are often optimized for each compound, especially when mild and/or selective reactions are required.

---

* Corresponding author.
[†] Checker.

3

The armed–disarmed concept, a useful tool in carbohydrate synthesis, usually refers to the relative ease or difficulty of activating a sugar as a glycosyl donor.[3] In spite of its importance in glycosylation chemistry,[4] this concept did not find wide application in acetolysis. To the best of our knowledge, the only example is the solvolysis of caged 1,6-anhydro-pyranoses governed by armed-disarmed effects.[5] With the protocol presented here, we furnish a selective conversion of methyl glycosides of 6-deoxysugars into 1-O-Ac derivatives, based on the armed–disarmed concept. The methyl glycoside is treated with 10:10:1 Ac_2O–AcOH–TFA at 70°C for 8–20 h. A slight modification of such conditions (100:100:7.5 Ac_2O/AcOH/TFA, 60°C) was already reported for the acetolysis of a single armed 3-C-methyl-rhamnose derivative.[6] When applied to a rhamnose (6-deoxymannose) building block derivatized with an arming protecting group, acetolysis afforded the corresponding 1-O-Ac derivative, whereas a rhamnose building block protected with disarming groups did not react at all (Table 1.1, entries 1 and 2). Acetolysis with Ac_2O–AcOH–TFA protocol afforded 1-O-acetylated armed rhamnoside in good yields, in spite of the tendency of rhamnose and some other deoxy sugars to follow an endocyclic acetolysis mechanism[2b–d] giving preferentially open-chain derivatives and/or 1-O-acetylated furanosides.[7]

The acetolysis protocol presented in this chapter can be extended to disaccharide and oligosaccharide derivatives. When the aglycone-bearing monosaccharide (unit A) was protected with arming protecting groups and the other one (unit B) carried disarming groups, the acetolysis proceeded selectively at the armed anomeric position to give the 1-O-Ac disaccharide (entry 3). When units A and B were both disarmed, no reaction was observed (entry 4), whereas an armed–armed disaccharide gave simultaneous cleavage of both glycosidic linkages as expected (entry 5). The hypothesis that the cleavage of the interglycosidic bond started only after the complete cleavage of the methyl aglycone was ruled out by quenching the acetolysis before the complete disappearance of the starting material: a high amount of monosaccharide compounds was obtained. A similar study of acetolysis with oligosaccharides containing 6-deoxy-sugars (rhamnose, fucose, quinovose) can be found in literature.[7d,e]

EXPERIMENTAL METHODS

GENERAL METHODS

^{1}H and ^{13}C NMR spectra were recorded on a Bruker DRX-400 ([1]H: 400 MHz, [13]C: 100 MHz) instrument in $CDCl_3$. Chemical shifts are reported relative to the signals of residual $CHCl_3$ at δ 7.26 and of $CDCl_3$ at δ 77.0. Assignment of proton chemical shifts was based on 1D HOHAHA experiments. Positive MALDI-MS spectra were recorded on an Applied Biosystem Voyager DE-PRO MALDI-TOF mass spectrometer in the positive mode: compounds were dissolved in CH_3CN at a concentration of 1 mg/mL and 1 μL of these solutions was mixed with 1 μL of a 20 mg/mL solution of 2,5-dihydroxybenzoic acid in 7:3 CH_3CN–water. Optical rotations were measured on a JASCO P-1010 polarimeter. Elemental analysis was performed on a Carlo Erba 1108 instrument. Analytical thin layer chromatography (TLC) was performed on aluminum plates coated with Merck Silica Gel 60 F_{254} as the adsorbent.

TABLE 1.1
Acetolysis Reactions on Rhamnose Building Blocks

Entry[a]	Methyl Glycoside	Time (h)	Products (% Yield)[b]
1	1	8	2 (61%; 62%[c])
2	3	48	No reaction[d]
3	4	20	5 (56%)
4	6	20	No reaction[d]
5	7	14	2 (46%) 8 (33%)

[a] Reaction conducted on 0.1 mmol scale, unless otherwise specified.
[b] Isolated yield.
[c] Yield on 1 mmol scale.
[d] Starting material recovered in >90% yield (measured by ^{1}H NMR).

Compounds were visualized by spraying with 10% H_2SO_4 in EtOH, and heating until permanent spots developed. Column chromatography was performed on Merck Kieselgel 60 (63–200 mesh).

Acetolysis Procedure

Methyl glycoside (100 µmol) was dissolved in Ac_2O (1.5 mL) and treated with AcOH (1.5 mL) and TFA (150 µL). The solution was stirred at 70°C in a round-bottom flask closed with a glass stopper. The reaction was stopped by cooling to rt (see Table 1.1 for typical reaction times). It is worth noting that a low amount (≤10%) of unchanged starting material could be still present in the reaction mixture; nevertheless, longer reaction times are detrimental for the yield, since the products can react further by debenzylation.

After cooling to rt, the mixture was diluted with CH_2Cl_2 (25 mL) and washed successively with water (25 mL) and 1M $NaHCO_3$ (25 mL).* The organic layer was dried over anhydrous Na_2SO_4, filtered, concentrated and the residue was chromatographed (7:1 pentane–ethyl acetate for entry 1; 5:2 pentane–ethyl acetate for entry 3; 7:1 pentane–ethyl acetate for entry 5).

1-O-Acetyl-2,3,4-Tri-O-Benzyl-α-L-Rhamnopyranose[8] (2)

(Yield obtained by acetylation of 2,3,4-tri-O-benzyl-L-rhamnopyranose: 55%)[8]—
$[\alpha]_D$ −4.6 (c 1.4; CH_2Cl_2) ($[\alpha]_D$ lit.[8] −9.2 (c 1.1; $CHCl_3$)); ^1H NMR (400 MHz, $CDCl_3$): δ 7.34–7.31 (m, 15H, H-Ar), 6.12 (d, 1H, $J_{1,2}$ 2.0 Hz, H-1), 4.96 (d, 1H, J_{gem} 10.8 Hz, OC*H*HPh), 4.78 (d, 1H, J_{gem} 12.3 Hz, OC*H*HPh), 4.74 (d, 1H, J_{gem} 12.3 Hz, OC*H*HPh), 4.67 (d, 1H, J_{gem} 10.8 Hz, OC*H*HPh), 4.62 (d, 1H, J_{gem} 11.7 Hz, OC*H*HPh), 4.58 (d, 1H, J_{gem} 11.7 Hz, OC*H*HPh), 3.82 (dd, 1H, $J_{3,4}$ 9.3 Hz, $J_{3,2}$ = 3.1 Hz, H-3), 3.79 (dq, 1H, $J_{5,4}$ 9.4 Hz, $J_{5,6}$ 6.1 Hz, H-5), 3.74 (dd, 1H, $J_{2,3}$ 3.1 Hz, $J_{2,1}$ 2.0 Hz, H-2), 3.68 (t, 1H, $J_{4,5}$=$J_{4,3}$ 9.4 Hz, H-4), 2.03 (s, 3H, CH_3CO), 1.34 (d, 3H, $J_{6,5}$ 6.1 Hz, H-6); ^{13}C NMR (100 MHz, $CDCl_3$) δ 169.1 (CO), 138.3, 138.2, 137.8 (3 C_{ipso}-Bn), 128.5–127.6 (C-Ar), 91.7 (C-1), 79.8, 79.2, 75.5, 73.6, 72.5, 72.1, 70.5 (C-2, C-3, C-4, C-5, 3 OCH_2Ph), 21.0 (CH_3CO), 18.0 (C-6). TOF-MS: $[M+H]^+$ calcd for $C_{29}H_{32}O_6$ (m/z), 476.22; found: 499.11 ($[M+Na]^+$). Anal. calcd for $C_{29}H_{32}O_6$: C, 73.09; H, 6.77. Found: C, 72.77; H, 6.53.

2,3,4-Tri-O-Acetyl-α-L-Rhamnopyranosyl-(1 → 3)-1-O-Acetyl-
2,4-Di-O-Benzyl-α-L-Rhamnopyranose (5)

$[\alpha]_D$ −28.8 (c 3.3; CH_2Cl_2); ^1H NMR (400 MHz, $CDCl_3$): δ 7.44–7.28 (m, 10H, H-Ar), 6.18 (d, 1H, $J_{1,2}$ 1.9 Hz, H-1^I), 5.38 (m, 2H, H-2^{II}, H-3^{II}), 5.06 (d, 1H, $J_{1,2}$ 1.3 Hz, H-1^{II}), 5.03 (t, 1H, $J_{4,5}$=$J_{4,3}$ 9.8 Hz, H-4^{II}), 4.84 (d, 2H, J_{gem} 11.2 Hz, 2 OC*H*HPh), 4.66 (d, 1H, J_{gem} 10.9 Hz, OC*H*HPh), 4.64 (d, 1H, J_{gem} 12.0 Hz, OC*H*HPh), 4.03 (d, 1H, $J_{3,4}$ 9.4 Hz, $J_{3,2}$ 3.2 Hz, H-3^I), 3.78 (m, 2H, H-5^I, H-5^{II}), 3.73 (dd, 1H, $J_{2,3}$ 3.2 Hz, $J_{2,1}$ 1.9 Hz, H-2^I), 3.70 (t, 1H, $J_{4,5}$=$J_{4,3}$ 9.4 Hz, H-4^I), 2.08 (s, 3H, CH_3CO), 2.07 (s, 3H, CH_3CO), 2.04 (s, 3H, CH_3CO), 2.00 (s, 3H, CH_3CO), 1.32 (d, 3H, $J_{6,5}$ 6.1 Hz, H-6^I), 1.07 (d, 3H, $J_{6,5}$ 6.3 Hz, H-6^{II}); ^{13}C NMR (100 MHz, $CDCl_3$) δ 169.9, 169.8, 169.7, 169.1 (4 CO), 137.8, 137.5 (2 C_{ipso}-Bn), 128.6–127.7 (C-Ar), 99.5 (C-1^{II}), 90.9 (C-1^I), 79.8, 78.3, 76.7,

---

* CAUTION: Significant pressure built up in the separatory funnel when $NaHCO_3$ was added.

75.5, 72.2, 70.8, 70.7, 69.8, 69.0, 66.9 (C-2^I, C-3^I, C-4^I, C-5^I, C-2^{II}, C-3^{II}, C-4^{II}, C-5^{II}, 2 OCH$_2$Ph), 20.9–20.7 (4 CH$_3$CO), 18.0, 17.4 (C-6^I, C-6^{II}). TOF-MS: [M+H]$^+$ calcd for C$_{34}$H$_{42}$O$_{13}$(m/z), 658.26; found: 681.19 ([M+Na]$^+$). Anal. calcd for C$_{34}$H$_{42}$O$_{13}$: C, 62.00; H, 6.43. Found: C, 61.75; H, 6.30.

1,3-Di-O-Acetyl-2,4-Di-O-Benzyl-α-L-Rhamnopyranose[7a] (8)

(Yield obtained by acetolysis of methyl 3-O-acetyl-2,4-di-O-benzyl-α-L-rhamnopyranoside with 10:1 v/v Ac$_2$O/TFA at rt for 48 h: 43%)[7a] [α]$_D$ +2.4 (c 1.9; CH$_2$Cl$_2$) ([α]$_D$ lit.[7a] −4.2 (c 0.5; CHCl$_3$)); ^{1}H NMR (400 MHz, CDCl$_3$): δ 7.33–7.22 (m, 10H, H-Ar), 6.12 (d, 1H, $J_{1,2}$ 2.0 Hz, H-1), 5.19 (dd, 1H, $J_{3,4}$ 9.5 Hz, $J_{3,2}$ 3.4 Hz, H-3), 4.74 (d, 2H, J_{gem} 11.7 Hz, 2 OCHHPh), 4.67 (d, 1H, J_{gem} 11.1 Hz, OCHHPh), 4.57 (d, 1H, J_{gem} 12.2 Hz, OCHHPh), 3.87 (m, 2H, H-2, H-5), 3.69 (t, 1H, $J_{4,5}=J_{4,3}$ 9.5 Hz, H-4), 2.11 (s, 3H, CH$_3$CO), 1.98 (s, 3H, CH$_3$CO), 1.36 (d, 3H, $J_{6,5}$ 6.2 Hz, H-6); ^{13}C NMR (100 MHz, CDCl$_3$) δ 170.2, 169.2 (2 CO), 138.0, 137.4 (2 C$_{ipso}$-Bn), 128.4–127.4 (C-Ar), 91.3 (C-1), 78.5, 75.1, 74.8, 73.1, 72.9, 70.2 (C-2, C-3, C-4, C-5, 2 OCH$_2$Ph), 21.0, 20.9 (2 CH$_3$CO), 18.0 (C-6). TOF-MS: [M+H]$^+$ calcd for C$_{24}$H$_{28}$O$_7$(m/z), 428.18; found: 450.96 ([M+Na]$^+$). Anal. calcd for C$_{24}$H$_{28}$O$_7$: C, 67.28; H, 6.59. Found: C, 67.00; H, 6.38).

ACKNOWLEDGMENTS

NMR and MS facilities of CIMCF (Centro di Metodologie Chimico-Fisiche) of Università di Napoli "Federico II" are gratefully acknowledged.

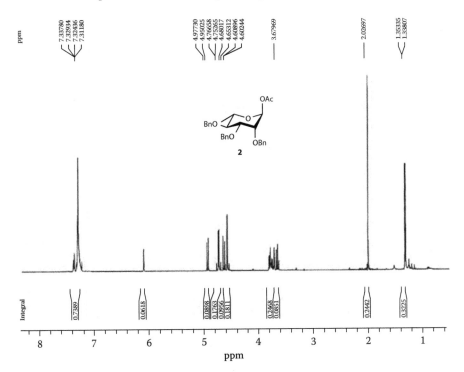

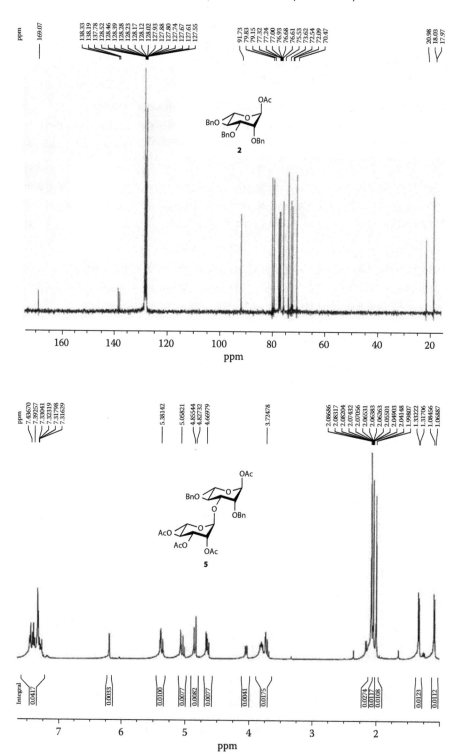

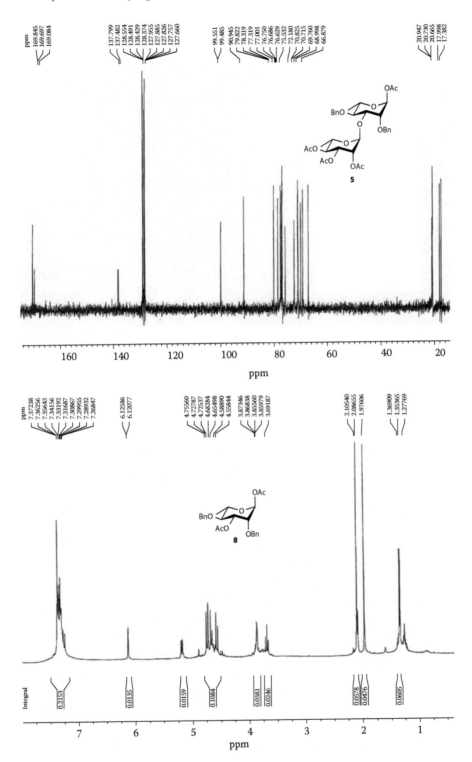

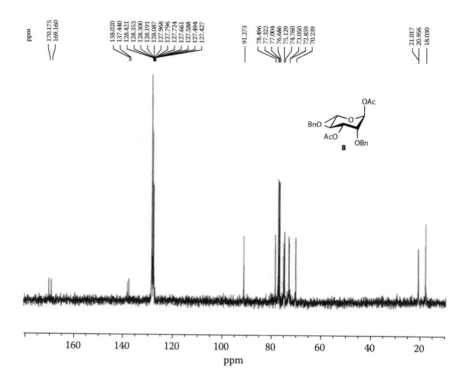

REFERENCES

1. Guthrie, R.D.; McCarthy, J.F. *Adv. Carbohydr. Chem. Biochem.* 1967, *22*, 11–23.
2. (a) Lichtenthaler, F.W.; Bambach, G. *Carbohydr. Res.* 1979, *68*, 305–312; (b) Dasgupta, F.; Singh, P.P.; Srivastava, H.C. *Ind. J. Chem.* 1988, *27B*, 527–529; (c) Kanie, O.; Takeda, T.; Ogihara, Y. *Carbohydr. Res.* 1990, *197*, 289–294; (d) McPhail, D.R.; Lee, J.R.; Fraser-Reid, B. *J. Am. Chem. Soc.* 1992, *114*, 1905–1906; (e) Kaczmarek, J.; Preyss, M.; Lönnberg, H.; Szafranek, J. *Carbohydr. Res.* 1995, *279*, 107–116; (f) Miljković, M.; Yeagley, D.; Deslongchamps, P.; Dory, Y.L. *J. Org. Chem.* 1997, *62*, 7597–7604; (g) Kaczmarek, J.; Kaczyński, Z.; Trumpakaj, Z.; Szafranek, J.; Bogalecka, M.; Lönnberg, H. *Carbohydr. Res.* 2000, *325*, 16–29.
3. (a) Mootoo, D.R.; Konradsson, P.; Udodong, U.E.; Fraser-Reid, B. *J. Am. Chem. Soc.* 1988, *110*, 5583–5584; (b) Fraser-Reid, B.; Wu, Z.; Udodong, U.E.; Ottosson, H. *J. Org. Chem.* 1990, *55*, 6068–6070; (c) Fraser-Reid, B.; Wu, Z.; Andrews, C.W.; Skowronski, E. *J. Am. Chem. Soc.* 1991, *113*, 1434–1435.
4. Garegg, P.J. *Adv. Carbohydr. Chem. Biochem.* 2004, *59*, 69–134.
5. Burgey, C.S.; Vollerthun, R.; Fraser-Reid, B. *Tetrahedron Lett.* 1994, *35*, 2637–2640.
6. Fekete, A.; Gyergyói, K.; Kövér, K.; Bajza, I.; Lipták, A. *Carbohydr. Res.* 2006, *341*, 1312–1321.
7. (a) Paulsen, H.; Lorentzen, J.P. *Carbohydr. Res.* 1987, *165*, 207–227; (b) Banaszek, A.; Ciunik, Z. *Tetrahedron Lett.* 1997, *38*, 273–276; (c) Banaszek, A. *Carbohydr. Res.* 1998, *306*, 379–385; (d) Bedini, E.; Comegna, D.; Di Nola, A.; Parrilli, M. *Tetrahedron Lett.* 2008, *49*, 2546–2551; (e) Cirillo, L.; Bedini, E.; Parrilli, M. *Eur. J. Org. Chem.* 2008, *2008*, 5704–5714.
8. Paulsen, H.; Kutschker, W.; Lockhoff, O. *Chem. Ber.* 1981, *114*, 3233–3241.

2 NaH/Im$_2$SO$_2$-Mediated Preparation of Hex-2- and Hex-3-Enopyranoside Enol Ethers

Emanuele Attolino, Giorgio Catelani,* Felicia D'Andrea, Lorenzo Guazzelli, and Marie-Christine Scherrmann†

CONTENTS

Experimental Methods 16
  General Methods 16
    Methyl 2,6-Di-*O*-Benzyl-4-Deoxy-3-*O*-Naphthylmethyl-β-D-*threo*-
    Hex-3-Enopyranoside (**13**) 16
    Methyl 2-*O*-Benzyl-4-Deoxy-3-*O*-*p*-Methoxybenzyl-6-*O*-
    Methoxymethyl-β-D-*threo*-Hex-3-Enopyranoside (**15**) 17
    3-Azidopropyl 2-Acetamido-3,6-Di-*O*-Benzyl-2,4-Dideoxy-β-
    D-*threo*-Hex-3-Enopyranosyl-(1 → 4)-2,3,6-Tri-*O*-Benzyl-β-D-
    Glucopyranosyl-(1 → 2)-3,4-Di-*O*-Benzyl-α-L-Rhamnopyranoside (**17**) 17
    Methyl 3,4,6-Tri-*O*-Benzyl-2-Deoxy-β-D-*threo*-Hex-2-
    Enopyranoside (**19**) 18
    2-Deoxy-3,4-*O*-Isopropylidene-6-*O*-Trityl-β-D-*threo*-Hex-2-
    Enopyranosyl-(1 → 4)-2,3:5,6-Di-*O*-Isopropylidene-*Aldehydo*-D-
    Glucose Dimethyl Acetal (**21**) 18
    Methyl 3,4-Di-*O*-Benzyl-2,6-Dideoxy-α-L-*threo*-Hex-2-
    Enopyranoside (**23**) 19
References 26

---

* Corresponding author.
† Checker.

One-pot activation–elimination of axial 4-OH group on some representative *O*-benzyl pro-tected derivatives belonging to the D-*galacto* and D-*talo* series. Reagent and conditions: (a) NaH (5 equiv)/DMF, room temperature, 30 min; (b) cooling to –30°C, Im_2SO_2 (1.5 equiv), 1 h; (c) warming to room temperature, stirring 2–6 h. a: X=β-OMe, R=OBn, R'=H, b: X=β-*O*-(2,3:5,6-di-*O*-isopropylidene-*aldehydo*-D-glucose dimethyl acetal)-4-yl, R=H, R'=OBn, c: X=β-OMe, R=NHAc, R'=H, d: X=α-OMe, R=OBn, R'=H, e: X=α-OMe, R=H, R'=OBn.

Unsaturated sugars are useful synthetic intermediates for the conversion of com-mon saccharides into complex carbohydrates,[1] as well as for the preparation of other types of enantiomerically pure derivatives.[1,2] Glycals, the cyclic vinyl ethers involv-ing the anomeric center, are the most popular class of unsaturated monosaccharide derivatives,[3] but other types of olefinic pyranosides are well known, for example, 2,3-dideoxy-hex-2-enopyranosides available from glycals through the Ferrier-I rear-rangement.[1,4] Less studied are other classes of cyclic pyranoside enol ethers having the double bond at different positions of the hexopyranose framework, with the exception of 6-deoxy-hex-5-enopyranosides, which are easily obtained by elimina-tion reaction on C-6-activated derivatives.[5] Preparation of pyranoside enol ethers by elimination of a leaving group from a secondary position has gained a preparative value only after the introduction of trifluoromethanesulfonates (triflates).[6] However, the use of triflates may be problematic, in particular (a) the difficult purification of the triflate intermediates by chromatography and (b) a side-reaction arising from the base attack at the sulfur atom, leading to the formation of the starting alcohol.

Recently, a substantial advance in the preparation of hex-3- and hex-4-enopyrano-side enol ethers has been achieved, formally arising from a water elimination involv-ing the axial OH-4 group and a vicinal antiperiplanar proton.[7] The standardized protocol for this unprecedented one-pot process is based (see opening scheme of this chapter) on initial deprotonation of the alcohol (**1**) with NaH in DMF, followed by treatment at low temperature (–30°C) of the alkoxide with *N,N'*-sulfuryldiimidazole (Im$_2$SO$_2$), and, finally, by warming up to room temperature. We have found only a reference to a similar elimination on a 4'-*O*-imidazolate lactoside affording an uncharacterized elimination product.[8]

The overall procedure is supposed to involve (Scheme 2.1), after initial deproto-nation of the alcohol (path a), formation of an imidazylsulfonate intermediate (**7**) (path b), spontaneously evolving through *1H*-imidazol-1-ide (**8**) promoted elimination (path c) to enol ethers (**9**), sodium *1H*-imidazole-1-sulfonate (**10**), and imidazole (**11**).

By analyzing the results obtained for some D-Gal*p*, D-Tal*p*, and D-TalNAc*p* deriva-tives,[7] a specific relationship between the regioselectivity of the activation–elimina-tion reaction and the configuration at C-2 of the starting alcohol was highlighted. In case of the *galacto* configured (C-2 equatorially substituted) alcohol **1b**, H-5 and H-3 (both antiperiplanar to the axial *1H*-imidazole-1-sulfonate group) were elimi-nated at about the same rate, giving rise to an 1.5:1 mixture of 4-deoxy-hex-3- (**2b**)

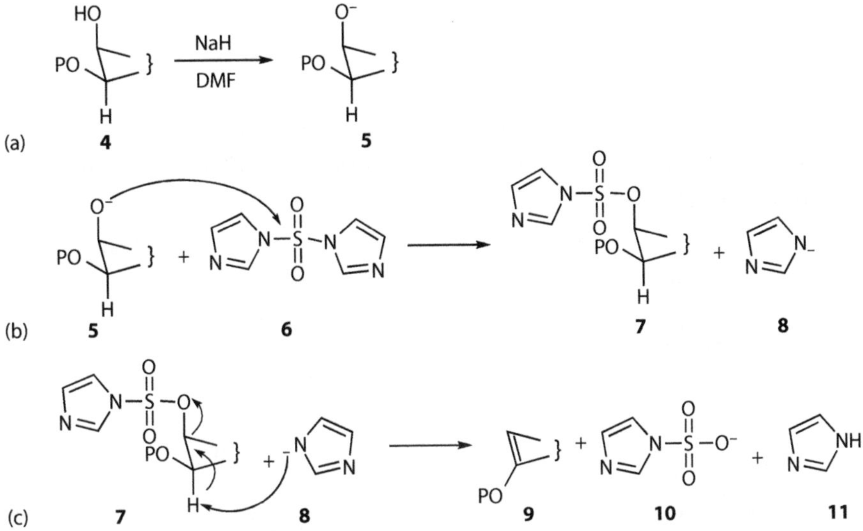

SCHEME 2.1 Pathways of the activation–elimination of axial hexopyranoside alcoholic groups.

and 4-deoxy-hex-4-enopyranoside (**3b**). Conversely, the presence of an axial group at C-2 (*talo* series) greatly facilitated the elimination of H-3, leading to the exclusive formation of hex-3-enopyranosides (**2**). The specific assistance of the C-2 axial electronegative group to the base-promoted elimination of the vicinal antiperiplanar H-3 has been attributed to stereoelectronic factors determining a borderline E2-E1cb mechanism.[7b] Furthermore, the anomeric configuration appreciably influences the rate of the elimination step. In the case of β-anomers (**1a–c**), TLC analysis showed that the elimination reaction takes place also at low temperature (–30°C, see step b of the opening scheme in this chapter), evidencing, even before the disappearance of the starting alcohol, the presence either of a lower-moving transient *1H*-imidazole-1-sulfonate or of faster-moving enol ethers (**2** and, in some cases, **3**). On the contrary, in the case of the α-anomers (**1d–e**) the disappearance of the starting alcohol is accompanied first by the sole formation of *1H*-imidazole-1-sulfonates,* which give enol ethers only when the reaction mixture is warmed to room temperature (see step c in the opening scheme of this chapter). In all cases, high yields of elimination products were obtained, with the sole exception of derivative **1e**, where the unfavorable configuration of both the anomeric center and the C-2 gives way to side reactions, greatly reducing the yield of the elimination product.[7b] The successful protocol for preparation of *talo* derivatives,[7b] where enol ethers **2** were isolated in more than 90% yield could be applied for the stereoselective synthesis of β-manno- and β-2-acetamido-2-deoxy-mannopyranosides,[9] which are difficult to obtain by common glycosidations.[10]

The effectiveness of this new method for the preparation of hexenopyranoside enol ethers has been further illustrated (Table 2.1) through some new examples involving (a)

---

* 4-O-1- imidazolylsulfonyl derivatives of **1d** and **1e** were isolated and fully characterized when the reaction was quenched before the final warming to room temperature.[7c]

TABLE 2.1

Activation–Elimination of the Axial 4-OH Group of D-Talopyranosides (12, 14, and 16), the Axial 2-OH of D-Talopyranosides (18 and 20) and of the 6-Deoxy-L-Talopyranoside (22)

Entry	Alcohol	Product (Yield %)

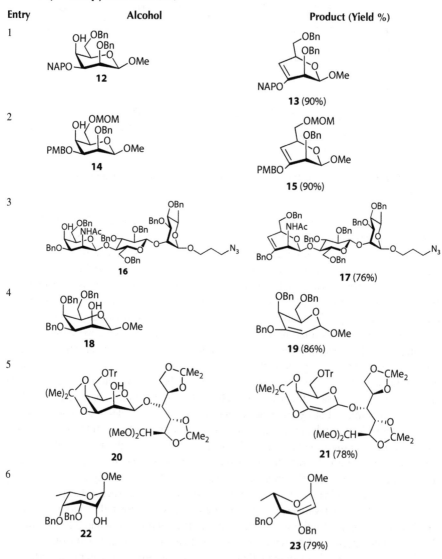

Entry 1: **12** → **13 (90%)**

Entry 2: **14** → **15 (90%)**

Entry 3: **16** → **17 (76%)**

Entry 4: **18** → **19 (86%)**

Entry 5: **20** → **21 (78%)**

Entry 6: **22** → **23 (79%)**

Tr, trityl; NAP, *p*-naphtylmethyl; MOM, methoxymethyl; PMB, *p*-methoxybenzyl.

the 4-OH group of two β-D-talopyranosides carrying different types of ether protecting groups (entries 1–2), (b) the 4-OH group of the D-TalNAc unit of a complex trisaccharide (entry 3), and (c) the 2-OH group of two β-D-talopyranosides (entry 4 and 5) and of a 6-deoxy-α-L-talopyranoside (entry 6). All compounds in Table 2.1 have the same structural feature, namely, a 1,2,3-*syn* relationship between a free axial OH group, a vicinal equatorial group, and an electronegative axial substituent. As expected, the extraction of the axially oriented H located on the intermediate C is selectively facilitated for stereoelectronic reasons, leading to the enol ethers with complete regioselectivity. Hexenopyranoside enol ethers **13**, **15**, and **19** (entries 1, 2, and 4) have been isolated pure in excellent yields, showing a very good compatibility of MOM, PMB, and NAP protecting groups with the reaction conditions. A slightly diminished yield has been observed in the preparation of the aminated trisaccharide enol ether **17** (76%) and the 6-deoxy-hex-2-α-enopyranoside **23** (79%). In both cases, TLC analysis revealed a decrease in the elimination rate, evidencing the presence of substantial amount of slower-moving *1H*-imidazole-1-sulfonate intermediates at the end of the activation step (−30°C, 1 h).

This result is not surprising for the activation–elimination of the α-configured alcohol **22**, where the axial anomeric methoxy group offers a steric hindrance during the attack of the imidazolate ion to the 1,3-*syn*-diaxial H-3. An appreciably deduced reaction rate was observed for the 3,4-*O*-isopropylidene disaccharide **20**, where the intermediate imidazylate was completely converted to the enol ether product **21** after 16 h at room temperature. In this case, the presence of the *cis*-3,4-fused dioxolane could contribute to a substantial deviation from the usual $^4C_1$ conformation of the pyranose ring, and prevent a good antiperiplanar disposition between the C-2 *1H*-imidazole-1-sulfonate leaving group and H-3. Furthermore, an appreciable degradation of **21** was observed during purification by chromatography, resulting in substantially reduced yield (44%). However, the yield increased to a satisfactory 78%, when packing and elution of the column were made in presence of 1% of Et$_3$N in the solvent mixture, rather than 0.1% used during purification of the other enol ethers. The observed instability of compound **21** could be attributed to the presence of the 3',4'-dioxolane fused ring, causing some strong bond angle deviation from the normal geometry, and, consequently, a greater susceptibility of the enol ether toward degradation by the acidity of silica gel.

In conclusion, the NaH/Im$_2$SO$_2$ system is a valuable tool for the one-pot dehydration of pyranosides having an axial OH group. The method presents several advantages with respect to the alternative use of triflates,[6] which requires (a) two distinct reactions, (b) purification of the intermediate triflate, and (c) use of more expensive and less stable reagent (triflic anhydride instead of the stable and crystalline *N,N'*-sulfuryldiimidazole). Moreover, the activation–elimination with NaH/Im$_2$SO$_2$ system requires short reaction times, generally permitting the preparation and purification of hexenopyranoside enol ethers in only 1 day. Furthermore, the presence of an axially oriented electronegative group in position 3 with respect to the free OH group greatly facilitates the elimination of the axial contiguous H, leading in high yields to a single enol ether. The method should be possible to apply to other pyranosides and to other six-membered polyoxygenated systems (e.g., inositols). The sole limitation is constituted by the combination of absence of stereoelectronic assistance and the presence of a steric hindrance to the imidazolate attack to the departing proton, as in the case of α-D-*galacto* alcohols (e.g., **1e** in the opening scheme of this chapter).

EXPERIMENTAL METHODS

GENERAL METHODS

Melting points were determined with a Kofler hot-stage apparatus and are uncorrected. Optical rotations were measured on a Perkin-Elmer 241 polarimeter at 20°C ±2°C. ^{1}H NMR and ^{13}C NMR spectra were recorded with a Bruker Avance II 250 instrument operating at 250.13 MHz (^{1}H) and 62.9 MHz (^{13}C) in the reported solvent (internal standard Me$_4$Si) and the assignments were made, when possible, with DEPT, HETCOR, and COSY experiments. All reactions were followed by TLC on Kieselgel 60 F$_{254}$ with detection by UV light and/or by charring with 10% sulfuric acid in ethanol. Kieselgel 60 (Merck, 230–400 mesh) was used for flash chromatography. Solvents were dried by distillation according to standard procedures,[11] and were stored over activated molecular sieves. Solutions in organic solvents were dried with MgSO$_4$. All reactions were performed under argon. Im$_2$SO$_2$ was purchased from Aldrich and used as received. Previously unreported starting alcohols **12**, **14**, **16**, **18**, **20**, and **22** have been prepared during other projects and their preparation will be reported in forthcoming papers.

Methyl 2,6-Di-O-Benzyl-4-Deoxy-3-O-Naphthylmethyl-β-D-*threo*-Hex-3-Enopyranoside (13)

Sodium hydride (396 mg of 60% dispersion in mineral oil, 9.90 mmol, 5.0 equiv) was washed with dry hexane (4 × 2 mL) and suspended in dry DMF (5 mL). A solution of **12** (1.02 g, 1.98 mmol) in dry DMF (41 mL) was added and the mixture was stirred at room temperature for 30 min. After cooling to −30°C, solid Im$_2$SO$_2$ (589 mg, 2.97 mmol, 1.5 equiv) was added and stirring at −30°C was continued for 1 h, when TLC (1:1 hexane–EtOAc) showed complete disappearance of the starting material (R_f 0.44) and formation of two UV active products (R_f 0.58 and 0.28). The mixture was allowed to warm to room temperature and stirred until TLC analysis (3 h, 1:1 hexane–EtOAc) revealed complete transformation of the compound with R_f 0.28 into the faster-moving product (R_f 0.58). The mixture was cooled to −30°C and the excess of NaH was destroyed with MeOH (2 mL). After 10 min, the solution was poured into a mixture of ice and ether (20 mL), the two layers were separated and the aqueous phase was further extracted with ether (2 × 20 mL). The collected ethereal extracts were dried, filtered, and concentrated under diminished pressure. The crude reaction product was chromatographed (4:1 hexane–EtOAc + 0.1% Et$_3$N), to give pure **13** (885 mg, 90%), mp 59–61°C (hexane); $[\alpha]_D$ +10.6 (c 1, CHCl$_3$), R_f 0.24 (4:1 hexane–EtOAc); ^{1}H NMR (CDCl$_3$) δ 7.85–7.75 (m, 4H, Ar-H), 7.51–7.19 (m, 13H, Ar-H), 4.96 (d, 1H, $J_{4,5}$ 1.6 Hz, H-4), 4.91, 4.82 (AB system, 2H, $J_{A,B}$ 12.4 Hz, CH$_2$Ph), 4.90, 4.84 (AB system, 2H, $J_{A,B}$ 12.4 Hz, CH$_2$Ph), 4.63, 4.55 (AB system, 2H, $J_{A,B}$ 12.4 Hz, CH$_2$Nap), 4.51 (d, 1H, $J_{1,2}$ 2.0 Hz, H-1), 4.42 (bt, 1H, spl 5.8 Hz, H-5), 3.93 (t, 1H, spl 1.8 Hz, H-2), 3.72 (dd, 1H, $J_{6a,6b}$ 9.8 Hz, $J_{5,6b}$ 6.2 Hz, H-6b), 3.59 (s, 3H, OCH$_3$), 3.54 (dd, 1H, $J_{5,6a}$ 5.8 Hz, H-6a); ^{13}C NMR (CDCl$_3$) δ 152.2 (C-3), 138.9, 138.1, 133.9, 133.1, 132.9 (5 × Ar-C), 128.3–125.3 (Ar-CH), 101.7 (C-1), 98.8 (C-4), 73.5, 73.2, 72.7 (2 × CH$_2$Ph, CH$_2$Nap), 72.6, 72.2 (C-2, C-5), 69.3 (C-6), 56.8 (OCH$_3$). Anal. Calcd for C$_{32}$H$_{32}$O$_5$: C, 77.40; H, 6.50. Found: C, 77.32; H, 6.47.

Methyl 2-*O*-Benzyl-4-Deoxy-3-*O*-*p*-Methoxybenzyl-6-*O*-Methoxymethyl-β-D-*threo*-Hex-3-Enopyranoside (15)

To a suspension of prewashed (hexane) 60% NaH in mineral oil (178 mg, 4.45 mmol, 5 equiv.) in dry DMF (4 mL) was added at room temperature a solution of **14** (400 mg, 0.89 mmol) in dry DMF (18 mL). The mixture was stirred for 30 min, cooled to −30°C and treated with Im$_2$SO$_2$ (264 mg, 1.33 mmol, 5 equiv) as described above for the preparation of **13**. After stirring for 1 h at −30°C, the starting material (R_f 0.52) was completely consumed (TLC, 1:4 hexane–EtOAc) and two new products (R_f 0.63 and 0.37) were formed. The mixture was warmed to room temperature and stirred until TLC analysis (2 h, 1:4 hexane–EtOAc) revealed the complete disappearance of the component with R_f 0.37. The crude product was purified by flash chromatography (1:1 hexane–EtOAc + 0.1% Et$_3$N) to give pure **15** (345 mg, 90%) as clear syrup, R_f 0.63 (1:4 hexane–EtOAc); [α]$_D$ +15 (*c* 1, CHCl$_3$); ^{1}H NMR (CDCl$_3$) δ 7.39–7.35 (m, 2H, Ar-H), 7.29–7.20 (m, 5H, Ar-H), 6.88 (AA'XX' system, 2H, *J* 8.6 Hz, Ar-H-PMB), 4.90 (d, 1H, $J_{4,5}$ 1.7 Hz, H-4), 4.85, 4.78 (AB system, 2H, $J_{A,B}$ 12.5 Hz, CH_2Ph), 4.69 (s, 2H, CH_2-MOM), 4.70, 4.63 (AB system, 2H, $J_{A,B}$ 11.1 Hz, CH_2Ph), 4.51 (d, 1H, $J_{1,2}$ 2.1 Hz, H-1), 4.39 (bt, 1H, spl 6.0 Hz, H-5), 3.95 (t, 1H, spl 1.7 Hz, H-2), 3.82 (s, 3H, OCH_3-PMB), 3.75 (dd, 1H, $J_{6a,6b}$ 10.1 Hz, $J_{5,6b}$ 6.4 Hz, H-6b), 3.62 (dd, 1H, $J_{5,6a}$ 5.6 Hz, H-6a), 3.59, 3.38 (2s, each 3H, OCH_3-1, OCH_3-MOM); ^{13}C NMR (CDCl$_3$) δ 159.3 (PMB-*C*), 152.5 (C-3), 138.9 (Ar-*C*), 129.1 (PMB-*C*H), 128.5 (PMB-*C*), 127.9–127.1 (Ar-*C*H), 113.7 (PMB-*C*H), 101.7 (C-1), 98.2 (C-4), 96.8 (*C*H$_2$-MOM), 72.6, 70.8 (*C*H$_2$-PMB, *C*H$_2$-MOM), 72.5, 72.1 (C-2, C-5), 69.0 (C-6), 56.8 (O*C*H$_3$-PMB), 55.3, 55.2 (O*C*H$_3$.1, O*C*H$_3$-MOM). Anal. Calcd for C$_{24}$H$_{30}$O$_7$: C, 66.96; H, 7.02. Found: C, 66.93; H, 7.01.

3-Azidopropyl 2-Acetamido-3,6-Di-*O*-Benzyl-2,4-Dideoxy-β-D-*threo*-Hex-3-Enopyranosyl-(1 → 4)-2,3,6-Tri-*O*-Benzyl-β-D-Glucopyranosyl-(1 → 2)-3,4-Di-*O*-Benzyl-α-L-Rhamnopyranoside (17)

To a stirred suspension of prewashed (hexane) 60% NaH in mineral oil (28 mg, 0.70 mmol, 5 equiv) in dry DMF (1 mL) was added at room temperature a solution of **16** (175 mg, 0.14 mmol) in dry DMF (4 mL). After 30 min, the mixture was cooled to −30°C and treated with Im$_2$SO$_2$ (41.6 mg, 0.21 mmol, 1.5 equiv) as described for the preparation of **13**. After 1 h at −30°C, the starting material (R_f 0.35) was completely consumed (TLC, 2:3 hexane–EtOAc) and a major (R_f 0.23) and a minor product (R_f 0.49) were formed. The mixture was allowed to warm to room temperature and stirred until TLC revealed complete disappearance of the component with R_f 0.23, and the presence of the sole product with R_f 0.49 (~2.5 h, 2:3 hexane–EtOAc). The mixture was cooled to −30°C and the reaction was quenched by addition of MeOH (2 mL). The resulting solution was diluted with CH$_2$Cl$_2$ (5 mL), washed with water (5 mL), and the aqueous phase was extracted with CH$_2$Cl$_2$ (3 × 5 mL). The combined organic layers were dried, filtered, concentrated, and chromatography (1:1 hexane–EtOAc + 0.1% Et$_3$N) of the residue gave pure **17** (130 mg, 76%) as clear syrup; R_f 0.49 (2:3 hexane–EtOAc); [α]$_D$ +14 (*c* 1.1, CHCl$_3$); ^{1}H NMR (CDCl$_3$) δ 7.39–7.01 (m, 35H, Ar-H), 5.83 (d, 1H, $J_{2,NH}$ 9.9 Hz, NH), 5.17, 4.73 (AB system, 2H, J_{AB} 11.2 Hz, CH_2Ph), 4.91 (m, 3H, H-1, CH_2Ph), 4.86 (d, 1H,

$J_{1,2}$ 1.9 Hz, H-1^{II}), 4.79, 4.45 (AB system, 2H, J_{AB} 10.9 Hz, CH_2Ph), 4.72–4.53 (m, 6H, 3×CH_2Ph), 4.70 (d, 1H, $J_{4,5}$ 2.0 Hz, H-4^{II}), 4.60 (d, 1H, $J_{1,2}$ 8.0 Hz, H-1^I), 4.41 (s, 2H, CH_2Ph), 4.62 (m, 1H, H-2^{II}), 4.55 (m, 1H, H-5^{II}), 4.00 (dd, 1H, $J_{1,2}$ 2.2 Hz, $J_{2,3}$ 2.9 Hz, H-2), 3.91 (t, 1H, $J_{3,4}=J_{4,5}$ 9.4 Hz, H-4^I), 3.86 (dd, 1H, H-3), 3.74 (dd, 1H, $J_{5,6b}$ 4.2 Hz, $J_{6a,6b}$ 11.3 Hz, H-6^{I}b), 3.70, 3.27 (2m, each 1H, CH_2O), 3.68–3.62 (m, 2H, H-6^{I}a,), H-5), 3.64 (t, 1H, $J_{2,3}$ 9.4 Hz, H-3^I), 3.55 (dd, 1H, $J_{2,3}$ 9.4 Hz, H-2^I), 3.49 (t, 1H, $J_{4,5}$ 9.5 Hz, H-4), 3.43–3.32 (m, 3H, H-5^I, H-6^{II}a, H-6^{II}b), 3.32 (t, 1H, J 6.8 Hz, CH_2N$_3$), 1.75 (s, 3H, CH_3CO), 1.73 (m, 2H, CH_2), 1.27 (d, 3H, $J_{5,6}$ 6.5 Hz, H-6); ^{13}C NMR (CDCl$_3$) δ 169.8 (CO), 152.2 (C-3^{II}), 139.3, 138.7, 138.3, 138.1, 138.2, 137.9, 136.4 (7×Ar-C), 128.3–126.8 (Ar-CH), 104.6 (C-1^I), 99.4 (C-1), 99.0 (C-1^{II}), 97.4 (C-4^{II}), 83.0 (C-3^I), 81.8 (C-2^I), 80.3 (C-4), 79.4 (C-3), 76.6 (C-4^I), 75.8 (C-2), 75.3, 74.7, 73.3, 73.2, 73.1, 72.4, 60.0 (7×CH_2Ph), 74.2 (C-5^I), 71.7 (C-5^{II}), 72.1 C-6^{II}), 68.6 (C-6^I), 67.9 (C-5), 64.0 (CH_2O), 48.9 (C-2^{II}), 48.2 (CH_2N$_3$), 28.8 (CH_2), 23.1 (CH_3CO), 17.9 (C-6). Anal. Calcd for C$_{72}$H$_{80}$N$_4$O$_{14}$: C, 70.57; H, 6.58; N, 4.57. Found: C, 70.51; H, 6.53; N, 4.53.

Methyl 3,4,6-Tri-O-Benzyl-2-Deoxy-β-D-threo-Hex-2-Enopyranoside (19)

The activation–elimination reaction with **18** (690 mg, 1.49 mmol) in dry DMF (50 mL) was performed as described for the preparation of **13**: the solution of **18** was added at room temperature to a suspension of prewashed (hexane) 60% NaH in mineral oil (298 mg, 7.45 mmol, 5 equiv) in dry DMF (10 mL). The mixture was stirred for 30 min and Im$_2$SO$_2$ (443 mg, 2.23 mmol, 1.5 equiv) was added at –30°C. After 1 h at the same temperature, TLC (1:1 hexane–EtOAc) showed complete disappearance of the starting material (R_f 0.36) and formation of two products (R_f 0.48 and 0.07). The mixture was allowed to warm to room temperature and stirred until TLC (~3 h, 1:1 hexane–EtOAc) revealed complete disappearance of the component with R_f 0.07. Purification of the crude product by flash chromatography (4:1 hexane–EtOAc + 0.1% Et$_3$N) gave pure **19** (573 mg, 86%) as clear syrup; R_f 0.48 (1:1 hexane–EtOAc); $[\alpha]_D$ –125 (c 1.2, CHCl$_3$); ^{1}H NMR (CDCl$_3$) δ 7.40–7.21 (m, 15H, Ar-H), 5.20 (bs, 1H, H-2), 4.86 (d, 1H, $J_{1,2}$ 1.3 Hz, H-1), 4.82, 4.77 (AB system, 2H, $J_{A,B}$ 11.6 Hz, CH_2Ph), 4.82, 4.63 (AB system, 2H, $J_{A,B}$ 12.0 Hz, CH_2Ph), 4.58, 4.51 (AB system, 2H, $J_{A,B}$ 11.9 Hz, CH_2Ph), 3.88–3.83 (m, 2H, H-4, H-5), 3.75 (m, 2H, H-6a, H-6b), 3.48 (s, 3H, OCH_3); ^{13}C NMR (CDCl$_3$) δ 156.5 (C-3), 138.5, 138.1, 136.2 (Ar-C), 128.5–127.4 (Ar-CH), 99.1, 99.0 (C-1, C-2), 74.6, 71.3 (C-4, C-5), 73.5, 72.4 (2×CH_2Ph), 69.4, 69.3 (C-6, CH_2Ph), 54.7 (OCH_3). Anal. Calcd for C$_{28}$H$_{30}$O$_5$: C, 75.31; H, 6.77. Found: C, 75.27; H, 6.74.

2-Deoxy-3,4-O-Isopropylidene-6-O-Trityl-β-D-threo-Hex-2-Enopyranosyl-(1 → 4)-2,3:5,6-Di-O-Isopropylidene-Aldehydo-D-Glucose Dimethyl Acetal (21)

To a stirred suspension of prewashed (hexane) 60% NaH in mineral oil (64 mg, 1.60 mmol, 5 equiv) in dry DMF (2.2 mL) was added at room temperature a solution of **20** (240 mg, 0.32 mmol) in dry DMF (6.5 mL). After 30 min, the solution was cooled to –30°C and treated with Im$_2$SO$_2$ (95 mg, 0.48 mmol, 1.5 equiv) as above described for the preparation of **13**. After 1 h at −30°C, TLC (EtOAc) showed complete disappearance of the starting material (R_f 0.69) and formation of a major (R_f 0.57) and a very minor, faster-moving product (R_f 0.74). The mixture was allowed to warm to room temperature and stirred until TLC (16 h, EtOAc) revealed complete disappearance of the component with R_f 0.57 and the presence of the sole product with R_f 0.74. The mixture was cooled to −30°C and the excess of NaH was destroyed by addition of MeOH (2 mL). After 10 min, the solution was poured into a mixture of ice and ether, the two layers were separated and the aqueous phase was further extracted with ether (2×15 mL). The collected ethereal extracts were dried, filtered and concentrated under diminished pressure. Chromatography (1:1 hexane–EtOAc containing 1% Et$_3$N) gave pure **21** (183 mg, 78%) as clear syrup; R_f 0.51 (1:1 hexane–EtOAc); $[\alpha]_D$ −1.5 (c 1.4, CHCl$_3$); ^{1}H NMR (CD$_3$CN) δ 7.46–7.21 (m, 15H, Ar-H), 5.40 (bs, 1H, H-1^I), 4.63 (m, 1H, H-2^I, H-4^I), 4.30 (m, 1H, H-5^I), 4.26 (d, 1H, $J_{1,2}$ 5.8 Hz, H-1), 4.18 (dt, 1H, $J_{4,5}$ 4.8 Hz, $J_{5,6a}$=$J_{5,6b}$ =6.4 Hz, H-5), 4.05 (dd, 1H, $J_{2,3}$ 7.5 Hz, H-2), 3.96 (dd, 1H, $J_{3,4}$ 2.1 Hz, H-3), 3.73 (dd, 1H, H-4), 3.89 (dd, 1H, $J_{6a,6b}$ 8.4 Hz, H-6b), 3.79 (dd, 1H, H-6a), 3.50 (dd, 1H, $J_{6a,6b}$ 10.3 Hz, $J_{5,6b}$ 4.0 Hz, H-6^{I}a), 3.39 (dd, 1H, $J_{5,6a}$ 6.6 Hz, H-6^{I}b), 3.36, 3.33 (2s, each 3H, 2×OCH$_3$), 1.43, 1.37, 1.28, 1.26, 1.22, 1.04 [6s, each 3H, 3×C(CH$_3$)$_2$]; ^{13}C NMR (CD$_3$CN) δ 152.4 (C-3^I), 145.2 (3×Ar-C), 129.6, 128.7, 128.0 (Ar-CH), 114.3, 110.3, 108.8 [3×C(CH$_3$)$_2$], 106.6 (C-1), 97.8 (C-1^I), 90.8 (C-2^I), 87.7 (CPh$_3$), 78.7 (C-3), 77.9 (C-4), 77.5 (C-5), 76.6 (C-2), 72.2 (C-4^I), 71.4 (C-5^I), 66.4 (C-6), 62.9 (C-6^I), 56.7, 54.8 (2×OCH$_3$), 27.2, 27.1, 26.8, 26.7, 25.2, 24.7 [3×C(CH$_3$)$_2$]. Anal. Calcd for C$_{42}$H$_{52}$O$_{11}$: C, 68.83; H, 7.15. Found: C, 68.78; H, 7.12.

Methyl 3,4-Di-*O*-Benzyl-2,6-Dideoxy-α-ʟ-*threo*-Hex-2-Enopyranoside (23)

To a stirred suspension of prewashed (hexane) 60% NaH in mineral oil (248 mg, 6.2 mmol, 1.5 equiv) in dry DMF (5 mL) was added at room temperature a solution of **22** (444 mg, 1.24 mmol) in dry DMF (19 mL). After 30 min, the mixture was cooled to −30°C and treated with Im$_2$SO$_2$ (369 mg, 1.86 mmol, 1.5 equiv) as described for the preparation of **13**. After 1 h at −30°C, TLC analysis (1:1 hexane–EtOAc) revealed complete disappearance of the starting material (R_f 0.40) and formation of two products (R_f 0.20 and 0.46). The mixture was allowed to warm to room temperature and stirred until TLC (2 h, 1:4 hexane–EtOAc) revealed complete disappearance of the component with R_f 0.20. Chromatography (7:3 hexane–EtOAc + 0.1% Et$_3$N) gave pure **23** (332 mg, 79%) as syrup, which spontaneously crystallized on standing but resisted all recrystallization attempts from common organic solvents: R_f 0.46 (1:1 hexane–EtOAc); mp 57–60°C.; $[\alpha]_D$ +67 (c 1.2, CHCl$_3$); ^{1}H NMR (CDCl$_3$) δ 7.36–7.22 (m, 10H, Ar-H), 5.12 (d, 1H, $J_{1,2}$ 3.3 Hz, H-2), 4.95 (d, 1H, H-1), 4.83, 4.65 (AB system, 2H, $J_{A,B}$ 11.7 Hz, CH$_2$Ph), 4.80 (s, 2H, CH$_2$Ph), 4.18 (dq, 1H, $J_{5,6}$ 6.7 Hz, $J_{4,5}$ 2.5 Hz, H-5), 3.56 (d, 1H, H-4), 3.42 (s, 3H, OCH$_3$), 1.32 (d, 3H, H-6); ^{13}C NMR (CDCl$_3$) δ 156.6 (C-3), 138.3, 136.3 (Ar-C), 128.5–127.5 (Ar-CH), 96.8, 96.7 (C-1, C-2), 72.9 (C-4), 72.9, 69.2 (2×CH$_2$Ph), 66.7 (C-5), 55.3 (OCH$_3$), 16.2 (C-6). Anal. Calcd for C$_{21}$H$_{24}$O$_4$: C, 74.09; H, 7.11. Found: C, 74.05; H, 7.09.

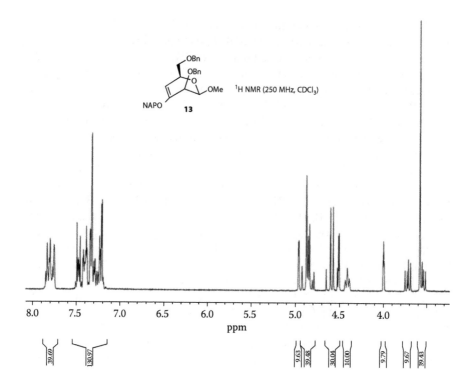

^{1}H NMR (250 MHz, CDCl$_3$)

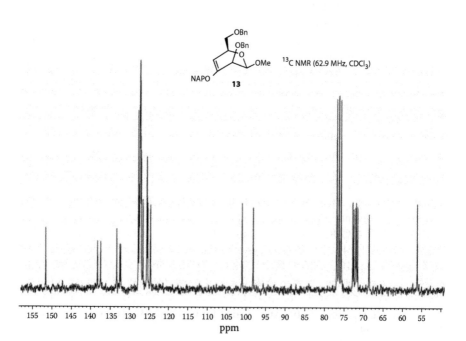

^{13}C NMR (62.9 MHz, CDCl$_3$)

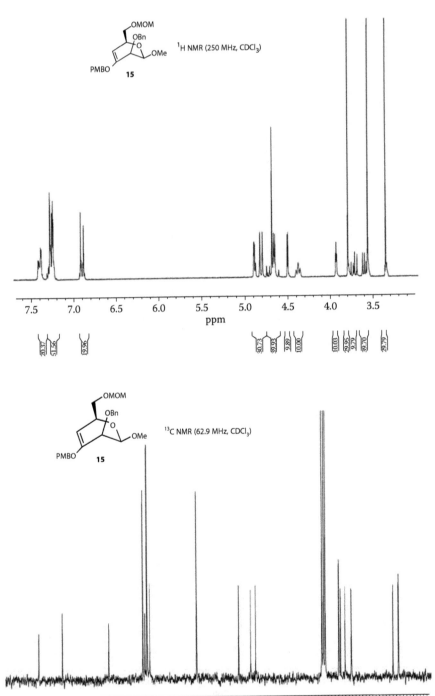

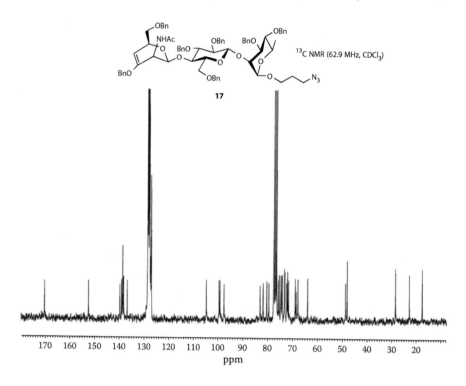

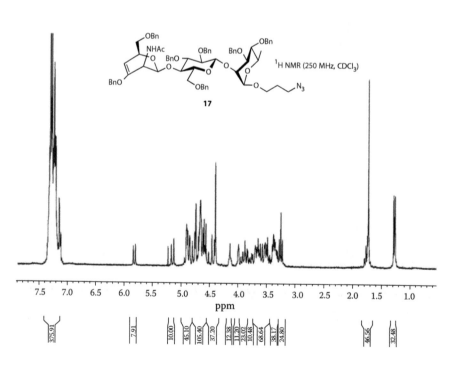

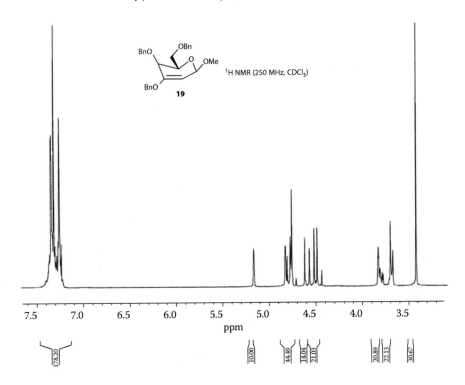

^{1}H NMR (250 MHz, CDCl$_3$)

19

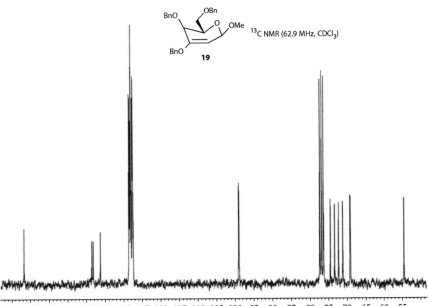

^{13}C NMR (62.9 MHz, CDCl$_3$)

19

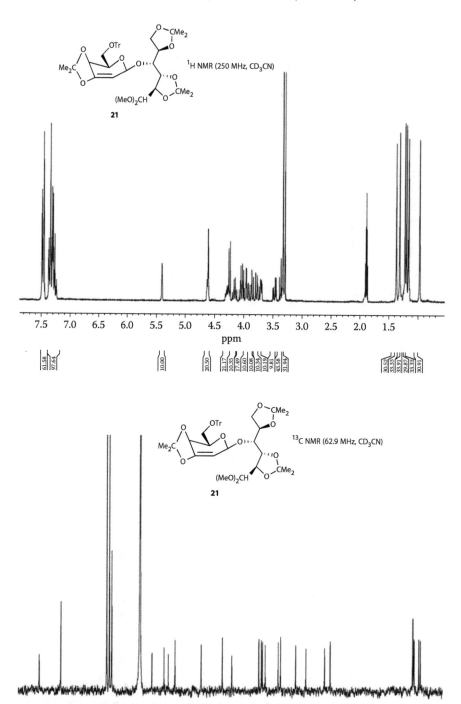

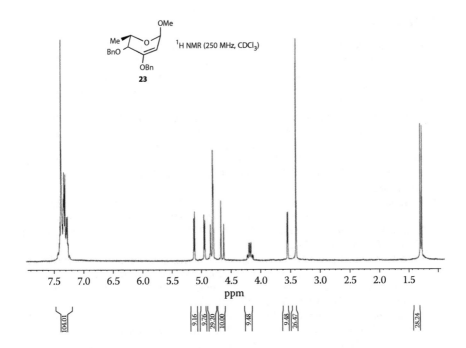

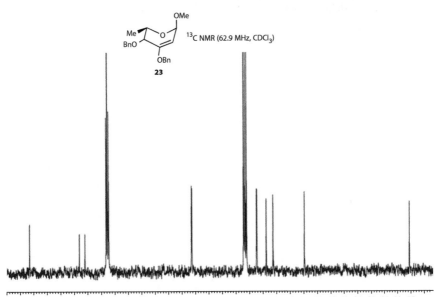

REFERENCES

1. (a) Ferrier, R. J. In *The Carbohydrates, Chemistry and Biochemistry*; Pigman, W.; Horton, D. Eds.; Academic Press: San Diego, CA, 1980; Vol. 1B, pp. 843–879; (b) Ferrier, R. J.; Hoberg, J. O. *Adv. Carbohydr. Chem. Biochem.* 2003, *58*, 55–119.
2. Hanessian, S. *Total Synthesis of Natural Products: The Chiron Approach*; Pergamon Press: Oxford, U.K., 1983.
3. Danishefsky, S. J.; Bilodeau, M. T. *Angew. Chem. Int. Ed. Engl.* 1996, *35*, 1380–1419.
4. Fraser-Reid, B. *Acc. Chem. Res.* 1996, *29*, 57–66.
5. (a) Chètrien, F. *Synth. Commun.* 1989, *19*, 1015–1024; (b) Khan, K. M.; Perveen, S.; Shah, S. T. A.; Shekhani, M. S.; Volter, W. *New. J. Chem.* 2001, *25*, 896–898; (c) Catelani, G.; Corsaro, A.; D'Andrea, F.; Mariani, M.; Pistarà, V.; Vittorino, E. *Carbohydr. Res.* 2003, *338*, 2349–2358.
6. (a) Binkley, R. W.; Ambrose, M. G. *J. Carbohydr. Chem.* 1984, *3*, 1–49; (b) El Nemr, A.; Tsuchiya, T.; Kobayashi, Y. *Carbohydr. Res.* 1996, *293*, 31–59; (c) El Nemr, A.; Tsuchiya, T. *Carbohydr. Res.* 1997, *303*, 267–281; (d) El Nemr, A.; Tsuchiya, T. *Carbohydr. Res.* 2001, *330*, 205–214.
7. (a) Attolino, E.; Catelani, G.; D'Andrea, F. *Tetrahedron Lett.* 2002, *43*, 1685–1688; (b) Attolino, E.; Catelani, G.; D'Andrea, F. *Eur. J. Org. Chem.* 2006, *23*, 5279–5292.
8. Bernabe, M.; Fernandez-Mayoralas, A.; Jimenez-Barbero, J.; Martin-Lomas, M. *J. Chem. Soc. Perkin Trans.* 1989, *2*, 1867–1873.
9. (a) Attolino, E.; Catelani, G.; D'Andrea, F. *Tetrahedron Lett.* 2002, *43*, 8815–8818; (b) Attolino, E.; Catelani, G.; D'Andrea, F.; Nicolardi, M. *J. Carbohydr. Chem.* 2004, *23*, 179–190; (c) Attolino, E.; Catelani, G.; D'Andrea, F.; Křenek, K.; Bezouška, K; Křen, V. *J. Carbohydr. Chem.* 2008, *27*, 156–171; (d) Attolino, E.; Bonaccorsi, F.; Catelani, G.; D'Andrea, F. *Carbohydr. Res.* 2008, *343*, 2545–2556.
10. Gridley, J. J.; Osborn, H. M. I. *J. Chem. Soc., Perkin Trans 1*, 2000, 1471–1491.
11. Armarengo, W. L. F.; Perrin, D. D. *Purification of Laboratory Chemicals*, 4th edn., Butterworth-Heinemann, Oxford, 1996.

3 Enhancement of the Rate of Purdie Methylation by Me$_2$S Catalysis

Shujie Hou, Thomas Ziegler,[†] and Pavol Kováč[*]

CONTENTS

Experimental Methods 29
  General Methods 29
    General Procedure 29
    Methylation of Methyl 3-*O*-Benzyl-β-D-Galactopyranoside (**1**) 30
    Methylation of Methyl 6-*O*-Trityl-β-D-Galactopyranoside (**3**) 31
    Methylation of Methyl 6-*O*-Trityl-α-D-Glucopyranoside (**5**) 32
    Methylation of Methyl 2,3-Di-*O*-Benzyl-6-*O*-Benzoyl-β-D-
    Glucopyranoside (**7**) 33
Acknowledgment 35
References 42

* Corresponding author.
[†] Checker.

Methylation with the Purdie reagent (MeI and Ag_2O, with or without addition of external solvent)[1] is a slow reaction; several treatments with the alkylating agent are often required to complete the task.[2] This method is, however, still useful when more powerful reagents cannot be applied because of synthon instability. Although its exact role has not been established, the addition of a catalytic amount of dimethyl sulfide to Purdie reagent has been shown[3,4] to affect the rate of O-methylation markedly and to yield permethylated product in cases where the standard Purdie procedure resulted in only partial methylation. It has been suggested[4] that the enhancement of the rate of O-methylation in the presence of dimethyl sulfide is due to a modification of silver oxide, for example, by complex formation, in such a manner as to convert it to a more efficient base.

Acyl groups present in the molecule may migrate or be removed when such compounds are methylated with Purdie reagent. The migration can be largely avoided by the use of 2,6-dimethoxybenzoyl protecting group.[5] Deacylation might be minimized when Me_2S is added to the Purdie reagent, as the rate of methylation may increase more relative to that of deacylation, compared to the situation in the absence of Me_2S. For example,[6] methylation of a partially acetylated disaccharide with Purdie reagent in the presence of Me_2S resulted in good yield of the desired product within a relatively short period of time, when other methylation protocols failed.

Purdie methylations in the presence of Me_2S have been most often carried out with MeI as solvent and reagent,[3] THF[6] or 1,2-dimethoxyethane[7-10] (DME). During this work, methylations of 1, 3, 5, and 7 were initially conducted in MeI as solvent and reagent (not described in the "Experimental methods" section), with and without addition of Me_2S. The addition of Me_2S enhanced the process in all cases but there was room for improvement. When carried out in CH_3CN as solvent in absence of Me_2S, the efficiency of Purdie methylation increased compared to methylations in other solvents (TLC, these experiments are not described in "Experimental methods" section), and when Me_2S-assisted Purdie methylation was carried out using MeCN as solvent, the efficiency of this type of methylation was unprecedented: a single treatment overnight with the reagent resulted in complete conversion of starting materials into the corresponding fully methylated product. Such was the case even with the galactose derivative 3, despite the presence of the bulky 6-O-triphenylmethyl and the poorly reactive, axially oriented HO-4 groups. Methyl sulfide-promoted Purdie methylation involving aprotic solvents may find application also in methylation of polysaccharides and other substances that are unstable at more basic conditions.

EXPERIMENTAL METHODS

GENERAL METHODS

Optical rotations were measured at ambient temperature in CHCl$_3$ with a Jasco automatic polarimeter, Model P-2000. All reactions were monitored by thin-layer chromatography (TLC) on silica gel 60 coated glass slides (Analtech, Inc.). Column chromatography was performed by elution from columns of silica gel with CombiFlash Companion Chromatograph (Isco., Inc.). Solvent mixtures less polar than those used for TLC were used at the onset of separations. Nuclear magnetic resonance (NMR) spectra were measured at 600 MHz (^{1}H) and 150 MHz (^{13}C) with a Bruker Avance 600 spectrometer in CDCl$_3$ as solvent. ^{1}H and ^{13}C chemical shifts are referenced to signals of TMS (0 ppm) and CDCl$_3$ (77.0 ppm). Assignments of NMR signals were made by homonuclear and heteronuclear two-dimensional correlation spectroscopy, run with the software supplied with the spectrometer. Silver oxide was prepared as described.[2] The yield of methyl 2,3-di-*O*-benzyl-6-*O*-benzoyl-β-D-glucopyranoside was increased to 83% by conducting the selective benzoylation[11] in more dilute solution (15 mL/g), mp 96°C–98°C (from ether-hexane), Ref. [11], yield, 63%, mp 96°C–98°C. ^{1}H NMR: δ 4.96–4.71 (4d, 4H, 4 CH_2Ph), 4.63 (dd, 1H, $J_{5,6}$=4.4, $J_{6a,6b}$=12.0 Hz, H-6$_a$), 4.58 (dd, 1H, $J_{5,6}$=2.1 Hz, H-6$_b$), 4.37 (d, 1H, $J_{1,2}$=7.7 Hz, H-1), 3.58 (t, partially overlapped, H-4), 3.57 (s, partially overlapped, OMe), 3.56 (m, partially overlapped, H-5), 3.50 (t, 1H, J=9.0 Hz, H-3), 3.43 (dd, 1H, $J_{2,3}$=9.1 Hz, H-2), 2.64 (bs, 1H, OH). ^{13}C NMR: δ 104.87 (H-1), 83.63 (H-3), 81.76 (C-2), 75.44, 74.65 (2 CH_2Ph), 73.57 (C-5), 69.93 (C-4), 63.69 (C-6), 57.17 (OCH$_3$). Solutions in organic solvents were dried with anhydrous Na$_2$SO$_4$ and concentrated at 40°C/2 kPa.

General Procedure

A. A mixture of the starting carbohydrate derivative to be methylated (1 mmol), methyl iodide (3.2 mL, 50 mmol), Ag$_2$O (2 mmol/OH), and Me$_2$S (0.1 mL) in CH$_3$CN (12 mL) was stirred in the dark and the reaction was monitored by TLC.* After 24 h, or 7 h for the conversion (**7 → 8**), the mixture was filtered through Celite 545, the solids were washed with EtOAc, the combined filtrate was concentrated, and the residue was chromatographed.

B. For comparison, a parallel reaction was run with the same proportion of reagents without addition of Me$_2$S (0.1 mL). After 7 and 24 h, the TLC profile of reactions in (A) and (B) were compared (see below), and the mixture was discarded.

---

* The rate of methylation with Purdie reagent may vary and formation of by-products may be affected by quality of MeI and Ag$_2$O. Freshly prepared Ag$_2$O[2] is dark brown; old, weathered preparations turn black and should not be used. Decomposition of MeI manifests itself by discoloration of the reagent. Purified, colorless material should be stored in the dark. Its shelf life can be extended by contact with small amount of mercury, powdered silver, or copper.[12]

Methylation of Methyl 3-*O*-Benzyl-β-D-Galactopyranoside (1)

As shown in Figure 3.1, Line 3, Purdie methylation with addition of Me$_2$S was almost complete after 7 h of reaction time, whereas a large amount of starting material and of products of undermethylation were present in the reaction mediated with Purdie reagent alone. After 24 h, only the target, fully methylated product was present in the mixture involving Me$_2$S. After the same reaction time, the mixture resulting from methylation with Purdie reagent contained mainly products of undermethylation, in addition to a small proportion of **2**. Chromatography of the mixture shown in Figure 3.1 (Line 5) gave methyl 3-*O*-benzyl-2,4,6-tri-*O*-methyl-β-D-galactopyranoside (307 mg, 94%), mp 58°C–59°C (hexane); [α]$_D$ −23.3° (c 1.06, CHCl$_3$); ^{1}H NMR: δ 7.33–7.19 (m, 5H, aromatic protons), 4.67 (s, 2H, PhCH_2), 4.07 (bd, 1H, $J_{1,2} \sim 7.0$ Hz, H-1), 3.55–3.51 (m, 8H, H-4, H-6$_a$, 2×OCH$_3$), 3.46 (dd, 1H, $J_{5,6a} = 5.6$ Hz, $J_{6a,b} = 9.4$ Hz, H-6$_b$), 3.44 (s, 3H, OCH$_3$), 3.39 (m, 1H, H-5), 3.35–3.30 (m, 5H, H-2, H-3, OCH$_3$); ^{13}C NMR: 138.4 (C$_q$), 128.3, 127.6, 127.5, 104.4 (C-1), 87.1 (C-2), 80.9 (C-3), 75.8 (C-4), 72.9 (C-5), 72.6 (PhCH_2), 70.7 (C-6), 61.2 (OCH$_3$), 60.8 (OCH$_3$), 59.1 (OCH$_3$), 56.7 (OCH$_3$); ESI-MS: [M + Na]$^+$calcd for C$_{17}$H$_{26}$O$_6$Na, 349.1627; found: 349.1631; Anal. calcd for C$_{17}$H$_{26}$O$_6$: C, 62.56; H, 8.03. Found: C, 62.35; H, 8.01.

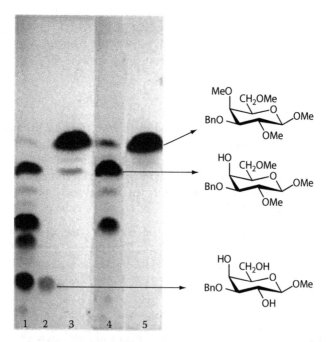

FIGURE 3.1 Monitoring of methylation of methyl 3-*O*-benzyl-β-D-galactopyranoside by TLC, 2:1 hexane–acetone. Line 1, 3: Reaction time, 7 h, methylation with Purdie reagent and methylation with Purdie reagent with addition of Me$_2$S, respectively. Line 2: Starting material. Line 4, 5: Reaction time 24 h, methylation with Purdie reagent and methylation with Purdie reagent with addition of Me$_2$S, respectively.

When the same reaction was carried out in MeI as solvent and reagent, the yield of **2** after 24h of reaction time was 74%, and the incompletely methylated product, methyl 3-O-benzyl-2,6-di-O-methyl-β-D-galactopyranoside, was also isolated. ^{1}H NMR: 7.39–7.26 (m, 5H, aromatic protons), 4.70 (s, 2H, PhCH_2), 4.17 (d, 1H, $J_{1,2}$=7.7 Hz, H-1), 3.99 (bs, 1H, H-4), 3.71 (dd, 1H, $J_{5,6a}$=5.6 Hz, $J_{6a,b}$=10.5 Hz, H-6$_a$), 3.63(dd, 1H, $J_{5,6b}$=6.0 Hz, H-6$_b$), 3.61 (s, 3H, OCH$_3$), 3.55 (s, 3H, OCH$_3$), 3.50 (t, 1H, J=5.8 Hz, H-5), 3.41 (s, 3H, OCH$_3$), 3.40 (dd, 1H, $J_{2,3}$=9.3 Hz, $J_{3,4}$=3.3 Hz, H-3), 3.34 (dd, 1H, $J_{1,2}$=7.7 Hz, $J_{2,3}$=9.3 Hz, H-2), 2.57 (s, 1H, 4-OH); ^{13}C NMR (CDCl$_3$ 150 MHz): 137.8 (C$_q$), 128.4, 127.8, 127.7, 104.4 (C-1), 80.6 (C-4), 80.4 (C-2), 72.8 (C-5), 72.2 (PhCH$_2$), 71.6 (C-6), 66.8 (C-4), 60.9 (OCH$_3$), 59.4 (OCH$_3$), 56.8 (OCH$_3$); ESI-MS: [M+Na]$^+$calcd for C$_{16}$H$_{24}$O$_6$Na, 335.1471; found: 35.1481.

Methylation of Methyl 6-O-Trityl-β-D-Galactopyranoside (3)

As shown in Figure 3.2 (Line 3), after 7h of reaction time, Purdie methylation with addition of Me₂S (Line 3) was almost complete, whereas a large amount of products of undermethylation were present in the reaction carried out with plain Purdie reagent (Line 1). After 24h, only the target, fully methylated product was present in the mixture involving Me₂S (Line 5). After the same reaction time, the mixture resulting from Purdie reagent-mediated methylation contained two products of

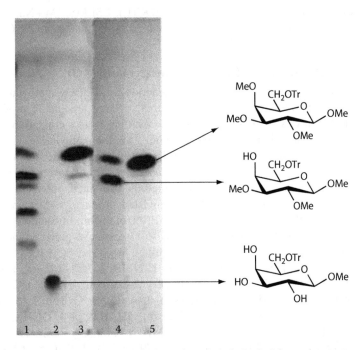

FIGURE 3.2 Monitoring of methylation of methyl 6-O-trityl-β-D-galactopyranoside by TLC, 3:2 hexane–acetone. Line 1, 3: Reaction time, 7h, methylation with Purdie reagent and methylation with Purdie reagent with addition of Me₂S, respectively. Line 2: Starting material. Line 4, 5: Reaction time 24h, methylation with Purdie reagent and methylation with Purdie reagent with addition of Me₂S, respectively.

which the product of undermethylation, methyl 2,3-di-O-methyl-6-O-trityl-β-D-galactopyranoside, predominated. Chromatography (9: 1: 0.02 hexane–acetone–Et$_3$N) of the mixture shown in Figure 3.2 (Line 5) gave methyl 2,3,4-tri-O-methyl-6-O-trityl-β-D-galactopyranoside (**4**) (420 mg, 88%) as a white foam, [α]$_D$ −44.1° (c 2.3); Ref. [13] [α]$_D$ −23° (c 2.2, CHCl$_3$). ^{1}H NMR: δ 4.11 (d, 1H, $J_{1,2}$=7.6 Hz, H-1), 3.76 (bd, 1H, $J_{3,4}$=3.0 Hz, H-4), 3.57, 3.55, 3.48, 3.38 (4 s, 3H each, 4×OCH$_3$), 3.46–3.41 (m, 2H, H-6$_a$,5), 3.27 (dd, partially overlapped, $J_{2,3}$=9.7 Hz, H-2), 3.24 (dd, partially overlapped, $J_{5,6b}$=6.9 Hz, H-6$_b$), 3.16 (dd, 1H, H-3). ^{13}C NMR: δ 104.38 (C-1), 86.80 (C-Ph$_3$), 83.98 (C-3), 80.71 (C-2), 74.91 (C-4), 73.09 (C-5), 61.75 (C-6), 61.07, 60.76, 58.33, 56.60 (4 OCH$_3$). ESI-MS: calcd for C$_{29}$H$_{34}$O$_6$Na, 501.2253; found: 501.2240; Anal. calcd for C$_{29}$H$_{34}$O$_6$: C, 72.78; H, 7.16. Found: C, 72.55; H, 7.24.

When the same reaction was carried out in MeI as solvent and reagent, the yield of **2** after 24 h of reaction time was 74%, and a small amount of incompletely methylated product, the amorphous methyl 2,3-di-O-methyl-6-O-trityl-β-D-galactopyranoside, was also isolated, [α]$_D$ −22.7° (c 0.6). ^{1}H NMR: δ 7.48–7.22 (m, 15H, aromatic protons), 4.16 (d, 1H, $J_{1,2}$=7.7 Hz, H-1), 4.05 (t, 1H, J=3.2 Hz, H-4), 3.58 (s, 3H, OCH$_3$), 3.57 (s, 3H, OCH$_3$), 3.49 (s, 3H, OCH$_3$), 3.47–3.44 (m, 2H, H-5 and H-6$_a$), 3.37 (dd, 1H, $J_{5,6}$=7.7 Hz, $J_{6a,b}$=11.6 Hz, H-6$_b$), 3.26 (dd, 1H, $J_{1,2}$=7.7 Hz, $J_{2,3}$=9.2 Hz, H-2), 3.15 (dd, 1H, $J_{3,4}$=3.3 Hz, $J_{2,3}$=9.2 Hz, H-3); ^{13}C NMR (CDCl$_3$ 150 MHz): 144.3 (C$_q$), 129.2, 128.4, 127.6, 104.9 (C-1), 87.4 (C$_q$), 83.4 (C-3), 80.8 (C-2), 73.8 (C-5), 66.6 (C-4), 63.6 (C-6), 61.4 (OCH$_3$), 58.3 (OCH$_3$), 57.2 (OCH$_3$); ESI-MS: [M + Na]$^+$calcd for C$_{28}$H$_{32}$O$_6$Na, 487.2097; found: 487.2088. Found: 35.1481. Anal. calcd for C$_{28}$H$_{32}$O$_6$: C, 72.39; H, 6.94. Found: C, 72.32; H, 6.97.

Methylation of Methyl 6-O-Trityl-α-D-Glucopyranoside (5)

Figure 3.3 (Line 3) shows that after 7 h of reaction time Purdie methylation with addition of Me$_2$S was almost complete whereas a large amount of products of undermethylation was present in the mixture resulting from methylation with the plain Purdie reagent (Figure 3.3, Line 1). After 24 h, the methylation in presence of Me$_2$S was complete: Only the target, fully methylated product **6** was present (Figure 3.3, Line 5). After the same reaction time, the mixture resulting from Purdie reagent-mediated methylation contained the fully methylated compound **6** as the main product and two partially methylated products were also present. Chromatography (9: 1: 0.02 hexane–acetone–Et$_3$N) of the mixture shown in Figure 3.3 (Line 5) gave methyl 2,3,4-tri-O-methyl-6-O-trityl-α-D-glucopyranoside (**6**, 448 mg, 93%), mp 106°C–108°C (EtOAc–hexane); [α]$_D$ +98.2° (c 1.1, CHCl$_3$), Ref. [14] mp 109°C, Ref. [14] [α]$_D$ not reported. ^{1}H NMR: δ 7.50–7.21 (m, 15H, aromatic protons), 4.91 (d, 1H, $J_{1,2}$=4.1 Hz, H-1), 3.62–3.60 (m, 4H, H-5, OCH$_3$), 3.56 (s, 3H, OCH$_3$), 3.48 (t, 1H, J=9.2 Hz, H-3), 3.44 (s, 3H, OCH$_3$), 3.40 (dd, 1H, $J_{5,6}$=1.8 Hz, $J_{6a,b}$=10.0 Hz, H-6$_a$), 3.31–3.28 (m, 5H, H-2, H-4, OCH$_3$), 3.11(dd, 1H, $J_{5,6}$=4.6 Hz, $J_{6a,b}$=10.0 Hz, H-6$_b$); ^{13}C NMR: δ 144.0 (C$_q$), 128.7, 127.7, 126.9, 97.2 (C-1), 86.2 (C$_q$), 83.7 (C-3), 81.8 (C-2), 79.9 (C-4), 70.0 (C-5), 62.4 (C-6), 60.9 (OCH$_3$), 60.3 (OCH$_3$), 59.0 (OCH$_3$), 54.9 (OCH$_3$); ESI-MS: [M + Na]$^+$calcd for C$_{29}$H$_{34}$O$_6$Na, 501.2231; found: 501.2241. Anal. calcd for C$_{29}$H$_{34}$O$_6$: C, 72.78; H, 7.16. Found: C, 72.86; H, 7.15.

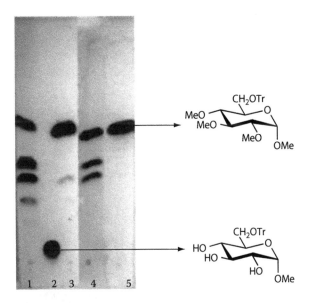

FIGURE 3.3 Monitoring of methylation of methyl 6-O-trityl-α-D-glucopyranoside by TLC, 2:1 hexane–acetone. Line 1, 3: Reaction time, 7 h, methylation with Purdie reagent and methylation with Purdie reagent with addition of Me₂S, respectively. Line 2: Starting material. Line 4, 5: Reaction time 24 h, methylation with Purdie reagent and methylation with Purdie reagent with addition of Me₂S, respectively.

Methylation of Methyl 2,3-Di-O-Benzyl-6-O-Benzoyl-β-D-Glucopyranoside (7)

After the first 7 h of reaction time, only little material other than the starting alcohol **7** was present in the mixture resulting from treatment with Purdie reagent (Figure 3.4A, Line 1). After 24 h, some progress of conversion was noted but the starting material **7** was still the main component of the mixture (Figure 3.4A, Line 2). Monitoring the treatment of **7** with Purdie reagent in presence of Me₂S by TLC (4:1 hexane–acetone) showed that all the starting material was consumed after 7 h (Figure 3.4B, Line 2). The reaction mixture contained one major and a number of very minor products. Using 4:1 hexane–EtOAc as elution solvent, TLC showed (Figure 3.4C, Line 2) that the mixture contained a by-product whose presence had not been revealed previously, having virtually the same chromatographic mobility as that of starting alcohol **7**, which was no longer present (Figure 3.4B, Line 2). After processing, chromatography (10:1 hexane–EtOAc) gave first methyl 6-benzoyl-2,3-di-O-benzyl-4-O-methyl-β-D-glucopyranoside (410 mg, 83%), mp 77°C–78°C (EtOH); [α]$_D$ +39.5° (c 1.1); ¹H NMR: δ 8.07–7.25 (m, 15H, aromatic protons), 4.93–4.71 (m, 4H, 2×PhCH_2), 4.64 (dd, ¹H, $J_{5,6a}$=2.3 Hz, $J_{6a,b}$=11.9 Hz, H-6$_a$), 4.47 (dd, 1H, $J_{5,6b}$=5.2 Hz, $J_{6a,b}$=11.9 Hz, H-6$_b$), 4.35 (d, 1H, $J_{1,2}$=7.7 Hz, H-1), 3.60 (t, 1H, J=9.0 Hz, H-3), 3.57–3.55 (m, 7H, H-5, 2×OCH₃), 3.43 (dd, 1H, $J_{2,3}$=9.2 Hz, H-2), 3.38 (t, J=9.2 Hz, H-4); ¹³C NMR: 166.3 (CO), 138.4, 138.3, 133.0, 129.6, 128.3, 128.0, 127.7, 127.6, 104.6 (C-1), 84.3 (C-3), 82.0 (C-2), 79.8 (C-4), 75.7 (PhCH₂), 74.7

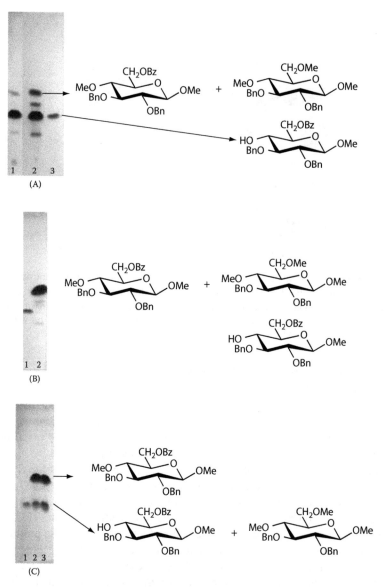

FIGURE 3.4 Monitoring of methylation of methyl 2,3-di-*O*-benzyl-6-*O*-benzoyl-β-D-glucopyranoside by TLC. (A) Methylation with Purdie reagent; 4:1 hexane–acetone. Line 1: Reaction time, 7 h. Line 2: Reaction time, 24 h. Line 3, Starting material. (B) Methylation with Purdie reagent with addition of Me₂S, 4:1 hexane–acetone. Line 1: Starting material. Line 2: Reaction time, 7 h. (C) Methylation with Purdie reagent with addition of Me₂S, 4:1 hexane–EtOACc. Line 1: Starting material. Line 2: Reaction time, 7 h. Line 3: Reaction time 7 h, with addition of starting material.

(PhCH_2), 72.9 (C-5), 63.5 (C-6), 60.8 (OCH$_3$), 57.1 (OCH$_3$); ESI-MS: [M+Na]$^+$calcd for C$_{29}$H$_{32}$O$_7$Na, 515.2046; found: 515.2046. Anal. calcd for C$_{29}$H$_{32}$O$_7$: C, 70.71; H, 6.55. Found: C, 70.79; H, 6.55.

Eluted next was methyl 2,3-di-O-benzyl-4,6-di-O-methyl-β-D-glucopyranoside (40 mg, 10%), resulting from the removal of the 6-O-benzoyl group and subsequent methylation. ^{1}H NMR: 7.35–7.25 (m, 10H, aromatic protons), 4.90–4.68 (m, 4H, 2×PhCH_2), 4.27 (d, 1H, $J_{1,2}$=7.8 Hz, H-1), 3.66 (dd, 1H, $J_{5,6a}$=1.9 Hz, $J_{6a,b}$=10.6 Hz, H-6$_a$), 3.58 (dd, 1H, $J_{5,6b}$=4.6 Hz, $J_{6a,b}$=10.6 Hz, H-6$_b$), 3.56 (s, 3H, OCH$_3$), 3.53 (s, 3H, OCH$_3$), 3.52 (dd, 1H, $J_{2,3}$=9.3 Hz, $J_{3,4}$=8.9 Hz, H-3), 3.41 (s, 3H, OCH$_3$), 3.36 (dd, 1H, $J_{1,2}$=7.8 Hz, $J_{2,3}$=9.3 Hz, H-2), 3.32 (m, 1H, H-5), 3.27 (dd, 1H, $J_{3,4}$=8.9 Hz, $J_{4,5}$=9.7 Hz, H-4); ^{13}C NMR (CDCl$_3$ 150 MHz): 138.6 (C$_q$), 138.5 (C$_q$), 128.3, 128.1, 127.9, 127.6, 104.7 (C-1), 84.4 (C-3), 82.1 (C-2), 79.6 (C-4), 75.5 (PhCH_2), 74.8 (C-5), 74.7 (PhCH_2), 71.3 (C-6), 60.6 (OCH$_3$), 59.4 (OCH$_3$), 57.1(OCH$_3$); ESI-MS: [M+NH$_4$]$^+$calcd for C$_{23}$H$_{34}$NO$_6$, 420.2386; found: 420.2393.

ACKNOWLEDGMENT

This chapter was supported by the Intramural Research Program of the NIH, NIDDK.

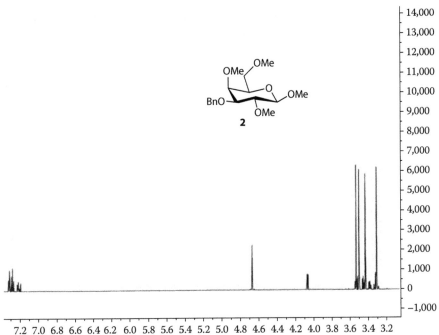

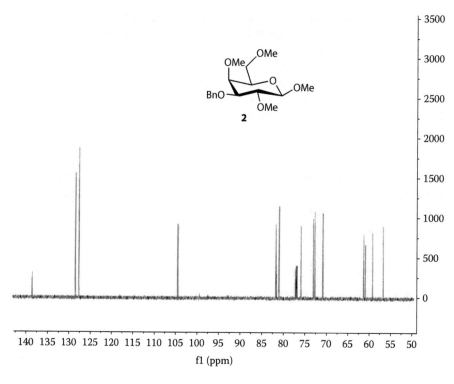

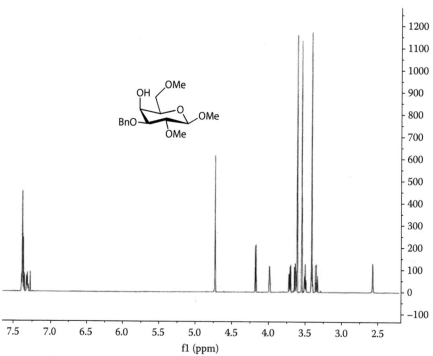

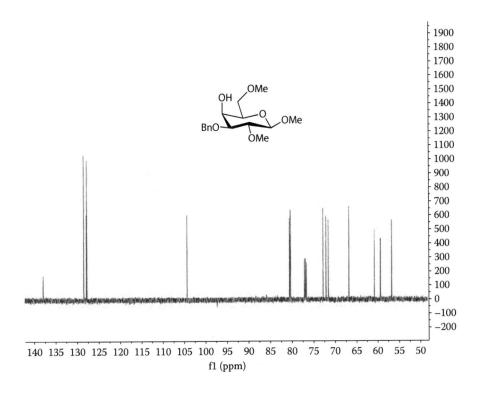

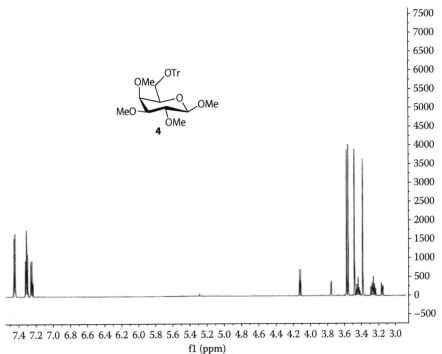

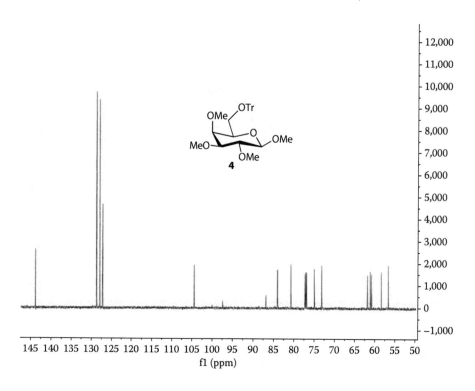

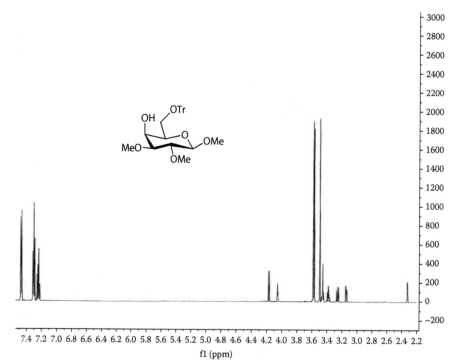

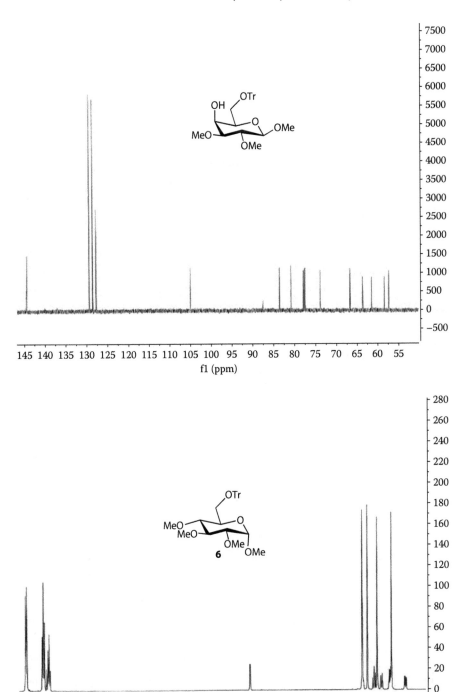

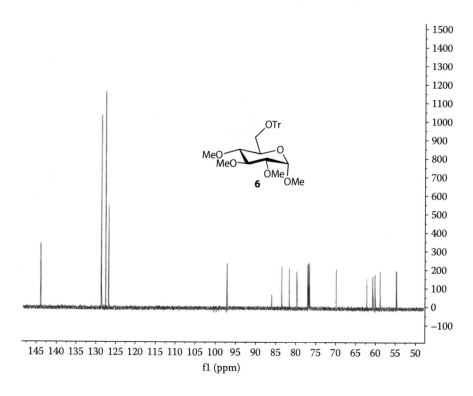

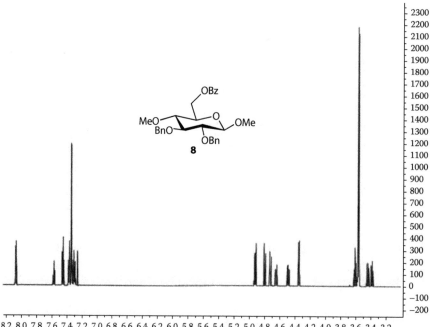

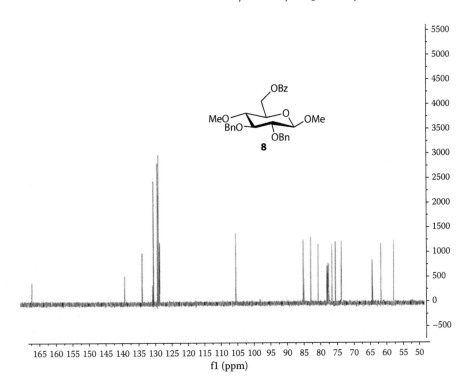

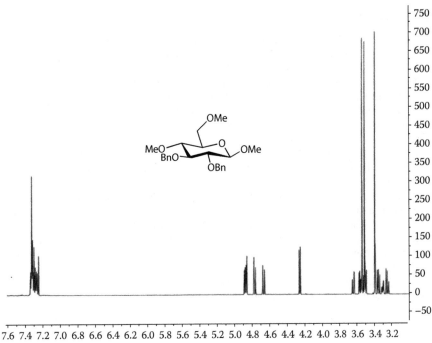

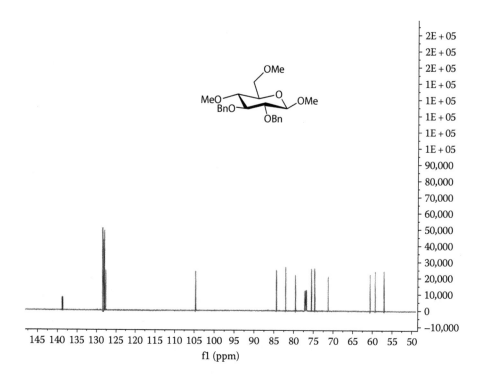

REFERENCES

1. Purdie, T.; Irvine, J. C. *J. Chem. Soc. Trans.* 1903, *83*, 1021–1037.
2. Hirst, E. L.; Percival, E. *Methods Carbohydr. Chem.* 1963, *2*, 145–150.
3. Kovacik, V.; Kováč, P. *Chem. Zvesti* 1973, *27*, 662–667.
4. Bannister, B.; Kováč, P. An examination of the catalytic effect of dimethyl sulfide in the Purdie O-alkylation of carbohydrates. *Proceedings of the VIIth International Symposium on Carbohydrate Chemistry, August 5–9, 1974*, Bratislava, Czechoslovakia, p. 8.
5. Abbas, S.; Haines, A. H. *Carbohydr. Res.* 1975, *41*, 298–303.
6. Werz, D. B.; Seeberger, P. H. *Angew. Chem. Int. Ed. Engl.* 2005, *44*, 6315–6318.
7. Kováč, P. *Carbohydr. Res.* 1972, *22*, 464–466.
8. Kováč, P.; Hirsch, J.; Palovčík, R.; Tvaroška, I.; Bystrický, S. *Collect. Czech. Chem. Commun.* 1976, *41*, 3119–3130.
9. Adamo, R.; Saksena, R.; Kováč, P. *Helv. Chim. Acta.* 2006, *89*, 1075–1089.
10. Saksena, R.; Adamo, R.; Kováč, P. *Carbohydr. Res.* 2005, *340*, 1591–1600.
11. Ittah, Y.; Glaudemans, C. P. J. *Carbohydr. Res.* 1981, *95*, 189–194.
12. Armarego, W. L. E.; Chai, C. L. L. Purification of laboratory chemicals, in: *Book Purification of Laboratory Chemicals*; 5th edn.; Elsevier, Amsterdam, the Netherlands, 2003.
13. Luckett, S.; Smith, F. *J. Chem. Soc.* 1940, 1506–1511.
14. Lehmann, J. *Carbohydr. Res.* 1966, *2*, 1–13.

4 Synthesis of Oligosaccharides by Preactivation-Based Chemoselective Glycosylation of Thioglycosyl Donors

Zhen Wang, Gilbert Wasonga, Benjamin M. Swarts,[†] and Xuefei Huang*

CONTENTS

Experimental Methods 45
  General Methods 45
    p-Toluenesulfenyl Chloride (**1**)[25] 46
    p-Tolyl 6-*O*-(2,3,4-Tri-*O*-Benzoyl-6-*O*-*Tert*-Butyldiphenylsilyl-β-D-
    Glucopyranosyl)-2,3,4-Tri-*O*-Benzyl-1-Thio-β-D-Glucopyranoside (**4**) 46
    Methyl 2-*O*-Benzoyl-3-*O*-Benzyl-4-*O*-*Tert*-Butyldimethylsilyl-6-*O*-
    p-Methoxybenzyl-β-D-Glucopyranosyl-(1 → 3)-4,6-*O*-Benzylidene-
    2-Deoxy-2-*N*-Phthalimido-β-D-Galactopyranosyl-(1 → 4)-2,3-Di-*O*-
    Benzyl-6-*O*-*p*-Methoxybenzyl-β-D-Glucopyranoside (**8**) 47
Acknowledgment 48
References... 50

---

* Corresponding author.
[†] Checker.

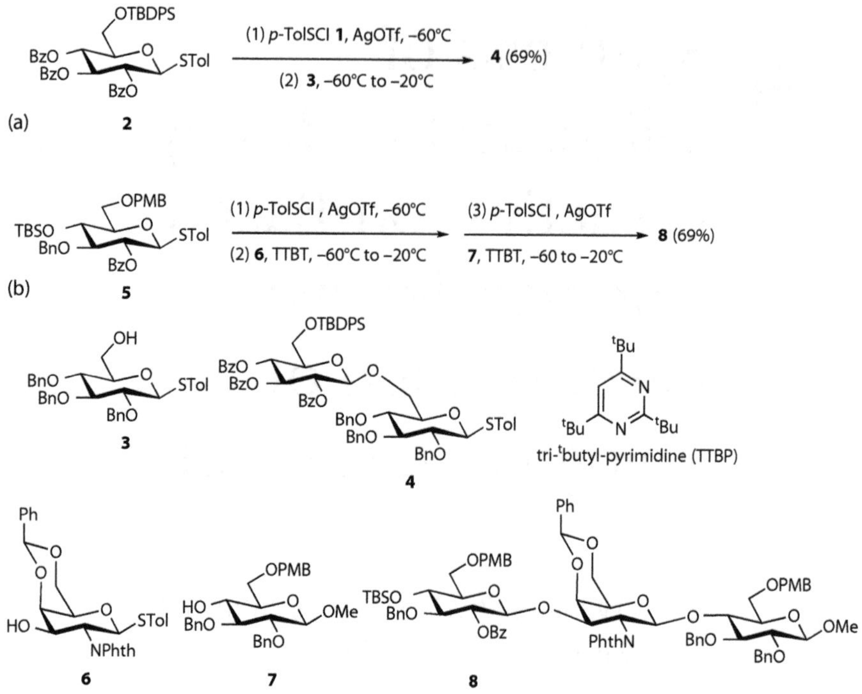

(a)

(1) p-TolSCl **1**, AgOTf, –60°C

(2) **3**, –60°C to –20°C

4 (69%)

(b)

(1) p-TolSCl , AgOTf, –60°C

(2) **6**, TTBT, –60°C to –20°C

(3) p-TolSCl , AgOTf

7, TTBT, –60 to –20°C

8 (69%)

tri-ᵗbutyl-pyrimidine (TTBP)

Increasing recognition of important biological functions of carbohydrates has stimulated the development of many innovative methodologies in carbohydrate synthesis during the past two decades.[1-4] In most glycosylation reactions, a promoter is added to a mixture of a glycosyl donor and an acceptor. The glycosyl donor is activated by the promoter, which undergoes an in situ nucleophilic addition or displacement reaction with the acceptor leading to the glycoside product. Alternatively, the glycosyl donor can be activated in the absence of an acceptor (preactivation).[5-12] Upon complete donor activation, the acceptor is added to the reaction mixture initiating glycoside formation. Using the preactivation strategy, unique stereochemical outcomes[5,9,11,13] and chemoselectivities[6-8,10,14] have been observed.

In recent years, we have developed a preactivation-based chemoselective glycosylation strategy using thioglycosides, which enables integration of several glycosylation processes to furnish the target oligosaccharides in one pot within a few hours (see opening scheme of this chapter).[7,15-20] This is realized by preactivating, for example, a monosaccharide thiotolyl glycosyl donor with a stoichiometric amount of the promoter p-toluenesulfenyl triflate (p-TolSOTf), generated in situ from p-toluenesulfenyl chloride (p-TolSCl, **1**) and silver triflate (AgOTf). Upon complete donor activation, a monosaccharide thioglycosyl acceptor is added to the reaction mixture. Nucleophilic attack on the activated donor intermediate(s) by the acceptor yields a disaccharide, which contains the same thiotolyl aglycon. The latter can be directly activated by the same promoter for the next glycosylation without any aglycon adjustment as typically required by other selective activation strategies. The same type of thioglycosides (i.e., p-tolyl thioglycosides) and the identical glycosylation conditions can be used throughout the synthetic sequence, rendering it conceptually and operationally simple. Furthermore, because activation of the donor and addition of the acceptor occur at two distinct stages, the anomeric reactivity of the thioglycosyl donor is independent of that of the thioglycosyl acceptor. This confers much freedom on protective group selection, greatly simplifying the overall synthetic design, and is in contrast to the popular reactivity-based armed–disarmed chemoselective glycosylation method,[21–23] where the glycosyl donor must possess much higher anomeric reactivity than the glycosyl acceptor,[21] as the donor is activated in the presence of the acceptor.

The preactivation-based one pot glycosylation strategy is a powerful method, which has been successfully applied to the assembly of a variety of complex oligosaccharides, including Globo-H,[17] Lewis X pentasaccharide,[18] dimeric Lewis X octasaccharide,[18] hyaluronan oligosaccharide,[16] and the complex type bi-antennary fucosylated N-glycan dodecasaccharide.[15] Herein, we present two examples of this strategy (see opening scheme of this chapter).

In the first example, although it is disarmed and not very reactive,[21] glycosyl donor **2** was cleanly preactivated within 1 min by the powerful promoter system p-TolSCl/AgOTf at −60°C (see part a in the opening scheme of this chapter).[7] Addition of the armed acceptor **3**, which contains benzyl protecting groups, led to disaccharide **4** in 69% yield. This reversal of anomeric reactivity, that is, the glycosyl donor is less reactive toward the thiophilic promoter than the acceptor, is not possible with the reactivity-based armed–disarmed chemoselective glycosylation strategy.

For the second example, preactivation of donor **5** was followed by addition of acceptor **6** at −60°C (see part b in the opening scheme of this chapter).[24] As 1 eq of triflic acid was generated during glycosylation and the donor contains an acid labile p-methoxybenzyl (PMB) group, the sterically hindered base tri-ᵗbutyl-pyrimidine (TTBP) was added together with the acceptor **6**. Upon warming up to −20°C over 2 h, the acceptor **6** was completely consumed and the reaction was cooled back down to −60°C. Addition of acceptor **7**, p-TolSCl, and AgOTf to the reaction mixture generated trisaccharide **8**, which was isolated by chromatography in 67% yield (three steps performed in one pot).

EXPERIMENTAL METHODS

GENERAL METHODS

Unless stated otherwise, all reactions were carried out in flame-dried glassware under nitrogen using anhydrous solvents. All glycosylation reactions were performed in the presence of 4 Å molecular sieves, which were flame-dried under high vacuum before the reaction. Solvents used for glycosylations were dried using solvent purification columns packed with activated alumina. Chemicals used were reagent grade, used as supplied, except where noted. Analytical thin-layer chromatography was performed using silica gel 60 F254 glass plates. Compounds were visualized by UV light (254 nm) and by staining with a yellow CAM solution containing $Ce(NH_4)_2(NO_3)_6$ (0.5 g) and $(NH_4)_6Mo_7O_{24} \cdot 4H_2O$ (24.0 g) in 6% H_2SO_4 (500 mL). CAM can be used to stain organic compounds containing a wide range of functional groups and is an alternative to the conventional charring solution (dilute sulfuric acid in alcohol).

Flash column chromatography was performed on silica gel 60 (230–400 Mesh). ^{1}H and ^{13}C NMR chemical shifts were referenced to signals of Me$_4$Si (0 ppm) and residual CHCl$_3$ (δ^1H-NMR 7.26 ppm, ^{13}C-NMR 77.0 ppm). Peak and coupling constant assignments are based on ^{1}H-NMR, ^{1}H–^{1}H gCOSY, and/or ^{1}H–^{13}C gHMQC experiments. Optical rotations were measured at 25°C. ESI mass spectra were recorded in positive ion mode. High-resolution mass spectra were recorded on a Micromass electrospray mass spectrometer equipped with an orthogonal electrospray source (Z-spray) operated in positive ion mode.

p-Toluenesulfenyl Chloride (1)[25]

Sulfuryl chloride (4.8 mL, 60 mmol) was added, at 0°C over 10 min, to a solution of 4-methylbenzenethiol (6.20 g, 50 mmol) in anhydrous hexane (25 mL), and the mixture was stirred at the same temperature for 1 h. The mixture was allowed to warm to room temperature over 1 h, and stirred at room temperature for one more hour. After removal of hexane and excess sulfuryl chloride under vacuum, *p*-TolSCl (**1**, 5.6 g, d = 1.1, 70%) was obtained as a red liquid by vacuum distillation (50°C/1 mmHg) using a short-path distillation apparatus.* ^{1}H-NMR (400 MHz, CDCl$_3$) δ 7.65–7.60 (m, 2H), 7.25–7.20 (m, 2H), 2.40 (s, 3H).

p-Tolyl 6-*O*-(2,3,4-Tri-*O*-Benzoyl-6-*O*-*Tert*-Butyldiphenylsilyl-β-D-Glucopyranosyl)-2,3,4-Tri-*O*-Benzyl-1-Thio-β-D-Glucopyranoside (4)

A mixture of donor **2** (0.050 mmol) and freshly activated molecular sieves 4 Å (150 mg) in CH$_2$Cl$_2$ (2 mL) was stirred at room temperature for 30 min, cooled to −60°C, and AgOTf (39 mg, 0.15 mmol) dissolved in Et$_2$O (1 mL) was added without the solution touching the wall of the flask. After 5 min, orange-colored *p*-TolSCl (7.9 μL, 0.060 mmol) was added through a microsyringe. Since the reaction temperature was lower than the freezing point of *p*-TolSCl, the reagent was added directly into the reaction mixture to prevent it from freezing on the flask wall. The characteristic yellow color of *p*-TolSCl in the reaction solution dissipated within a few seconds, indicating depletion of *p*-TolSCl.† When the donor was completely consumed (TLC, ~5 min at −60°C), a solution of acceptor **9** (28 mg, 0.050 mmol) in CH$_2$Cl$_2$ (0.2 mL) was added slowly and dropwise along the flask wall with the aid of a syringe. The reaction mixture was stirred and allowed to warm to −10°C within 2 h. CH$_2$Cl$_2$ (20 mL) was added, and the mixture was filtered (Celite pad). The Celite was washed with CH$_2$Cl$_2$ until no organic compounds were present in the filtrate (TLC). The combined CH$_2$Cl$_2$ solutions were washed successively with a saturated aqueous solution of NaHCO$_3$ (2 × 20 mL) and water (2 × 10 mL). The organic phase was dried (Na$_2$SO$_4$) and concentrated, and chromatography gave the desired, amorphous oligosaccharide **4** (42 mg, 34.7 μmol, 69% yield). $[\alpha]_D^{20}$ +10.0 (c = 1, CH$_2$Cl$_2$); ^{1}H-NMR

---

* Compound **1** (*p*-TolSCl) is moisture sensitive and should be kept in a dessicator at −20°C, in small round bottoms flasks capped with rubber septa. The compound is corrosive to rubber. Therefore, the inside of the rubber septum should be wrapped with TEFLON tape. *p*-TolSCl is stable for more than six months when properly stored. When frozen as a solid at −20°C, *p*-TolSCl **1** is orange. It should be discarded when the solid turns green.

† The temperature at which preactivation occurs is not crucial as long as it does not exceed −50°C.

(500 MHz, CDCl$_3$) δ 7.90–7.08 (m, 44H, aromatic), 5.78 (t, 1H, J=9.6 Hz, H-3′), 5.65 (t, 1H, J=9.6 Hz, H-4′), 5.56 (dd, 1H, J=8.0, 9.6 Hz, H-2′), 4.89 (d, 1H, J=8.0 Hz, H-1′), 4.85 (d, 1H, J= 10.4 Hz, CH$_2$Ph), 4.82 (d, 1H, J= 10.4 Hz, CH$_2$Ph), 4.72 (d, 1H, J= 10.4 Hz, CH$_2$Ph), 4.65 (d, 1H, J= 10.4 Hz, CH$_2$Ph), 4.54 (d, 1H, J= 10.4 Hz, CH$_2$Ph), 4.52 (d, 1H, J=9.6 Hz, H-1), 4.41 (d, 1H, J=11.0 Hz, CH$_2$Ph), 4.18 (d, 1H, J=11.2 Hz, H-6a), 3.88–3.82 (m, 2H, H-6′a, H-6′b), 3.78 (dd, 1H, J=4.2, 11.2 Hz, H-6b), 3.77–3.72 (m, 1H, H-5′), 3.61 (t, 1H, J=9.6 Hz, H-3), 3.45 (dd, 1H, J=3.6, 9.6 Hz, H-5), 3.41 (d, 1H, J=9.6 Hz, H-2), 3.39 (d, 1H, J=9.6 Hz, H-4), 2.34 (s, 3H, SPhCH$_3$), 1.04 (s, 9H,C(CH$_3$)$_3$Si); ^{13}C-NMR (100 MHz, CDCl$_3$) δ 166.15, 165.26, 138.63, 138.40, 138.18, 138.15, 135.92, 135.74, 133.41, 133.38, 133.30, 133.22, 133.04, 130.13, 130.03, 130.01, 129.99, 129.90, 129.87, 129.82, 129.66, 129.53, 129.31, 128.64, 128.59, 128.53, 128.49, 128.43, 128.09, 128.04, 127.96, 127.88, 101.21 ($^1J_{13C,1H}$= 163.0 Hz, C-1′), 87.88 ($J_{C-1,H-1}$= 157.7 Hz, C-1), 86.87 (C-3), 80.67 (C-4), 79.19 (C-5′), 77.64 (C-2), 75.84 (CH$_2$Ph), 75.52 (CH$_2$Ph), 75.42 (C-5), 75.00 (CH$_2$Ph), 73.73 (C-3′), 72.41 (C-2′), 69.58 (C-4′), 67.88 (C-6), 63.07 (C-6′), 26.92 (C(CH$_3$)$_3$), 21.83 (SPhCH$_3$), 19.41 (SiC(CH$_3$)$_3$); HRMS C$_{77}$H$_{76}$NaO$_{13}$SSi [M + Na]$^+$ calcd 1291.4674; found: 1291.4651; Anal. calcd C$_{77}$H$_{76}$NaO$_{13}$SSi: C, 72.85; H, 6.03. Found: C,72.78, H, 5.85.

Methyl 2-*O*-Benzoyl-3-*O*-Benzyl-4-*O*-*Tert*-Butyldimethylsilyl-6-*O*-*p*-Methoxybenzyl-β-ᴅ-Glucopyranosyl-(1 → 3)-4,6-*O*-Benzylidene-2-Deoxy-2-*N*-Phthalimido-β-ᴅ-Galactopyranosyl-(1 → 4)-2,3-Di-*O*-Benzyl-6-*O*-*p*-Methoxybenzyl-β-ᴅ-Glucopyranoside (8)

Compound **8** was synthesized by a three-component one-pot synthesis procedure. After the donor **5** (50 mg, 69.93 μmol) and activated molecular sieves MS-4 Å (500 mg) were stirred for 30 min at room temperature in CH$_2$Cl$_2$ (5 mL), the solution was cooled to −60°C, followed by addition of AgOTf (54 mg, 209 μmol) in Et$_2$O (1.5 mL). The mixture was stirred for 5 min at −60°C and *p*-TolSCl (11.1 μL, 69.9 μmol) was added to the solution (for precautions, see the procedure for synthesis of **4**). The mixture was vigorously stirred for 10 min, followed by addition of a solution of building block **6** (28.2 mg, 56.0 μmol) and TTBP (17.4 mg, 69.9 μmol) in CH$_2$Cl$_2$ (1 mL) slowly along the flask wall. The reaction mixture was stirred for 2 h, while the temperature of the mixture was allowed to rise slowly from −60°C to −20°C. The mixture was cooled down to −60°C, followed by sequential addition of AgOTf (18 mg, 69.9 μmol) in Et$_2$O (1 mL) and a mixture of acceptor **7** (20.8 mg, 42.0 μmol) and TTBP (17.4 mg, 69.9 μmol) in CH$_2$Cl$_2$ (1 mL). After the mixture was stirred for 5 min at −60°C, *p*-TolSCl (8.9 μL, 56.0 μmol) was added, and the mixture was stirred for 2 h while it was allowed to warm up from −60°C to −20°C. The reaction was quenched with Et$_3$N (50 μL) and concentrated to dryness under vacuum. The residue was dissolved in CH$_2$Cl$_2$ (20 mL) and, after filtration through Celite, the filtrate was processed as described above for preparation of **4**. Chromatography (3:1:1 hexanes–ethyl acetate–CH$_2$Cl$_2$) followed by freeze-drying of a solution of the desired compound in benzene afforded **8** (41.2 mg, 67%). [α]$_D^{20}$+30.4 (*c* = 1, CH$_2$Cl$_2$); ^{1}H-NMR (600 MHz, CDCl$_3$): δ 7.50–7.34 (m, 7H, aromatic), 7.31–7.16 (m, 16H, aromatic), 7.12–7.00 (m, 8H, aromatic), 6.92–6.90 (m, 2H, aromatic), 6.83–6.79 (m, 4H, aromatic), 5.40 (s, 1H, CHPh), 5.30 (d, 1H, J=8.4 Hz, H-1′), 5.12 (t, 1H, J=7.8 Hz, H-2″), 5.02 (d, 1H, J=11.4 Hz, CH$_2$Ph), 4.85 (d, 1H, J= 12.0 Hz, CH$_2$Ph), 4.76

(d, 1H, $J = 11.4$ Hz, CH$_2$Ph), 4.70 (d, 1H, $J = 7.2$ Hz, H-1′), 4.66–4.64 (m, 1H, H-2′), 4.60–4.57 (m, 2H, H-4′, CH$_2$Ph), 4.46–4.32 (m, 5H, H-3′, H-6a′, H-6b′, CH$_2$Ph), 4.10 (d, 1H, $J = 7.8$ Hz, H-1), 4.09–4.07 (s, 3H, OCH$_3$), 3.99–3.97 (d, 1H, $J = 10.4$ Hz, CH$_2$Ph), 3.78–3.76 (m, 6H, OCH$_3$, H-4, H-5′, CH$_2$Ph,), 3.65–3.64 (m, 1H, H-4″), 3.59–3.55 (m, 2H, H-3, CH$_2$Ph), 3.53–3.46 (m, 3H, H-6a, H-3″, CH$_2$Ph), 3.43–3.37 (m, 4H, OCH$_3$, H-6a″), 3.32–3.28 (m, 2H, H-2, H-5″), 3.14–3.10 (m, 2H, H-6b, H-6b″), 2.96 (m, 1H, H-5), 0.78 (s, 9H, (CH$_3$)$_3$CSi), −0.11(s, 3H, CH$_3$Si), −0.15 (s, 3H, CH$_3$Si); ^{13}C-NMR (150 MHz, CDCl$_3$): δ 169.4, 167.3, 164.4, 159.5, 159.1, 139.6, 138.7, 138.3, 137.8, 133.8, 133.6, 132.7, 131.4, 131.2, 130.7, 130.2, 129.6 (×2), 129.1, 128.7, 128.4 (×2), 128.3, 128.2 (×2), 128.1, 127.7, 127.5, 127.3 (×2), 127.1, 126.7, 123.4, 122.6, 114.0, 113.7, 104.5 ($J_{\text{C-1,H-1}} = 162.2$ Hz, C-1), 101.8 ($J_{\text{C-1,H-1}} = 159.3$ Hz, C-1″), 100.7, 98.5 ($J_{\text{C-1,H-1}} = 162.2$ Hz, C-1′), 83.6, 83.3, 82.3, 76.5, 76.3, 76.0, 75.1, 74.9, 74.8, 74.7, 74.3, 74.1, 73.3, 72.4, 71.3, 70.0, 69.0, 68.2, 67.0, 57.1, 55.5 (×2), 52.5, 26.1, 18.1, −3.7, −4.5; HRMS: [M + Na]$^+$ calcd for C$_{84}$H$_{93}$NNaO$_{20}$Si 1486.5958; found: 1486.5946; Anal. calcd for C$_{90}$H$_{99}$NO$_{20}$Si.C$_6$H$_6$: C, 70.06; H, 6.47; N, 0.91. Found: C, 70.02; H, 6.63; N, 0.99.

ACKNOWLEDGMENT

We are grateful for financial support from the National Institutes of Health (R01-GM-72667) and a CAREER award from the National Science Foundation (CHE 0547504).

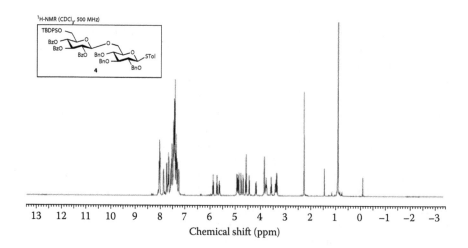

Synthesis of Oligosaccharides

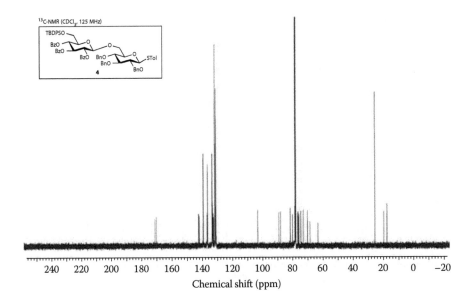

^{13}C-NMR (CDCl$_3$, 125 MHz)

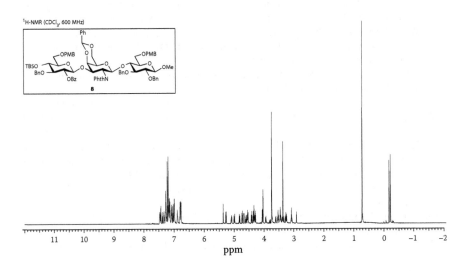

^{1}H-NMR (CDCl$_3$, 600 MHz)

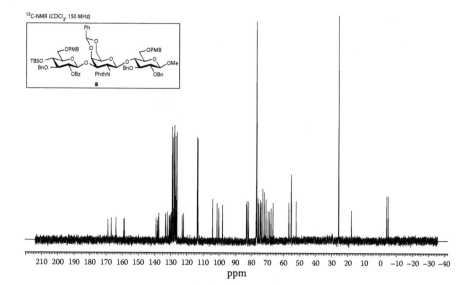

REFERENCES

1. Huang, X.; Wang, Z. In *Comprehensive Glycoscience from Chemistry to Systems Biology*; Kamerling, J. P., Ed.; Elsevier: New York, 2007; Vol. 1, pp. 379–413.
2. Wang, Y.; Ye, X.-S.; Zhang, L.-H. *Org. Biomol. Chem.* 2007, *5*, 2189–2200.
3. Codée, J. D. C.; Litjens, R. E. J. N.; van den Bos, L. J.; Overkleeft, H. S.; van der Marel, G. A. *Chem. Soc. Rev.* 2005, *34*, 769–782.
4. Ernst, B.; Hart, G. W.; Sinaÿ, P., Eds. *Carbohydrates in Chemistry and Biology*; Wiley-VCH: Weinheim, Germany, 2000.
5. Kim, J.-H.; Yang, H.; Park, J.; Boons, G.-J. *J. Am. Chem. Soc.* 2005, *127*, 12090–12097.
6. Yamago, S.; Yamada, T.; Maruyama, T.; Yoshida, J.-I. *Angew. Chem. Int. Ed.* 2004, *43*, 2145–2148.
7. Huang, X.; Huang, L.; Wang, H.; Ye, X.-S. *Angew. Chem. Int. Ed.* 2004, *42*, 5221–5224.
8. Codée, J. D. C.; van den Bos, L. J.; Litjens, R. E. J. N.; Overkleeft, H. S.; van Boeckel, C. A. A.; van Boom, J. H.; van der Marel, G. A. *Tetrahedron* 2004, *60*, 1057–1064.
9. Kim, K. S.; Kim, J. H.; Lee, Y. J.; Lee, Y. J.; Park, J. *J. Am. Chem. Soc.* 2001, *123*, 8477–8481.
10. Nguyen, H. M.; Poole, J. L.; Gin, D. Y. *Angew. Chem. Int. Ed.* 2001, *40*, 414–417.
11. Crich, D.; Sun, S. *Tetrahedron* 1998, *54*, 8321–8348.
12. Kahne, D.; Walker, S.; Cheng, Y.; van Engen, D. *J. Am. Chem. Soc.* 1989, *111*, 6881–6882.
13. Lu, Y.-S.; Li, Q.; Zhang, L.-H.; Ye, X.-S. *Org. Lett.* 2008, *10*, 3445–3448.
14. Yamago, S.; Yamada, T.; Ito, H.; Hara, O.; Mino, Y.; Maruyama, T.; Yoshida, J.-I. *Chem. Eur. J.* 2005, *11*, 6159–6194.
15. Sun, B.; Srinivasan, B.; Huang, X. *Chem. Eur. J.* 2008, *14*, 7072–7081.
16. Huang, L.; Huang, X. *Chem. Eur. J.* 2007, *13*, 529–540.
17. Wang, Z.; Zhou, L.; El-Boubbou, K.; Ye, X.-S.; Huang, X. *J. Org. Chem.* 2007, *72*, 6409–6420.
18. Miermont, A.; Zeng, Y.; Jing, Y.; Ye, X.-S.; Huang, X. *J. Org. Chem.* 2007, *72*, 8958–8961.
19. Teumelsan, N.; Huang, X. *J. Org. Chem.* 2007, *72*, 8976–8979.

20. Huang, L.; Wang, Z.; Li, X.; Ye, X.-S.; Huang, X. *Carbohydr. Res.* 2006, *341*, 1669–1679.
21. Koeller, K. M.; Wong, C.-H. *Chem. Rev.* 2000, *100*, 4465–4493 and references cited therein.
22. Fraser-Reid, B.; Wu, Z.; Udodong, U. E.; Ottosson, H. *J. Org. Chem.* 1990, *55*, 6068–6070.
23. Paulsen, H. *Angew. Chem. Int. Ed. Engl.* 1982, *21*, 155–173.
24. Zeng, Y.; Wang, Z.; Whitfield, D.; Huang, X. *J. Org. Chem.* 2008, *73*, 7952–7962.
25. Barrett, A. G. M.; Dhanak, D.; Graboski, G. G.; Taylor, S. J. *Org. Syn. Coll.*, 1993, *8*, 550–552.

5 The Use of Hypophosphorous Acid in Radical Chain Deoxygenation of Carbohydrates

Karsten Krohn, Ivan Shuklov,
Ishtiaq Ahmed, and Alice Voss†*

CONTENTS

Experimental Methods 56
General Methods 56
Methyl 2,3-*O*-Isopropylidene-4-*O*-[(Methylsulfanyl)thiocarbonyl]-6-*O*-
Triphenylmethyl-α-D-Mannopyranoside (**2**) 57
Methyl 4-Deoxy-2,3-*O*-Isopropylidene-6-*O*-Triphenylmethyl-α-D-
Lyxo-Hexopyranoside (**3**) 57
1,2:5,6-Di-*O*-Isopropylidene-3-*O*-[(Methylsulfanyl)thiocarbonyl]-α-D-
Glucofuranose (**5**)...58
3-Deoxy-1,2:5,6-Di-*O*-Isopropylidene-α-D-*Ribo*-Hexofuranose (**6**) 58
1,2:4,5-Di-*O*-Isopropylidene-3-*O*-[(Methylsulfanyl)thiocarbonyl]-β-D-
Fructopyranose (**8**) 58
3-Deoxy-1,2:4,5-Di-*O*-Isopropylidene-β-D-*Erythro*-Hex-2-
Ulopyranose (**9**) 59
1,6-Anhydro 4-*O*-Benzyl-2-Deoxy-2-*C*-Methyl-3-*O*-[(Methylsulfanyl)
thiocarbonyl]-β-D-Glucopyranose (**11**) 59
1,6-Anhydro 4-*O*-Benzyl-2,3-Dideoxy-2-*C*-Methyl-β-D-*Ribo*-
Hexopyranose (**12**) 59
References...63

* Corresponding author.
† Checker.

The selective replacement of hydroxyl groups by hydrogen is an important functional group transformation in organic synthesis. In the pioneering work of Barton and coworkers on radical chain reductions of thiocarbonyl compounds, easily prepared from the parent alcohols, it has been demonstrated that radical processes can be carried out more effectively than the relatively more drastic ionic reactions, which are also more susceptible to steric retardation and rearrangements (reviews: [1–4]). In the initial work by Barton and McCombie, tributyltin hydride was used as the hydrogen source.[5,6] A broad range of compound classes with great functional group tolerance have been deoxygenated in generally good yields using this tin hydride. Examples of this very efficient deoxygenation in the sugar area were presented as procedures in Org. Syntheses.[7] However, the toxic nature and the need to remove relatively large amounts of tin compounds prompted the search for improvement. Thus, a catalytic variant[8,9] or the use of polymer-bound tin hydrides were proposed.[9,10] Alternatively, a number of less toxic silicon compounds such as tris(trimethylsilyl)silane,[11] phenyl-silane,[12] diphenylsilane,[13–16] triphenylsilane,[17] or even triethylsilane[18] were suggested as reducing agents. Other sources of hydrogen were the formate ion[19] or magnesium in methanol.[20] Irradiation of thiocarbonyl compounds in the sugar series also led to deoxygenation in good yields.[21]

Shortly after their first communications concerning the tin hydride reduction, Barton and coworkers proposed dialkyl phosphites[22,23] and hypophosphorous acid[23,24] as reducing agents for thiocarbonyl compounds. Although a number of other phosphorous-based reagents such as di-n-butylphospane oxide,[25] diphenylphosphane oxide,[26] and phosphane-boranes[27] were later recommended for special cases, both the simple and inexpensive dialkyl phosphites[22,23,28] or hypophosphorous acid[23,24,28,29–31] found the most widespread application, particularly in the deoxygenation of nucleotides[28,32,33] and sugars.[34–38] Inspection of the literature showed that the yield obtained with either dialkyl phosphites or hypophosphorous acid is comparable. It should be noted that triethylamine, used as a base to buffer the hypophosphorous acid, was replaced by other bases such as N-ethylpiperidine.[33,36,39] For reaction in water, the addition of a transfer catalyst and 4,4-azobis(4-cyanovaleric acid) (ABCVA) and a water-soluble radical initiator was recommended.[40] Also, in the absence of acid-sensitive groups, hypophosphorous acid without buffering by addition of bases gave good results.[39]

Although the deoxygenation of sugars has been reviewed by Barton et al.,[4] hypophosphorous acid as the hydrogen source has not been applied as much in the current literature as the tin hydrides. In a recent example, we compared the two reagents in the reduction of the xanthogenate **2**, prepared in 98% yield from the mannose derivative **1**.[38]

It turned out that the use of hypophosphorous acid, buffered by addition of triethylamine, gave better yields and was operationally much easier because no organic tin compounds had to be removed by chromatography, in addition to avoiding the use of toxic and expensive tin compounds. The same result was obtained by Vasella et al.[34] Attempted deoxygenation with tin compounds did not give the desired reduction product but the use of hypophosphorous acid using the modified procedure[38] resulted in 90% reduction. Four to eight equivalents of triethyl amine were used without noticeable differences in yield of deoxygenation products. We also found

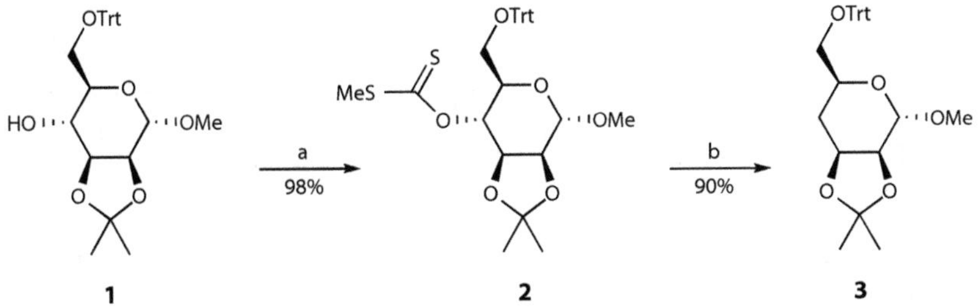

SCHEME 5.1   Reagents and conditions: (a) 1. NaH, 2. CS$_2$, 3. MeI, THF; (b) H$_3$PO$_2$/AIBN, Et$_3$N, dioxane, reflux.

that maintenance of a constant concentration of the radical initiator azobisisobu-tyronitrile (AIBN) by slow addition with a syringe pump had advantages over the batch-wise addition.[38] This procedure entirely suppressed the formation of alcoholic side products, observed by Barton et al.[23]

Concerning functional group compatibility, the example in Scheme 5.1 showed that in the triethylamine buffered reaction, the acid-sensitive acetonides, methyl gly-cosides, and even trityl ethers are perfectly stable.

To probe the stability of two different acetonide groups in one molecule and to compare the efficiency of our variation of the deoxygenation with literature yields, we subjected diacetone glucose [1,2:5,6-di-O-isopropylidene-α-D-glucofuranose (**4**)] to the conversion to xanthogenate **5** and reduction to **6**.[41] This example was extensively investigated by Barton et al. using tributyltin hydride,[5] and both dialkyl phosphites and hypophosphorous acid/base.[22–24] Yields were generally good with all hydrogen sources (ca. 90%). However, with hypophosphorous acid/base always some of the starting alcohol **4** was detected in the reaction mixture even with a larger excess (20 equiv.) of the base. In our experiments, applying a constant concentration of the radi-cal starter AIBN by slow addition with a syringe pump and 5 equiv. of triethylamine, we could not detect the presence of alcohol **4** by thin-layer chromatography (TLC), and the yield of isolated deoxgenation product **6** was 97% (95% from **4**) under the optimized conditions (Scheme 5.2).

Next, the related fructose diacetonide **7** was subjected to the xanthogenate forma-tion (**8**) and radical replacement reaction to **9**. Deoxygenation of this compound using n-tributyltin hydride has been extensively described in the literature and the yield ranged from 55%,[42] 65%,[43] to 87%.[44] In our experiment, employing hypophosphorous

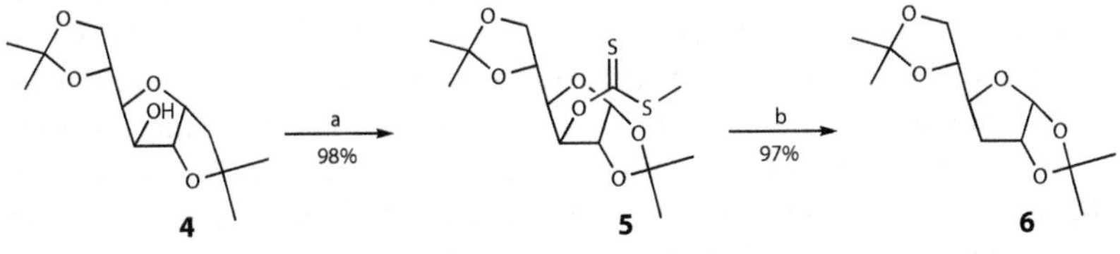

SCHEME 5.2   Reagents and conditions: (a) 1. NaH, 2. CS$_2$, 3. MeI, THF; (b) H$_3$PO$_2$/AIBN, Et$_3$N, dioxane, reflux.

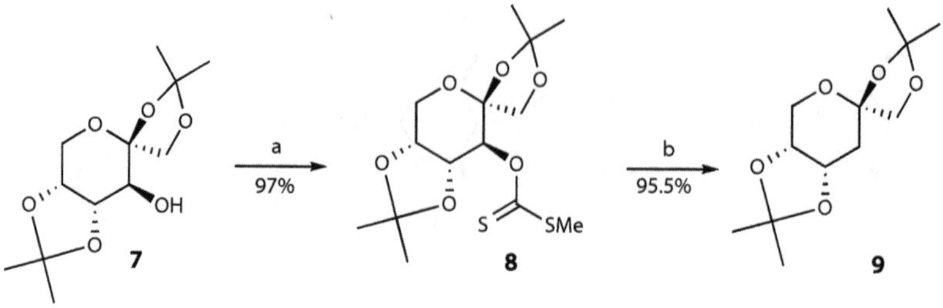

SCHEME 5.3 Reagents and conditions: (a) 1. NaH, 2. CS$_2$, 3. MeI, THF; (b) H$_3$PO$_2$/AIBN, Et$_3$N, dioxane, reflux.

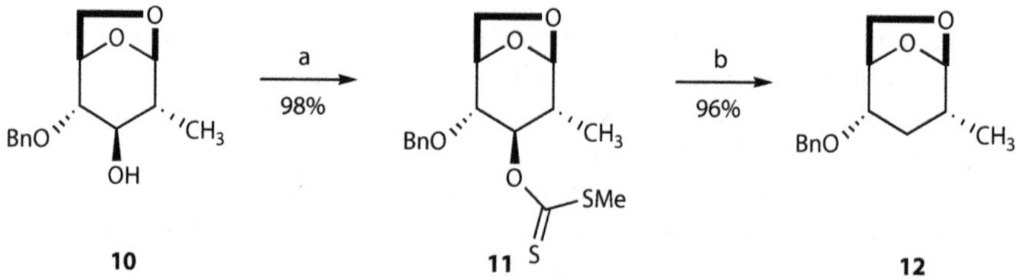

SCHEME 5.4 Reagents and conditions: (a) 1. NaH, 2. CS$_2$, 3. MeI, THF; (b) H$_3$PO$_2$/AIBN, Et$_3$N, dioxane, reflux.

acid/triethylamine, the combined yield of 93% was clearly superior and again no alcohol **7** was detected in the reaction mixture (Scheme 5.3).

Finally, we wanted to probe the deoxygenation of the anhydro sugar **10** (4-*O*-benzyl-2-methyl-1,6-anhydro-β-D-glucopyranose)[45] via **11** to the highly deoxygenated sugar **12**. In this experiment, the stability of the anhydro bridge and the benzyl ether under the reaction conditions could be tested. In fact, not surprisingly, both groups were perfectly stable and the deoxygenation product was isolated in 94% yield over the two steps (Scheme 5.4).

EXPERIMENTAL METHODS

GENERAL METHODS

TLC was performed on precoated TLC plates (silica gel). Melting points were measured with a Gallenkamp apparatus and are corrected. Nuclear magnetic resonance (NMR) spectra were recorded on Bruker Avance 500 at the following frequencies: 500.13 MHz (^{1}H) and 125.76 MHz. (^{13}C). Chemical shifts of ^{1}H and ^{13}C NMR spectra are reported in parts per million (ppm) downfield from TMS as an internal standard. Elemental analyses were performed with a Perkin-Elmer Elemental Analyzer 2400. Optical rotations were measured at 25°C on a Perkin-Elmer Polarimeter 241. Mass spectra were recorded using a Finnigan MAT 8430 spectrometer in the electron-impact mode at 70 eV and chemical ionizations are given as *m/z* values and relative abundances. The infrared spectra were recorded using a FT-IR Spectrometer Nicolet 510 P.

Methyl 2,3-*O*-Isopropylidene-4-*O*-[(Methylsulfanyl)thiocarbonyl]-6-*O*-Triphenylmethyl-α-D-Mannopyranoside (2)

A 250 mL three-necked round-bottomed flask equipped with a magnetic stirring bar, nitrogen-inlet adapter, pressure-equalizing addition funnel, and stopper was charged with methyl mannopyranoside **1**[46] (5.05 g, 10.6 mmol), imidazole (0.025 g, 4 mmol), and anhydrous THF (100 mL). The reaction vessel was flushed with nitrogen and a nitrogen atmosphere was maintained during the ensuing steps. Over a 5 min period, a 50% sodium hydride dispersion (0.76 g, 15 mmol) was added. Vigorous gas evolution was observed. After the reaction mixture was stirred for 20 min, CS_2 (2.3 mL, 15.0 mmol) was added all at once. Stirring was continued for 30 min, after which time iodomethane (1.2 mL, 17.7 mmol) was added in a single portion. The reaction mixture was stirred for another 15 min, and acetic acid (5.0 mL) was added dropwise to destroy the excess of sodium hydride. The solution was filtered and the filtrate was concentrated on a rotary evaporator. The semisolid residue was extracted with $CHCl_3$ (3 × 150 mL), and the combined organic extracts were washed successively with saturated $NaHCO_3$ (2 × 200 mL) and water (2 × 200 mL). The organic phase was dried over $MgSO_4$, filtered, and the filtrate was concentrated to ~20 mL. Addition of ether provided nearly pure xanthate **2** (6.0 g, 94%). An analytical sample was obtained by column chromatography. R_f = 0.85 (CH_2Cl_2); mp 204°C ($CHCl_3$–Et_2O). $[\alpha]_D$ +22.0 (*c* 1.2, $CHCl_3$). IR (KBr): 1630, 1265. ^1H NMR (500 MHz, $CDCl_3$) δ 1.26 (s, 3H, CCH_3), 1.47 (s, 3H, $CC'H_3$), 2.31 (s, 3H, SCH_3), 2.97 (dd, 1H, $J_{6a,5}$ = 2.2 Hz, J_{gem} = 10.4, H-6a), 3.16 (dd, 1H, $J_{6b,5}$ = 7.1 Hz, J_{gem} = 10.4, H-6b), 3.47 (s, 3H, OCH_3), 3.85 (ddd, $J_{5,6a}$ = 2.2 Hz, $J_{5,6b}$ = 7.1 Hz, $J_{5,4}$ = 10.4 Hz, 1H, H-5), 4.11 (d, 1H, $J_{2,3}$ = 5.6 Hz, H-2), 4.25 (m, 1H, H-3), 4.95 (s, 1H, H-1), 5.78 (dd, 1H, $J_{4,3}$ = 7.4, $J_{4,5}$ = 10.4, H-4), 7.11–7.16 (m, 3H, H_p, Trt), 7.17–7.21 (m, 6H, H_o, Trt), 7.37–7.39 (m, 6H, H_m, Trt); ^{13}C NMR (125 MHz, $CDCl_3$) δ 19.2 (CCH_3), 26.4 ($CC'H_3$), 27.6 (SCH_3), 55.0 (OCH_3), 63.2 (C-6), 68.1 (C-5), 75.8 (C-3), 76.0 (C-2), 78.4 (C-4), 86.8 (CPh_3), 98.0 (C-1), 110.1, 126.9, 127.8, 128.0, 128.8, 143.8, 215.6 (7 × $C_{Ar, Tr}$); MS (70 eV) *m/z* (%): 566 (0.1) $[M]^+$, 551 (10) $[M-CH_3]^+$, 458 (71) $[M-C_2H_4OS_2]^+$, 398 (32) $[M-C_8H_5S_2]^+$, 323 (19) $[M-CPh_3]^+$, 243 (100) $[Ph_3C]^+$, 228 (59) $[M-CH_3-CPh_3]^+$, 185 (94) $[M-CH_4O-CPh_3-C_2H_4OS_2]^+$, 165 (98). Anal. Calcd for $C_{31}H_{34}O_6S_2$: C; 65.7; H, 6.05. Found: C, 65.4; H 5.83.

Methyl 4-Deoxy-2,3-*O*-Isopropylidene-6-*O*-Triphenylmethyl-α-D-*Lyxo*-Hexopyranoside (3)[38]

A solution of xanthate **2** (0.7 g, 1.25 mmol), hypophosphorous acid (50% solution in water, 0.64 mL, 6.2 mmol), and triethylamine (0.69 mL, 4.96 mmol) in dioxane (15 mL) was degassed and then refluxed under an argon atmosphere for 0.25 h. A 0.2 M solution of AIBN in dioxane (~1 mL) was added slowly at a rate of 1 mL/h by means of a syringe pump to the refluxing mixture, until TLC shows that the starting material is consumed. The mixture was cooled and poured into water, extracted with ether, and chromatography through a short column of silica gel (5 g) eluted with CH_2Cl_2 afforded compound **3** as colorless oil (0.55 g, 95%); R_f = 0.55 (CH_2Cl_2); mp 186°C (CH_2Cl_2); $[\alpha]_D^{20}$ +15 (*c* 0.6, $CHCl_3$); IR (KBr): 1730, 1599, 1433, 1267, 1153, 1043, 1020, 922; ^1H NMR (500 MHz, $CDCl_3$) δ 1.36 (s, 3H, CCH_3). 1.50 (s, 3H, $CC'H_3$), 1.52–1.57 (m, 1H, H-4a), 1.85–1.89 (m, 1H, H-4b), 3.04 (dd, 1H,

$J_{6a,5}=4.2\,Hz$, $J_{gem}=9.6$, H-6a), 3.35 (dd, 1H, $J_{6b,5}=6.8\,Hz$, $J_{gem}=9.6$, H-6b), 3.50 (s, 3H, OCH_3), 3.87–3.91 (m, 1H, H-5), 3.9 (d, 1H, $J_{2,3}=5.7\,Hz$, H-2), 4.25 (m, 1H, H-3), 5.00 (s, 1H, H-1), 7.25–7.28 (m, 3H, Hp, Trt), 7.30–7.36 (m, 6H, Ho, Trt), 7.50–7.52 (m, 6H, Hm, Trt); ^{13}C NMR (125.76 MHz, $CDCl_3$) δ 26.3 (CCH_3), 28.1 ($CC'H_3$), 31.1 (C-4), 54.9 (C-5), 66.6 (C-6), 70.9 (C-3), 73.2 (C-2), 86.6 (CPh_3), 98.7 (C-1), 108.9 (CMe_2), 127.0, 127.3, 127.8, 127.9, 128.8, 144.1 ($6 \times C_{Ar,\,Trt}$). MS (EI, 70eV): m/z (%)=458 (10) $[M-H_2]^+$, 243 (100) $[CPh_3^+]$, 215 (10) $[M-H_2-CPh_3]^+$, 185 (80) $[M-CH_3OH-CPh_3]^+$. Anal. Calcd for $C_{29}H_{32}O_5$: C; 75.6; H, 7.00. Found: C, 75.4; H 6.87.

1,2:5,6-Di-O-Isopropylidene-3-O-[(Methylsulfanyl)thiocarbonyl]-α-D-Glucofuranose (5)

The reaction, yielding **5** as a yellow oil (13.7 g, 98%), was conducted as described for **2** using 1,2:5,6-di-O-isopropylidene-α-D-glucofuranose (**4**)[41] (10.40 g, 40 mmol), imidazole (65 mg, 0.96 mmol), and anhydrous tetrahydrofuran (160 mL), sodium hydride dispersion (2.9 g, 72.50 mmol), carbon disulfide (8.3 mL, 138 mmol), and iodomethane (4.3 mL, 69 mmol). ^{1}H NMR (500 MHz, $CDCl_3$) δ 1.29 (s, 6H), 1.38 (s, 3H), 1.51 (s, 3H), 2.56 (s, 3H), 3.98–4.04 (m, 2H, H-6, H-3), 4.26–4.27 (m, 2H, H-4, H-6′), 4.61 (d, J=3.9, 1H, H-5), 5.85–5.86 (m, 2H, H-2, H-1); ^{13}C NMR (125 MHz, $CDCl_3$) δ 19.2 (SCH_3), 25.2 (CH_3), 26.2 (CH_3), 26.6 (CH_3), 26.7 (CH_3), 66.9 (C-6), 72.3 (C-5), 79.7 (C-3), 82.7 (C-4), 84.2 (C-2), 105.0 (C-1), 109.2 ($C(CH_3)_2$), 112.3 ($C(CH_3)_2$), 214 (C=S).

3-Deoxy-1,2:5,6-Di-O-Isopropylidene-α-D-*Ribo*-Hexofuranose (6)[41]

The reaction was conducted as described for **3**, using xanthate **5** (3.50 g, 10 mmol), hypophosphorous acid (50% solution in water, 5 mL, 48.25 mmol), and triethylamine (5.40 mL, 39 mmol) in dioxane (80 mL) and a 0.2 M solution of AIBN in dioxane (2 mL). Yield of **6** (colorless oil), 2.37 g (97%); R_f=0.38 (3:1 heptane–ethyl acetate); ^{1}H NMR (500 MHz, $CDCl_3$) δ 1.24 (s, 3H), 1.29 (s, 3H), 1.33 (s, 3H), 1.42 (s, 3H), 1.64–1.70 (m, 1H, H-3), 2.07–2.13 (dd, J=13.4, 4.4, 1H, H-3′), 3.71–3.76 (m, 1H, H-6), 3.99–4.09 (m, 3H, H-6′, H-2, H-4), 4.66 (t, J=4.4, 1H, H-5), 5.72 (d, J=3.7, 1H); ^{13}C NMR (125 MHz, $CDCl_3$) δ 25.1 (CH_3), 26.0 (CH_3), 26.4 (CH_3), 26.7 (CH_3), 35.2 (C-3), 67.1 (C-6), 76.8 (C-4), 78.5 (C-5), 82.7 (C-4), 80.3 (C-2), 105.5 (C-1), 109.4 ($C(CH_3)_2$), 111.1 ($C(CH_3)_2$)

1,2:4,5-Di-O-Isopropylidene-3-O-[(Methylsulfanyl)thiocarbonyl]-β-D-Fructopyranose (8)

The reaction was conducted as described for **2**, using 1,2:4,5-di-O-isopropylidene-D-erythro-2,3-hexodiuro-2,6-pyranose (**7**) (10.40 g, 40 mmol), imidazole (65 mg, 0.96 mmol), 60% sodium hydride dispersion (2.9 g, 72.50 mmol), carbon disulfide (8.3 mL, 138 mmol), and iodomethane (4.3 mL, 69 mmol). Yield of xanthate **8** as yellow oil, 13.6 g (97%). ^{1}H NMR (500 MHz, $CDCl_3$) δ 1.35 (s, 3H), 1.39 (s, 3H), 1.48 (s, 3H), 1.54 (s, 3H), 2.58 (s, 3H, SCH_3), 3.93 (s, 2H, H-1, H-1′), 4.10 (d, $J_{6,6'}=13.5$, 1H, H-6), 4.14 (dd, $J_{6',6}=13.5$, $J_{6',5}=2.6$, 1H, H-6′), 4.22–4.27 (m, 1H, H-5), 4.45 (dd, $J_{4,5}=5.3$, $J_{4,3}=7.9$, 1H, H-4), 6.03 (d, J=7.9, 1H, H-3); ^{13}C NMR (125 MHz, $CDCl_3$) δ 19.2 (SCH_3), 26.3 (CH_3), 26.5 (CH_3), 26.6 (CH_3), 27.7 (CH_3), 60.2 (C-6), 71.3 (C-1), 73.9 (C-4), 74.8 (C-5), 78.3 (C-3), 103.6 (C-2), 109.8 ($C(CH_3)_2$), 112.2 ($C(CH_3)_2$), 217.0 (C=S).

3-Deoxy-1,2:4,5-Di-*O*-Isopropylidene-β-D-Erythro-Hex-2-Ulopyranose (9)[42–44]

The reaction was conducted as described for **3**, using xanthate **8** (3.50 g, 10 mmol), hypophosphorous acid (50% solution in water, 5 mL, 48.25 mmol), triethylamine (5.4 mL, 39 mmol) in dioxane (80 mL), 0.2 M solution of AIBN in dioxane (2 mL), to give compound **9** (colorless oil), 2.33 g (95.5%); R_f = 0.25 (3:1 heptane–EtOAc); ^{1}H NMR (500 MHz, CDCl$_3$) δ 1.22 (s, 3H), 1.26 (s, 3H), 1.36 (s, 3H), 1.37 (s, 3H), 1.87–1.98 (m, 2H, H-3, CH$_2$), 3.72 (d, J = 8.8, 1H, H-1'), 3.74–3.81 (m, 2H, H-6, H-6') 3.94 (d, J = 7.8, 1H, H-1), 4.03 (dt, J = 1.7, 1H, H-5), 4.34–4.37 (m, 1H, H-4); ^{13}C NMR (125 MHz, CDCl$_3$) δ 25.2 (CH$_3$), 26.4 (CH$_3$), 26.5 (CH$_3$), 27.0 (CH$_3$), 34.1 (C-3), 62.1 (C-6), 70.0 (C-4), 71.8 (C-5), 76.0 (C-1), 103.1 (C-2), 108.5 (C(CH$_3$)$_2$), 109.8 (C(CH$_3$)$_2$).

1,6-Anhydro 4-*O*-Benzyl-2-Deoxy-2-*C*-Methyl-3-*O*-[(Methylsulfanyl)thiocarbonyl]-β-D-Glucopyranose (11)

The reaction was conducted as described for **2**, using 4-*O*-benzyl-2-methyl-1,6-anhydro-β-D-glucopyranose (**10**)[45] (1.00 g, 4 mmol), imidazole (10 mg, 0.14 mmol), anhydrous tetrahydrofuran (30 mL), 60% sodium hydride dispersion (0.3 g, 7.5 mmol), carbon disulfide (0.8 mL, 13.3 mmol), and iodomethane (0.45 mL, 7.2 mmol). Yield of xanthate **11** as yellow oil, 1.33 g (97.7%); R_f = 0.27 (5:1 heptane–EtOAc); [α]$_D$ = −28.2 (*c* 1.0, CH$_2$Cl$_2$); IR (Film): 2948, 1604, 1531, 1454, 1374, 1216, 1172 cm^{-1}; ^{1}H NMR (500 MHz, CDCl$_3$) δ 1.28 (d, $J_{7,2}$ = 7.6 Hz, 3H, CH$_3$), 2.05–2.10 (m, 1H, H-2), 2.59 (s, 1H, SCH$_3$), 3.47 (brs, 1H, H-4), 3.78 (dd, $J_{6,6'}$ = 7.4 Hz, $J_{6,5}$ = 6.8 Hz 1H, H-6), 4.01 (d, $J_{6',5}$ = 6.8 Hz, 1H, H-6'), 4.59 (d, $J_{3,4}$ = 5.7 Hz, 1H, H-3), 4.73 (d, $J_{8,8'}$ = 12.2 Hz, 1H, CH$_2$Ph), 4.83 (d, $J_{8',8}$ = 12.2 Hz, 1H, CH$_2$Ph), 5.37 (s, 1H, H-5), 5.57 (d, 4.73 (d, $J_{1,2}$ = 12.2 Hz, 1H, H-1), 7.30–7.41 (m, 5H, Ar-H); ^{13}C-NMR (125 MHz, CDCl$_3$) δ 14.5 (CH$_3$), 18.9 (SCH$_3$), 38.0 (C-2), 64.7 (C-6), 71.5 (C-8, CH$_2$Ph), 74.3 (C-3), 74.9 (C-5), 80.1 (C-4), 103.5 (C-1), 127.7, 127.8, 128.8 (d, C-Ar), 137.7 (s, C-Ar), 214.5 (s, C=S); MS (EI): *m/z* (%) = 341 (2) [M + H]$^+$, 325 (4), 307 (6), 293 (3), 232 (15), 189 (35), 186 (14), 132 (18), 91 (100), 65 (18), 29 (2); MS (CI, 70 eV): *m/z* (%) = 341 (42) [M + H]$^+$, 289 (6), 233 (46), 189 (2), 143 (2), 91 (2), 57 (100), 43 (10).

1,6-Anhydro 4-*O*-Benzyl-2,3-Dideoxy-2-*C*-Methyl-β-D-*Ribo*-Hexopyranose (12)

The reaction was conducted as described for **3**, using xanthate **11** (0.8 g, 2.3 mmol), hypophosphorous acid (50% solution in water, 1.2 mL, 11.5 mmol), triethylamine (1.3 mL, 9.3 mmol) in dioxane (20 mL), and a 0.2 M solution of AIBN in dioxane (1 mL). Yield of the reduced compound **12**: colorless oil, 0.518 g (96.2%). [α]$_D$ = −51.8 (*c* 1.0, CH$_2$Cl$_2$); IR (Film): 2935, 1454, 1417, 1361, 1299 cm^{-1}; ^{1}H NMR (200 MHz, CDCl$_3$) δ 1.20 (d, $J_{7,2}$ = 8.3 Hz, 3H, CH$_3$), 1.58–1.63 (m, 1H, H-3), 1.74–1.80 (m, 1H, H-3'), 1.93–1.98 (m, 1H, H-2), 3.36 (t, $J_{4,3}$ = 2.3 Hz 1H, H-4), 3.73–3.77 (m, 2H, H-6, H-6'), 4.57–4.64 (m, 3H, H-5, CH$_2$Ph), 5.29 (s, 1H, H-1), 7.26–7.38 (m, 5H, Ar-H); ^{13}C-NMR (125 MHz, CDCl$_3$) δ 16.9 (CH$_3$), 26.0 (C-2), 33.3 (C-3), 65.9 (C-6), 70.3 (C-8, CH$_2$Ph), 73.7 (C-4), 75.0 (C-5), 105.4 (C-1), 127.4, 127.5, 128.3 (d, C-Ar), 138.4 (s, C-Ar); MS (EI): *m/z* (%) = 234 (3) [M$^+$], 216 (1), 191 (6), 173 (1), 164 (2), 143 (3), 114 (12), 107 (5), 91 (100), 65 (7), 55 (15), 28 (2). HRMS: *m/z* [M]$^+$ Calcd for C$_{14}$H$_{18}$O$_3$: 234.12560. Found: 234.12567.

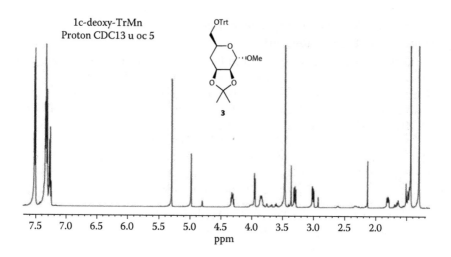

1c-deoxy-TrMn
Proton CDC13 u oc 5

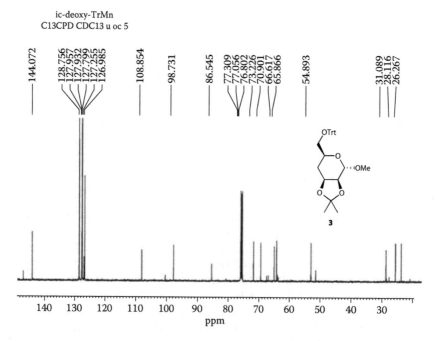

ic-deoxy-TrMn
C13CPD CDC13 u oc 5

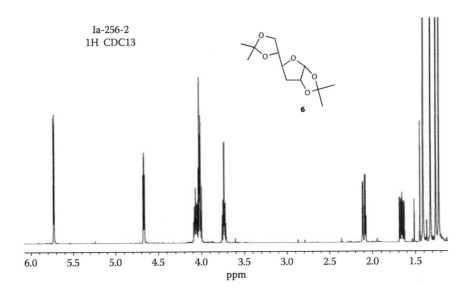

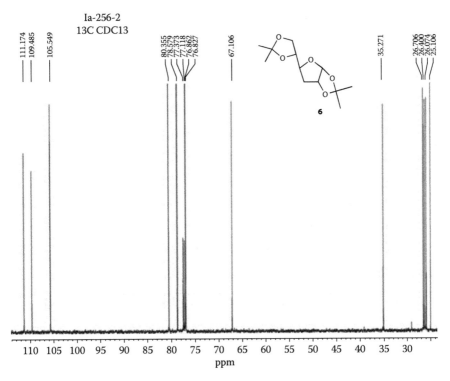

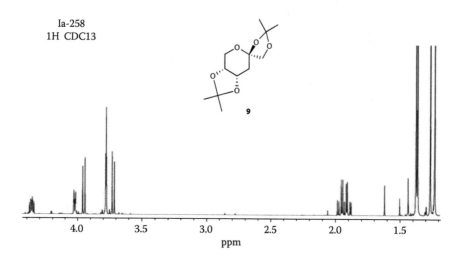

Ia-258
1H CDC13

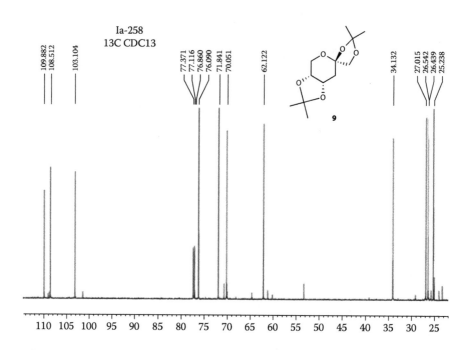

Ia-258
13C CDC13

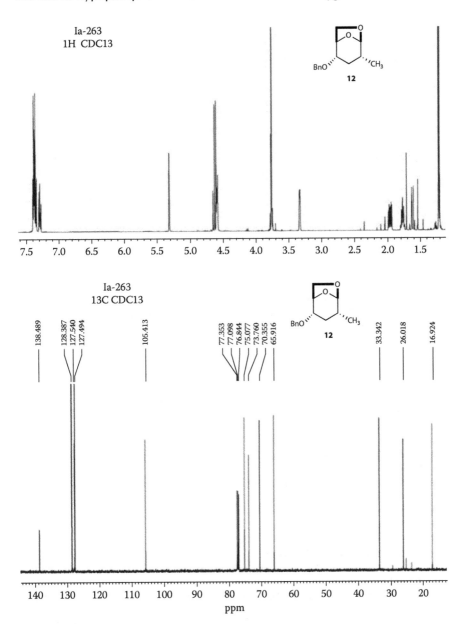

REFERENCES

1. Barton, D. H. *Aldrichimica Acta* 1990, *23*, 3–10.
2. Hartwig, W. *Tetrahedron* 1983, *39*, 2609.
3. Lundt, I. *Glycosci.* 2001, *1*, 501–531.
4. Barton, D. H. R.; Ferreira, J. A.; Jaszberenyi, J. C. Free radical deoxygenation of thiocarbonyl derivatives of alcohols., In: *Preparative Carbohydrate Chemistry*, Hanessian, S. (Ed.); Marcel Dekker, New York, 1997, pp. 151–172.

5. Barton, D. H. R.; McCombie, S. W. *J. Chem. Soc. Perkin Trans. 1* 1975, 1574.

6. Barton, D. H. R.; Subramanian, R. *J. Chem. Soc. Chem. Commun.* 1976, 867–868.

7. Iacono, S.; Rasmussen, J. R. *Org. Syntheses* 1986, *64*, 57; *Org. Synth. Coll.* 1990, *7*, 139.

8. Lopez, R. M.; Hays, D. S.; Fu, G. C. *J. Am. Chem. Soc.* 1997, *119*, 6949–6950.

9. Boussaguet, P.; Delmond, B.; Dumartin, G.; Pereyre, M. *Tetrahedron Lett.* 2000, *41*, 3377–3380.

10. Neumann, W. P.; Peterseim, M. *Synlett* 1992, 801–802.

11. Schummer, D.; Höfle, G. *Synlett* 1990, *11*, 705–706.

12. Barton, D. H. R.; Jang, D. O.; Jaszberenyi, J. C. *Synlett* 1991, 435–438.

13. Barton, D. H. R.; Jang, D. O.; Jaszberenyi, J. C. *Tetrahedron Lett.* 1990, *31*, 4681–4684.

14. Barton, D. H. R.; Jang, D. O.; Jaszberenyi, J. C. *Tetrahedron* 1993, *49*, 7193–7214.

15. Jang, D. O.; Kim, J.; Cho, D. H.; Chung, C. M. *Tetrahedron Lett.* 2001, *42*, 1073–1075.

16. (a) Joselevich, M.; Ghini, A. A.; Burton, G. *Org. Biomol. Chem.* 2003, *1*, 939–943; (b) Parra, A.; Lopez, P. E.; Garcia-Granados, A. *Nat. Prod. Res.* 2010, *24*, 177–196.

17. Barton, D. H. R.; Blundell, P.; Dorchak, J.; Jang, D. O.; Jaszberenyi, J. C. *Tetrahedron* 1991, *47*, 8969–8984.

18. Kirwan, J. N.; Roberts, B. P.; Willis, C. R. *Tetrahedron Lett.* 1990, *35*, 5093–5096.

19. Park, H. S.; Lee, H. Y.; Kim, Y. H. *Org. Lett.* 2005, *7*, 3187–3190.

20. Rho, H. S.; Ko, B. S. *Synth. Commun.* 1999, *29*, 2875–2880.

21. Collins, P. M.; Munasinghe, V. R. *J. Chem. Soc. Chem. Commun.* 1977, 927–928.

22. Barton, D. H. R.; Jang, D. O.; Jaszberenyi, J. C. *Tetrahedron Lett.* 1992, *33*, 2311–2314.

23. Barton, D. H. R.; Jang, D. O.; Jaszberenyi, J. C. *J. Org. Chem.* 1993, *58*, 6838–6842.

24. Barton, D. H. R.; Jang, D. O.; Jaszberenyi, J. C. *Tetrahedron Lett.* 1992, *33*, 5709–5712.

25. Jang, D. O.; Cho, D. H.; Barton, D. H. R. *Synlett* 1998, *9*, 39–40.

26. Jang, D. O.; Cho, D. H.; Kim, J. *Synth. Commun.* 1998, *28*, 3559–3565.

27. Barton, D. H. R.; Jacob, M. *Tetrahedron Lett.* 1998, *39*, 1331–1334.

28. Takamatsu, S.; Katayama, S.; Hirose, N.; Naito, M.; Izawa, K. *Tetrahedron Lett.* 2001, *42*, 7605–7608.

29. Yorimitsu, H.; Shinokubo, H.; Oshima, K. *Synlett* 2002, *5*, 674–686.

30. Jang, D. O. *Tetrahedron Lett.* 1996, *37*, 5367–5368.

31. Nambu, H.; Alinejad, A. H.; Hata, K.; Fujioka, H.; Kita, Y. *Tetrahedron Lett.* 2004, *45*, 8927–8929.

32. Takayoshi Torii, T. O., Shigehisa T., Kunisuke I. *Nucleos Nucleot Nucl Acids* 2005, *24*, 1051–1054.

33. Azhayev, A.; Guzaev, A.; Hovinen, J.; Mattinen, J.; Sillanpaeae, R.; Loennberg, H. *Synthesis* 1994, *25*, 396–400.

34. Pathak, R.; Perez-Fernandez, D.; Nandurdikar, R.; Kalapala, S. K.; Böttger, E. C.; Vasella, A. *Helv. Chim. Acta* 2008, *91*, 1533–1552.

35. Izquierdo, I.; Plaza, M. T.; Rodriguez, M.; Tamayo, J. A. *Eur. J. Org. Chem.* 2002, *2*, 309–317.

36. Torii, T.; Izawa, K.; Cho, D. H.; Jang, D. O. *Nucleos Nucleot Nucl Acids* 2007, *26*, 985–988.

37. (a) Zlatev, I.; Vasseur, J.-J.; Morvan, F. *Tetrahedron Lett.* 2008, *49*, 3288–3290; (b) Perchyonok, V. T.; Tuck, K. L.; Langford, S. J.; Hearn, M. W. *Tetrahedron Lett.* 2008, *49*, 4777–4779.

38. Krohn, K.; Shuklov, I. *J. Carbohydr. Chem.* 2006, *25*, 331–343.

39. Jang, D. O.; Song, S. H. *Tetrahedron Lett.* 2000, *41*, 247–249.

40. Jang, D. O.; Cho, D. H. *Tetrahedron Lett.* 2002, *43*, 5921–5924.

41. Brady, R. F. Jr. *Carbohydr. Res.* 1970, *15*, 35–40.

42. Dills, Jr., W. L. *Carbohydr. Res.* 1990, *208*, 276–279.

43. Rasrnussen, J. R.; Slinger, C. J.; Kordish, R. J.; Newman-Evans, D. D. *J. Org. Chem.* 1981, *46*, 4843–4846.

44. Szarek, W. A.; Rafka, R. J.; Yang, T. F.; Martin, O. R. *Can. J. Chem.* 1995, *73*, 1639–1644.
45. Kochetov, N. K.; Sviridov, A. F.; Ermolenko, M. S. *Tetrahedron Lett.* 1981, *22*, 4315–4318.
46. Tennant-Eyles, R. J.; Davis, B. G.; Fairbanks, A. J. *Tetrahedron: Asymmetry* 2000, *11*, 231–243.

6 Diphenylsulfoxide-Trifluoromethanesulfonic Anhydride: A Potent Activator for Thioglycosides

Jeroen D.C. Codée, Thomas J. Boltje,†
and Gijsbert A. van der Marel*

CONTENTS

Experimental Methods 68
   General Methods 68
      Methyl (4-*O*-Acetyl-2,3-Di-*O*-Benzyl-β-D-
      Mannopyranosyl)-(1 → 6)-(Methyl 2,3,4-Tri-*O*-Benzyl-α-D-
      Glucopyranosid)uronate (**6**) 69
Acknowledgments 70
References 71

* Corresponding author.
† Checker.

Thioglycosides are among the most popular glycosyl donors for the formation of interglycosidic linkages.[1] This popularity stems from the fact that the anomeric thiofunction is stable to most conditions used for protection and functional group manipulations. When treated with an appropriate electrophile, the anomeric thiofunction can be activated to provide a glycosylating species. The stability of thioglycosides, particularly to Lewis acids, has put them at the heart of several sequential glycosylation strategies.[2] They can be employed in an orthogonal condensation sequence in which they are combined with other glycosyl donors such as anomeric fluorides and imidates. Alternatively, the difference in reactivity of differentially functionalized thioglycosides can be exploited in a chemoselective glycosylation strategy. Recently, iterative glycosylation procedures have been introduced,[2] which are based on the preactivation of thioglycosidic donors. In a preactivation protocol, the thioglycoside donor is transformed into a reactive glycosylating species before the addition of the appropriate acceptor, which in turn can be a second thioglycoside. In 2001, Crich and coworkers introduced the 1-benzenesulfinyl piperidine (BSP, **1a**)-trifluoromethanesulfonic anhydride (**2**) (Tf$_2$O) reagent for the (pre-)activation of thioglycosides, which has become a popular thiophilic activating system.[3] Subsequently, our laboratory introduced the analogous diphenylsulfoxide (Ph$_2$SO, **1b**)-triflic anhydride (**2**) combination.[4] This reagent couple was originally developed by Gin and coworkers for the activation of 1-hydroxyl donors,[3b,5] and we applied it for the activation of disarmed thioglycosides.[4] BSP and Ph$_2$SO are commercially available at €3.3/mmol and €0.23/mmol, respectively. Although the sulfonium *bis*-triflate systems **3a** and **3b** are rather similar in reactivity,[6] the latter is a stronger electrophile and has been shown to activate thioglycosides, which were not reactive enough toward sulfonium triflate **3a**.[4,7] The Ph$_2$SO-Tf$_2$O reagent combination (**3b**) has been used in condensation reactions of a variety of thioglycosidic donors, including several uronate esters[8] and sialic acids.[7a,d] Activator **3b** can also be used in an iterative glycosylation sequence combining 1-hydroxyl donors and thioglycosides.[9] Furthermore, **3b** is effective in the stereoselective construction of the challenging β-mannosidic bond using Crich's benzylidene mannose system[6,7b,c] or mannuronate ester donors as recently disclosed by our laboratory.[10] The opening scheme of this chapter depicts a representative example in which mannuronate ester **4** is preactivated by treatment with diphenylsulfonium *bis*(triflate) **3b** and subsequently coupled to glucoside (**5**) to provide the β-linked disaccharide **6** in 94% yield.

EXPERIMENTAL METHODS

GENERAL METHODS

Dichloromethane (DCM) was refluxed with P$_2$O$_5$ and distilled before use. Tf$_2$O was distilled from P$_2$O$_5$ and stored in a Schlenk flask.* TLC analysis was conducted on silica gel-coated aluminum TLC sheets (Merck, silica gel 60, F$_{245}$). Compounds were visualized by UV absorption (245 nm), by spraying with 20% H$_2$SO$_4$ in ethanol or

---

* The Schlenk flask containing Tf$_2$O was stored in a desiccator over silica blue (2–5 mm). Depending on usage, the quality of the Tf$_2$O remained good for several weeks.

with a solution of $(NH_4)_6Mo_7O_{24}\cdot4H_2O$ 25 g/L, $(NH_4)_4Ce(SO_4)_4\cdot2H_2O$ 10 g/L, 10% H_2SO_4 in H_2O followed by charring at ~140°C. Flash chromatography was performed on silica gel (Screening Devices, 40–63 μm 60 Å, www.screeningdevices. com) using petroleum ether 40–60 (PE) and ethyl acetate (EtOAc), technical grade, distilled. NMR spectra were recorded on a Bruker AV400. For solutions in $CDCl_3$ chemical shifts (δ) are reported relative to tetramethylsilane (^{1}H) or $CDCl_3$ (^{13}C). Peak assignments were made based on HH-COSY and HSQC measurements. The stereochemistry of the newly formed glycosidic bond was assigned based on the $J_{C1'-H1'}$ coupling constant.[11]

Methyl (4-O-Acetyl-2,3-Di-O-Benzyl-β-D-Mannopyranosyl)-(1 → 6)-(Methyl 2,3,4-Tri-O-Benzyl-α-D-Glucopyranosid)uronate (6)

A solution of methyl (phenyl 4-O-acetyl-2,3-di-O-benzyl-1-thio-β-D-mannopyranosyl) uronate[10b] (4) (300 mg, 0.575 mmol), tri-tert-butylpyrimidine (TTBP)* (2.5 equivalents, 355 mg, 1.44 mmol) and Ph_2SO (1.2 equivalents, 139 mg, 0.689 mmol), which had been co-evaporated† with dry toluene three times, in DCM (11.5 mL) and stirred over molecular sieves (Fluka, type UOP, 3Å, flame dried) for 30 min under argon atmosphere. After cooling to −60°C,‡ Tf_2O (1.1 equivalents, 105 μL, 0.631 mmol) was added, causing the mixture to turn bright yellow. The mixture was stirred for 20 min and allowed to warm to −45°C.§ After cooling to −60°C, methyl 2,3,4-tri-O-benzyl-α-D-glucopyranoside[13] (5) (396 mg, 0.857 mmol, which had been coevaporated with toluene (thrice), in DCM (1.7 mL) was added dropwise, during which the reaction mixture decolorized. The mixture was allowed to reach slowly 0°C (~3 h),¶ after which Et_3N (5 equivalents, 0.4 mL, 2.9 mmol) was added. The mixture was filtered and the filtrate was diluted with DCM (10 mL) and washed with saturated aqueous $NaHCO_3$ (10 mL). The aqueous layer was extracted with DCM (2 × 10 mL) and the combined organic layers were dried ($MgSO_4$), filtered, and concentrated. Silica gel column chromatography (5:1 toluene–EtOAc) provided the pure disaccharide (6, 475 mg, 0.542 mmol, 94%)**; TLC: 30% EtOAc in PE: R_f 0.15; 40% EtOAc in PE: R_f 0.40; $[α]_D$ −11 (c 0.6, $CHCl_3$); ^{1}H NMR (400 MHz, $CDCl_3$) δ 7.39–7.20 (m, 25H,

---

* TTBP was synthesized according to Crich et al.[12]

† TTBP is slightly volatile and can sublime. Prolonged coevaporation or exposure to high vacuum is therefore not advised.

‡ At this temperature, some of the TTBP precipitates resulting in a cloudy reaction mixture.

§ The activation of the donor glycoside can be followed by TLC analysis, which reveals the formation of the corresponding 1-OH species (TLC: 30% EtOAc in PE: R_f 0.15; 40% EtOAc in PE: R_f 0.30). However, care should be taken with the interpretation of this analysis given the large temperature difference between the reaction temperature and the temperature at which the TLC analysis is executed. The minute amount of the reaction mixture in the capillary used warms up quickly, thereby giving a possibly false representation of the reaction mixture.

¶ Reaction progress can be monitored by TLC, taking into account the precautions described in the above footnote. The relative amount of the 1-OH compound decreases and that of the desired product increases. TLC analysis also shows the formation of the methyl 2,3,4-tri-O-benzyl-6-O-trifluoromethanesulfonyl-α-D-glucopyranoside (TLC: 30% EtOAc in PE: R_f 0.8).

** If separation difficulties are encountered during the purification process, the unresolved mixture can be acetylated using Ac_2O in pyridine (1/3 v/v) which allows the more facile separation of the disaccharide and the 6-O-acetyl acceptor. Alternatively the disaccharide product and excess acceptor can be separated using size exclusion chromatography (Sephadex LH-20, eluent: MeOH/DCM 1:1).

H arom), 5.50 (t, 1H, $J_{4',3'}=J_{4',5'}=9.6\,$Hz, H-4'), 5.02 (d, 1H, $J_{vic}=11.2\,$Hz, CHH Bn), 4.91 (d, 1H, $J_{vic}=12.4\,$Hz, CHH Bn), 4.84–4.75 (m, 4H, 4 × CHH Bn), 4.66 (d, 1H, $J_{vic}=12.0\,$Hz, CHH Bn), 4.58 (d, 1H, $J_{1,2}=3.2\,$Hz, H-1), 4.50 (d, 1H, $J_{vic}=11.6\,$Hz, CHH Bn), 4.48 (d, 1H, $J_{vic}=12.4\,$Hz, CHH Bn), 4.37 (d, 1H, $J_{vic}=12.4\,$Hz, CHH Bn), 4.14 (m, 2H, H-1' and H-6), 4.02 (t, 1H, $J_{3,2}=J_{3,4}=9.2\,$Hz, H-3), 3.79 (m, 1H, H-5), 3.75 (d, 1H, $J_{5',4'}=9.6\,$Hz, H-5'), 3.71 (m, 4H, CH$_3$ CO$_2$Me and H-2'), 3.51 (dd, 1H, $J_{2,1}=3.6\,$Hz, $J_{2,3}=9.6\,$Hz), 3.45–3.35 (m, 3H, H-4, H-6 and H-3'), 3.31 (s, 3H, CH$_3$ C-1-OMe), 2.00 (s, 3H, CH$_3$ Ac); ^{13}C NMR (100 MHz, CDCl$_3$) δ 169.3 (C=O, Ac or CO$_2$Me), 167.7 (C=O, Ac or CO$_2$Me), 138.6 (C$_q$ Bn), 138.1 (2×C$_q$ Bn), 137.9 (C$_q$ Bn), 137.6 (C$_q$ Bn), 128.3–127.2 (CH arom), 101.4 ($J_{C-1', H-1'}=156\,$Hz, C-1'), 97.6 (C-1), 81.9 (C-3), 79.7 (C-2), 78.0 (C-3'), 77.4 (C-4), 75.5 (CH$_2$ Bn), 74.5 (CH$_2$ Bn), 73.5 (C-5'), 73.4 (CH$_2$ Bn), 73.1 (CH$_2$ Bn), 72.7 (C-2'), 71.4 (CH$_2$ Bn), 69.6 (C-5), 68.8 (C-4'), 68.6 (C-6), 54.9 (CH$_3$ C-1-OMe), 52.3 (CH$_3$ CO$_2$Me), 20.6 (CH$_3$ Ac); HRMS: [M+NH$_4$]$^+$ calcd for C$_{51}$H$_{60}$O$_{13}$N, 894.4065; found: 894.4053.

ACKNOWLEDGMENTS

We thank the Netherlands Organisation for Scientific Research (NWO) for financial support (VENI fellowship to J.D.C.C.)

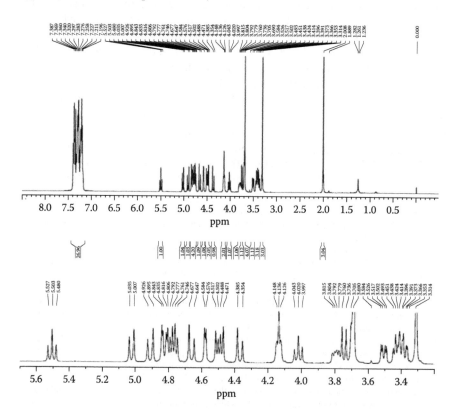

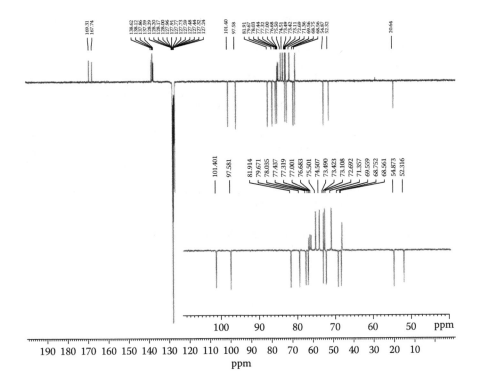

REFERENCES

1. (a) *The Organic Chemistry of Sugars*, Levy, D.E., Fügedi, P. Eds., CRC Press, Boca Raton, 2006. (b) *Handbook of Chemical Glycosylation*, Demchenko, A. V. Ed., Wiley-VCH, Weinheim, Germany, 2008.
2. Codée, J. D. C., Litjens, R. E. J. N., Van den Bos, L. J., Overkleeft, H. S., Van der Marel, G. A., *Chem. Soc. Rev.* 2005, *34*, 769.
3. (a) Crich, D., Smith, M., *J. Am. Chem. Soc.* 2001, *123*, 9015. (b) *Handbook of Reagents for Organic Synthesis. Reagents for Glycoside, Nucleotide and Peptide Synthesis*, Crich, D., Ed., John Wiley and Sons Ltd, Chichester, U.K., 2005.
4. (a) Codée, J. D. C., Van den Bos, L. J., Litjens, R. E. J. N., Overkleeft, H. S., Van Boom, J. H., Van der Marel, G. A., *Org. Lett.* 2003, *5*, 1519. (b) Codée, J. D. C., Litjens, R. E. J. N., Van den Bos, L. J., Overkleeft, H. S., Van Boom, J. H., Van der Marel, G. A., *Tetrahedron* 2004, *60*, 1057.
5. (a) Garcia, B. A., Poole, J. L., Gin, D. Y., *J. Am. Chem. Soc.* 1997, *119*, 7597. (b) Garcia, B. A., Gin, D. Y., *J. Am. Chem. Soc.* 2000, *122*, 4269.
6. Crich, D., De la Mora, M., Vinod, A. U., *J. Org. Chem.* 2003, *68*, 8124.
7. (a) Crich, D., Li, W., *Org. Lett.* 2006, *8*, 959. (b) Crich, D., Bowers, A. A., *J. Org. Chem.* 2006, *71*, 3452. (c) Crich, D., Banerjee, A., *J. Am. Chem. Soc.* 2006, *128*, 8078. (d) Crich, D., Wu, B., *Tetrahedron* 2008, *64*, 2042.
8. (a) Van den Bos, L. J., Codée, J. D. C., Van der Toorn, J. C., Boltje, T. J., Van Boom, J. H., Overkleeft, H. S., Van der Marel, G. A., *Org. Lett.* 2004, *6*, 2165. (b) Codée, J. D. C., Stubba, B., Schiattarella, M., Overkleeft, H. S., Van Boeckel, C. A. A., Van Boom, J. H.,

Van der Marel G. A., *J. Am. Chem. Soc.* 2005, *127*, 3767. (c) Litjens, R. E. J. N., Van den Bos, L. J., Codée, J. D. C., Van den Berg, R. H. J. B. N., Overkleeft, H. S., Van der Marel G. A., *Eur. J. Org. Chem.* 2005, *2005*, 918.

9. (a) Codée, J. D. C., Van den Bos, L. J., Litjens, R. E. J. N., Overkleeft, H. S., Van Boom, J. H., Van der Marel, G. A., *Org. Lett.* 2003, *5*, 1947. (b) Litjens, R. E. J. N., Hoogerhout, P., Filippov, D. V., Codée, J. D. C., Van den Bos, L. J., Van den Berg, R. H. J. B. N., Overkleeft, H. S., Van Boom, J. H., Van der Marel, G. A., *J. Carbohydr. Chem.* 2005, *24*, 755.

10. (a) Van den Bos, L. J., Dinkelaar, J., Overkleeft, H. S., Van der Marel, G. A., *J. Am. Chem. Soc.* 2006, *128*, 13066. (b) Codée, J. D. C., Van den Bos, L. J., De Jong, A. R., Dinkelaar, J., Lodder, G., Overkleeft, H. S., Van der Marel, G. A., *J. Org. Chem.* 2009, *74*, 38.

11. (a) Bock, K., Pedersen, C., *J. Chem. Soc. Perkin Trans. 2*, 1974, 293. (b) Juaristi, E., Cuevas, G., *Acc. Chem. Res.* 2007, *40*, 961. (c) Crich, D., Sun, S., *Tetrahedron* 1998, *54*, 8321.

12. Crich, D., Smith, M., Yao, Q., Picione, J., *Synthesis* 2001, 323.

13. Jaramillo, C., Chiara, J.-L., Martín-Lomas, M., *J. Org. Chem.* 1994, *59*, 3135.

7 Preparation of Glycosyl Chlorides from Glycopyranoses/ Glycofuranoses under Mild Conditions

Chih-Wei Chang, Chin-Sheng Chao,
Chang-Ching Lin,† and Kwok-Kong T. Mong*

CONTENTS

Introduction..73
General TCT/DMF Chlorination Protocols 75
Experimental Methods...75
    General Methods 75
    TCT/DMF Chlorination Protocol A for Preparation of Glycosyl Chlorides
    1a and **2a**..76
    TCT/DMF Chlorination Protocol B for Preparation of Glycosyl Chlorides
    3a and **4a**..76
        2,3,4,6-Tetra-*O*-Acetyl-α-D-Glucopyranosyl Chloride (**1a**)..........76
        2,3,4,6-Tetra-*O*-Acetyl-α-D-Mannopyranosyl Chloride (**2a**).....77
        2,3,4,6-Tetra-*O*-Benzyl-α-D-Galactopyranosyl Chloride (**3a**) 77
        2,3:5,6-Di-*O*-Isopropylidene-α-D-Mannofuranosyl Chloride (**4a**) 77
Acknowledgment 78
References..81

INTRODUCTION

Glycosyl chlorides constitute an important class of glycosyl donors for synthesis of oligosaccharides,[1] *O*-glycosides,[2] *C*-glycosides,[3a] *N*-glycosides,[3b] and glycals.[4] Typical preparation of glycosyl chlorides involves treatment of glycosyl derivatives

---

* Corresponding author.
† Checker.

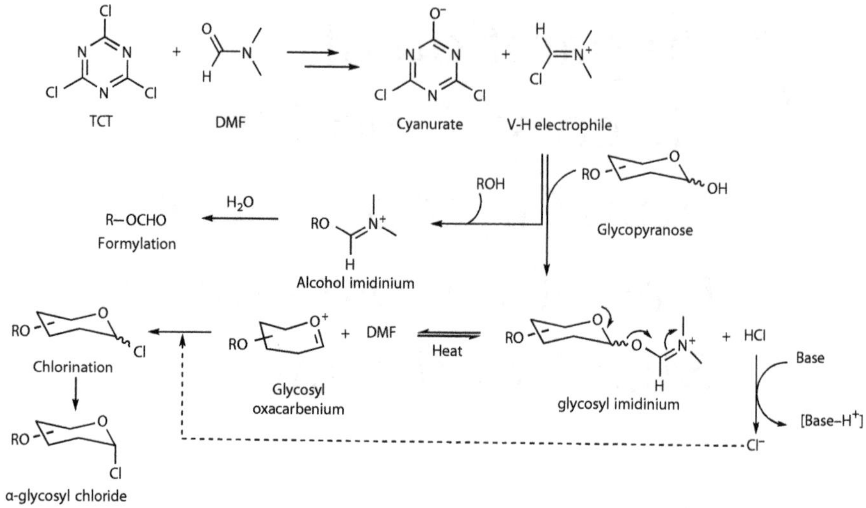

SCHEME 7.1 Proposed mechanism for TCT/DMF chlorination of glycopyranoses.

with acidic chlorinating reagents. However, strongly acidic conditions are incompatible with many acid-labile protecting functions; consequently, application of this methodology is limited.[5,6] Although there are milder reagents for chlorination of glycopyranoses such as PPh₃-CCl₄,[7a] Viehe's salt,[7b] chloroenamine,[7c] chlorodiphenyl phosphate,[7d] triphosgene,[7e] and dichloromethyl methyl ether,[7f,g] each of these methods has its limitations. For example, the use of Viehe's salt or chloroenamine needs additional preparatory steps,[7b,7c] while triphosgene chlorination reagent is less effective for disarmed glycosyl substrates.[7e] Accordingly, developing milder and more general chlorination methods remains desirable.

Applications of noncorrosive 2,4,6-trichlorotriazine (TCT) have long been employed in functional group transformations. For recent reviews and applications for uses of TCT in synthetic chemistry, see Ref. [8]. Particularly noteworthy is the use of TCT and dimethylformamide (DMF) in formylation of aliphatic alcohols.[8c] This reaction involves the initial formation of Vilsmeier-Haack (V-H) electrophile, followed by reaction with aliphatic hydroxyl function and subsequent hydrolysis, leading to formation of formylated product. Given the stereoelectronic features of anomeric hydroxyl function, glycospyranoses should react with V-H electrophile in a different pathway as shown in Scheme 7.1.

V-H electrophile formed from TCT and DMF is first coupled with the glycopyranose to form glycosyl imidinium intermediate. Unlike the alcohol imidinium counterpart, the glycosyl imidinium undergoes elimination to form an oxacarbenium ion with the departure of a DMF molecule. Such a facile elimination is attributed to the presence of ring oxygen atom, which is capable of donating lone electron pair. It promotes the elimination by (1) a "push and pull" mechanism to facilitate the departure of DMF and (2) stabilization of resulting oxacarbenium ion via delocalization of lone electron pair from ring oxygen. Subsequent coupling of oxacarbenium ion with chloride nucleophile and anomerization leads to the production of α-glycosyl chloride.

GENERAL TCT/DMF CHLORINATION PROTOCOLS

To apply the above concept, two TCT/DMF chlorination protocols are designed (Scheme 7.2). In these, TCT (1.1 equiv) and DMF (4 equiv) are first mixed together to form V-H electrophile. Note that when DMF was used as solvent, such conditions promoted formation of formylated product via glycosyl imidinium and thus reduced the yield of chlorination.

According to the first chlorination protocol (protocol A), a stoichiometric amount of diazabicyclo[5,4,0]undec-7-ene (DBU) is employed and the reaction is conducted in dichloroethane (DCE) at 60°C. This protocol is suitable for "disarmed" glycopyranoses such as **1** and **2** (Scheme 7.2a)[9] and the corresponding glycosyl chlorides **1a** and **2a** are produced in excellent yields (~90%) within 2–4 h. Alternatively, (protocol B), 5 equiv of K_2CO_3 is used as acid scavenger and the reaction is performed in dichloromethane (CH_2Cl_2) at 45°C. Such conditions are suitable for more reactive substrates such as armed glycopyranose and glycofuranose **3** and **4**, respectively (Scheme 7.2b).[10] It should be noted that both K_2CO_3- and TCT-derived by-products in the chlorination protocol B readily precipitate in Et_2O and thus can be removed by filtration.

As glycosyl chlorides are generally acid-labile, their purification needs precautions. Prolonged contact with silica gel leads to substantial product decomposition; consequently rapid elution from a short pad of silica gel or preactivation of silica gel at high temperature (160°C) is recommended for purification of all glycosyl chlorides.[5c,10]

EXPERIMENTAL METHODS

GENERAL METHODS

ACS reagent grade DMF, CH_2Cl_2 (purchased from J.T. Baker), and DCE (purchased from Mallinckrodt) were distilled over CaH_2 before use. Reagent grade TCT and

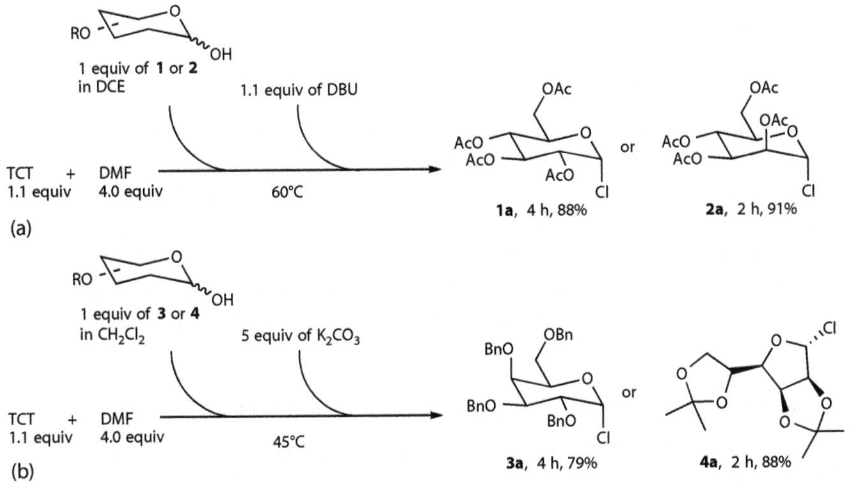

SCHEME 7.2 (a) TCT/DMF chlorination protocol A for substrates **1** and **2**; (b) TCT/DMF chlorination protocol B for substrates **3** and **4**.

DBU were purchased from Acros and used as supplied. K_2CO_3 (purchased from Fisher Scientific or Acros) was dried in vacuo at 80°C for 2–3 h before use. Optical rotations were measured with a JASCO DIP-1000 polarimeter at 27°C. Flash column chromatography was performed on silica gel 60 (70–230 mesh, Merck). Silica gel was activated by heating at high temperature (>100°C overnight) before use. ^{1}H and ^{13}C NMR spectra were recorded at 300 and 75 MHz, respectively with Bruker or Varian Unity-300 spectrometers. Chemical shifts δ (ppm) are reported relative to the residual proton and the ^{13}C signal of $CDCl_3$. Coupling constants (Hz) are based on first-order analysis of ^{1}H NMR spectra. Compounds **1**–**4** were co-evaporated with toluene and dried in vacuo for 2–3 h before use. In our studies, glycosyl hemiacetals for chlorination are dried under vacuo for couple of hours before use; while the checker recommends co-evaporating glycosyl substrates with toluene and drying under vacuo.

TCT/DMF Chlorination Protocol A for Preparation of Glycosyl Chlorides 1a and 2a

DMF (1.55 mL, 20.0 mmol) was added to TCT (1.00 g, 5.5 mmol) and the suspension was stirred at RT for 15 min under N_2. A solution of glycopyranose (**1** or **2**, 5.0 mmol, prepared by literature procedures)[11] in DCE (50 mL) was added, followed by addition of DBU (0.80 mL, 5.5 mmol). The mixture was stirred at 60°C and progress of the reaction was monitored by thin layer chromatography (ca. 1 vol% of Et_3N was added to developing solution to prevent product degradation). When the chlorination was complete (~4 h for substrate **1**, ~2 h for substrate **2**), the mixture was allowed to cool to RT and Et_2O (ca. 100 mL) was added to precipitate the side products. After filtration, the filtrate was concentrated to give crude glycosyl chloride, which, after short-path chromatography (15 g gel per gram glycosyl chloride), gave glycosyl chloride **1a** or **2a**.

TCT/DMF Chlorination Protocol B for Preparation of Glycosyl Chlorides 3a and 4a

DMF (1.55 mL, 20.0 mmol) was added to TCT (1.00 g, 5.5 mmol) and the suspension was stirred at RT for 15 min under N_2. A solution of glycopyranose or glycofuranose (**3** or **4**, 5.0 mmol, prepared by literature procedures)[12] in CH_2Cl_2 (50 mL) was added, followed by K_2CO_3 (3.50 g, 25 mmol). The mixture was stirred at 45°C and the progress of the reaction was monitored by TLC (ca 1 vol% of Et_3N was added to developing solution to prevent product degradation). When the reaction was complete (~4 h for substrate **3**, ~2 h for substrate **4**), work up procedure as described in protocol A, was followed to furnish glycosyl chloride **3a** or **4a**.

2,3,4,6-Tetra-*O*-Acetyl-α-ᴅ-Glucopyranosyl Chloride (1a)

Prepared from glucopyranosyl hemiacetal **1** (0.46 g, 1.3 mmol), TCT (0.27 g, 1.5 mmol) and DMF (0.4 mL, 5.0 mmol); reaction time, 4 h, 60°C as described in chlorination protocol A with DBU as acid scavenger. Chromatography (1:2 EtOAc–hexane) gave glucopyranosyl chloride **1a** as white amorphous solid.

Yield, 0.43 g, 88%; R_f 0.42, 1:2 EtOAc–hexane; ^{1}H NMR (CDCl$_3$) δ 6.24 (d, 1H, $J = 4.0$ Hz, H-1), 5.50 (t, 1H, $J = 9.8$ Hz, H-3), 5.08 (t, 1H, $J = 9.6$ Hz, H-4), 4.96 (dd, 1H, $J = 10.1$, 4.0 Hz, H-2), 4.34–4.19 (m, 2H, H-6, H-6′), 4.07 (dd, 1H, $J = 14.1$, 3.7 Hz, H-5), 2.04 (s, 3H, CH$_3$CO), 2.03 (s, 3H, CH$_3$CO), 1.99 (s, 3H, CH$_3$CO), 1.98 (s, 3H, CH$_3$CO); ^{13}C NMR (CDCl$_3$) δ 170.4 (CO), 169.8 (CO), 169.7 (CO), 169.3 (CO), 90.0 (C-1), 70.6, 70.3, 69.3, 67.3, 61.0, 20.6 (CH$_3$CO), 20.5 (CH$_3$CO), 20.5 (CH$_3$CO), 20.4 (CH$_3$CO). The spectroscopic data of **1a** were consistent with literature values.[13]

2,3,4,6-Tetra-O-Acetyl-α-D-Mannopyranosyl Chloride (2a)

Prepared from mannopyranosyl hemiacetal **2** (0.43 g, 1.2 mmol), TCT (0.25 g, 1.37 mmol) and DMF (0.40 mL, 5 mmol) according to the chlorination protocol A with DBU as acid scavenger; reaction time of 2 h, 60°C. Chromatography (1:2 EtOAc–hexane) gave mannopyranosyl chloride **2a** as white amorphous solid. Yield, 0.41 g, 91%; R_f 0.40, 1:2 EtOAc–hexane; ^{1}H NMR (CDCl$_3$) δ 5.96 (d, 1H, $J = 0.9$ Hz, H-1), 5.59 (dd, 1H, $J = 10.1$, 3.3 Hz, H-3), 5.42–5.25 (m, 2H, H-2, H-4), 4.37–4.04 (m, 3H, H-5, H-6, H-6′), 2.16 (s, 3H, CH$_3$CO), 2.09 (s, 3H, CH$_3$CO), 2.05 (s, 3H, CH$_3$CO), 1.99 (s, 3H, CH$_3$CO); ^{13}C NMR (CDCl$_3$) δ 170.8 (CO), 170.0 (CO), 169.9 (CO), 169.8 (CO), 89.0 (C-1), 71.8, 71.5, 68.0, 65.5, 61.9, 21.0 (CH$_3$CO), 21.0 (CH$_3$CO), 20.9 (CH$_3$CO), 20.8 (CH$_3$CO). The spectroscopic data of **2a** were consistent with literature values.[13]

2,3,4,6-Tetra-O-Benzyl-α-D-Galactopyranosyl Chloride (3a)

Prepared from galactopyranosyl hemiacetal **3** (0.54 g, 1.0 mmol), TCT (0.22 g, 1.1 mmol) and DMF (0.31 mL, 4.0 mmol) according to the chlorination protocol B with K$_2$CO$_3$ as acid scavenger; reaction time of 4 h, 45°C. Chromatography (1:9 EtOAc–hexane) gave galactopyranosyl chloride **3a** as colorless syrup. Yield, 0.44 g, 79%; R_f 0.35, 1:9 EtOAc–hexane; ^{1}H NMR (CDCl$_3$) δ 7.48–7.25 (m, 20H, Ar-H), 6.17 (d, 1H, $J = 3.8$ Hz, H-1), 4.97 (d, 1H, $J = 11.3$ Hz, OCH$_2$Ph), 4.88 (d, 1H, $J = 11.7$ Hz, OCH$_2$Ph), 4.81–4.70 (m, 3H, OCH$_2$Ph), 4.58 (d, 1H, $J = 11.3$ Hz, OCH$_2$Ph), 4.50 (d, 1H, $J = 11.8$ Hz, OCH$_2$Ph), 4.42 (d, 1H, $J = 11.8$ Hz, OCH$_2$Ph), 4.27–4.20 (m, 2H, H-2, H-4), 4.04–3.96 (m, 2H, H-3, H-5), 3.56 (d, 2H, $J = 6.7$ Hz, H-6, H-6′); ^{13}C NMR (CDCl$_3$) δ 138.4, 138.2, 137.8, 137.6, 128.4, 128.3, 128.2, 127.9, 127.8, 127.8, 127.7, 127.6, 127.5, 94.9 (C-1), 78.3, 76.2, 75.0, 74.3, 73.4, 73.3, 73.0, 72.3, 67.9. The spectroscopic data of **3a** were consistent with literature values.[14]

2,3:5,6-Di-O-Isopropylidene-α-D-Mannofuranosyl Chloride (4a)

Prepared from mannofuranosyl hemiacetal **4** (0.44 g, 1.7 mmol), TCT (0.34 g, 1.9 mmol) and DMF (0.53 mL, 6.8 mmol) according to the chlorination protocol B with K$_2$CO$_3$ as acid scavenger; reaction time of 2 h, 45°C. Chromatography (1:9 EtOAc–hexane) gave mannofuranosyl chloride **4a** as colorless syrup. Yield, 0.51 g, 88%; R_f 0.30, 1:9 EtOAc–hexane; ^{1}H NMR (CDCl$_3$) δ 6.02 (s, 1H, H-1), 4.91 (d, 1H, $J = 5.8$ Hz, H-2), 4.84 (dd, 1H, $J = 5.8$, 3.6 Hz, H-3), 4.40–4.38 (m, 1H, H-5), 4.16 (dd, 1H, $J = 11.0$, 3.6 Hz, H-4), 4.05 (dd, 1H, $J = 8.9$, 6.1 Hz, H-6), 3.97 (dd, 1H, $J = 8.8$, 4.4 Hz, H-6′), 1.42 (s, 6H, CH$_3$), 1.33 (s, 3H, CH$_3$), 1.28 (s, 3H, CH$_3$); ^{13}C NMR (CDCl$_3$) δ 113.2 (C(CH$_3$)$_2$), 109.4 (C(CH$_3$)$_2$), 97.5 (C-1), 89.1, 82.3,

78.4, 72.2, 66.6, 26.8, 25.7, 25.0, 24.5. The spectroscopic data of **4a** were consistent with literature values.[4]

ACKNOWLEDGMENT

We thank the National Science Council of Taiwan for financial support (Grant no. 97-2113-M-009-007).

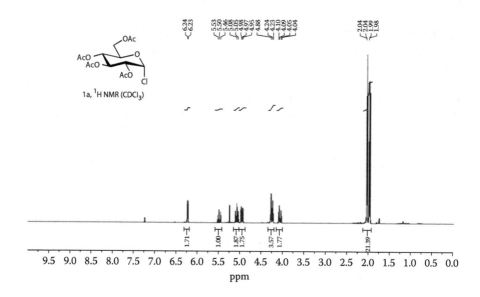

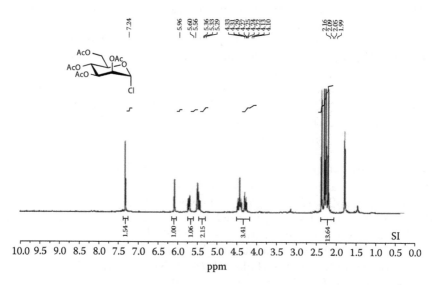

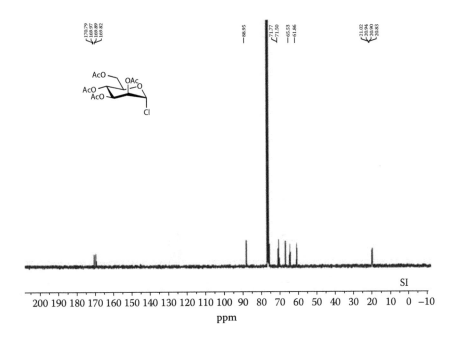

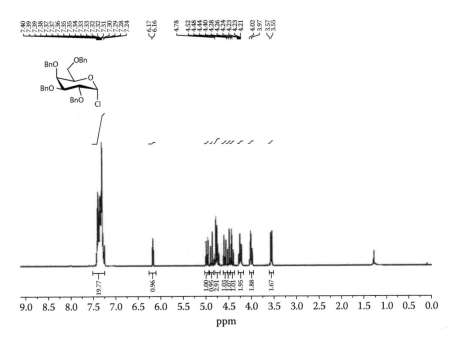

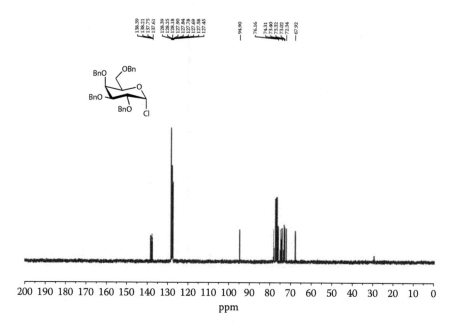

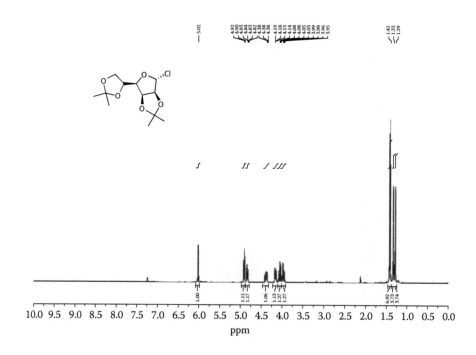

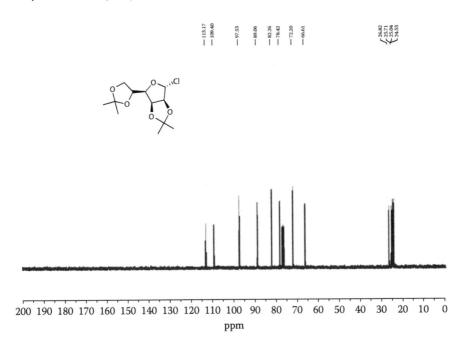

REFERENCES

1. (a) Igarashi, K. *Adv. Carbohydr. Chem. Biochem.* 1977, *34*, 243–283. (b) Kováč, P.; Taylor, R.B.; Glaudemans, C.P.J. *J. Org. Chem.* 1985, *50*, 5323–5333. (c) Matsuo, I.; Wada, M.; Manabe, S.; Yamaguchi, Y.; Otake, K.; Kato, K.; Ito, Y. *J. Am. Chem. Soc.* 2003, *125*, 3402–3403.
2. Toshima, K. In *Glycoscience*; Fraser-Reid, B., Tatsuta, K., Thiem, J., Eds.; Springer: Berlin, Germany, 2008; pp. 429–449.
3. (a) Demchenko, A. V. In *Handbook of Chemical Glycosylation*; Wiley-VCH: Weinheim, Germany, 2008; pp. 29–85. (b) Brito-Arias, M. In *Synthesis and Characterization of Glycosides*; Springer: Berlin, Germany, 2006; pp. 151–161.
4. Kim, C.; Hoang, R.; Theodorakis, E. A. *Org. Lett.* 1999, *1*, 1295–1297.
5. (a) Haynes, L. J.; Newth, F. H. *Adv. Carbohydr. Chem. Biochem.* 1955, *10*, 207–256. (b) Peromo, G. R.; Krepinsky, J. J. *Tetrahedron Lett.* 1987, *28*, 5595–5598. (c) Kováč, P.; Edgar, J. J. *J. Org. Chem.* 1992, *57*, 2455–2467. (d) Montero, J.-L.; Winum, J.-Y.; Leydet, A.; Kamal, M.; Pavia, A. A.; Roque, J.-P. *Carbohydr. Res.* 1997, *297*, 175–180. (e) Pozsgay, V.; Dubois, E. P.; Pannell, L. *J. Org. Chem.* 1997, *62*, 2832–2846. (f) Ghosh, R.; Chakraborty, A.; Maiti, S. *Tetrahedron Lett.* 2004, *45*, 9631–9634. (g) Wang, Q. B.; Fu, J.; Zhang, J. B. *Carbohydr. Res.* 2008, *343*, 2989–2991.
6. Kocieński, P. J. In *Protecting Groups*; Georg Thieme: Leipzig, Germany, 2005; pp. 187–350.
7. (a) Ohrui, H.; Fox, J.-J. *Tetrahedron Lett.* 1973, *14*, 1951–1954. (b) Copeland, C.; McAdam, D. P.; Stick, R. V. *Aust. J. Chem.* 1983, *36*, 1239–1247. (c) Ernst, B.; Winkler, T. *Tetrahedron Lett.* 1989, *30*, 3081–3084. (d) Hung, S.-C.; Wong, C.-H. *Tetrahedron Lett.* 1996, *37*, 4903–4906. (e) Cicchillo, R. M.; Norris, P. *Carbohydr. Res.* 2000, *328*, 431–434. (f) Gross, H.; Farkas, I.; Bognár, R. *Z. Chem.* 1978, *18*, 201–210. (g) Kováč,

P. Synthesis of glycosyl halides for oligosaccharide synthesis using dihalogenomethyl methyl ethers. In *Modern Methods in Carbohydrate Synthesis*; Khan, S. H., O'Neill, R. A., Eds.; Harwood Academic Publishers: Amsterdam, the Netherlands, 1996; pp. 55–81.

8. (a) Giacomelli, G.; Porcheddu, A. *Curr. Org. Chem.* 2004, *8*, 1487–1519. (b) Blotny, G. *Tetrahedron* 2006, *62*, 9507–9522. (c) De Luca, L.; Giacomelli, G.; Porcheddu, A. *J. Org. Chem.* 2002, *67*, 5152–5155. (d) Giacomelli, G.; Porcheddu, A.; Salaris, M. *Org. Lett.* 2003, *5*, 2715–2717.

9. Mootoo, D. R.; Konradsson, P.; Udodong, U. E.; Fraser-Reid, B. *J. Am. Chem. Soc.* 1988, *110*, 5583–5584.

10. Ruttens, B.; Saksena, R.; Kováč, P. *Eur. J. Org. Chem.* 2007, *26*, 4366–4375.

11. Mori, M.; Ito, Y.; Ogawa, T. *Carbohydr. Res.* 1990, *195*, 199–224.

12. Oshitar, T.; Shibasaki, M.; Yoshizawa, T.; Tomita, M.; Takao, K.-I.; Kobayashi, S. *Tetrahedron* 1997, *53*, 10993–11006.

13. Zhang, Z.-Y.; Magnusson, G. *Carbohydr. Res.* 1996, *295*, 41–55.

14. Sugiyama, S.; Diakur, J. M. *Org. Lett.* 2000, *2*, 2713–2715.

8 C-Glycosylation Starting from Unprotected O-Glycosides

Barbara La Ferla, Laura Cipolla, Wouter Hogendorf,† and Francesco Nicotra*

CONTENTS

Experimental Methods 84
   General Methods 84
      3-(α-D-Galactopyranosyl)prop-1-Ene (**2**) 85
      Bicyclic Iodoethers (**3**) 85
      Methyl (2R)-2-Acetamido-3-(α-D-Galactopyranosylpropylthio)
      propanoate (**4**) 85
Acknowledgments 86
References 89

(a) CH_3CN, BTSFA (6 equiv.), 80°C then TMSOTf (0.5 equiv.), AllTMS (1.5 equiv.), 0°C to rt overnight (85%); (b) NIS (1.5 equiv.), DMF, 12 h (90%); (c) N-acetyl-L-cysteine methyl ester (2 equiv.), $MeOH/H_2O$ 1/1, $h\nu = 254$ nm, 1 h (84%); (d) N-acetyl-L-cysteine methyl ester, AIBN 20 mol %, THF/H_2O, 70°C, 2 h, 98%.

---

* Corresponding author.
† Checker.

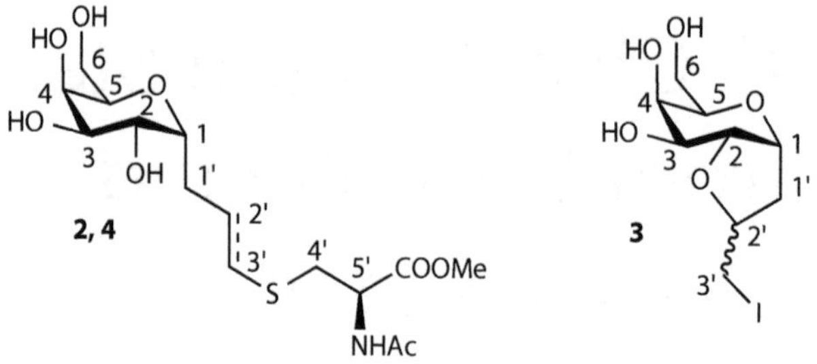

FIGURE 8.1   NMR skeleton numbering.

The use of carbohydrates as structural scaffolds for the design and synthesis of new drugs has found growing interest in the last decade. The main drawback of existing syntheses of carbohydrate scaffolds is the tedious protecting group manipulation necessary for the introduction of orthogonality of protecting groups. In this chapter, we describe a direct approach for generation of monocyclic and bicyclic C-galactosyl compounds from commercially available methyl α-D-galactopyranoside without the use of protecting groups.

Commercially available methyl α-D-galactopyranoside (**1**) was silylated, using bis(trimethylsilyl)trifluoroacetamide (BTSFA), and treated with allyltrimethylsilane and catalytic amount of trimethylsilyl trifluoromethanesulfonate, to afford 3-(α-D-galactopyranosyl)prop-1-ene (**2**) as a single diastereoisomer.[1,2] Iodocyclization of compound **2** (N-iodosuccinimide in DMF) provided an inseparable mixture (the composition varies from 3:2 to 4:1) of diastereomeric iodides **3**,[3] the ratio of which can be determined by ^{1}H-NMR. The cysteine derivative compound **4**[4] was synthesized exploiting the chemoselective reaction between a thiol group and a terminal olefinic double bond. This reaction was carried out by irradiation ($hv = 254\,nm$) of compound **2** and N-acetyl-L-cysteine methyl ester in degassed 1:1 MeOH–H$_2$O. The conversion can also be achieved (~98%) without UV irradiation, using AIBN as radical initiator (20 mol %) (Figure 8.1).

EXPERIMENTAL METHODS

GENERAL METHODS

All solvents were dried with molecular sieves, for at least 24 h prior to use. Thin layer chromatography (TLC) was performed on silica gel 60 F254 plates (Merck) with detection by UV light, by charring with mixture of concd. H$_2$SO$_4$:EtOH:H$_2$O (5:45:45) or with a solution of (NH$_4$)$_6$Mo$_7$O$_{24}$ (21 g), Ce(SO$_4$)$_2$ (1 g), concentrated H$_2$SO$_4$ (31 mL) in water (500 mL). Flash column chromatography was performed on silica gel 230–400 mesh (Merck). ^{1}H and ^{13}C NMR spectra were recorded at 25°C with a Varian Mercury 400 MHz instrument. Chemical shifts are reported in ppm, relative to the corresponding solvent peaks. Mass spectra were recorded with an ESI positive Fourier Transform Ion Ciclotron Resonance Mass Spectrometer APEX II (Bruker Daltonics) equipped with a 4.7T magnet (Magnex). Optical rotations were measured at room temperature using a Krüss P3002 electronic polarimeter.

3-(α-D-Galactopyranosyl)prop-1-Ene (2)

To a suspension of methyl α-D-galactopyranoside (2.00 g, 10 mmol) in acetonitrile (2.0 mL), BTSFA (8.20 mL, 31 mmol) was added and the mixture was heated at reflux for 1 h, during which time a clear solution was formed. Allyltrimethylsilane (2.40 mL, 15 mmol) was added at 0°C, followed by trimethylsilyl trifluoromethane-sulfonate (0.92 mL, 5.00 mmol), and the mixture was stirred overnight at rt. The mixture was poured (CAUTION!) into ice-cold water and stirred for 3 h, prior to neutralization (pH = 7) with IRN 78 resin (OH⁻ form). The mixture was filtered, the filtrate was concentrated under reduced pressure, and chromatography (15:1 EtOAc–MeOH) afforded **2** (1.78 g, 85%), mp 127°C–131°C (EtOAc), $[\alpha]_D$ = +88.0 (c = 1.0, MeOH), R_f = 0.4, (4:1 EtOAc–MeOH,), ¹H NMR (400 MHz, D₂O): δ 5.74–5.56 (m, 1H, CH=CH₂), 5.07–4.86 (m, 2H, CH=CH_2), 3.98–3.85 (m, 1H, H(1)), 3.84–3.72 (m, 2H), 3.70–3.56 (m, 2H), 3.54–3.41 (m, 2H), 2.40–2.24 (m, 1H, H(1′a)), 2.24–2.10 (m, 1H, H(1′b)); ¹³C NMR (100 MHz, D₂O, 25°C) δ = 137.6 (CH), 120.1 (CH₂), 77.63 (CH), 74.31 (CH), 72.32 (CH), 71.70 (CH), 70.90 (CH), 63.62 (CH₂), 31.47 (CH₂); MS-ESI m/z 227.0889 [(M + Na)⁺ calcd for $C_9H_{14}O_5Na$ 227.0898].

Bicyclic Iodoethers (3)

NIS (3.66 mmol) was added to a solution of compound **2** (500 mg, 2.44 mmol) in DMF (5 mL) and the mixture was stirred at rt for 12 h. After concentrated under reduced pressure, and chromatography of the material in the residue (gradient, 100:0 → 95:5 EtOAc-MeOH) afforded **3** (725 mg, 90%) as a pale yellow solid. R_f = 0.5, (EtOAc-MeOH, 4:1). ¹H NMR (6:4 mixture of diastereomers, asterisk denotes resonances from the minor anomer, 400 MHz, CD₃OD, 25°C) δ = 4.57–4.52 (m, 1H, H(1), H(1*)), 4.19–4.13 (m, 0.6H, H(2′)), 4.15–4.07 (m, 1H, H, H*), 3.97–3.86 (m, 2.4H, H, H*)), 3.83–3.76 (m, 2H, H(5), H(5*), H(6), H(6*)), 3.70–3.66 (m, 0.6H, H(6*)), 3.67–3.64 (m, 0.4H, H(6)), 3.36–3.33 (m, 2H, H(3′a,b), H(3′a,b*)), 2.33–2.17 (m, 1H, H(1a′), H(1a′*)), 1.97–1.87 (ddd, J = 4.5, 5.8, 13.6 Hz, 0.4H, H(1b′*)), 1.86–1.79 (ddd, J = 5.8, 8.2, 13.7 Hz, 0.6H, H(1b′)); ¹³C NMR (100 MHz, D₂O, 25°C) δ = 83.0* (CH), 81.6 (CH), 80.0 (CH), 79.3* (CH), 77.4* (CH), 76.9 (CH), 76.6 (CH), 75.8* (CH), 74.4 (CH), 72.2* (CH), 70.7 (CH), 70.5* (CH), 62.9 (CH₂), 62.3* (CH₂), 37.6* (CH₂), 37.0 (CH₂), 13.5* (CH₂), 12.6 (CH₂); MS-ESI m/z 352.9856 [(M + Na)⁺ calcd for $C_9H_{15}IO_5Na$ 352.9846].

Methyl (2R)-2-Acetamido-3-(α-D-Galactopyranosylpropylthio)propanoate (4)

Photochemical Reaction

A solution of compound **2** (100 mg, 0.49 mmol) and N-acetyl-L-cysteine methyl ester (174 mg, 0.98 mmol) in degassed* 1:1 MeOH–H₂O (3 mL) in an open glass beaker and was irradiated from above (10 cm) with a standard, 4 W, hν = 254 nm UV lamp.† After 1 h, the solvent was removed under reduced pressure and the crude material was chromatographed (4:1 AcOEt–MeOH) to afford **4** (156 mg, 84%) as amorphous white solid.

---

* Degassing was done by bubbling argon through the solvent mixture for 20 min.
† A UV lamp which is normally employed for TLC detection was used.

Non-Photochemical Reaction

A solution of compound **2** (100 mg, 0.49 mmol), *N*-acetyl-L-cysteine methyl ester (174 mg, 0.98 mmol) and 2,2'-azobis(2-methylpropionitrile, AIBN, 16 mg, 0.098 mmol) in 1:1 THF–H_2O was stirred under argon for 15 min at room temperature and then at 70°C for 2 h. After concentration, chromatography (8:2 AcOEt–MeOH) afforded **4** (183 mg, 98%) as amorphous white solid. $[\alpha]_D^{25}$ +65.3 (c = 0.15, CH_3OH); R_f = 0.3 (8:1.5:0.5 EtOAc–MeOH–H_2O,), ^{1}H NMR (400 MHz, D_2O) δ: 4.61 (dd, J = 8.2, 4.9 Hz, 1H, H(5')), 4.05–3.97 (m, 1H, H(1)), 3.96–3.91 (m, 2H), 3.76–3.71 (m, 5H), 3.70–3.65 (m, 2H), 3.07 (dd, J = 14.0, 4.9 Hz, 1H, H(4'a)), 2.90 (dd, J = 14.0, 8.3 Hz, 1H, H(4'b)), 2.64–2.61 (m, 2H, H(3'a,b)), 2.03 (s, 3H, NHCOCH_3), 1.80–1.50 (m, 4H, H(1'a,b), H(2'a,b)); ^{13}C NMR (100 MHz) δ: 174.3 (C), 172.9 (C), 75.13 (CH), 71.72 (CH), 69.74 (CH), 69.17 (CH), 68.33 (CH), 61.22 (CH_2), 53.15, 52.67 (CH, CH_3), 32.28 (CH_2), 31.41 (CH_2), 24.89 (CH_2), 22.61 (CH_2), 21.66 (CH_3); HRMS calcd for $C_{15}H_{27}NO_8S$ (MNa$^+$) 404.1349; found: 404.1348.

ACKNOWLEDGMENTS

We thank CINMPIS Consortium for the financial support.

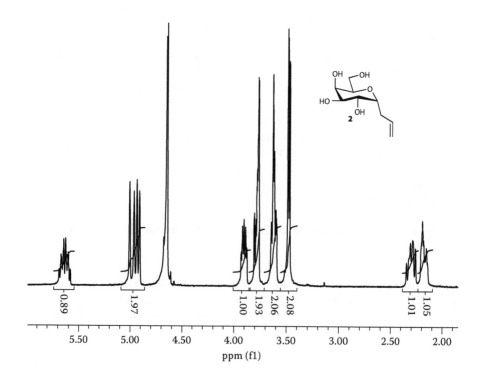

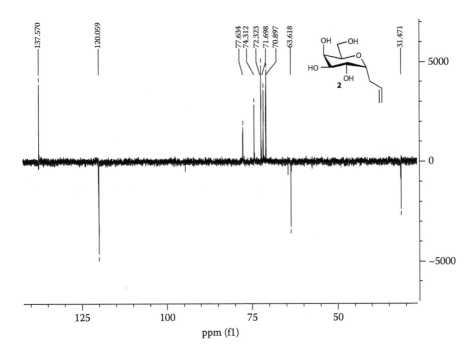

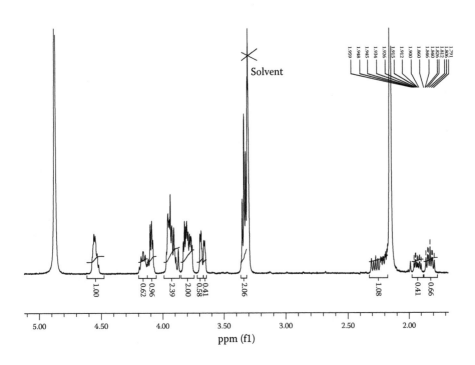

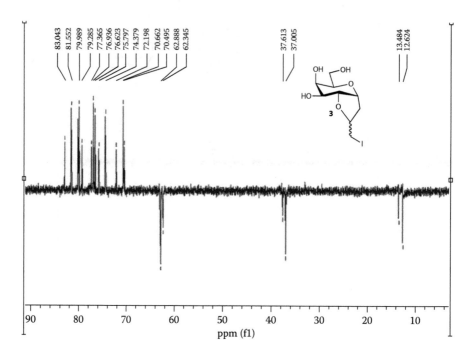

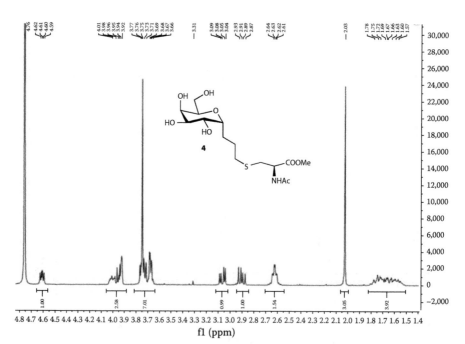

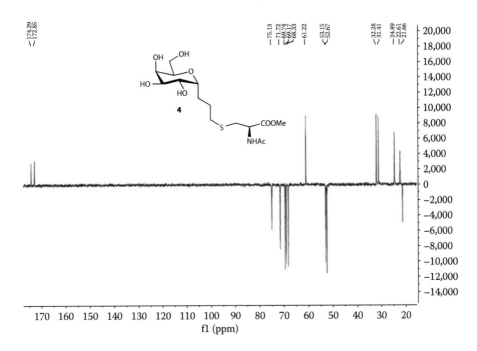

REFERENCES

1. Bennek, J. A.; Gray, G. R., *J. Org. Chem.* 1987, *52*, 892–897.
2. Mari, S.; Cañada, J. F.; Jiménez-Barbero, J.; Bernardi, A.; Marcou, G.; Motto, I.; Velter, I.; Nicotra, F.; La Ferla, B., *Eur. J. Org. Chem.* 2006, *13*, 2925–2933.
3. La Ferla, B.; Cardona, F.; Perdigão, I.; Nicotra, F., *Synlett* 2005, *17*, 2641–2642.
4. Cardona, F.; La Ferla, B., *J. Carbohydr. Chem.* 2008, *27*(4), 203–213.

9 Palladium-Catalyzed Sonogashira Coupling on *p*-Iodophenyl α-D-Mannopyranoside

Tze Chieh Shiao, Jacques Rodrigue,[†]
*and Mohamed Touaibia**

CONTENTS

Experimental Methods 92
   General Methods 92
      3-[4-(2,3,4,6-Tetra-*O*-Acetyl-α-D-Mannopyranosyloxy)
      phenyl]prop-2-Yn-1-ol (**2**) 92
Acknowledgments 93
References 94

Transition metal–catalyzed cross-coupling reactions of organometallic compounds with organic electrophiles rank among the most useful processes for forming carbon–carbon bonds.[1] The palladium-catalyzed coupling of terminal acetylenes with aryl or vinyl halides (Sonogashira reaction) is one of the important and widely used procedures for the preparation of terminal and internal alkynes in organic syntheses.[2]

    In carbohydrate chemistry, the mono or multiple Sonogashira coupling represents a versatile approach to the synthesis of more rigid simple glycosides[3] or

---

* Corresponding author.
[†] Checker.

glycodendrimers.[4,5] Decreased flexibility should improve the interaction with receptors or enzymes by reducing the entropy of binding. Indeed, considerable effort has been allocated to the synthesis of conformationally rigid oligosaccharide analogues for the investigation of carbohydrate–protein binding.[3-5]

This methodology has been successfully applied by Al-Mughaid and Grindley for the preparation of a nonavalent glycodendrimer.[4] More recently, we have described a synthesis of libraries of mannoside clusters[5] constructed for the establishment of a quantitative structure activity relationship (QSAR) model toward *E. coli* FimH lectin,[6] the adhesin portion of type 1 fimbria. As preliminary results, the family of clusters indicated that they were shown to be much faster in cross-linking the tetravalent lectin ConA than the positive control, the mannan polysaccharide from yeast. Considering the wide variety of possible applications offered by new glycosides and glycodendrimers, development of more adaptable methodologies to specific needs is necessary. Based on our previous work,[5] we here describe synthesis of mannopyranoside **2** from *p*-iodophenyl 2,3,4,6-tetra-*O*-acetyl-α-D-mannopyranoside **1**[7] and by palladium-catalyzed Sonogashira cross-coupling, as shown above.

EXPERIMENTAL METHODS

GENERAL METHODS

The reaction was carried out under nitrogen using freshly distilled solvent. After workup, the organic layer was dried over anhydrous $MgSO_4$, filtered, and concentrated under reduced pressure. The progress of the reaction was monitored by thin-layer chromatography using silica gel 60 F_{254} precoated plates (E. Merck). Optical rotation was measured with a JASCO P-1010 polarimeter. NMR spectra were recorded on a Varian Gemini 300 spectrometer. Proton and carbon chemical shifts are reported in ppm relative to the signal of $CDCl_3$. Coupling constants (J) are reported in Hertz and the following abbreviations are used: singlet (s), doublet (d), doublet of doublets (dd), triplet (t), multiplet (m), and broad (b). Assignments were made by COSY, DEPT, and HETCOR experiments. High-resolution mass spectra (HRMS) were taken by Plateforme analytique pour molécules organiques de l'UQAM (Université du Québec à Montréal, Canada).

3-[4-(2,3,4,6-Tetra-*O*-Acetyl-α-D-Mannopyranosyloxy) phenyl]prop-2-Yn-1-ol (2)

To a solution of *p*-iodophenyl 2,3,4,6-tetra-*O*-acetyl-α-D-mannopyranoside **1** (125 mg, 0.227 mmol, 1.0 equiv.), dichlorobis(triphenylphosphane)palladium(II) (($PPh_3)_2PdCl_2$,* 10 mg, 0.011 mmol (5 mol%)) and CuI† (1.0 mg, 0.005 mmol) in 3 mL of dry DMF was degassed under nitrogen atmosphere[8] using ultrasonic cleaner. After 5 min, propargyl alcohol (30 μL, 0.454 mmol, 2 equiv.) and triethylamine (3 mL) were added into the solution. The reaction mixture was stirred at

---

* The reaction was tested in the absence of Cu(I) and heating (60°C, 12 h), the yields varied considerably from one attempt to the other. We also tried $Pd_2(dba)_3$ and $Pd(PPh_3)_4$ with varied success as well.
† Addition of copper(I) iodide as cocatalyst allowed the reaction to proceed at room temperature with high and reproducible yield.

room temperature. The TLC (hexane/AcOEt 1:1) showed the complete disappearance of the starting material (R_f=0.61, 3 h). The solvent and triethylamine were evaporated under reduced pressure. AcOEt (30 mL) was added to the reaction mixture and washed with saturated aqueous NH_4Cl^* (3 × 50 mL), brine (3 × 50 mL), and water (3 × 50 mL). The organic layers were dried over $MgSO_4$ and evaporated under reduced pressure, leaving a yellow oil; the resulting crude product was purified by flash chromatography on silica gel (hexane/AcOEt 1:1) to give 3-[4-(2,3,4,6-tetra-O-acetyl-α-D-mannopyranosyloxy)phenyl]prop-2-yn-1-ol **2** as yellow foam (106 mg, 0.222 mmol, 98%). The desired compound was crystallized in petroleum ether with a little amount of dichloromethane and EtOH (100%). R_f=0.28 (1:1 hexane–AcOEt); mp 63°C–64°C (from CH_2Cl_2/EtOH/EP 1:0.5:30); $[α]_D$ +70.3 (c 1.0, $CHCl_3$). ^{1}H NMR ($CDCl_3$) δ 7.38 (d, 2H, $J_{H,H}$ 8.8 Hz, H_{ar}-meta), 7.03 (d, 2H, $J_{H,H}$ 8.8 Hz, H_{ar}-ortho), 5.54 (dd, 1H, $J_{2,3}$ 3.3 Hz, $J_{3,4}$ 10.0 Hz, H-3), 5.52 (d, 1H, $J_{1,2}$ 1.9 Hz, H-1), 5.43 (dd, 1H, $J_{1,2}$ 1.9 Hz, $J_{2,3}$ 3.3 Hz, H-2), 5.35 (t, 1H, $J_{3,4}$=$^3J_{4,5}$ 10.0 Hz, H-4), 4.48 (d, 2H, J_{H-OH} 6.1 Hz, CCH_2O), 4.27 (dd, 1H, $J_{6a,6b}$ 5.9 Hz, $J_{5,6}$ 12.6 Hz, H-6a), 4.08–4.03 (m, 2H, H-5 and H-6b), 1.94 (t, 1H, J_{OH-H} 6.1 Hz, OH), 2.20, 2.05, 2.04, 2.03 ppm (4s, 4 × 3H, $COCH_3$); ^{13}C NMR ($CDCl_3$) δ 170.5, 170.0, 169.9, 169.7 (CO), 155.5, ($C_{q-ar}O$), 133.2 (C_{ar}-meta), 117.2 ($C_{q-ar}C$), 116.4 (C_{ar}-ortho), 95.6 (C-1), 86.7 ($C_{q-alcyn}C_{ar}$), 84.9 ($C_{q-alcyn}CH_2$), 69.2 (C-5), 69.2 (C-2), 68.7 (C-3), 65.8 (C-4), 62.0 (C-6), 51.5 (CH_2OH), 20.8–20.6 ppm (4 × CH_3). ESI$^+$-HRMS: $[M+H]^+$ calcd for $C_{23}H_{27}O_{11}$, 479.1548; found: 479.1544.

ACKNOWLEDGMENTS

M.T. acknowledges the financial contribution of the New Brunswick Innovation Foundation and The Medical Research Fund of New Brunswick.

---

* Incomplete removal of paramagnetic copper salts from the organic phase is readily seen by signal broadening in the ^{1}H-NMR spectra. The washing of the organic phase with NH_4Cl or EDTA usually eliminates the problem.

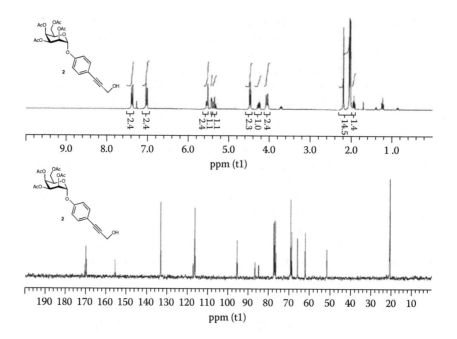

REFERENCES

1. (a) Sonogashira, K. In: *Comprehensive Organic Synthesis*, Eds. Trost, B. M. and Fleming, L. Pergamon Press, Elmsford, NY, 1991, vol. 3, pp. 521–549; (b) Miyaura, N.; Suzuki, A. *Chem. Rev.*, 1995, *95*, 2457–2483.
2. (a) Nicolaou, K. C.; Dai, W.-M. *Angew. Chem. Int. Ed.*, 1991, *30*, 1387–1416; (b) de Kort, M.; Correa, V.; Valentijin, A. R.; Van der Marel, G.A.; Potter, B. V. L.; Taylor, C. W.; Van Boom, J. H. *J. Med. Chem.*, 2000, *43*, 3295–3303.
3. a) Todd Lowary, T.; Meldal, M.; Helmboldt, A.; Vasella, A.; Bock, K. *J. Org. Chem.*, 1998, *63*, 9657–9668; (b) Franzyk, H.; Christensen, M. K.; Jørgensen, M.; Meldal, M.; Cordes, H.; Mouritsen, S.; Bock, K. *Bioorg. Med. Chem.*, 1997, *5*, 21–40.
4. Al-Mughaid, H.; Grindley, T. B. *J. Org. Chem.*, 2006, *71*, 1390–1398.
5. Touaibia, M.; Roy, R. *J. Org. Chem.*, 2008, *73*, 9292–9302.
6. Touaibia, M.; Roy, R. Application of multivalent mannosylated dendrimers in glycobiology. *Carbohydrate-Protein and Carbohydrate–Carbohydrate Interactions; Comprehensive Glycoscience*, Ed. Kamerling, J. P. Elsevier, New York, USA, 2007, vol. 3, pp. 781–829.
7. Roy, R.; Trono, M. C.; Giguère, D. *ACS Symp. Ser.*, 2004, *896*, 137–150.
8. Siemsen, P.; Livingston, R. C.; Diederich, F. *Angew. Chem. Int. Ed.*, 2000, *39*, 2632–2657.

10 Synthesis by "Click Chemistry" of an α-D-Mannopyranoside Having a 1,4-Disubstituted Triazole as Aglycone

Tze Chieh Shiao, Denis Giguère,[†]
and Mohamed Touaibia*

CONTENTS

Experimental Methods 96
  General Methods 96
    Methyl 2-{[4-(2,3,4,6-Tetra-*O*-Acetyl-α-D-Mannopyranosyloxy)
    methyl]-1*H*-1,2,3-Triazol-1-yl]}Acetate (**2**) 96
Acknowledgments..97
References..98

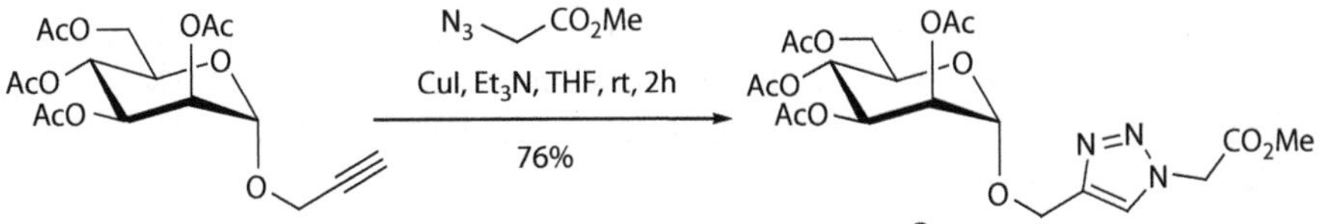

Triazoles are important five-member ring nitrogen heterocycles involved in a wide range of industrial applications such as agrochemicals, corrosion inhibitors, dyes, optical brighteners, as well as biologically active agents.[1] Since Sharpless and Meldal's independent reports in 2002,[2] this chemoselective [3+2] cycloaddition,

---

* Corresponding author.
[†] Checker.

95

providing only the 1,4-disubstituted 1,2,3-triazoles, has opened the way toward the synthesis of new glycoside and oligosaccharide mimetics, glyco-macrocycles, gly-copeptides, glyco-clusters, and carbohydrate microarrays.[3] The copper (I)-catalyzed 1,3-cycloaddition owes its usefulness in part to its high compatibility with a broad range of functional groups in different solvent systems.

In a recent study, we have elaborated libraries of mannosides and mannoside clusters constructed for the establishment of a quantitative structure activity relationship (QSAR) model toward *E. coli* FimH lectin,[4] the adhesin portion of type 1 fimbria. The library included several C- and O-linked mannopyranoside analogs as well as new glycodendrimers. The family of clusters indicated that they were approximately 100 times more efficient in the inhibition of agglutination of *E. coli* x7122[5] by baker's yeast than D-mannose. Considering the wide variety of possible applications offered by glycoclusters and glycodendrimers, development of a versatile methodology to render the synthesis of these macromolecules more adaptable to specific needs is necessary for their eventual commercialization. Preliminary data identified monosaccharides that bind in nanomolar concentration to *E. coli* FimH. Consequently, and on the basis of our expertise,[4,5] the synthesis of mannopyranoside **2** from prop-2-ynyl 2,3,4,6-tetra-*O*-acetyl-α-D-mannopyranoside **1**,[6] methyl azidoacetate,[7] by copper(I)-catalyzed 1,3-cycloaddition is proposed herein.

EXPERIMENTAL METHODS

General Methods

The reaction was carried out under nitrogen using freshly distilled solvent. After workup, the organic layer was dried over anhydrous $MgSO_4$, filtered, and concentrated under reduced pressure. Progress of the reaction was monitored by thin-layer chromatography using silica gel 60 F_{254} precoated plates (E. Merck). Optical rotation was measured with a JASCO P-1010 polarimeter. NMR spectra were recorded on a Varian Gemini 300 spectrometer. Proton and carbon chemical shifts are reported in ppm relative to the signal of $CDCl_3$. Coupling constants (J) are reported in Hertz and the following abbreviations are used: singlet (s), doublet (d), doublet of doublets (dd), triplet (t), multiplet (m), and broad (b). Assignments were made by COSY, DEPT, and HETCOR experiments. High-resolution mass spectra (HRMS) were taken by Plateforme analytique pour molécules organiques de l'UQAM (Université du Québec à Montréal, Canada).

Methyl 2-{[4-(2,3,4,6-Tetra-*O*-Acetyl-α-D-Mannopyranosyloxy) methyl]-1*H*-1,2,3-Triazol-1-yl]}Acetate (2)

To a solution of prop-2-ynyl 2,3,4,6-tetra-*O*-acetyl-α-D-mannopyranoside **1** (100 mg, 0.258 mmol), methyl azidoacetate,* (45 mg, 0.414 mmol, 1.6 equiv.), and CuI† (5 mg, 0.025 mmol, 0.1 equiv.) in anhydrous THF[2] (4 mL) was added triethylamine

---

* Organic azides are potentially explosive substances, safety precautions must be taken.

† The reaction was tested with the $CuSO_4$ and sodium ascorbate in THF-H_2O and t-BuOH-H_2O but the yields were systematically less than 40%.

(44 μL, 0.31 mmol, 1.2 equiv.). The reaction mixture was stirred at room temperature* for 2 h. TLC (hexane/AcOEt 1:1) indicated complete consumption of **1** ($R_f = 0.53$, 2 h). After solvent evaporation, the crude product was dissolved in ethyl acetate (30 mL), washed with $NH_4Cl^\dagger$ solution (3 × 10 mL), brine (3 × 10 mL), and concentrated. The yellow oil was purified by flash chromatography on silica gel (99:1 CH_2Cl_2–MeOH) to give **2** as colorless foam (99 mg, 0.197 mmol, 76%), $R_f = 0.55$ (AcOEt 100%); $[\alpha]_D$ +44.8 (*c* 1.0, $CHCl_3$); ^1H NMR ($CDCl_3$) δ 7.73 (s, 1H, C=CH), 5.30–5.27 (m, 2H, H-3 and H-4), 5.23 (dd, 1H, $J_{1,2}$ 1.7 Hz, $J_{2,3}$ 3.4, H-2), 5.19 (s, 2H, NCH_2CO), 4.96 (d, 1H, $J_{1,2}$ 1.7 Hz, H-1), 4.86 (d, 1H, J_{H-H} 12.4 Hz, OCH_2), 4.71 (d, 1H, J_{H-H} 12.4 Hz, OCH_2), 4.28 (dd, 1H, $J_{6a,6b}$ 5.2 Hz, $J_{5,6}$ 12.3 Hz, H-6a), 4.10–4.02 (m, 2H, H-6b and H-5), 3.81 (s, 3H, OCH_3), 2.14, 2.10, 2.02, 1.97 ppm (4×s, 12H, CH_3); ^{13}C NMR ($CDCl_3$) δ 170.6, 169.9, 169.8, 169.6, 166.5 (CO), 144.0 (C_q-triazol), 124.3 (CH-triazol), 96.9 (C-1), 69.3 (C-2), 68.9 (C-5), 68.6 (C-3), 65.9 (C-4), 62.2 (OCH_2), 61.0 (C-6), 53.0 (OCH_3), 50.6 (NCH_2CO), 20.8, 20.7, 20.6, 20.6 ppm ($COCH_3$). ESI$^+$-HRMS: $[M+H]^+$ calcd for $C_{20}H_{28}N_3O_{12}$, 502.1667; found: 502.1662; ESI$^+$-HRMS: $[M+Na]^+$ calcd for $C_{20}H_{27}N_3O_{12}Na$, 524.1487; found: 524.1484.

ACKNOWLEDGMENTS

M.T. acknowledges the financial contribution of the New Brunswick Innovation Foundation and The Medical Research Fund of New Brunswick.

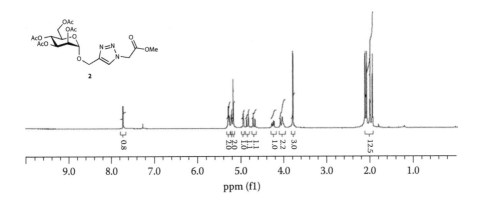

---

* Heating is not recommended as it can cause cycloaddition to occur with the ensuing mixture of 1,4 plus 1,5-regioisomers.
† Incomplete removal of paramagnetic copper salts from the organic phase is readily seen by signal broadeing in the ^1H-NMR spectra. Washing of the organic phase with NH_4Cl or EDTA usually eliminates the problem.

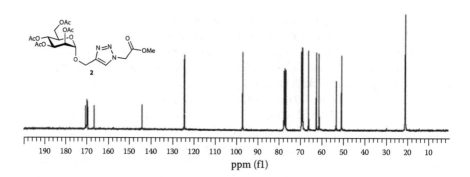

ppm (f1)

REFERENCES

1. Dehne, H. In *Methoden der Organischen Chemie (Houben-Weyl)*; M. Schumann, Ed.; Thieme: Stuttgart, Germany, 1994, Vol. E8d, pp. 305–320.
2. Rostovtsev, V. V.; Green, L. G.; Fokin, V. V.; Sharpless, K. B. *Angew. Chem. Int. Ed.*, 2002, *41*, 2596–2599; Tornøe, C. W.; Christensen, C.; Meldal, M. *J. Org. Chem.*, 2002, *67*, 3057–3064.
3. Dedola, S.; Nepogodiev, S. A.; Field, R. A. *Org. Biomol. Chem.*, 2007, *5*, 1006–1017; Santoyo-González, F.; Hernández-Mateo, F. *Top Heterocycl. Chem.*, 2007, *7*, 133–177; Meldal, M.; Wenzel Tornoe, C. W. *Chem. Rev.*, 2008, *108*, 2952–3015.
4. Touaibia, M.; Roy, R. *Mini-Rev. Med. Chem.*, 2007, *7*, 1270–1283.
5. Touaibia, M.; Shiao, T. C.; Papadopoulos, A.; Vaucher, J.; Wang, Q.; Benhamioud, K.; Roy, R. *Chem. Commun.*, 2007, *4*, 380–382.
6. Das, S. K.; Trono, M. C.; Roy, R. *Methods Enzymol.*, 2003, *362*, 3–17.
7. Sechi, M.; Derudas, M.; Dallocchio, R.; Dessi, A.; Bacchi, A.; Sannia, L.; Carta, F.; Palomba, M.; Ragab, O.; Chan, C.; Shoemaker, R.; Sei, S.; Dayam, R.; Neamati, N. *J. Med. Chem.*, 2004, *47*, 5298–5310.

11 Synthesis of Methyl Glycuronates by Chemo- and Regioselective TEMPO/BAIB-Oxidation

Marthe T.C. Walvoort, Deepak Sail,[†] Gijsbert A. van der Marel, and Jeroen D.C. Codée*

CONTENTS

Experimental Methods 101
    General Methods 101
        Phenyl 3-*O*-Benzoyl-2-Deoxy-2-Phthalimido-1-Thio-β-D-
        Glucopyranosyluronic Acid (**2**) 102
        Methyl (Phenyl 3-*O*-Benzoyl-2-Deoxy-2-Phthalimido-1-Thio-β-D-
        Glucopyranoside) Uronate (**3**) 102
Acknowledgments 103
References 104

TEMPO/BAIB-mediated oxidation and ensuing methylation of **1**. Reagents and conditions: (i) 0.2 eq TEMPO, 2.5 eq BAIB, DCM/H$_2$O (2/1); (ii) 3 eq MeI, 3 eq K$_2$CO$_3$, DMF.

Uronic acids are widely present in natural polysaccharides. Synthetic methods to obtain uronic acid-containing oligosaccharides involve either a post- or pre-glycosylation oxidation step. For a recent review on oxidation strategies towards uronic acids, see Ref. [1]. Since the carboxylic acid/ester moiety can have a profound influence on both the reactivity[1] and selectivity (see for an example, Ref. [2])

---

* Corresponding author.
† Checker.

in a glycosylation, the most applicable strategy has to be selected carefully (for an example of post-glycosylation oxidation, see Ref. [3]).

Thioglycosides are frequently used as building blocks in the assembly of oligo-saccharides, but 1-thioglycuronate esters are relatively scarcely employed. Next to the challenge to distinguish between primary and secondary hydroxyls, the oxidation of thioglycosides can lead to oxidation of the thio functionality to the sulfoxide/sulfone. Although various chemo- (see for example, Ref. [4]) or regioselective (see for example, Ref. [5]) oxidation protocols exist, only few deal simultaneously with the chemo- and regioselectivity required for 1-thioglycuronides. For a chromium-based chemo- and regioselective oxidation, see Ref. [6].

We here describe an efficient oxidation protocol for the preparation of diversely protected thioglycuronic acids, based on the use of 2,2,6,6-tetramethylpiperidin-1-yloxyl (TEMPO) (see for the first application of TEMPO in carbohydrate oxidation, Ref. [7]) together with [bis(acetoxy)iodo]benzene (BAIB) as the co-oxidant.[8,9] As depicted in Scheme 11.1, diol **1** is treated with a catalytic amount of TEMPO and an excess of BAIB in DCM/H_2O at ambient temperature. The starting compound **1** was synthesized from known phenyl 4,6-benzylidene-2-deoxy-2-phthalimido-1-thio-β-D-glucopyranoside[16] by benzoylation (2 eq. BzCl, 0.5 M pyridine), followed by cleavage of the benzylidene group by hydrolysis (cat. pTsOH, 0.12 M MeOH/DCM, 5/1). Compound **1** (74% over two steps) was obtained as a white foam after flash chromatography (1:4, PE:EtOAc). Filtration through a syringe filter (0.45 μm) gave material showing $[\alpha]_D$ +141.6° (c 1, $CHCl_3$). IR (neat, cm^{-1}): 710, 1022, 1069, 1265, 1381, 1713; ^{1}H NMR ($CDCl_3$, 400 MHz, HH-COSY) δ 7.65–7.88 (m, 6H, CH_{arom}), 7.50 (dt, 1H, J = 1.2, 7.4 Hz, CH_{arom}), 7.38–7.42 (m, 2H, CH_{arom}), 7.34 (t, 2H, J = 7.8 Hz, CH_{arom}), 7.27–7.30 (m, 3H, CH_{arom}), 5.90 (dd, 1H, J = 8.9, 10.3 Hz, H-3), 5.84 (d, 1H, J = 10.5 Hz, H-1), 4.51 (t, 1H, J = 10.4 Hz, H-2), 4.03 (dd, 1H, J = 3.1, 12.0 Hz, H-6), 3.87–3.96 (m, 2H, H-4, H-6), 3.76 (ddd, 1H, J = 3.4, 4.7, 9.7 Hz, H-5), 3.17 (bs, 1H, 4-OH), 2.12 (bs, 1H, 6-OH); ^{13}C-APT NMR ($CDCl_3$, 100 MHz, HSQC) δ 167.7, 166.9 (C=O NPhth), 166.2 (C=O Bz), 134.0, 133.8, 133.0, 132.0 (CH_{arom}), 131.5 (C_q SPh), 131.1, 130.1 (C_q NPhth), 129.4, 128.7 (CH_{arom}), 128.6 (C_q Bz), 128.0, 127.7, 123.3, 123.1 (CH_{arom}), 82.8 (C-1), 79.8 (C-5), 74.7 (C-3), 69.3 (C-4), 61.8 (C-6), 53.6 (C-2); ESI-MS: 505.8 $[M+H]^+$. Calcd for $C_{27}H_{23}NO_7S$: C, 64.15; H, 4.59; N, 2.77. Found: C, 63.95; H, 4.57; N, 2.80. Thin-layer chromatography (TLC) analysis shows the disappearance of **1** to be quite fast (~20 min) and the formation of the product acid as near-base-line material. In addition, an unidentified, nonpolar by-product is also formed. Prolonged reaction time results in formation of another by-product and a decreased yield. After work-up, crude **2** is methylated using iodomethane under basic conditions, to obtain the corresponding methyl uronate **3** in 82% yield.

This oxidation protocol was successfully applied to various carbohydrates containing thio-alkyl and thio-aryl, azido, benzyl, benzoyl, silyl, and phthaloyl protecting groups (Table 11.1).

TABLE 11.1

Overview of Chemo- and Regioselectively Oxidized Thioglycosides with the TEMPO/BAIB Method

Ref. [10]   Ref. [10]   R = Et, Ph

Ref. [11]   Ref. [10]   Ref. [12]

Ref. [10]   Ref. [10]   Ref. [10]   Ref. [11]

Ref. [13]   Ref. [14]   Ref. [15]

EXPERIMENTAL METHODS

GENERAL METHODS

Dichloromethane (stabilized with amylene, Baker, p.a.) was used as received. Water used in the reaction was demineralized. Technical grade, distilled petroleum ether (PE) 40°C–65°C was used. TLC analysis was conducted using silica gel-coated aluminum sheets (Merck, silica gel 60, F_{245}). Compounds were visualized by UV light (245 nm) and by spraying with 20% H_2SO_4 in ethanol or with a solution of $(NH_4)_6Mo_7O_{24} \cdot 2H_2O$ (25 g/L), $(NH_4)_4Ce(SO_4)_4 \cdot 2H_2O$ (10 g/L), and 10% H_2SO_4 in H_2O, followed by charring at ~140°C. Flash chromatography was performed on pre-packed columns of silica gel (Analogix Si35) connected to a Biotage Isolera flash chromatograph. TEMPO, iodobenzene diacetate (BAIB), and iodomethane were purchased from Acros. Nuclear magnetic resonance (NMR) spectra were recorded for solutions in $CDCl_3$ on a Bruker AV400 with the chemical shift (δ) relative to tetramethylsilane (^{1}H) or CHCl$_3$ (^{13}C). Signal nuclei assignments were done by one- and two-dimensional experiments (^{1}H-^{1}H COSY, ^{1}H-^{13}C HSQC), using software supplied with the spectrometer. Optical rotation was measured using a Propol automatic polarimeter. The infrared (IR) absorbance was recorded using a Shimadzu FTIR-83000 spectrometer. Mass analysis was performed using a PE/SCIEX API 165 with an Electrospray Interface (Perkin-Elmer).

Phenyl 3-O-Benzoyl-2-Deoxy-2-Phthalimido-1-Thio-β-D-Glucopyranosyluronic Acid (2)

A 25 mL round bottom flask is charged with compound **1** (0.51 g, 1 mmol) and DCM/H$_2$O (5 mL, 2/1). The starting compound **1** was synthesized from known phenyl 4,6-benzylidene-2-deoxy-2-phthalimido-1-thio-β-D-glucopyranoside[16] by benzo-ylation (2 eq. BzCl, 0.5 M pyridine), followed by cleavage of the benzylidene group by hydrolysis (cat. pTsOH, 0.12 M MeOH/DCM, 5/1). Compound **1** (74% over two steps) was obtained as a white foam after flash chromatography (1:4, PE:EtOAc). Filtration through a syringe filter (0.45 μm) gave material showing [α]$_D$ +141.6° (c 1, CHCl$_3$). IR (neat, cm^{-1}): 710, 1022, 1069, 1265, 1381, 1713; ^{1}H NMR (CDCl$_3$, 400 MHz, HH-COSY) δ 7.65–7.88 (m, 6H, CH$_{arom}$), 7.50 (dt, 1H, J = 1.2, 7.4 Hz, CH$_{arom}$), 7.38–7.42 (m, 2H, CH$_{arom}$), 7.34 (t, 2H, J = 7.8 Hz, CH$_{arom}$), 7.27–7.30 (m, 3H, CH$_{arom}$), 5.90 (dd, 1H, J = 8.9, 10.3 Hz, H-3), 5.84 (d, 1H, J = 10.5 Hz, H-1), 4.51 (t, 1H, J = 10.4 Hz, H-2), 4.03 (dd, 1H, J = 3.1, 12.0 Hz, H-6), 3.87–3.96 (m, 2H, H-4, H-6), 3.76 (ddd, 1H, J = 3.4, 4.7, 9.7 Hz, H-5), 3.17 (bs, 1H, 4-OH), 2.12 (bs, 1H, 6-OH); ^{13}C-APT NMR (CDCl$_3$, 100 MHz, HSQC) δ 167.7, 166.9 (C=O NPhth), 166.2 (C=O Bz), 134.0, 133.8, 133.0, 132.0 (CH$_{arom}$), 131.5 (C$_q$ SPh), 131.1, 130.1 (C$_q$ NPhth), 129.4, 128.7 (CH$_{arom}$), 128.6 (C$_q$ Bz), 128.0, 127.7, 123.3, 123.1 (CH$_{arom}$), 82.8 (C-1), 79.8 (C-5), 74.7 (C-3), 69.3 (C-4), 61.8 (C-6), 53.6 (C-2); ESI-MS: 505.8 [M + H]$^+$. Calcd for C$_{27}$H$_{23}$NO$_7$S: C, 64.15; H, 4.59; N, 2.77. Found: C, 63.95; H, 4.57; N, 2.80. While stirred at ~7°C,* TEMPO (31.3 mg, 0.2 mmol) and iodobenzene diacetate (0.81 g, 2.5 mmol) are added. The flask is stoppered and allowed to warm to room temperature. The resulting clear emulsion is stirred vigorously until TLC analysis indicates complete consumption of the starting material (~30 min, R$_f$ 0.42, 1:2 hexane–EtOAc, +1% AcOH). After additional 15 min, the reaction is quenched with saturated aqueous Na$_2$S$_2$O$_3$ (5 mL), diluted with EtOAc (25 mL), and washed with saturated aqueous NaCl (2 × 25 mL). The combined aqueous layers are extracted with EtOAc (25 mL), the organic layers are dried over Na$_2$SO$_4$, filtered, and concentrated in vacuo. The crude product is used without purification in the methylation step.

Methyl (Phenyl 3-O-Benzoyl-2-Deoxy-2-Phthalimido-1-Thio-β-D-Glucopyranoside) Uronate (3)

The crude uronic acid **2** is transferred to a 25 mL round bottom flask and dissolved in dry DMF† (5 mL). Iodomethane (0.19 mL, 3 mmol) and potassium carbonate (0.42 g, 3 mmol) are added and the mixture is stirred in a closed flask at room temperature

---

* Temperature is measured in the ice-containing water bath.
† DMF was dried using 4 Å molecular sieves >24 h prior to use.

until TLC analysis* revealed complete consumption of the starting material (~2 h). The reaction mixture is transferred to a separatory funnel containing EtOAc (25 mL) and washed with saturated aqueous NaCl (3 × 25 mL). The combined aqueous layers are extracted with EtOAc (25 mL), the organic layers are dried over Na_2SO_4, filtered, and concentrated *in vacuo*. Chromatography (silica gel, 4:1 → 2:1 hexane–EtOAc) afforded the title compound, 0.44 g (82% over two steps); R_f 0.42 (1:1 PE–EtOAc); mp 94°–97° (from ether, twice); $[\alpha]_D$ +119° (c 1, $CHCl_3$); IR (neat, cm⁻¹) 725, 905, 1250, 1385, 1717; ¹H NMR ($CDCl_3$, 400 MHz): δ 7.55–7.90 (m, 6H, CH_{arom}), 7.38–7.49 (m, 3H, CH_{arom}), 7.20–7.30 (m, 5H, CH_{arom}), 6.09 (t, 1H, $J_{3,2}=J_{3,4}=9.6$ Hz, H-3), 5.99 (d, 1H, $J_{1,2}=10.8$ Hz, H-1), 4.54 (t, 1H, $J_{2,1}=J_{2,3}=10.4$ Hz, H-2), 4.38 (d, 1H, $J_{5,4}=10.0$ Hz, H-5), 4.18 (t, 1H, $J_{4,3}=J_{4,5}=9.6$ Hz, H-4), 3.82 (bs, 4H, $CH_3\,CO_2Me$, 4-OH); ¹³C NMR ($CDCl_3$, 100 MHz): δ 168.6 (C=O CO_2Me), 167.9, 166.8 (C=O Phth), 166.3 (C=O Bz), 134.1, 133.2, 132.6 (CH_{arom}), 131.2 (C_q Phth), 131.0 (C_q SPh), 130.9 (C_q Phth), 129.6, 128.8 (CH_{arom}), 128.5 (C_q Bz), 128.1, 123.4 (CH_{arom}), 83.7 (C-1), 78.3 (C-5), 73.8 (C-3), 70.8 (C-4), 53.1 (C-2), 52.7 ($CH_3\,CO_2Me$); ESI MS: 534.1 [M + H]⁺; Calcd for $C_{28}H_{23}NO_8S$: C, 63.03; H, 4.34; N, 2.63. Found: C, 63.12; H, 4.37; N, 2.61.

ACKNOWLEDGMENTS

We thank the Netherlands Organization for Scientific Research (NWO) and Top Institute Pharma (TIP) for financial support.

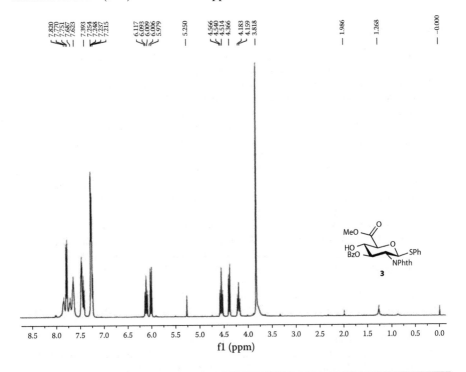

---

* To execute TLC analysis, an aliquot of the reaction mixture was diluted with EA and a fivefold amount of water and mixed vigorously. The organic layer was then used for the analysis.

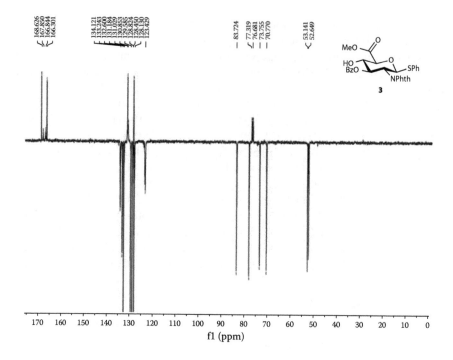

REFERENCES

1. Van den Bos, L. J.; Codée, J. D. C.; Litjens, R. E. J. N.; Dinkelaar, J.; Overkleeft, H. S.; Van der Marel, G. A. *Eur. J. Org. Chem.* 2007, *24*, 3963.
2. Codée, J. D. C.; Van den Bos, L. J.; De Jong, A. -R.; Dinkelaar, J.; Lodder, G.; Overkleeft, H. S.; Van der Marel, G. A. *J. Org. Chem.* 2009, *74*, 38.
3. Dinkelaar, J.; Van den Bos, L. J.; Hogendorf, W. F. J.; Lodder, G.; Overkleeft, H. S.; Codée, J. D. C.; Van der Marel, G. A. *Chem. Eur. J.* 2008, *14*, 9400; for an example of pre-glycosylation oxidation, Van den Bos, L. J.; Dinkelaar, J.; Overkleeft, H. S.; Van der Marel, G. A. *J. Am. Chem. Soc.* 2006, *128*, 13066.
4. Magaud, D.; Grandjean, C.; Doutheau, A.; Anker, D.; Sheychik, V.; Cotte-Pattat, N.; Robert-Baudouy, J. *Tetrahdron Lett.* 1996, *38*, 241; Liu, D.; Chen, R.; Hong, L.; Sofia, M. J. *Tetrahedron Lett.* 1998, *39*, 4951; Tully, S. E.; Mabon, R.; Gama, C.I.; Tsai, S. M.; Liu, X. L.; Hsieh-Wilson, L. C. J. *Am. Chem. Soc.* 2004, *126*, 7736.
5. Lichtenthaler, F. W.; Klotz, J.; Nakamura, K. *Tetrahedron: Asymm.* 2003, *14*, 3973; Martin, D.; Lichtenthaler, F.W. *Tetrahedron: Asymm.* 2006, *17*, 756; Breton, T.; Bashiardes, G.; Leger, J. -M.; Kokoh, K. B. *Eur. J. Org. Chem.* 2007, *10*, 1567.
6. Kakarla, R.; Ghosh, M.; Anderson, J. A.; Dulina, R. G.; Sofia, M. J. *Tetrahedron Lett.* 1999, *40*, 5.
7. Davis, N. J.; Flitsch, S. L. *Tetrahedron Lett.* 1993, *34*, 1181.
8. De Mico, A.; Margarita, R.; Parlanti, L.; Vescovi, A.; Piancatelli, G. J. *Org. Chem.* 1997, *62*, 6974.
9. Epp, J. B.; Widlanski, T. S. *J. Org. Chem.* 1999, *64*, 293.
10. Van den Bos, L. J.; Codée, J. D. C.; Van der Toorn, J. C.; Boltje, T. J.; Van Boom, J. H.; Overkleeft, H. S.; Van der Marel, G. A. *Org. Lett.* 2004, *6*, 2165.

11. Codée, J. D. C.; Stubba, B.; Schiattarella, M.; Overkleeft, H. S.; Boeckel, C. A. A.; Van Boom, J. H.; Van der Marel, G. A. *J. Am. Chem. Soc.* 2005, *127*, 3767.
12. Yamamoto, K.; Watanabe, N.; Matsuda, H.; Oohara, K.; Araya, T.; Hashimoto, M.; Miyairi, K.; Okazaki, I.; Saito, M.; Shimizu, T.; Kato, H.; Okuno, T. *Bioorg. Med. Chem. Lett.* 2005, *15*, 4932.
13. Van den Bos, L. J.; Dinkelaar, J.; Overkleeft, H. S.; Van der Marel, G. A. *J. Am. Chem. Soc.* 2006, *128*, 13066.
14. Van den Bos, L. J.; Duivendoorden, B. A.; De Koning, M. C.; Filippov, D. V.; Overkleeft, H. S.; Van der Marel, G. A. *Eur. J. Org. Chem.* 2007, *1*, 116.
15. Dinkelaar, J.; Van den Bos, L. J.; Hogendorf, W. F. J.; Lodder, G.; Overkleeft, H. S.; Codée, J. D. C.; Van der Marel, G. A. *Chem. Eur. J.* 2008, *14*, 9400.
16. Ogawa, T.; Nakabayashi, S.; Sasajima, K. *Carbohydr. Res.* 1981, *95*, 308.

12 Synthesis of Sugar Nucleotides: A Phosphoramidite Approach

Henrik Gold, Karine Descroix,[†]
Jeroen D.C. Codée, and Gijsbert
A. van der Marel*

CONTENTS

Experimental Methods 109
  General Methods 109
    Uridine 5′-(2-Acetamido-2-Deoxy-α-D-Glucopyranosyl Diphosphate)
    Disodium Salt (**5**) 109
References 112

* Corresponding author.
[†] Checker.

(i) 4,5-Dicyanoimidazole (DCI) (2 eq) and sugar phosphate **2** (1.2 eq), MeCN, rt, 30 min. (ii) *t*-BuOOH (5.5 M in nonane, 4 eq), rt, 30 min. (iii) DBU (5 eq), rt, 30 min. (iv) triethylamine (16 eq) and Et$_3$N · (HF)$_3$ (8 eq), rt, 4 h. (v) NH$_4$OH (25% in water, 30 eq), rt, o.n. (vi) workup and purification by ion-exchange chromatography. (vii) Amberlite-Na$^+$.

Glycans are a ubiquitous, structurally diverse class of biopolymers, the biosynthesis of which is catalyzed by glycosyltransferases.[1] These enzymes utilize nucleoside diphosphate saccharides as substrates for the transfer of a saccharide unit to acceptors such as (oligo)saccharides, lipids, or proteins.[2] Eukaryotic glycosyltransferases employ a limited number of sugar nucleotides as glycosyl donors (UDP-Glc, UDP-GlcNAc, UDP-GlcUA, UDP-Gal, UDP-GalNAc, GDP-Fuc, GDP-Man, and CMP-Neu5Ac),[3] while the structures of sugar nucleotides in prokaryotes are both numerous and diverse. For the assembly of glycans using glycosyl transferases, an efficient synthesis of (non)natural nucleoside diphosphate saccharides is imperative. Numerous strategies for the synthesis of pyrophosphates have previously been reported in the literature,[4,5] of which the morpholidate method of Moffatt and Khorana is the most frequently used.[6] In this chapter we present a convenient approach for the preparation of sugar nucleotides using a nucleotide phosphoramidite, as exemplified by the synthesis of UDP-*N*-acetylglucosamine (UDP-GlcNAc, **5**). Phosphoramidites have long been used as powerful phosphorylating agents in the synthesis of nucleic acid oligomers.[7] Utilizing this property in combination with a suitable phosphate nucleophile (i.e., glycosyl-phosphate) enables the facile construction of sugar nucleotides. As seen in the opening scheme of this chapter activation of phosphoramidite **1**[8] in presence of glycosyl phosphate **2**[8] leads to the formation of two diastereomeric phosphate–phosphite intermediates **3**. ^{31}P NMR [$\delta = 130.3$ (d, $J = 5.8$ Hz), 128.3 (d, $J = 4.5$ Hz), -10.9 (d, $J = 4.5$ Hz), -11.0 (d, $J = 5.8$ Hz) ppm]. Subsequent oxidation and ensuing deprotection produces the required sugar nucleotide **5**. The method described herein is attractive for a number of reasons: First, the high reactivity of phosphoramidites enables rapid and efficient formation of sugar nucleotides. Second, the accidental presence of moisture does not give rise to homocoupling, under the used reaction conditions. This type of side reaction can occur when methods involving activated forms of phosphates are applied. Hydrolysis of the reactive phosphorous (V) species with concurrent homocoupling results in a complex reaction mixture, which makes purification cumbersome.[9] Finally, the stereochemistry of the final product is ensured and retained throughout the reaction by the use of diastereomerically pure glycosyl phosphates.

EXPERIMENTAL METHODS

GENERAL METHODS

Acetonitrile (DNA reagent grade, Biosolve) was stored over 3 Å molecular sieves (Acros Organics, 8-12 mesh, 60 g/L solvent; the molecular sieves were dried in a vacuum oven at 80°C overnight). Triethylamine was distilled from CaH_2 and stored over potassium hydroxide pellets. 4,5-Dicyanoimidazole (DCI) and $Et_3N \cdot (HF)_3$ (97%) were obtained from Acros Organics. Diaza(1,3)bicyclo[5.4.0]undecane (DBU) and ammonium hydroxide (~25% in H_2O) were purchased from Sigma-Aldrich and t-BuOOH (~5.5 M in nonane) was acquired from Fluka. The synthesized pyrophosphates were purified by ion exchange chromatography (Q-Sepharose, 50 mM—0.5 M ammonium acetate, with a flow rate of 4 mL per minute). Detection was performed with UV light at 280 nm and fractions were collected at 1 min intervals. ^{1}H, ^{13}C, and ^{31}P nuclear magnetic resonance (NMR) spectra were recorded on a Bruker AV400 MHz spectrometer at 400.2, 100.6, and 162.0 MHz, respectively. Chemical shifts are reported as δ values (ppm) and indirectly referenced to H_3PO_4 (0.00 ppm) in D_2O via the solvent residual signal. Peak assignments were based on HH-COSY and HSQC measurements.

Uridine 5′-(2-Acetamido-2-Deoxy-α-ᴅ-Glucopyranosyl Diphosphate) Disodium Salt (5)

In a 10 mL round bottom flask, a solution of phosphoramidite **1**[8] (53 mg, 0.1 mmol, 1 eq) in anhydrous acetonitrile (6 mL) was concentrated and the flask was filled with argon.* The mono-tetrabutylammonium salt[†] of sugar phosphate **2**[8] (87 mg, 0.12 mmol, 1.2 eq)[‡] and DCI (24 mg, 0.2 mmol, 2 eq) were weighed into a 10 mL cone-shaped flask and coevaporated with anhydrous acetonitrile (6 mL). The residue was dissolved in anhydrous acetonitrile (2 mL) and added via syringe to the

---

* Rigorously anhydrous conditions are essential, since presence of water results in the formation of hydrogen phosphonate, upon activation of the phosphoramidite. This is manifested by the occurrence of a doublet at ~10 ppm in the ^{31}P NMR spectrum of the reaction mixture.

† The use of 1 equivalent of the tetrabutylammonium counter ion increased both the speed and efficiency of the reaction compared to the use of glycosyl phosphate in its free acid form. More than 1 eq of the tetrabutylammonium ion lowers the efficiency.

‡ Application of more than 1.2 eq of the glycosyl phosphate as acceptor does not seem to improve yields, but tends to make the final purification more difficult (see footnote on page 110).

phosphoramidite.* The reaction mixture was stirred for 30 min at ambient temperature after which t-BuOOH (73 μL, 0.4 mmol, 4 eq) was added by means of a micro
syringe.[†,‡] After 30 min, DBU (75 μL, 0.5 mmol, 5 eq) was added and the reaction
was stirred for an additional 30 min at ambient temperature. Silyl deprotection was
accomplished by addition of triethylamine (0.23 mL, 1.6 mmol, 16 eq), followed by
Et_3N·$(HF)_3$ (130 μL, 0.8 mmol, 8 eq).[§] After 4 h at ambient temperature, NH_3 (25%
in water, 0.43 mL, 3 mmol, 30 eq) was added and the reaction was stirred for 12 h
to ensure complete deacetylation.[¶] The reaction mixture was diluted with Milli Q
(4 mL) and washed with dichloromethane (2 × 6 mL). The organic layers were then
extracted with Milli Q (6 mL). The combined aqueous layers were concentrated in a
50 mL round bottom flask under reduced pressure at 25°C.** The crude product was
dissolved in Milli Q (6 mL) and filtered through a syringe equipped with a GRACE,
HPLC syringe filter (13 mm, 0.45 μM, PTFE). The flask and filter were rinsed with
additional Milli Q (6 mL). The filtrate was applied to a column packed with strong
anion exchange material and eluted with a gradient of ammonium acetate [0.05 M
(pH 7.0)–0.5 M (pH 7.1) over 20 CV] at 4 mL per minute.[††] The fractions containing
the product were collected and lyophilized.[‡‡] The purified sugar nucleotide was dissolved in Milli Q (5 mL) and filtered through a short Amberlite Na^+ column (~3 mL),[§§]
which then was rinsed with additional Milli Q (10 mL). The combined filtrate was
lyophilized, giving the title compound as a white powder (41–49 mg, 64%–76%).[¶¶] ^1H
NMR (400 MHz, D_2O) δ 8.02 (d, 1H, $J_{5,6}$ 8.1 Hz, H-6), 6.05 (d, 1 H, $J_{1,2}$ 4.9 Hz, H-1^I),
6.03 (d, 1H, $J_{5,6}$ 8.1 Hz, H-5), 5.59 (dd, 1H, $J_{1,2}$ 3.3 Hz, $J_{1,P}$ 7.3 Hz, H-1^{II}), 4.48–4.41
(m, 2H, H-2^I, H-3^I), 4.36 (m, 1H, H-4^I), 4.32 (m, 1H, H-5a^I), 4.26 (m, 1H, H-5b^I), 4.06
(ddd, 1H, $J_{2,P}$ 3.1 Hz, $J_{1,2}$ 3.3 Hz, $J_{2,3}$ 10.4 Hz, H-2^{II}), 4.00 (ddd, 1H, $J_{5,6a}$ 2.4 Hz, $J_{5,6b}$
4.5 Hz, $J_{4,5}$ 9.7 Hz, H-5^{II}), 3.95 (dd, 1H, $J_{5,6a}$ 2.4 Hz, $J_{6a,6b}$ 12.4 Hz, H-6a^{II}), 3.92–3.84
(m, 2H, H-6b^{II}, H-3^{II}), 3.62 (t, 1H, $J_{4,5}$ 9.7 Hz, H-4^{II}), 2.15 (s, 3H, Ac); ^{13}C NMR
(101 MHz, D_2O) δ 174.9 (CO, Ac), 166.3 (C4), 151.9 (C2), 141.7 (C6), 102.8 (C5), 94.6
(d, $J_{1,P}$ 6.3 Hz, C-1^{II}), 88.6 (C-1^I), 83.4 (d, $J_{4,P}$ 9.1 Hz, C-4^I), 73.9 (C-3^I), 73.1 (C-5^{II}),

---

* The reaction was stirred under an overpressure of argon by means of an argon balloon.
† Anhydrous t-BuOOH was used as oxidant, due to the presumed (hydrolytic) instability of interme-
diate **3**.
‡ Progress of the reactions could be monitored by ^{31}P NMR using an NMR capillary filled with acetone-
d_6. The yield of the reaction was determined using optimized conditions without monitoring of the
reaction progress.
§ Triethylamine was added prior to addition of Et_3N $(HF)_3$ to ensure basic reaction conditions.
¶ The use of NH_4OH ensures full deacetylation with minimum degradation of the product (although
extended reaction times do result in degradation of the product). The more commonly used deprotection mixture Et_3N/MeOH/H_2O (3:7:1) resulted in degradation of the sugar nucleotide, due to the long
reaction time required.
** Low temperature prevents degradation of the product. Some water added to the receiving flask
increased rate of evaporation.
†† With 20 mL of Q-sepharose material, the crude mixture was applied to the column in four consecutive
runs with 3 mL (~0.025 mmol) crude product per run. The sugar nucleotide has a slightly longer retention time as compared to the excess sugar phosphate. The fractions containing pure product were collected and lyophilized. The slightly impure fractions were collected and repurified for higher yields.
‡‡ Repeated lyophilization (3–4 times) is required to remove excess ammonium acetate. The removal of
acetate can be monitored after each lyophilization by ^1H NMR.
§§ Dowex Na^+ can be used instead of Amberlite Na^+ without any decrease in efficiency.
¶¶ The yields reported correspond to the minimum and maximum yields acquired in the reaction.

71.1 (C-3^{II}), 69.8 (C-2^{I}), 69.7 (C-4^{II}), 65.1 (d, $J_{5,P}$ 5.3 Hz, C-5^{I}), 60.5 (C-6^{II}), 53.8 (d, $J_{2,P}$ 8.5 Hz, C-2^{II}), 22.2 (CH$_3$, Ac); ^{31}P NMR (162 MHz, D$_2$O) δ −10.77 (d, 1P, $J = 21.1$ Hz), −12.48 (d, 1P, $J = 21.1$ Hz); HRMS Calcd for [C$_{17}$H$_{27}$N$_3$O$_{17}$P$_2$ + H]$^+$: 608.0888. Found: 608.0889.

Uridine 5′–(2-acetamido-2-deoxy-α-D-glucopyranosyl diphosphate) disodium salt (5).

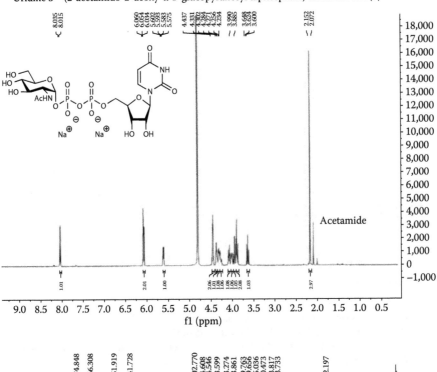

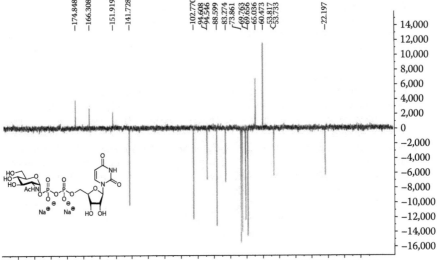

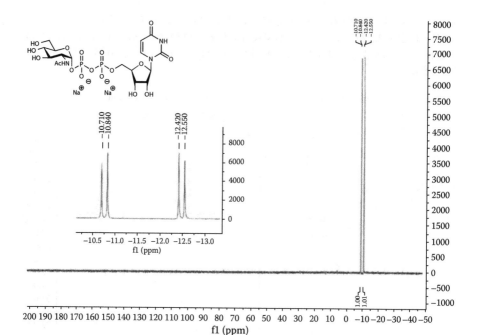

REFERENCES

1. Watkins, W. *Carbohydr. Res.* 1986, *149*, 1–12.
2. Reuter, G.; Gabius, H.-J. *Cell. Mol. Life. Sci.* 1999, *55*, 368–422.
3. Ohtsubo, K.; Marth, J. D. *Cell* 2006, *126*, 855–867.
4. (a) Freel Meyers, C. L.; Borch, R. F. *Org. Lett.* 2001, *23*, 3765–3768. (b) Ohkubo, A.; Aoki, K.; Seio, K.; Sekine, M. *Tetrahedron Lett.* 2004, *45*, 979–982. (c) Marlow, A. L.; Kiessling, L. L. *Org. Lett.* 2001, *3*, 2517–2519. (d) Timmons, S. C.; Jakeman, D. L. *Carb. Res.* 2008, *343*, 865–875. (e) Yamazaki, T.; Warren, C. D.; Herscovics, A.; Jeanloz, R. W. *Can. J. Chem.* 1981, *59*, 2247–2252. (f) Nunez, H. A.; O'Connor, J. V.; Rosevear, P. R.; Barker, R. *Can. J. Chem.* 1981, *59*, 2086–2095. (g) Imperiali, B.; Zimmerman, J. W. *Tetrahedron Lett.* 1990, *31*, 6485–6488.
5. (a) Timmons, S. C.; Jakeman, D. L. *Org. Lett.* 2007, *9*, 1227–1230. (b) Uchiyama, T.; Hindsgaul, O. *J. Carb. Chem.* 1998, *17*, 1181. (c) Ernst, C.; Klaffke, W. *J. Org. Chem.* 2003, *68*, 5780–5783. (d) Hanessian, S.; Lu, P.-P.; Ishida, H. *J. Am. Chem. Soc.* 1998, *120*, 13296–13330.
6. (a) Moffatt, J. G.; Khorana, H. G. *J. Am. Chem. Soc.* 1958, *80*, 3756–3761. (b) Roseman, S.; Distler, J. J.; Moffatt, J. G.; Khorana, H. G. *J. Am. Chem. Soc.* 1961, *83*, 659–663.
7. Caruthers, M. H.; Barone, A. D.; Beaucage, S. L.; Dodds, D. R.; Fisher, E. F.; McBride, L. J.; Matteucci, M.; Stabinsky, Z.; Tang, J-Y. *Methods Enzymol.* 1987, *154*, 287–313.
8. Gold, H.; van Delft, P.; Meeuwenoord, N.; Codée, J. D. C.; Filippov, D. V.; Eggink, G.; Overkleeft, H. S.; van der Marel, G. A. *J. Org. Chem.* 2008, *73*, 9458–9460.
9. Liemann, S.; Klaffke, W. *Liebigs Ann.* 1995, 1779–1787.

13 Conversion of *N*-2,2,2-Trichloroethoxycarbonyl-Protected 2-Aminoglycosides into *N*-Alkylated 2,3-*N,O*-Carbonyl Glycosides

Thomas Honer, Siegfried Förster,[†]
and Thomas Ziegler*

CONTENTS

Experimental Methods 115
   General Methods 115
   General Procedure 115
      2-Trimethylsilylethyl 4,6-*O*-Benzylidene-2-Deoxy-2-(2,2,2-
      Trichlorethoxycarbamido)-β-D-Glucopyranoside (**1**) 115
      2-Trimethylsilylethyl 2-Amino-2-*N*-Benzyl-4,6-*O*-Benzylidene-2,3-
      N,O-Carbonyl-2-Deoxy-β-D-Glucopyranoside (**2**) 116
      Phenyl 4,6-*O*-Benzylidene-2-Deoxy-1-Thio-2-(2,2,2-
      Trichlorethoxycarbamido)-β-D-Glucopyranoside (**3**) 116
      Phenyl 2-Amino-2-*N*-Benzyl-4,6-*O*-Benzylidene-2,3-*N,O*-Carbonyl-2-
      Deoxy-1-Thio-β-D-Glucopyranoside (**4**) 117
      Phenyl 2-Amino-4,6-*O*-Benzylidene-2,3-*N,O*-Carbonyl-2-Deoxy-2-*N*-
      (4-Nitrobenzyl)-1-Thio-β-D-Glucopyranoside (**5**) 117
      Phenyl 2-Amino-4,6-*O*-Benzylidene-2,3-*N,O*-Carbonyl-2-Deoxy-2-*N*-
      (4-Methoxybenzyl)-1-Thio-β-D-Glucopyranoside (**6**) 117
      Phenyl 2-Amino-4,6-*O*-Benzylidene-2,3-*N,O*-Carbonyl-2-Deoxy-2-*N*-
      (Prop-2-Enyl)-1-Thio-β-D-Glucopyranoside (**7**) 118

---

* Corresponding author.
[†] Checker.

Phenyl 2-Amino-4,6-*O*-Benzylidene-2,3-*N,O*-Carbonyl-2-Deoxy-2-*N*-
(Prop-2-Ynyl)-1-Thio-β-D-Glucopyranoside (**8**).. 118
Phenyl 4,6-*O*-Benzylidene-2-Deoxy-1-Thio-2-(2,2,2-
Trichlorethoxycarbamido)-β-D-Galactopyranoside (**9**) 118
Phenyl 2-Amino-2-*N*-Benzyl-4,6-*O*-Benzylidene-2,3-*N,O*-Carbonyl-2-
Deoxy-1-Thio-β-D-Galactopyranoside (**10**) 119
References.. 127

N-2,2,2-Trichloroethoxycarbonyl (Troc)-protected glycosamine derivatives are versatile glycosyl donors in oligosaccharide syntheses. The Troc protecting group can easily be introduced via its acid chloride; it is stable under acidic conditions but is base labile. It can be selectively cleaved under reductive conditions. As a protecting group for the amino function in glycosamine donors, Troc behaves like a neighbor group active protecting group leading, upon Koenigs–Knorr type glycosylation,[1-5] predominately to the corresponding 1,2-*cis* glycosides.

Under basic alkylating conditions, *N*-Troc-protected 4,6-*O*-benzylidene-glycosamines undergo loss of trichloro-EtOH with concomitant formation of a cyclic 2,3-urethane (oxazolidinone) and *N*-alkylation of the urethane moiety.[6,7] The resulting 2,3-*N,O*-carbonyl-protected glycosamine derivatives are useful glycosyl donors for the preparation of α-linked aminoglycosides in the *gluco* and *galacto* series.[6,8] For example, Troc-protected 2-aminoglycosyl donors in the *gluco* and *galacto* series give predominately β-linked glycosides upon glycosylation. In contrast, the corresponding *N*-alkylated 2,3-*N*,*O*-carbonyl-protected glycosyl donors predominately afford α-linked glycosides. Accordingly, the conversion of *N*-Troc-protected 2-aminoglycosyl donors into *N*-alkylated 2,3-*N*,*O*-carbonyl-protected glycosyl donors provides for a significant extension of the Troc group in carbohydrate chemistry. Under the optimized conditions described here, the *N*-Troc-protected 4,6-*O*-benzylidene-aminoglycosides are conveniently converted into various *N*-alkylated 4,6-*O*-benzylidene-2,3-*N*,*O*-carbonyl-aminoglycosides in high yield.

EXPERIMENTAL METHODS

GENERAL METHODS

All solvents were dried and distilled. Reactions were performed under Ar and monitored by thin-layer chromatography (TLC) on Polygram Sil G/UV silica gel plates (Machery and Nagel). Detection was affected by charring with H_2SO_4 (5% in EtOH) or by UV light. Nuclear magnetic resonance (NMR) spectra were recorded on a Bruker Avance 400 spectrometer (400 MHz for ^{1}H and 100 MHz for ^{13}C). Tetramethylsilane was used as the internal standard. Assignments of NMR signals were made by first-order analysis and by homonuclear and heteronuclear two-dimensional correlation spectroscopy. Melting points were determined on a Büchi, Model B-540 apparatus, and were uncorrected. Elemental analyses were performed on a Hekatech, Model Euro 3000 CHN analyzer. Optical rotations were measured with a Perkin-Elmer Polarimeter, Model 341 at 589 nm and 20°C in a quartz cuvette of 10 cm length. Preparative chromatography was performed on silica gel (0.032–0.063 mm, Machery and Nagel). Solutions in organic solvents were concentrated by rotary evaporation below 45°C.

GENERAL PROCEDURE

The *N*-Troc-protected glycoside (1.0 mol eq.) and the alkyl bromide (1.01 mol eq.) are dissolved in DMF, and the solution is cooled to 0°C. NaH (1.2 mol eq.) is added in 2–3 portions to the stirred solution in a stream of Ar. After each addition, stirring at 0°C is continued until the evolution of hydrogen ceases. The mixture is warmed to room temperature and stirred until a clear solution is formed. The solution is cooled to 0°C, and the next portion of NaH is added. After the addition of NaH is complete, MeOH (1 mL) is added with stirring followed by dichloromethane (50 mL). The solution is washed with 1 N aqueous HCl solution, dried with Na_2SO_4, filtered, and concentrated in vacuo. Chromatography of the residue with 10:1—20:1 toluene–acetone and crystallization from EtOH affords the *N*-alkylated 2,3-*N*,*O*-carbonyl-protected glycosides.

2-Trimethylsilylethyl 4,6-*O*-Benzylidene-2-Deoxy-2-(2,2,2-Trichlorethoxycarbamido)-β-D-Glucopyranoside (1)

A 1 N solution of NaOMe in MeOH (1 mL) is added at room temperature to a suspension of 2-trimethylsilylethyl 3,4,6-tri-*O*-acetyl-2-deoxy-2-(2,2,2-trichlorethoxycarbamido)-β-D-glucopyranoside[4] (2.17 g, 3.74 mmol) in MeOH (20 mL), and the mixture is stirred for 4 h until a clear solution is formed. The solution is neutralized with Dowex ion exchange resin (H$^+$) form and filtered. Concentration of the filtrate affords crude 2-trimethylsilylethyl 2-deoxy-2-(2,2,2-trichlorethoxycarbamido)-β-D-glucopyranoside (1.68 g), which is directly used for the next step. A solution of 2-trimethylsilylethyl 2-deoxy-2-(2,2,2-trichlorethoxycarbamido)-β-D-glucopyranoside (1.68 g, 3.69 mmol), benzaldehyde dimethyl acetal (2.25 mL, 15.0 mmol), and p-toluenesulfonic acid (110 mg) in MeCN (40 mL) is stirred at room temperature for 24 h. Triethylamine (0.3 mL) is added, the mixture is poured into water (100 mL) and extracted with ethyl acetate (3 × 75 mL). The combined extracts are dried, filtered, and concentrated. Chromatography of the residue (10:1 toluene–acetone) affords the title compound 1 (1.49 g, 73%); mp 143°C (EtOH); $[\alpha]_D^{20} = -35.2$ (c 1.0, CHCl$_3$). ^{1}H NMR (CDCl$_3$): δ = 5.33 (s, 1H, CH-Ph), 5.22 (bs, 1H, NH), 4.55 (bs, 2H, NCH$_2$), 4.40 (d, 1H, $J_{1,2} = 7.6$ Hz, 1-H), 4.15 (dd, 1H, $J_{5,6a} = 4.9$ Hz, $J_{6a,6b} = -10.5$ Hz, 6a-H), 3.89–3.86 (m, 1H, 3-H), 3.79–3.72 (m, 1H, OCH$_2$CH$_2$Si), 3.58 (t, 1H, $J_{5,6b} = 10.5$ Hz, 6b-H), 3.39–3.32 (m, 2H, 4-H, OCH$_2$CH$_2$Si), 3.27–3.21 (m, 1H, 5-H), 3.17–3.14 (m, 1H, 2-H), 0.81–0.69 (m, 2H, OCH$_2$CH$_2$Si), −0.17 (s, 9H, Si(CH$_3$)$_3$). ^{13}C NMR (CDCl$_3$): δ = 154.5 (NCO), 101.8 (CH-Ph), 100.3 (C-1), 95.4 (CCl$_3$), 81.4 (C-4), 74.5 (NCH$_2$), 70.5 (C-3), 68.6 (C-6), 67.7 (OCH$_2$CH$_2$Si), 66.0 (C-5), 58.8 (C-2), 18.1 (OCH$_2$CH$_2$Si), −1.45 (Si(CH$_3$)$_3$). Anal. Calcd for C$_{21}$H$_{30}$Cl$_3$NO$_7$Si (542.91): C 46.46, H5.57, N 2.58. Found: C 46.56, H5.59, N 2.42.

2-Trimethylsilylethyl 2-Amino-2-N-Benzyl-4,6-O-Benzylidene-2,3-N,O-Carbonyl-2-Deoxy-β-D-Glucopyranoside (2)

Treatment of compound 1 (0.50 g, 0.91 mmol) and benzyl bromide (0.12 mL, 1.01 mmol) in DMF (5 mL) with NaH (29 mg, 1.20 mmol) followed by workup and chromatography (20:1 toluene–acetone) affords compound 2 (0.40 g, 90%); mp 182°C (EtOH); $[\alpha]_D^{20} = -76.0$ (c 1.0, CHCl$_3$). ^{1}H NMR (CDCl$_3$): δ = 5.59 (s, 1H, CH-Ph), 4.68–4.64 (m, 2H, 1-H, NCH$_2$-Ph), 4.49 (d, 1H, $J = -25.2$ Hz, NCH$_2$-Ph), 4.34 (dd, 1H, $J_{5,6a} = 4.6$ Hz, $J_{6a,6b} = -10.5$ Hz, 6a-H), 4.28 (t, 1H, $J_{2,3} = J_{3,4} = 10.7$ Hz, 3-H), 3.98 (bt, 1H, 4-H), 3.92–3.84 (m, 2H, 6b-H, OCH$_2$CH$_2$Si), 3.56–3.50 (m, 1H, 5-H), 3.37–3.30 (m, 2H, 2-H, OCH$_2$CH$_2$Si), 1.00–0.88 (m, 2H, OCH$_2$CH$_2$Si), −0.06 (s, 9H, Si(CH$_3$)$_3$). ^{13}C NMR (CDCl$_3$): δ = 158.7 (NCO), 101.7 (C-1), 101.1 (CH-Ph), 78.6 (C-4) 76.3 (C-3), 69.2, (C-5), 68.3 (C-6), 67.6 (OCH$_2$CH$_2$Si), 61.5 (C-2), 47.9 (NCH$_2$-Ph), 18.1 (OCH$_2$CH$_2$Si), −1.7 (3 C, Si(CH$_3$)$_3$). Anal. Calcd for C$_{26}$H$_{33}$NO$_6$Si (483.63): C 64.57, H 6.88, N 2.90. Found: C 64.21, H 6.95, N 3.19.

Phenyl 4,6-O-Benzylidene-2-Deoxy-1-Thio-2-(2,2,2-Trichlorethoxycarbamido)-β-D-Glucopyranoside (3)

Treatment of phenyl 2-deoxy-1-thio-2-(2,2,2-trichlorethoxycarbamido)-β-D-glucopyranoside[9] (8.0 g, 18.03 mmol) with benzaldehyde dimethyl acetal (11.14 mL, 73.92 mmol) and p-toluenesulfonic acid (360 mg) in MeCN (75 mL) followed by workup and chromatography (15:1 toluene–acetone) affords compound 3 (7.42 g, 77%); mp 175°C (EtOH); $[\alpha]_D^{20} = -36.7$ (c 1.0, CHCl$_3$). ^{1}H NMR (acetone-d$_6$): δ = 5.62 (s, 1H, CH-Ph), 5.07 (d, 1H, $J_{1,2} = 10.6$ Hz, 1-H), 4.91 (d, 1H, $J = -12.3$ Hz, CH$_2$-Ph), 4.72 (d, 1H, NCH$_2$CCl$_3$), 4.29 (dd, 1H, $J_{5,6a} = 5.1$ Hz, $J_{6a,6b} = -10.3$ Hz, 1H, 6a-H),

3.99–394 (m, 1H, 3-H), 3.81–3.77 (m, 1H, 6b-H), 3.64–3.61 (m, 1H, 2-H), 3.59–3.51 (m, 2H, 4-H, 5-H), 2.89 (s, 1H, OH). ^{13}C NMR (acetone-d$_6$): δ = 155.4 (NCO), 102.1 (CH-Ph), 97.0 (CCl$_3$), 88.4 (C-1), 82.4 (C-4), 74.9 (N$\underline{C}$H$_2$CCl$_3$), 73.3 (C-3), 71.3 (C-5), 69.0 (C-6), 58.5 (C-2). Anal. Calcd for C$_{22}$H$_{22}$Cl$_3$NO$_6$S (534.84): C 49.40, H 4.15, N 2.62, S 6.00. Found: C 49.64, H 4.07, N 2.40, S 5.76.

Phenyl 2-Amino-2-*N*-Benzyl-4,6-*O*-Benzylidene-2,3-*N,O*-Carbonyl-2-Deoxy-1-Thio-β-D-Glucopyranoside (4)

Treatment of compound **3** (0.80 g, 1.51 mmol) and benzyl bromide (0.20 mL, 1.66 mmol) in DMF (20 mL) with NaH (47 mg, 2.00 mmol) followed by workup and chromatography (15:1 toluene–acetone) affords compound **4** (0.66 g, 92%); mp 177°C (EtOH); [α]$_D^{20}$ = −76.0 (*c* 1.0, CHCl$_3$). ^{1}H NMR (CDCl$_3$): δ = 5.63 (s, 1H, CH-Ph), 4.90–4.83 (m, 3H, 1-H, NCH$_2$-Ph, NCH$_2$-Ph), 4.39–4.34 (m, 2H, 3-H, 6a-H), 4.07 (bt, 1H, 4-H), (t, 1H, $J_{5,6b}$ = 11.0 Hz, $J_{6a,6b}$ = −11.0 Hz, 6b-H), 3.63–3.54 (m, 2H, 2-H, 5-H). ^{13}C NMR (CDCl$_3$): δ = 158.9 (NCO), 101.4 (CH-Ph), 87.7 (C-1), 78.9 (C-3), 78.3 (C-4), 72.8, (C-5), 68.2 (C-6), 61.5 (C-2), 47.7 (NCH$_2$-Ph). Anal. Calcd for C$_{27}$H$_{25}$NO$_5$S (475.56): C 68.19, H 5.30, N 2.95, S 6.74. Found: C 68.25, H 5.36, N 2.79, S 6.53.

Phenyl 2-Amino-4,6-*O*-Benzylidene-2,3-*N,O*-Carbonyl-2-Deoxy-2-*N*-(4-Nitrobenzyl)-1-Thio-β-D-Glucopyranoside (5)

Treatment of compound **3** (0.50 g, 0.94 mmol) and 4-nitrobenzyl bromide (0.22 mg, 1.03 mmol) in DMF (20 mL) with NaH (29 mg, 1.22 mmol) followed by workup and chromatography (15:1 toluene–acetone) affords compound **5** (0.41 g, 85%); mp 183°C (EtOH); [α]$_D^{20}$ = −66.0 (*c* 1.0, CHCl$_3$). ^{1}H NMR (CDCl$_3$): δ = 5.66 (s, 1H, CH-Ph), 5.01 (d, 1H, *J* = −16.4 Hz, NCH$_2$-Ph), 4.90 (d, 1H, $J_{1,2}$ = 9.9 Hz, 1-H), 4.82 (d, 1H, NCH$_2$-Ph), 4.45–4.37 (m, 3H, 3-H, 6a-H), 4.12 (bt, 1H, 4-H), 3.96 (t, 1H, $J_{5,6b}$ = 10.4 Hz, $J_{6a,6b}$ = −10.4 Hz, 6b-H), 3.68–3.55 (m, 2H, 2-H, 5-H). ^{13}C NMR (CDCl$_3$): δ = 158.7 (NCO), 101.5 (CH-Ph), 87.2 (C-1), 79.0 (C-3), 78.2 (C-4), 72.9, (C-5), 68.2 (C-6), 62.1 (C-2), 47.6 (NCH$_2$-Ph). Anal. Calcd for C$_{27}$H$_{24}$N$_2$O$_7$S (520.55): C 62.30, H 4.65, N 5.38, S 6.16. Found: C 62.32, H 4.54, N 5.39, S 5.92.

Phenyl 2-Amino-4,6-*O*-Benzylidene-2,3-*N,O*-Carbonyl-2-Deoxy-2-*N*-(4-Methoxybenzyl)-1-Thio-β-D-Glucopyranoside (6)

Treatment of compound **3** (0.50 g, 0.94 mmol) and 4-methoxybenzyl bromide (0.15 mL, 1.03 mmol) in DMF (10 mL) with NaH (29 mg, 1.22 mmol) followed by workup and chromatography (30:1 toluene–acetone) affords compound **6** (0.47 g, 99%); mp 175°C (EtOH); [α]$_D^{20}$ = −62.9 (*c* 1.0, CHCl$_3$). ^{1}H NMR (CDCl$_3$): δ = 5.61 (s, 1H, CH-Ph), 4.92 (d, 1H, $J_{1,2}$ = 9.6 Hz, 1-H), 4.82 (d, 1H, *J* = −15.4 Hz, NCH$_2$-Ph), 4.74 (d, 1H, NCH$_2$-Ph), 4.37–4.30 (m, 3H, 3-H, 6a-H), 4.04 (bt, 1H, 4-H), 3.92 (t, 1H, $J_{5,6b}$ = 10.4 Hz, $J_{6a,6b}$ = −10.4 Hz, 6b-H), 3.85 (s, 3H, CH$_3$), 3.62–3.50 (m, 2H, 2-H, 5-H). ^{13}C NMR (CDCl$_3$): δ = 159.0 (NCO), 101.3 (CH-Ph), 87.7 (C-1), 78.8 (C-3), 78.4 (C-4), 72.7, (C-5), 68.2 (C-6), 61.2 (C-2), 55.2 (CH$_3$), 47.0 (NCH$_2$-Ph). Anal. Calcd for C$_{28}$H$_{27}$NO$_6$S (505.58): C 66.52, H 5.38, N 2.77, S 6.34. Found: C 66.48, H 5.35, N 2.76, S 6.14.

Phenyl 2-Amino-4,6-O-Benzylidene-2,3-N,O-Carbonyl-2-Deoxy-2-N-(Prop-2-Enyl)-1-Thio-β-D-Glucopyranoside (7)

Treatment of compound **3** (0.50 g, 0.94 mmol) and allyl bromide (87 μL, 1.03 mmol) in DMF (10 mL) with NaH (29 mg, 1.22 mmol) followed by workup and chromatography (15:1 toluene–acetone) affords compound **7** (0.38 g, 99%); mp 169°C (EtOH); $[\alpha]_D^{20}=-78.5$ (c 1.0, CHCl$_3$). ^{1}H NMR (CDCl$_3$): δ = 5.93–5.64 (m, 1H, NCH$_2$C**H**CH$_2$), 5.60 (s, 1H, CH-Ph), 5.45–5.34 (m, 2H, NCH$_2$CHC**H**$_2$), 4.90 (d, 1H, $J_{1,2}$=9.9 Hz, 1-H), 4.33 (dd, 1H, $J_{5,6a}$=4.7 Hz, $J_{6a,6b}$=−10.4 Hz, 6a-H), 4.28–4.17 (m, 3H, 3-H, NC**H**$_2$CHCH$_2$), 4.01 (bt, 1H, 4-H), 3.90 (t, 1H, $J_{5,6b}$=10.4 Hz, 6b-H), 3.57–3.50 (m, 2H, 2-H, 5-H). ^{13}C NMR (CDCl$_3$): δ = 158.1 (NCO), 133.3 (NCH$_2$**C**HCH$_2$), 119.1 (NCH$_2$CH**C**H$_2$), 100.9 (CH-Ph), 88.9 (C-1), 78.3 (C-3), 78.0 (C-4), 72.3 (C-5), 67.9 (C-6), 60.7 (C-2), 46.1 (N**C**H$_2$CHCH$_2$). Anal. Calcd for C$_{23}$H$_{23}$NO$_5$S (425.50): C 64.92, H 5.45, N 3.29, S 7.54. Found: C 64.84, H 5.52, N 3.26, S 7.39.

Phenyl 2-Amino-4,6-O-Benzylidene-2,3-N,O-Carbonyl-2-Deoxy-2-N-(Prop-2-Ynyl)-1-Thio-β-D-Glucopyranoside (8)

Treatment of compound **3** (1.00 g, 1.87 mmol) and propargyl bromide (0.22 mL, 2.06 mmol) in DMF (20 mL) with NaH (58 mg, 2.43 mmol) followed by workup and chromatography (30:1 toluene–acetone) affords compound **8** (0.70 g, 88%); mp 174°C (EtOH); $[\alpha]_D^{20}=-72.5$ (c 1.0, CHCl$_3$). ^{1}H NMR (CDCl$_3$): δ = 5.63 (s, 1H, Ch-Ph), 4.97 (d, 1H $J_{1,2}$=9.9 Hz, 1-H), 4.44 (dd, 1H, J=2.3 Hz, J=−17.5 Hz, C**H**$_2$CCH), 4.38–4.24 (m, 3H, 3-H, 6a-H, C**H**$_2$CCH), 4.09 (bt, 1H, 4-H), 3,93 (t, 1H, $J_{5,6b}$=10.4 Hz, $J_{6a,6b}$=−10.4 Hz, 6b-H), 3.67 (bt, 1H, 2-H), 3.62–3.56 (m, 1H, 5-H), 2.36 (bs, 1H, CH$_2$CC**H**). ^{13}C NMR (CDCl$_3$): δ = 158.3 (NCO), 101.3 (CH-Ph), 87.0 (C-1), 78.4 (C-4), 78.3 (C-3), 76.4 (CH$_2$**C**CH), 74.6 (CH$_2$C**C**H), 72.7 (C-5), 68.2 (C-6), 60.2 (C-2), 34.8 (**C**H$_2$CCH). Anal. Calcd for C$_{23}$H$_{21}$NO$_5$S (423.48): C 65.23, H 5.00, N 3.31, S 7.57. Found: C 65.30, H 4.95, N 3.02, S 7.48.

Phenyl 4,6-O-Benzylidene-2-Deoxy-1-Thio-2-(2,2,2-Trichlorethoxycarbamido)-β-D-Galactopyranoside (9)

A solution of phenyl 2-deoxy-1-thio-2-(2,2,2-trichlorethoxycarbamido)-β-D-galactopyranoside[10] (0.78 g, 1.74 mmol), benzaldehyde dimethyl acetal (1.03 mL, 6.96 mmol), and p-toluenesulfonic acid (37 mg) in MeCN (20 mL) is stirred at room temperature for 48 h. Triethylamine (0.50 mL) is added, the mixture poured into water (100 mL) and extracted with ethyl acetate (3 × 50 mL). The combined extracts are dried, filtered, and concentrated in vacuo. Chromatography of the residue (10:1 toluene–acetone) affords the title compound **9** (0.65 g, 70%); mp 113°C (EtOH); $[\alpha]_D^{20}=-67.7$ (c 1.0, CHCl$_3$). ^{1}H NMR (acetone-d$_6$): δ = 5.66 (s, 1H, CH-Ph), 4.98 (d, 1H, $J_{1,2}$=9.6 Hz, 1-H), 4.85 (d, 1H, J=−12.4 Hz, NCH$_2$), 4.72 (d, 1H, NCH$_2$), 4.34 (bs, 1H, 4-H), (dd, 1H, $J_{5,6a}$=2.2 Hz, $J_{6a,6b}$=−12.4 Hz, 6a-H), 4.15–4.12 (m, 1H, 6b-H), 3.95–3.91 (m, 2H, 2-H, 3-H), 3.72 (bs, 1H, 5-H). ^{13}C NMR (acetone-d$_6$): δ = 155.4 (NCO), 101.5 (CH-Ph), 97.0 (CCl$_3$), 87.3 (C-1), 76.6 (C-4), 74.8 (NCH$_2$), 72.3 (C-3), 70.9 (C-5), 69.9 (C-6), 54.3 (C-2). Anal. Calcd for C$_{22}$H$_{22}$Cl$_3$NO$_6$S (534.84): C 49.40, H 4.15, N 2.62, S 6.00. Found: C 49.42, H 4.30, N 2.52, S 5.61.

Phenyl 2-Amino-2-N-Benzyl-4,6-O-Benzylidene-2,3-N,O-Carbonyl-2-Deoxy-1-Thio-β-D-Galactopyranoside (10)

Treatment of compound **9** (0.27 g, 0.51 mmol) and benzyl bromide (66 μL, 0.56 mmol) in DMF (20 mL) with NaH (16 mg, 0.66 mmol) followed by workup and chromatography (10:1 toluene–acetone) affords compound **10** (0.21 g, 86%); $[\alpha]_D^{20} = -82.3$ (*c* 1.0, CHCl$_3$); ^{1}H NMR (CDCl$_3$): δ = 5.52 (s, 1H, 1-H), 4.76–4.71 (m, 2H, 1-H, NCH$_2$-Ph), 4.60 (d, 1H, $J = -15.7$ Hz, NCH$_2$-Ph), 4.47 (bs, 1H, 4-H), 4.31–4.28 (m, 1H, 6a-H), 4.17–4.08 (m, 2H, 2-H, 3-H), 4.02–3.99 (m, 1H, 6b-H), 3.46 (bs, 1H, 5-H). ^{13}C NMR (CDCl$_3$): δ = 158.8 (NCO), 100.1 (CH-Ph), 85.5 (C-1), 79.3 (C-3), 70.6 (C-4), 69.7 (C-6), 69.7 (C-5), 55.5 (C-2), 47.9 (NCH$_2$-Ph). Anal. Calcd for C$_{27}$H$_{25}$NO$_5$S (475.56): C 68.19, H 5.30, N 2.95, S 6.74. Found: C 67.99, H 5.33, N 2.81, S 6.56.

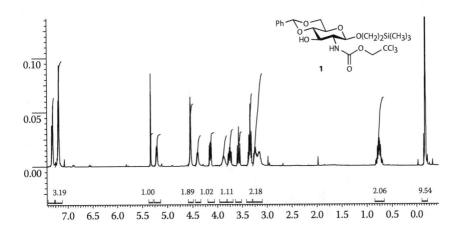

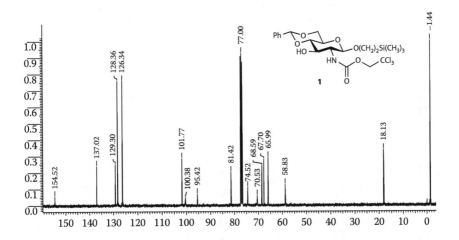

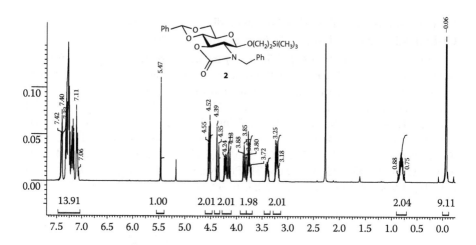

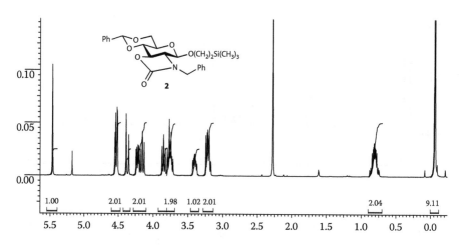

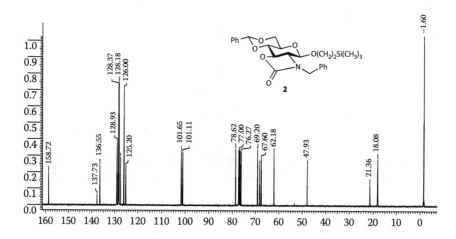

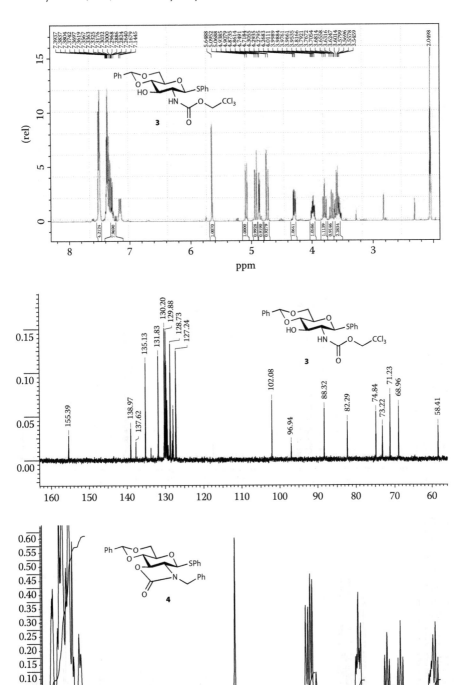

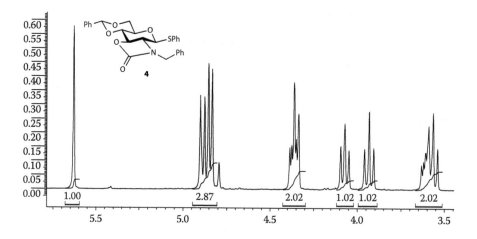

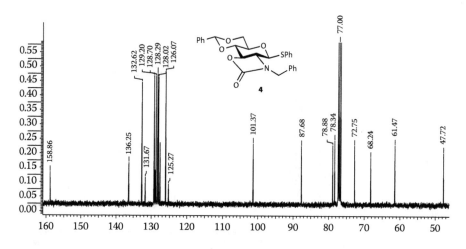

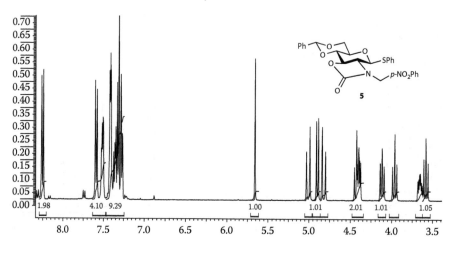

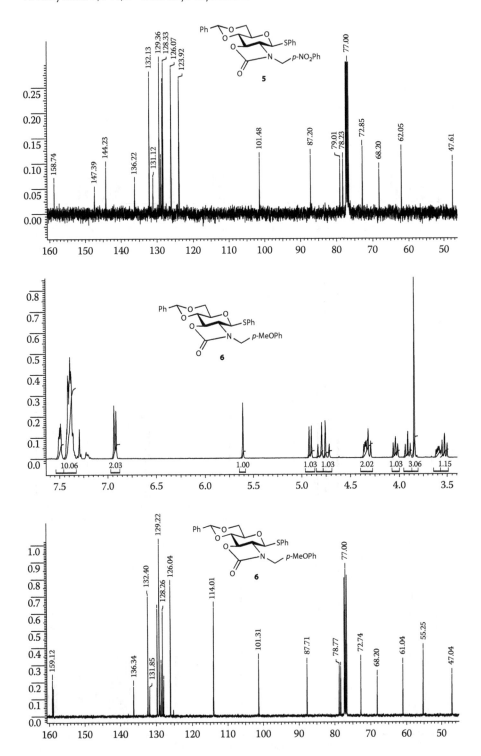

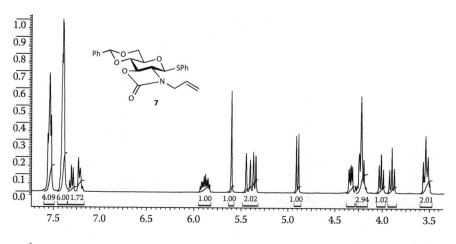

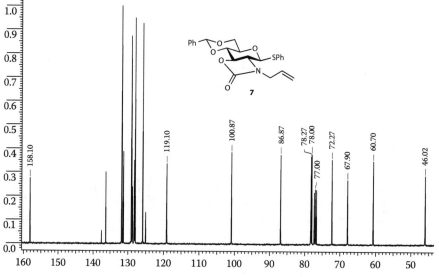

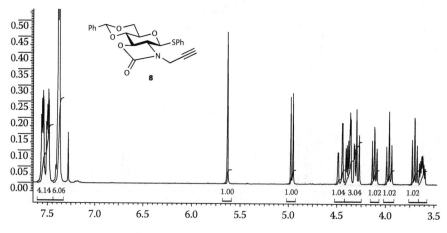

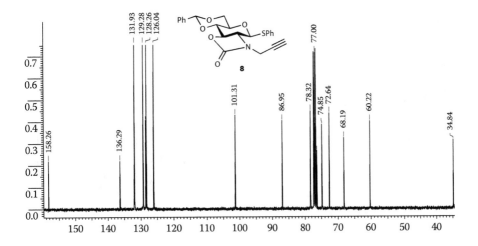

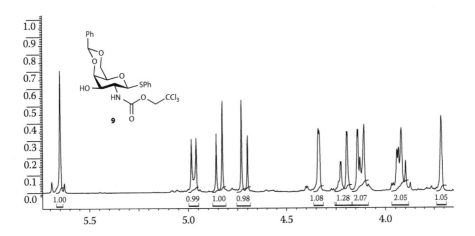

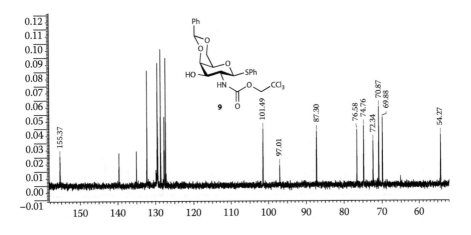

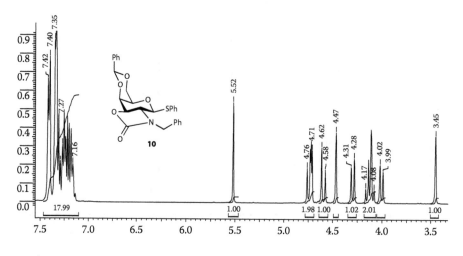

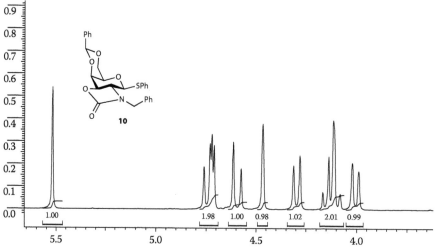

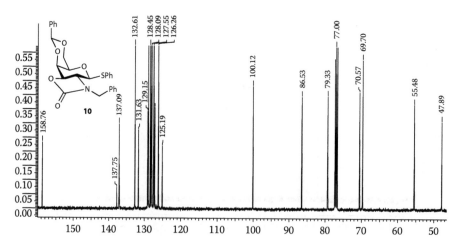

REFERENCES

1. Paulsen, H.; Helpap, B. *Carbohydr. Res.* 1991, *216*, 289–313.
2. Blatter, G.; Beau, J.-M.; Jacquinet, J.-C. *Carbohydr. Res.* 1994, *260*, 189–202.
3. Ziegler, T. *Carbohydr. Res.* 1994, *262*, 195–212.
4. Ellervik, U.; Magnusson, G. *Carbohydr. Res.* 1996, *280*, 251–260.
5. Dullenkopf, W.; Castro-Palomino, J. C.; Manzoni, L.; Schmidt, R. R. *Carbohydr. Res.* 1996, *296*, 135–147.
6. Manabe, S.; Ishii, K.; Ito, Y. *J. Am. Chem. Soc.* 2006, *128*, 10666–10667.
7. Honer, T. Dissertation, University of Tuebingen, Tuebingen, Germany, 2009.
8. Benakli, K.; Zha, C.; Kerns, R. J. *J. Am. Chem. Soc.* 2001, *123*, 9461–9462.
9. Yan, F.; Mehta, S.; Eichler, E.; Wakarchuk, W. W.; Gilbert, M.; Schur, M. J.; Whitfield, D. M. *J. Org. Chem.* 2003, *68*, 2426–2431.
10. Imamura, A.; Ando, H.; Ishida, H.; Kiso, M. *Org. Lett.* 2005, *7*, 4415–4418.

14 TIBAL-Induced Rearrangement: Synthesis of *gem*-Difluorocarbagalactose

João Sardinha, Amélia Pilar Rauter,
Matthieu Sollogoub,* and Yves Bleriot†

CONTENTS

Experimental Methods 131
    General Methods 131
        Rearrangement of 1 into 2,3,4-Tri-*O*-Benzyl-6,7,8-Trideoxy-
        5a-Difluoro-5a-Carba-α-D-*Galacto*-Oct-6-Ynopyranose (**4**) and
        2,3,4-Tri-*O*-Benzyl-6,7,8-Trideoxy-5a-Difluoro-5a-Carba-β-D-*Galacto*-
        Oct-6-Ynopyranose (**5**).. 132
Acknowledgment 132
References.. 135

(i) Co$_2$(CO)$_8$, CH$_2$Cl$_2$, rt, 1 h; (ii) 10 eq 1 M soln TIBAL in toluene, CH$_2$Cl$_2$, −78°C to rt, 1 h; (iii) CAN, Et$_3$N, acetone, rt, 1 h, **4** (35%) and **5** (29%) over three steps.

---

* Corresponding author.
† Checker.

The TIBAL-mediated rearrangement of cyclic sugars was introduced[1] as an alternative to Ferrier-II rearrangement for preparation of carbocyclic products. The advantage of the former methodology lies in the retention of the anomeric integrity (both aglycon and stereochemistry) of the starting sugar (Scheme 14.1).

The key step in this transformation is the *endo*-cleavage of the glycosidic bond to form an acyclic oxonium ion intermediate **9** (Scheme 14.2), which then undergoes intramolecular recyclization through a chair-like six-membered ring intermediate **11**, followed by reduction of the formed ketone to yield the carbocyclic product **7**.

Later studies demonstrated that this type of reactions were favored in the presence of an electron donating group that is α to the endocyclic oxygen that stabilizes the positive charge formed after the endocleavage.[2] This methodology was extended to preparation of *gem*-difluorocarbasugars using an original cobalt cluster as electron donating group.[3,4] The foregoing strategy allows replacement of the endocyclic oxygen by other functionalities leading to sugar analogues, which may be of interest for studies of enzyme–carbohydrate interactions.

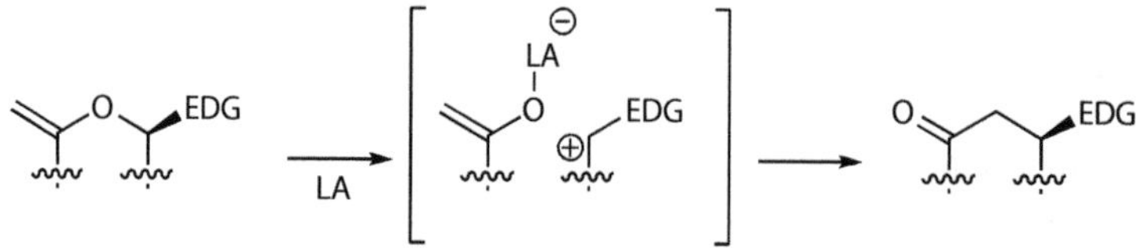

EDG = Electron-donating group
LA = Lewis acid

SCHEME 14.1

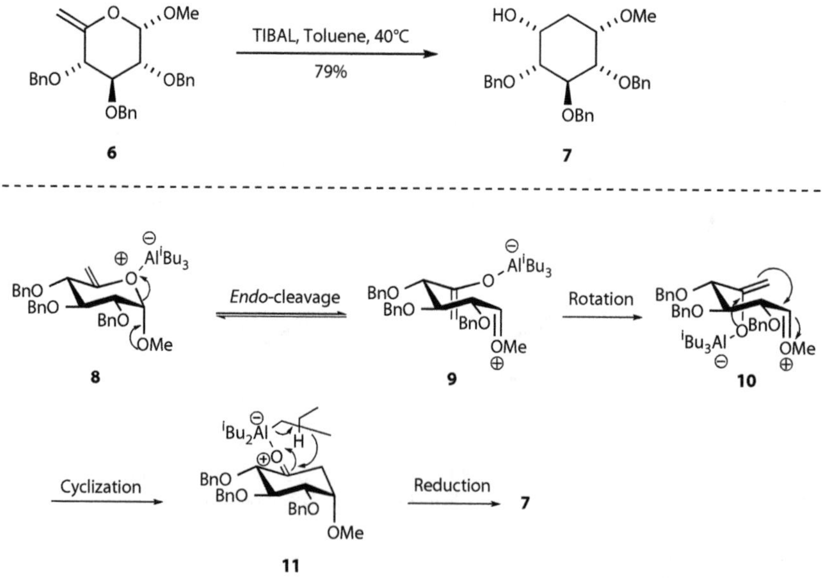

SCHEME 14.2

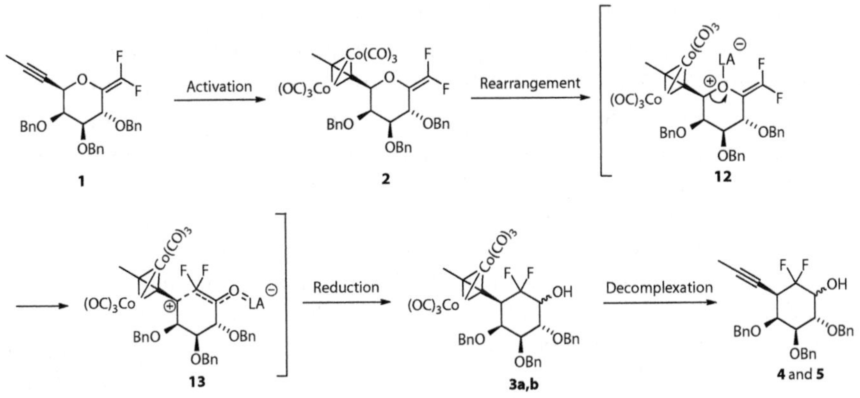

SCHEME 14.3

The conversion (Scheme 14.3) is based on a two-step one-pot process, which begins with the activation of the triple bond by the cobalt octacarbonyl, followed by the reductive rearrangement induced by the Lewis acid. Decomplexation of the cobalt cluster by ammonium cerium (IV) nitrate (CAN) affords the carbocyclic products as a mixture of anomers.

This methodology was applied successfully also to D-mannose[4] and D-glucose[3] scaffolds, which makes it a valuable and reliable strategy for the preparation of such *gem*-difluorinated analogues.

EXPERIMENTAL METHODS

GENERAL METHODS

Solvents and reagents were purchased from Sigma-Aldrich or Acros. Anhydrous CH_2Cl_2 was freshly distilled under argon from P_2O_5. Solvents for column chromatography (cyclohexane and EtOAc) were distilled before use. All transfers (reagents in solution and solvents) were carried out with oven-dried syringes. Reactions were monitored by thin-layer chromatography (TLC) on plates precoated with Silica Gel 60 F_{254} (layer thickness 0.2 mm; E. Merck, Darmstadt, Germany) and detection with UV light (254 nm), by charring with a 10% ethanolic H_2SO_4 or with a solution of 0.2% w/v cerium sulfate and 5% ammonium molybdate in 2 M H_2SO_4. Flash chromatography was performed using silica gel 60 (230–400 mesh, E. Merck). Optical rotations ($[\alpha]_D$) were measured at 20°C ± 2°C with a Perkin Elmer Model 241 digital polarimeter, using a 10 cm, 1 mL cell. ^1H nuclear magnetic resonance (NMR) spectra (400 MHz) were recorded at room temperature for solutions in $CDCl_3$, with a Bruker Avance 400. Assignments were confirmed by COSY experiments. ^{13}C NMR spectra were recorded at 100.6 MHz with a Bruker Avance 400 spectrometer. Assignments were confirmed by J-mod technique and HMQC experiment. Solutions in organic solvents were dried with anhydrous $MgSO_4$ and concentrated at reduced pressure.

Rearrangement of 1 into 2,3,4-Tri-*O*-Benzyl-6,7,8-Trideoxy-5a-Difluoro-5a-Carba-α-D-*Galacto*-Oct-6-Ynopyranose (4) and 2,3,4-Tri-*O*-Benzyl-6,7,8-Trideoxy-5a-Difluoro-5a-Carba-β-D-*Galacto*-Oct-6-Ynopyranose (5)

$Co_2(CO)_8$ (150.0 mg, 0.45 mmol, 1.5 equiv) was added under argon to a stirred solution of difluoroalkene **1** (150.0 mg, 0.30 mmol, 1 equiv) in dry CH_2Cl_2 (15 mL). After 1 h, TLC (4:1 cyclohexane–EtOAc) indicated complete complexation of the starting material. The mixture was cooled to −78°C and TIBAL (1 M in toluene, 3.00 mL, 3.00 mmol, 10 equiv) was added dropwise over a period of 15 min. The mixture was allowed to reach room temperature and stirred for an additional 1 h until TLC showed that the reaction was complete. The mixture was diluted with CH_2Cl_2 (20 mL) and washed with a saturated solution of $NaHCO_3$ (15 mL). The organic phase was filtered through a pad of Celite®, and the solids were washed with CH_2Cl_2 (2 × 15 mL). The combined solutions in CH_2Cl_2 were washed with saturated $NaHCO_3$ and concentrated. The crude product was dissolved in acetone (10 mL) and Et_3N (30.0 μL, 0.30 mmol, 1 equiv) and CAN (820.0 mg, 1.50 mmol, 5 equiv) were added. After stirring at room temperature for 30 min, TLC (4:1 cyclohexane–EtOAc) showed that the reaction was complete and that two products were formed. After concentration, chromatography (8:1 cyclohexane–EtOAc) gave compounds **4** and **5** as amorphous solids.

Compound **4**: Yield 52.1 mg (35%); $[\alpha]_D = +33.5$ (*c* 1, CHCl$_3$); ^{1}H NMR (CDCl$_3$, 250 MHz): δ 7.37–7.20 (m, 15H, H$_{arom.}$ Ph), 4.89 (s, 2H, 2×CHPh), 4.79 (d, 1H, ^2J 11.2 Hz, CHPh), 4.75 (s, 2H, 2×CHPh), 4.67 (d, 1H, ^2J 11.2 Hz, CHPh), 4.21 (dt, 1H, $J_{1,2} = J_{1,Feq}$ 3.0 Hz, $J_{1,Fax}$ 7.1 Hz, H-1), 4.09 (dd, 1H, $J_{1,2}$ 3.2 Hz, $J_{2,3}$ 8.9 Hz, H-2), 4.02 (app t, 1H, $J_{3,4} = J_{4,5}$ 2.8 Hz, H-4), 3.83 (dd, 1H, $J_{3,4}$ 3.0 Hz, $J_{2,3}$ 8.9 Hz, H-3), 3.25 (br d, 1H, $J_{5,Fax}$ 28.5 Hz, H-5), 2.62 (br s, 1H, OH), 1.82 (d, 3H, $J_{5,8}$ 2.2 Hz, H-8); ^{13}C NMR (C$_6$D$_6$, 100 MHz): δ 139.42, 139.26, 138.54 (3×C$_{arom.}$ quat. Ph), 128.62–127.66 (15×CH$_{arom.}$ Ph), 120.32 (t, $^1J_{C,F} = 251.5$ Hz, CF$_2$), 80.59 (C alcyn.), 78.29 (C-3), 77.50 (br s, C-2), 76.35 (d, $^3J_{C,F} = 6.5$ Hz, C-4), 75.66 (CH$_2$Ph), 73.35 (2×CH$_2$Ph), 72.78 (C alcyn.), 70.36 (br s, C-1), 36.94 (t, $^2J_{C,F} = 20.8$ Hz, C-5), 3.41 (C-8); HRCI MS [M + NH$_4$]$^+$ Calcd for $C_{30}H_{34}O_4NF_2$, 510.2456; found, 510.2441.

Compound **5** Yield 42.2 mg (29%); $[\alpha]_D = -15.1$ (*c* 0.8, CHCl$_3$); ^{1}H NMR (CDCl$_3$, 400 MHz): δ 7.37–7.29 (m, 15H, H$_{arom.}$ Ph), 4.92 (br d, 3H, ^2J 10.3 Hz, 3×CHPh), 4.79 (d, 1H, ^2J 11.1 Hz, CHPh), 4.75 (d, 1H, *J* 12.0 Hz, CHPh), 4.71 (d, 1H, *J* 11.9 Hz, CHPh), 4.07–4.02 (m, 2H, H-2, H-4) 3.74 (ddd, 1H, $J_{1,Feq}$ 6.8 Hz, $J_{1,2}$ 8.7 Hz, $J_{1,Fax}$ 15.3 Hz, H-1), 3.53 (dd, 1H, $J_{3,4}$ 2.0 Hz, $J_{2,3}$ 8.7 Hz, H-3), 2.90 (br d, 1H, $J_{5,Fax}$ 23.6 Hz, H-5), 1.84 (d, 3H, $J_{5,8}$ 2.4 Hz, H-8); ^{13}C NMR (CDCl$_3$, 100 MHz): δ 138.83, 138.56, 138.32 (3×C$_{arom.}$ quat. Ph), 128.92–127.89 (15×CH$_{arom.}$ Ph), 119.50 (dd, $^1J_{C,F} = 245.1$ Hz, $^1J_{C,F} = 255.4$ Hz, CF$_2$), 81.50 (C alcyn.), 81.17 (C-3), 79.36 (d, $^3J_{C,F} = 6.3$ Hz, C-2 or C-4), 75.87 (d, $^3J_{C,F} = 6.8$ Hz, C-2 or C-4), 75.81 (CH$_2$Ph), 75.09 (CH$_2$Ph), 74.22 (br s, C-1), 73.41 (CH$_2$Ph), 71.48 (C alcyn.), 38.72 (t, $^2J_{C,F} = 21.0$ Hz, C-5), 4.15 (C-8); HRCI MS [M + NH$_4$]$^+$. Calcd for $C_{30}H_{34}O_4NF_2$, 510.2456; found, 510.2463.

ACKNOWLEDGMENT

The authors thank Fundação para a Ciência e Tecnologia (FCT Portugal) for the research grant (João Sardinha) and financial support.

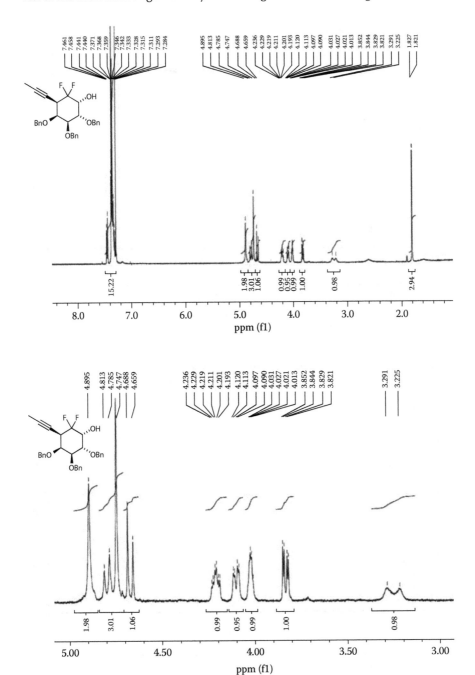

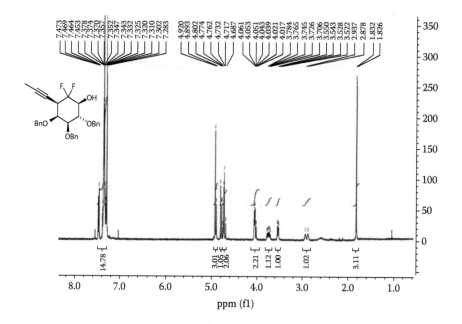

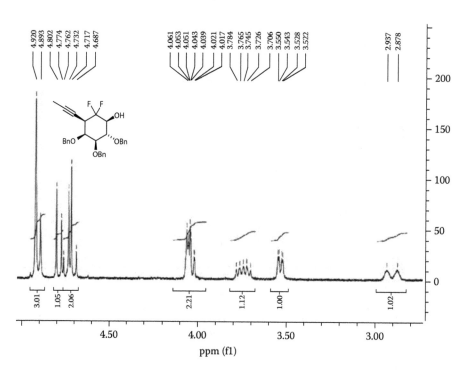

REFERENCES

1. Das, S. K.; Mallet, J.-M.; Sinaÿ, P. *Angew. Chem. Int. Ed.* 1997, *36*, 493–496.
2. Sollogoub, M.; Mallet, J.-M.; Sinaÿ, P. *Angew. Chem. Int. Ed.* 2000, *39*, 362–364.
3. Deleuze, A.; Menozzi, C.; Sollogoub, M.; Sinaÿ, P. *Angew. Chem. Int. Ed.* 2004, *43*, 6680–6683.
4. Sardinha, J.; Guieu, S.; Deleuze, A.; Fernández-Alonso, M. C.; Rauter, A. P.; Sinaÿ, P.; Marrot, J.; Jiménez-Barbero, J.; Sollogoub, M. *Carbohydr. Res.* 2007, *342*, 1689–1703.

REFERENCES

15 Pyranose-Fused Butenolides: An Expedient Preparation from Furanose Synthons

Nuno M. Xavier, Sebastian Kopitzki,[†]
and Amélia Pilar Rauter*

CONTENTS

Experimental Methods 140
    General Methods 140
        1,2:5,6-Di-*O*-Isopropylidene-α-D-*Ribo*-Hexofuranosid-3-Ulose (**1**) 141
        3-Deoxy-3-*C*-[(*Z*)-(Ethoxycarbonyl)methylene]-
        1,2:5,6-Di-*O*-Isopropylidene-α-D-*Ribo*-Hexofuranose (**2**) and
        3-Deoxy-3-*C*-[(*E*)-(Ethoxycarbonyl)methylene]-1,2:5,6-Di-*O*-
        Isopropylidene-α-D-*Ribo*-Hexofuranose (**3**) 141
        3-*C*-(Carboxymethylene)-3-Deoxy-D-*Ribo*-Hexopyranose-
        3′,2-Lactone (**4**) 141
        3-Deoxy-3-*C*-[(*Z*)-(Ethoxycarbonyl)methylene]-1,2-*O*-Isopropylidene-
        α-D-*Ribo*-Hexofuranose (**5**) 142
        3-Deoxy-3-*C*-[(*Z*)-(Ethoxycarbonyl)methylene]-1,2-*O*-
        Isopropylidene-6-*O*-Pivaloyl-α-D-*Ribo*-Hexofuranose (**6**) and
        3-Deoxy-3-*C*-[(*Z*)-(Ethoxycarbonyl)methylene]-1,2-*O*-Isopropylidene-
        5,6-Di-*O*-Pivaloyl-α-D-*Ribo*-Hexofuranose (**7**) 142
        3-*C*-(Carboxymethylene)-3-Deoxy-6-*O*-Pivaloyl-D-*Ribo*-
        Hexopyranose-3′,2-Lactone (**8**) 143
        1,4,6-Tri-*O*-Acetyl-3-*C*-(Carboxymethylene)-3-Deoxy-D-*Ribo*-
        Hexopyranose-3′,2-Lactone (**9**) 143
        5-*O*-*Tert*-Butyldimethylsilyl-1,2-*O*-Isopropylidene-α-D-*Erythro*-
        Pentofuranos-3-Ulose (**10**) 144

---

* Corresponding author.
[†] Checker.

5-*O*-*Tert*-Butyldimethylsilyl-3-Deoxy-3-*C*-[(*Z*)-(Ethoxycarbonyl)
methylene]-1,2-*O*-Isopropylidene-α-D-*Erythro*-Pentofuranose (**11**)
and 5-*O*-*Tert*-Butyldimethylsilyl-3-Deoxy-3-*C*-[(*E*)-(Ethoxycarbonyl)
methylene]-1,2-*O*-Isopropylidene-α-D-*Erythro*-Pentofuranose (**12**)........... 144
3-*C*-(Carboxymethylene)-3-Deoxy-D-*Erythro*-Pentopyranose-3′,2-
Lactone (**13**) 145
Acknowledgment... 145
References.. 157

Synthesis of hexopyranose-fused butenolides.

The α,β-unsaturated γ-lactone moiety, that is, butenolide and α-methylene-γ-lactone, represents an essential fragment in numerous bioactive compounds, including natural products.[1] Their conjugated carbonyl system, which is prone to nucleophilic attack by enzymes' nucleophiles, especially by Michael addition, frequently determines their bioactivity.[2] Because of a wide variety of their biological properties, including cytotoxic[3] and antimicrobial activities,[4] much progress has been made in the development of synthetic approaches toward such structural motifs.[5] Particularly, the insertion of α,β-unsaturated γ-lactone in sugar scaffolds has provided access to a series of bicyclic compounds exhibiting significant antifungal properties[6] and potent and selective insecticidal activity.[7] Therefore, sugar derivatives containing α,β-unsaturated γ-lactones are potential targets for the synthesis of sugar-based bioactive substances and valuable precursors for further derivatization, taking advantage of the ability of the conjugated system to undergo a variety of reactions.[8] Examples of pyranose-fused butenolides include intermediates for important sugar derivatives, such as the mycotoxin patulin,[9] or a 2-*C*-branched-chain sugar.[10] Their synthesis involved pyran-2-uloses as precursors, which are generally obtained in low yield by chemical synthesis. Our research group used this type of compounds for the synthesis of the sugar moiety of miharamycins.[11] This antibiotic is a potent inhibitor of *Pyricularia oryzae*, which causes the rice blast disease and is also considered a potential biological weapon. A prerequisite for efficient transformation into other analogues requires easy access to bicyclic structures comprising pyranose-fused five-membered ring lactones. In view of the synthetic utility and the biological profile of α,β-unsaturated γ-lactones, we report herein a full experimental procedure for an efficient and stereoselective access to pyranose-fused butenolides, starting from readily available furanos-3-uloses. The methodology is based on the stereoselective Wittig olefination of 1,2-*O*-isopropylidene-α-D-pento- or -hexofuranos-3-uloses containing acid-labile protecting groups. The subsequent acid hydrolysis of the intermediate (Z)-α,β-unsaturated esters allows intramolecular transesterification and furanose–pyranose isomerization, resulting in ready formation of the bicyclic fused butenolide–pyranose system.

For the synthesis of butenolides fused to hexopyranoses, as depicted in the opening scheme of this chapter, the 3-keto sugar **1**,[12] which was prepared by oxidation of diacetone-D-glucose (DAG) with pyridinium dichromate (PDC) in the presence of acetic anhydride, was subjected to Wittig reaction with the stabilized ylide, [(ethoxycarbonyl)methylene]triphenylphosphorane, in refluxing chloroform, providing stereoselectively the (Z)[13]-**2** and (E)[13]-**3**-α,β-unsaturated esters in 59%–68% and 12% yield, respectively. The reaction outcome is solvent/temperature dependent: When solvent was changed to dichloromethane, compounds **2** and **3** were obtained in 45% and 11% yield, respectively. Treatment of **2** with Amberlite IR-120 H$^+$ resin in refluxing MeOH–H$_2$O mixture, effected acetonide deprotection, furanose–pyranose isomerization, and intramolecular lactonization to afford the target compound **4** as a solid in 90% yield. When dry methanol was used as solvent, α-methyl glycoside was also obtained in 35% yield. The experimentally simple three-step sequence (DAG → **1** → **2** → **4**) could be carried out in an overall yield of 58%.

The regioselective 6-*O*-protection of derivative of **4** was then studied, in order to allow further selective derivatization on the carbohydrate moiety, enhancing thus the synthetic potential of these bicyclic compounds. The bulky pivaloyl group, stable under a broad range of reaction conditions, was chosen for partial protection of **4**. The diol **5**, which was obtained by selective hydrolysis of the primary acetonide in **2** (90%–95%) with aq. acetic acid (60%), was the substrate for pivaloylation, giving the monoprotected derivative **6** as the major product (57%), together with the 5,6-di-*O*-pivaloyl derivative **7** (27%). Treatment of **6** with aq. 70% acetic acid under reflux provided the 6-*O*-pivaloyl hexopyranose-fused butenolide **8** in 83% yield. On the other hand, the intermediate diol **5** was transformed into the triacetate-derived butenolide **9** by successive deacetonation/cyclization and acetylation.

To further explore the feasibility of the above-described methodology, preparation of a butenolide fused to a pentopyranose unit was also investigated (Scheme 15.1). Thus, the pentofuran-3-ulose **10**, easily synthesized by selective silylation of the commercially available 1,2-*O*-isopropylidene-α-D-xylofuranose, followed by oxidation of the resulting 5-*O*-silyl ether with PDC/Ac$_2$O, was converted into the

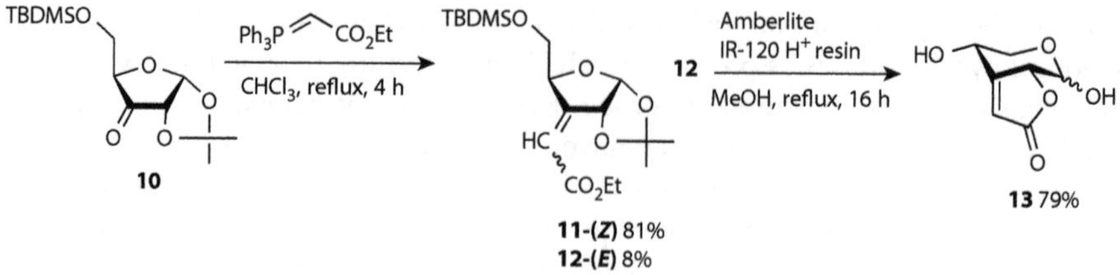

SCHEME 15.1   Synthesis of a pentopyranose-fused butenolide.

(Z)-α,β-unsaturated ester **11** in a stereoselective manner (81%) by Wittig olefination. The synthesis of **10** was reported by Swern oxidation of 5-*O*-TBDMS-1,2-*O*-isopropylidene-α-D-xylofuranose,[14a] and by oxidation of the latter with the system CrO_3/pyridine, Ac_2O.[14b] See, respectively.[14] The corresponding (*E*)-isomer **12**, formed concomitantly (8%), was also obtained. We performed the Wittig olefination of **10** with [(ethoxycarbonyl)methylene]-triphenylphosphorane in refluxing chloroform, which allowed the completion of the reaction in 2 h. The reported procedure required 16 h for complete transformation.[15] Treatment of **11** with Amberlite IR-120 resin, as described for **2**, furnished the desired bicyclic fused compound **13** in 79% yield.

In summary, a concise methodology is described for generation of pyranose-fused butenolides starting from readily accessible furan-3-uloses. The key steps are the stereoselective formation of the (Z)-α,β-unsaturated esters by Wittig olefination and the hydrolysis step, which effects simultaneous protecting group removal, ring expansion, and intramolecular lactonization. The structure of these molecules not only renders them attractive targets for biological investigations but also opens possibilities for further derivatization, either on the carbohydrate moiety or by exploring the reaction potential of the conjugated lactone unit.

EXPERIMENTAL METHODS

GENERAL METHODS

1,2:5,6-di-*O*-Isopropylidene-α-D-glucofuranose (DAG) and 1,2-*O*-isopropylidene-α-D-xylofuranose were purchased from Sigma-Aldrich. Melting points were determined with a Stuart Scientific SMP 3 apparatus and are uncorrected. Optical rotations were measured on a Perkin–Elmer 343 polarimeter at 20°C. ¹H and ¹³C nuclear magnetic resonance (NMR) spectra were recorded with a BRUKER Avance 400 spectrometer operating at 400.13 MHz for ¹H or 100.62 MHz for ¹³C. Chemical shifts are expressed in parts per million and are reported relative to internal tetramethylsilane (TMS) or relative to the respective solvent peak. Signal assignments were made with the help of DEPT, COSY, HMQC, and HMBC experiments. HRMS spectra were acquired with an Apex Ultra FTICR mass spectrometer equipped with an Apollo II Dual ESI/MALDI ion source (Bruker Daltonics), and a 7T actively shielded magnet (Magnex Scientific). Elemental analyses were performed at the Microanalyses Service of Instituto Superior Técnico-Universidade Técnica de Lisboa.

All reactions were monitored by thin-layer chromatography (TLC) on Merck 60 F_{254} silica gel-coated aluminum plates with detection under UV light

(254 nm) and/or by charring with 10% H_2SO_4 in EtOH. Column chromatography was performed on silica gel 60 G (0.040–0.063 mm, E. Merck). Concentration of solutions was done at reduced pressure.

1,2:5,6-Di-O-Isopropylidene-α-D-*Ribo*-Hexofuranosid-3-Ulose (1)

A solution of DAG (4.00 g, 15.4 mmol) in dry CH_2Cl_2 (24 mL) was added under argon to a mixture of PDC (4.32 g, 11.4 mmol) and Ac_2O (4.4 mL, 46.5 mmol) in dry CH_2Cl_2 (48 mL). The mixture was stirred under reflux for 2 h, cooled to rt, and concentrated. The gummy residue was triturated with Et_2O (3 × 150 mL), and the ethereal extract was filtered through Florisil. The eluate was concentrated to afford the title compound as a colorless oil (3.78 g, 95%); R_f 0.37 (2:3 EtOAc-petroleum ether); [^1]H NMR (CDCl$_3$) δ 6.15 (d, 1H, $J_{1,2}$ 4.3 Hz, H-1), 4.42–4.34 (m, 3H, H-2, H-4, H-5), 4.06–4.01 (m, 2H, H-6a, H-6b), 1.46 (s, 3H, Me), 1.44 (s, 3H, Me), 1.34 (s, 6H, 2×Me).

3-Deoxy-3-C-[(Z)-(Ethoxycarbonyl)methylene]-1,2:5,6-Di-O-Isopropylidene-α-D-*Ribo*-Hexofuranose (2) and 3-Deoxy-3-C-[(E)-(Ethoxycarbonyl) methylene]-1,2:5,6-Di-O-Isopropylidene-α-D-*Ribo*-Hexofuranose (3)

[(Ethoxycarbonyl)methylene]triphenylphosphorane (5.23 g, 15 mmol) was added to a solution of 3-ulose **1** (2.27 g, 8.78 mmol) in dry CHCl$_3$ (70 mL), and the mixture was stirred under reflux for 2 h. After concentration, the residue was chromatographed (1:9 EtOAc-petroleum ether) to afford **2**-(Z) as a white solid (1.70–1.95 g, 59%–68%) and its (E)-isomer as a colorless oil (0.34 g, 12%). Physical data were in agreement with those reported.[12]

Data for 2

R_f 0.27 (1:9 EtOAc-cyclohexane). [^1]H NMR (CDCl$_3$) δ 6.34 (brd, 1H, H-3′), 5.85 (d, 1H, $J_{1,2}$ 4.3 Hz, H-1,), 5.75 (brd, 1H, H-2), 4.68 (brdd, 1H, H-4), 4.25 (q, 2H, J 7.1 Hz, CH_2CH_3), 4.13–3.98 (m, 3H, H-5, H-6a, H-6b), 1.50, 1.45, 1.41, 1.37 (4s, 4×3H, 4×Me), 1.32 (t, 3H, CH_2CH_3).; [^13]C NMR (CDCl$_3$) δ 165.1 (CO), 155.7 (C-3), 117.9 (C-3′), 112.8, 110.1, (2×Cq, isop), 104.9 (C-1), 79.9 (C-4), 78.4 (C-2), 76.8 (C-5), 67.3 (C-6), 60.7 (CH_2CH_3), 27.3, 27.1, 26.7, 25.4 (4×Me), 14.2 (CH_2CH_3).

Data for 3

R_f 0.35 (1:9 EtOAc-cyclohexane); [^1]H NMR (CDCl$_3$) δ 6.23 (brd, 1H, H-3′), 5.94 (d, 1H, $J_{1,2}$ 4.8 Hz, H-1), 5.76 (brd, 1H, H-4), 5.11 (brdd, 1H, H-2), 4.35 (ddd, 1H, $J_{4,5}$ 2.3 Hz, H-5,), 4.19 (qd, 2H, CH_2CH_3), 3.97 (dd, 1H, $J_{5,6a}$ 6.3 Hz, H-6a,), 3.57 (t, 1H, $J_{6a,6b}$ 8.6 Hz, H-6b), 1.43, 1.39, 1.33, 1.32 (4s, 4×3H, 4×Me), 1.31 (t, 3H, J 7.1 Hz, CH_2CH_3); [^13]C NMR (CDCl$_3$) δ 165.6 (CO), 158 (C-3), 118.1 (C-3′), 113.7, 109.1 (2×Cq, isop), 103.8 (C-1), 82.3 (C-2), 80.0 (C-4), 79.0 (C-5), 65.4 (C-6), 60.8 (CH_2CH_3), 27.9, 27.9, 26.2, 25.7 (4×Me), 14.2 (CH_2CH_3).

3-C-(Carboxymethylene)-3-Deoxy-D-*Ribo*-Hexopyranose-3′,2-Lactone (4)

Amberlite IR-120 H⁺ resin (100 mg) was added to a solution of 3-deoxy-3-C-[(Z)-(ethoxycarbonyl)methylene]- 1,2:5,6-di-O-isopropylidene-α-D-*ribo*-hexofuranose (**2**, 0.3 g, 0.913 mmol) in MeOH–H_2O (5:1, 12 mL). The mixture was gently stirred under reflux for 16 h, the resin was filtered, and the solvent was evaporated. The crude product was chromatographed using AcOEt as eluent to afford **4** as a white solid (165 mg, 90%). R_f 0.22 (EtOAc); mp 168°C–174°C (AcOEt); ^{1}H NMR (DMSO-d_6) δ 7.56 (d, J 5.6, OH-1β), 7.04 (d, J 4.6, OH-1α), 6.00 (d, J 5.8 Hz, OH-4β), 5.95–5.87 (m, H-3'α, H-3'β, OH-4α), 5.47 (t, H-1α), 4.96 (d, $J_{1,2\,(α)}$ 4.1 Hz, H-2α), 4.89 (t, OH-6β), 4.79 (t, OH-6α), 4.65 (d, $J_{1,2\,(β)}$ 7.1 Hz, H-2β), 4.37–4.30 (m, H1-β, H-4α, H-4β), 3.79–3.52 (m, $J_{5,6a\,(β)}$ 5.3 Hz, $J_{6a,6b\,(β)}$ 12.1 Hz, $J_{5,6a\,(α)}$ 5.3 Hz, $J_{6a,6b\,(α)}$ 11.6 Hz, H-6aα, H-6aβ, H-6bα, H-6bβ, H-5α), 3.12 (ddd, H-5β). ^{13}C NMR (DMSO-d_6) δ 172.9, 172.6, 172.4 171.1 (CO-α, CO-β, C-3α, C-3β), 111.7 (C-3'α, C-3'β), 98.7 (C-1β), 90.4 (C-1α), 82.0 (C-2β), 80.2 (C-5β), 78.6 (C-2α), 74.4 (C-5α), 66.1 (C-4β), 65.7 (C-4α), 60.1 (C-6a, C-6β); HRMS: calcd for $C_8H_{10}O_6$ [M+H]$^+$ 203.0550; found: 203.0550; calcd for [M+Na]$^+$ 225.0370; found: 225.0369; calcd for [M+K]$^+$ 241.0109; found: 241.0109. Anal. calcd for $C_8H_{10}O_6$: C, 47.53; H, 4.99. Found: C, 47.60; H, 4.90.

3-Deoxy-3-C-[(Z)-(Ethoxycarbonyl)methylene]-1,2-O-Isopropylidene-α-D-*Ribo*-Hexofuranose (5)

A solution of 3-deoxy-3-C-[(Z)-(ethoxycarbonyl)methylene]-α,D-1,2:5,6-di-O-isopropylidene-α-D-*ribo*-hexofuranose (**2**, 0.79 g, 2.41 mmol) in 60% aq. AcOH (9.6 mL) was stirred at rt for 20 h. The mixture was concentrated, the residue was coevaporated with toluene (3×), and the crude product was chromatographed (2:3 EtOAc-petroleum ether) to afford the title compound as a colorless oil (0.66 g, 95%). R_f 0.25 (2:3 EtOAc-petroleum ether); [α]$_D$ +165 (c 1.2, CH$_2$Cl$_2$); ^{1}H NMR (CDCl$_3$) δ 6.30 (brdd, 1H, H-3'), 5.87 (d, 1H, $J_{1,2}$ 4.0 Hz, H-1,), 5.73 (brd, 1H, H-2), 4.80 (brd, 1H, H-4), 4.24 (q, 2H, CH$_2$CH$_3$), 3.79–3.70 (m, 3H, H-5, H-6a, H-6b), 1.49 (s, 3H, Me), 1.41 (s, 3H, Me), 1.31 (t, 3H, J 7.1 Hz, CH$_2$CH$_3$); ^{13}C NMR (CDCl$_3$) δ 165.3 (CO), 155.7 (C-3), 117.6 (C-3'), 113.0 (Cq, isop), 104.8 (C-1), 79.9 (C-4), 78.4 (C-2), 73.5 (C-5), 63.4 (C-6), 60.9 (CH$_2$CH$_3$), 27.3 (Me), 27.2 (Me), 14.2 (CH$_2$CH$_3$).

3-Deoxy-3-C-[(Z)-(Ethoxycarbonyl)methylene]-1,2-O-Isopropylidene-6-O-Pivaloyl-α-D-*Ribo*-Hexofuranose (6) and 3-Deoxy-3-C-[(Z)-(Ethoxycarbonyl)methylene]-1,2-O-Isopropylidene-5,6-Di-O-Pivaloyl-α-D-*Ribo*-Hexofuranose (7)

A solution of pivaloyl chloride (2.12 mmol, 0.26 mL) in dry CH$_2$Cl$_2$ (1 mL) was added under argon to a solution of 3-deoxy-3-C-[(Z)-(ethoxycarbonyl)methylene]-1,2-O-isopropylidene-α-D-*ribo*-hexofuranose (**5**, 0.24 g, 0.85 mmol) in dry pyridine (2.5 mL). The solution was stirred at rt for 1 h and concentrated. The residue was partitioned between water (10 mL) and CH$_2$Cl$_2$ (3×5 mL). Organic layers were washed with a sat. aq. NaHCO$_3$ solution, water, and brine and dried over MgSO$_4$. After filtration and evaporation of the solvent, the residue was chromatographed (1:4 EtOAc-cyclohexane) to afford **6** and **7** as white solids [0.18 g (57%) and 0.10 g (27%), respectively].

Data for 6

R_f 0.35 (1:4 EtOAc-cyclohexane); [α]$_D$ +87 (c 0.8, CH$_2$Cl$_2$); mp 97°C–99°C (cyclohexane); 1 H NMR (CDCl$_3$) δ 6.32 (brs, 1H, H-3'), 5.88 (d, 1H, J1,2 4.3 Hz, H-1), 5.74 (brd, 1H, H-2), 4.78 (brd, 1H, $J_{4,5}$ 6.6 Hz, H-4), 4.33, 4.32, 4.30, 4.29 (part AX of

ABX system, $J_{5,6a}$ 3.0 Hz, $J_{6a,6b}$ 11.6 Hz, H-6a,), 4.27–4.21 (m, 3H, H-6b, CH$_2$CH$_3$), 3.89 (ddd, H-5), 2.79 (d, $J_{5,OH}$ 3.8 Hz, OH-5), 1.49 (s, 3H, Me), 1.42 (s, 3H, Me), 1.31 (t, 3H, J 7.1 Hz, CH$_2$CH$_3$), 1.22 (9H, Me, Piv); ^{13}C NMR (CDCl$_3$) δ 179.4 (CO, Piv), 165.2 (CO), 155.3 (C-3), 117.9 (C-3′), 113.0 (Cq, isop), 105.0 (C-1), 79.6 (C-4), 78.5 (C-2), 72.3 (C-5), 65.8 (C-6), 60.8 (CH$_2$CH$_3$), 39.0 (Cq, Piv), 27.5 (Me, isop), 27.3 (Me, isop), 27.3 (Me, Piv), 14.3 (CH$_2$CH$_3$); Anal. calcd for C$_{18}$H$_{28}$O$_8$: C, 58.05; H, 7.58. Found: C, 57.92; H, 7.91.

Data for 7

R_f 0.24 (1:9 EtOAc-cyclohexane); $[\alpha]_D$ +91 (c 1, CH$_2$Cl$_2$); mp 94°C–96°C (hexane); ^{1}H NMR (CDCl$_3$) δ 6.03 (t, 1H, H-3′), 5.89 (d, 1H, $J_{1,2}$ 4.3 Hz, H-1,), 5.72 (brd, 1H, H-2), 5.12 (ddd, 1H, H-5), 4.98 (brd, 1H, H-4), 4.34, 4.33, 4.31, 4.30, (part AX of ABX system, $J_{5,6a}$ 3.0 Hz, $J_{6a,6b}$ 12.1 Hz, H-6a), 4.28–4.15 (m, 3H, $J_{5,6b}$ 6.8 Hz, J 7.1 Hz, H-6b, CH$_2$CH$_3$), 1.48 (s, 3H, Me), 1.43 (s, 3H, Me), 1.30 (t, 3H, CH$_2$CH$_3$), 1.23 (9H, Me, Piv), 1.18 (9H, Me, Piv); ^{13}C NMR (CDCl$_3$) δ 178.1 (CO, Piv), 177.6 (CO, Piv), 164.6 (CO), 154.4 (C-3), 118.1 (C-3′), 113.2 (Cq, isop), 105.2 (C-1), 78.8 (C-4), 78.3 (C-2), 72.4 (C-5), 62.0 (C-6), 61.0 (CH$_2$CH$_3$), 39.0 (Cq, Piv), 38.9 (Cq, Piv), 27.5 (Me, isop), 27.3 (Me, isop), 27.2 (Me, Piv), 27.2 (Me, Piv) 14.2 (CH$_2$CH$_3$); Anal. calcd for C$_{23}$H$_{36}$O$_9$: C, 60.51; H, 7.95. Found: C, 60.48; H, 8.39.

3-C-(Carboxymethylene)-3-Deoxy-6-O-Pivaloyl-D-Ribo-Hexopyranose-3′,2-Lactone (8)

A solution of 3-deoxy-3-C-[(Z)-(ethoxycarbonyl)methylene]-1,2-O-isopropylidene-6-O-pivaloyl-α-D-ribo-hexofuranose (6, 0.08 g, 0.22 mmol) in 70% aq. AcOH (1.2 mL) was stirred under reflux for 1 h 45 min. After concentration, the residue was coevaporated with toluene (3×) and the crude product was chromatographed (3:2 EtOAc-petroleum ether) to afford the title compound as a colorless oil (51 mg, 83%). R_f 0.33 (3:2 EtOAc-petroleum ether); ^{1}H NMR (CDCl$_3$) δ 6.13 (brs, H-3′), 5.66 (d, $J_{1,2(\alpha)}$ 4.2 Hz, H-1α,), 4.88 (dd, $J_{2,3'(\alpha)}$ 1.3 Hz, H-2α,), 4.67 (dd, $J_{1,2(\beta)}$ 7.1 Hz, $J_{2,3'(\beta)}$ 1.3, H-2β), 4.57–4.47 (m, $J_{5,6a(\alpha)}$ 3.5 Hz, $J_{6a,6b(\alpha)}$ 12.5 Hz, H-1β, H-6aα, H-6aβ), 4.46–4.35 (m, H-6bα, H-4α, H-4β, H-6bβ), 3.97 (ddd, H-5α), 3.47 (ddd, H-5β), 1.23 (s, Me, Piv, α, Me, Piv, β); ^{13}C NMR (CDCl$_3$) δ 180.0 (CO, Piv, β), 179.8 (CO, Piv, α), 174.3 (CO, lact., α), 173.6 (CO, lact., β), 169.3 (C-3β), 168.0 (C-3α), 113.8 (C-3′α, C-3′β), 99.0 (C-1β), 90.9 (C-1α), 82.4 (C-2β), 79.1 (C-2α), 78.2 (C-5β), 72.2 (C-5α), 67.2 (C-4β), 66.9 (C-4α), 62.9 (C-6β), 62.7 (C-6α), 39.2 (Cq, Piv), 27.3 (Me, Piv). HRMS: calcd for C$_{13}$H$_{18}$O$_7$ [M+H]$^+$ 287.1125; found: 287.1127; calcd for [M+Na]$^+$ 309.0945; found: 309.0947; calcd for [M+K]$^+$ 325.0684; found: 325.0684.

1,4,6-Tri-O-Acetyl-3-C-(Carboxymethylene)-3-Deoxy-D-Ribo-Hexopyranose-3′,2-Lactone (9)

A solution of 3-deoxy-3-C-[(Z)-(ethoxycarbonyl)methylene]-1,2-O-isopropylidene-α-D-ribo-hexofuranose (5, 0.07 g, 0.23 mmol) in 70% aq. AcOH (1.2 mL) was stirred under reflux for 1 h. After concentration, acetic anhydride (1 mL) and pyridine (2 mL) were added to the residue, and the mixture was stirred for 5 min. After coevaporation with toluene (3×), the crude product was chromatographed (1:1 EtOAc-petroleum ether) to afford the title compound as a colorless oil (0.06 g, 78%); R_f 0.32 (1:1 EtOAc-petroleum ether). $[\alpha]_D$ +178 (c 1.2, CH_2Cl_2); ^{1}H NMR (CDCl$_3$) δ 6.60 (d, $J_{1,2}$ 4.6 Hz, H-1α), 6.02–5.96 (m, 3'α-H, 3'β-H), 5.71 (dd, $J_{3',4\,(\alpha)}$ 1.5 Hz, $J_{4,5\,(\alpha)}$ 9.6 Hz, H-4α), 5.66 (dd, $J_{3',4\,(\beta)}$ 1.5 Hz, $J_{4,5\,(\beta)}$ 9.6, H-4β), 5.40 (d, $J_{1,2\,(\beta)}$ 7.6 Hz, H-1β), 5.10 (dd, $J_{2,3'\,(\alpha)}$ 1.5 Hz, H-2α), 4.90 (dd, $J_{2,3'(\beta)}$ 1.5 Hz, H-2β), 4.40–4.32 (m, H-6aα, H-6aβ) 4.28–4.19 (m, H-6bα, H-6bβ), 4.00 (ddd, H-5α), 3.77 (ddd, H-5β), 2.22 (s, Me, Ac, α, Me, Ac, β), 2.21 (s, Me, Ac, β), 2.11 (s, Me, Ac, α, Me, Ac, β), 2.09 (s, Me, Ac, α); ^{13}C NMR (CDCl$_3$) δ 171.0 (CO, Ac, α), 170.6 (CO, Ac, β, CO, lact., α, CO, lact., β), 169.1 (CO, Ac, β), 169.1 (CO, Ac, α), 168.7 (CO, Ac, β), 168.2 (CO, Ac, α), 163.2 (C-3β), 161.6 (C-3α), 115.3 (C-3'α), 114.7 (C-3'β), 95.4 (C-1β), 88.8 (C-1α), 78.9 (C-2β), 76.4 (C-2α), 76.2 (C-5β), 71.9 (C-5α), 66.4 (C-4β), 66.0 (C-4α), 61.4 (C-6α), 61.3 (C-6β), 20.9, 20.8, 20.7, 20.6 (Me, Ac); HRMS: calcd for $C_{14}H_{16}O_9$ [M + H]$^+$ 329.0867; found: 329.0864; calcd for [M + Na]$^+$ 351.0687; found: 351.0690; calcd for [M + K]$^+$ 367.0426; found: 367.0417.

5-*O-Tert*-Butyldimethylsilyl-1,2-*O*-Isopropylidene-α-D-*Erythro*-Pentofuranos-3-Ulose (10)[13]

A solution of 5-*O*-TBDMS-1,2-*O*-isopropylidene-α-D-xylofuranose[13a,b] (1.05 g, 3.47 mmol) in dry CH_2Cl_2 (6 mL) was added under argon to a mixture of PDC (0.96 g, 2.57 mmol) and acetic anhydride (1.1 mL, 11.6 mmol) in dry CH_2Cl_2 (12 mL), under argon. The mixture was stirred under reflux for 1 h 30 min, cooled to rt, and concentrated. The gummy residue was triturated with Et$_2$O (3 × 50 mL) and the extract was filtered through Florisil. The eluate was concentrated to afford the title compound as a waxy white solid (0.872 g, 97%). ^{1}H NMR (CDCl$_3$) δ 6.14 (d, 1H, $J_{1,2}$ 4.6 Hz, H-1), 4.37 (bd, 1H, H-4), 4.28 (d, 1H, H-2), 3.91, 3.90, 3.88, 3.87 (part A of ABX system, $J_{4,5a}$ 1.8 Hz, $J_{5a,5b}$ 10.9 Hz, H-5a), 3.84, 3.83, 3.81, 3.80 (part B of ABX system, $J_{4,5b}$ 2.0 Hz, H-5b), 1.46 (s, 3H, Me), 1.45 (s, 3H, Me), 0.86 (s, 9H, *t*-Bu, TBDMS), 0.06 (s, 3H, Me, TBDMS), 0.03 (s, 3H, Me, TBDMS); ^{13}C NMR (CDCl$_3$) δ 211.2 (CO), 114.2 (Cq, isop), 103.9 (C-1), 81.9 (C-4), 77.2 (C-2), 64.0 (C-5), 27.8 (Me), 27.3 (Me), 25.9 (3 × Me, *t*-Bu), 18.3 (Cq, *t*-Bu), −5.4 (Me, TBDMS), −5.6 (Me, TBDMS).

5-*O-Tert*-Butyldimethylsilyl-3-Deoxy-3-*C*-[(*Z*)-(Ethoxycarbonyl) methylene]-1,2-*O*-Isopropylidene-α-D-*Erythro*-Pentofuranose (11) and 5-*O-Tert*-Butyldimethylsilyl-3-Deoxy-3-*C*-[(*E*)-(Ethoxycarbonyl) methylene]-1,2-*O*-Isopropylidene-α-D-*Erythro*-Pentofuranose (12)

[(Ethoxycarbonyl)methylene]triphenylphosphorane (1.63 g, 4.67 mmol) was added to a solution of 3-ulose (**14**, 0.83 g, 2.7 mmol) in dry CHCl$_3$ (22 mL) and the mixture was stirred under reflux for 2 h. After concentration, the residue was chromatographed (1:9 EtOAc-cyclohexane) to afford the (*Z*)-adduct **11** and its (*E*)-isomer **12** as colorless oils [0.806 g, (81%), and 0.084 g (8%), respectively]. Spectral data were in full agreement with those reported.[14b]

3-*C*-(Carboxymethylene)-3-Deoxy-D-*Erythro*-Pentopyranose-3′,2-Lactone (13)

5-*O*-TBDMS-3-deoxy-3-*C*-[(*Z*)-(ethoxycarbonyl)methylene]-1,2-*O*-isopropylidene-α-D-*erythro*-pentofuranose (**11**, 0.11 g, 0.29 mmol) was treated with Amberlite IR-120 H⁺ resin as described for preparation of **4**. After filtration and concentration of the filtrate, the crude product was chromatographed (4:1 EtOAc-petroleum ether) to afford the title compound (39 mg, 79%, anomeric mixture) as a white solid. R_f = 0.32 (4:1 EtOAc-petroleum ether); mp 143°C–147°C (Et₂O); ¹H NMR (DMSO-d_6) δ 7.56 (d, *J* 6.6 Hz, OH-1β), 6.99 (d, *J* 4.6 Hz, OH-1α), 5.99 (d, *J* 5.1 Hz, OH-4β), 5.94–5.89 (m, H-3′β, OH-4α), 5.88 (brs, H-3′α), 5.44 (t, H-1 α), 4.96 (d, $J_{1,2\,(\alpha)}$ 3.5 Hz, H-2α), **4.63** (d, $J_{1,2\,(\beta)}$ 6.8 Hz, H-2β,), 4.56–4.55 (m, H-4α, H-4β), 4.27 (t, H-1β), 4.05 (dd, $J_{4,5a(\beta)}$ 8.1 Hz, $J_{5a,5b(\beta)}$ 10.2 Hz, H-5aβ), 3.75 (dd, $J_{4,5a(\alpha)}$ 8.1 Hz, $J_{5a,5b(\alpha)}$ 9.4 Hz, H-5aα,), 3.42 (t, $J_{4,5b\,(\alpha)}$ 10.1 Hz, H-5bα), 3.02 (t, H-5bβ); ¹³C NMR (DMSO-d_6, major anomer) δ 172.8 (CO), 170.4 (C-3), 111.1 (C-3′), 90.3 (C-1), 78.4 (C-2), 65.5 (C-4), 62.6 (C-5); HRMS: calcd for $C_7H_8O_5$ [M + H]⁺ 173.0445; found: 173.0443.

ACKNOWLEDGMENT

The authors thank Fundação para a Ciência e Tecnologia (FCT) for financial support of the project POCI/QUI/59672/2004-PPCDT/QUI/59672/2004 and for the PhD grant SFRH/BD/39251/2007 (N. M. Xavier).

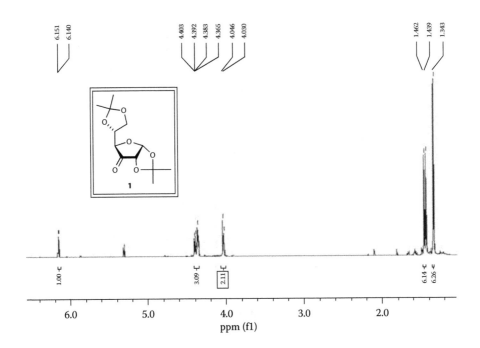

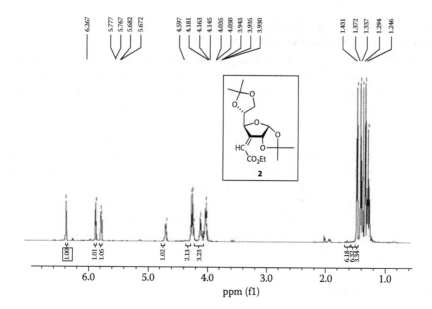

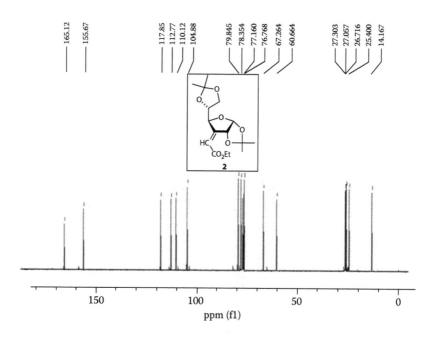

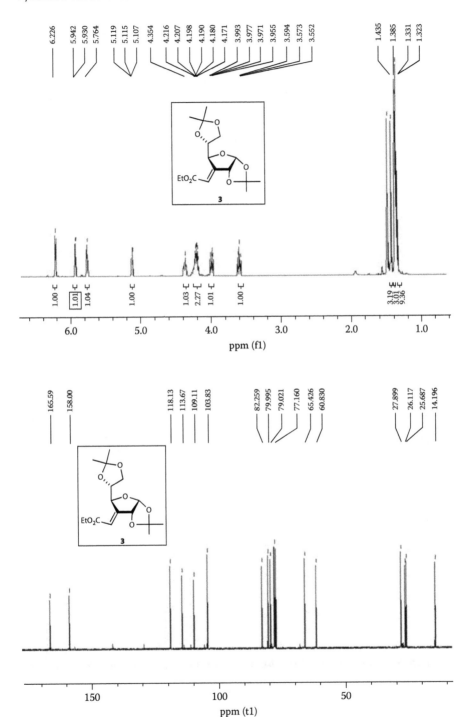

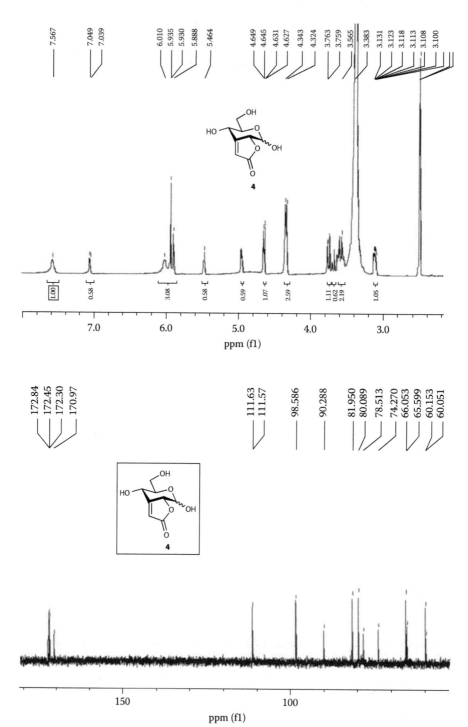

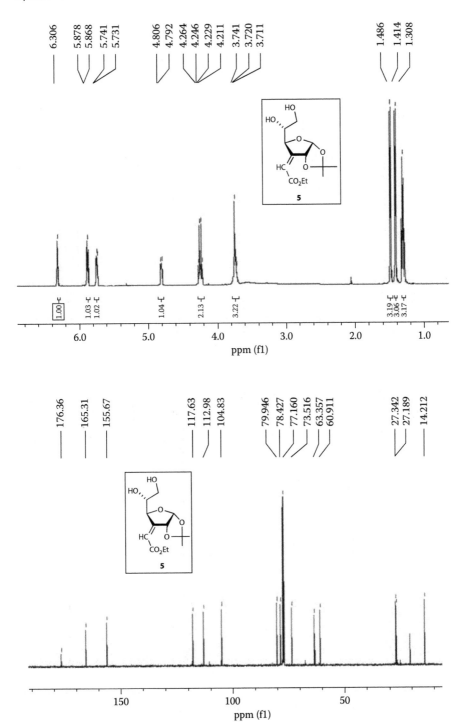

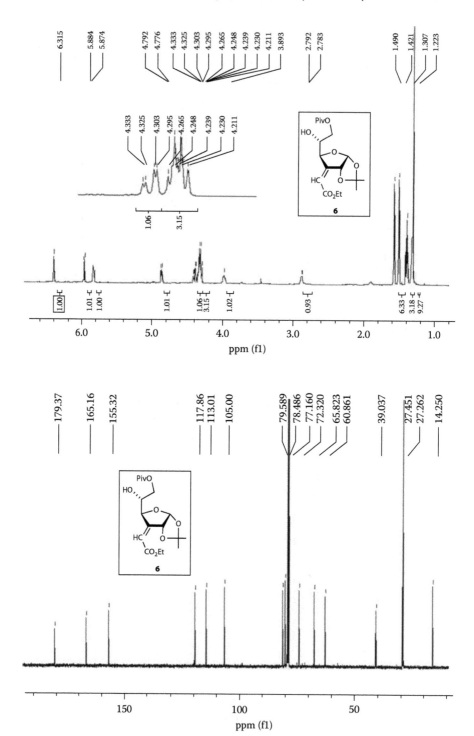

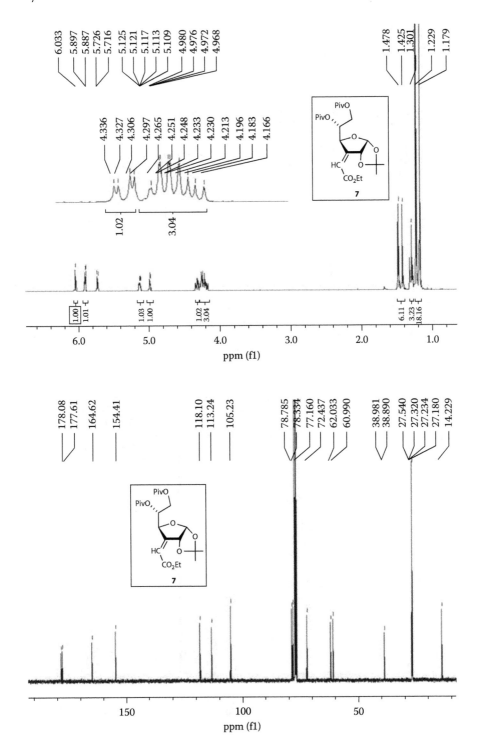

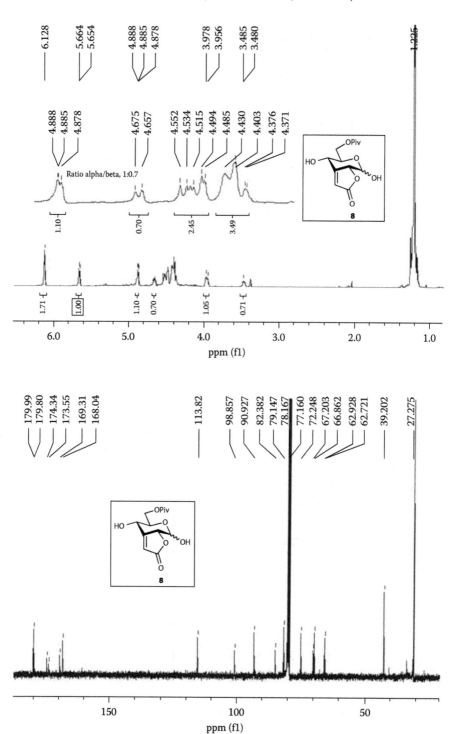

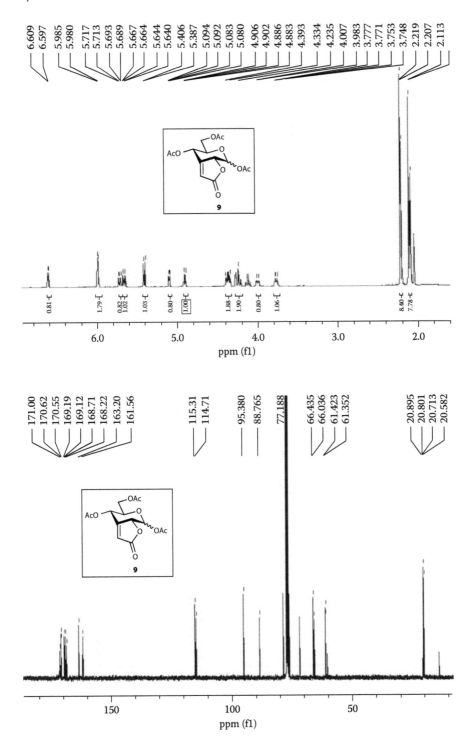

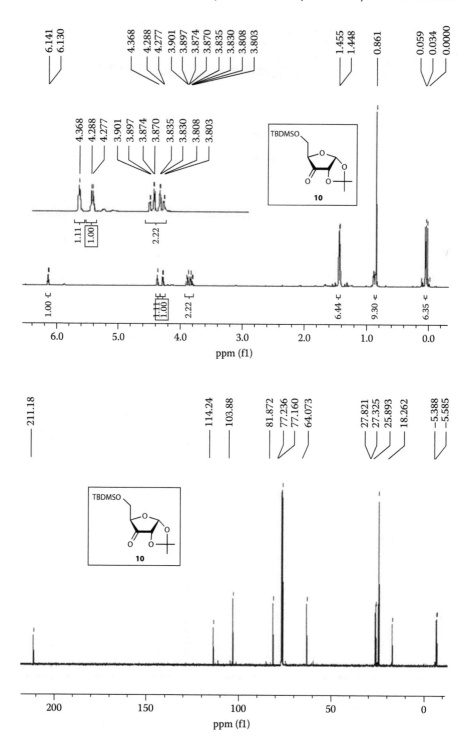

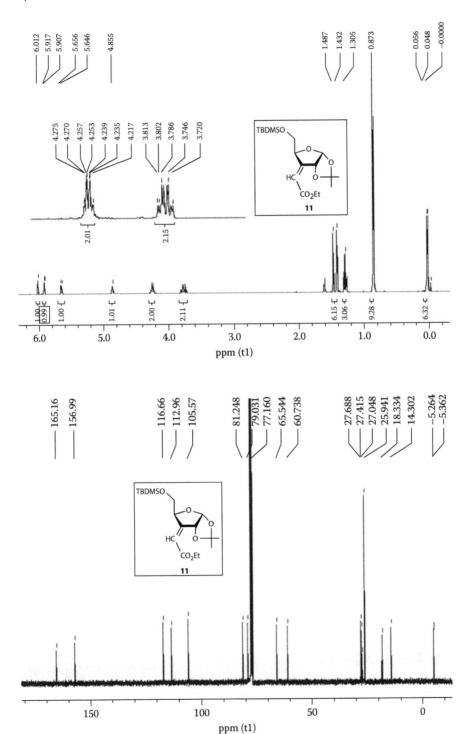

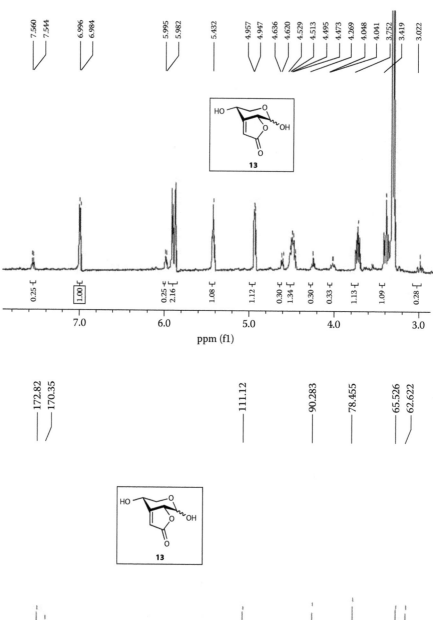

REFERENCES

1 (a) Alali, F. W.; Liu, X.-X.; McLaughlin, J. L. *J. Nat. Prod.* 1999, *62*, 504–540; (b) Hanson, J. R. *Nat. Prod. Rep.* 2002, *19*, 381–389; (c) Parvatkar, R. R.; D'Souza, C.; Tripathi, A.; Naik, C. G. *Phytochemistry* 2009, *70*, 128–132.

2. Rungeler, P.; Castro V.; Mora, G.; Goren, N.; Vichnewski, W.; Pahl, H. L.; Merfort, I.; Schmidt, T. *J. Bioorg. Med. Chem.* 1999, *7*, 2343–2352.

3. See, for example: (a) Oh, S.; Jeong, I. H.; Shin, W.-S.; Wang, Q.; Lee, S. *Bioorg. Med. Chem. Lett.* 2006, *16*, 1656–1659; (b) Li, D.-H.; Zhu, T.-J.; Liu, H.-B.; Fang, Y.-C.; Gu, Q.-Q.; Zhu, W.-M. *Arch. Pharm. Res.* 2006, 29(8), 624–626; (c) Cateni, F.; Zilic, J.; Zacchigna, M.; Bonivento, P.; Frausin, F.; Scarcia, V. *Eur. J. Med. Chem.* 2006, 41, 192–200.

4. Husain, A.; Hasan, S. M.; Lal, S.; Alam, M. M. *Indian J. Pharm. Sci.* 2006, *68*(4), 536–538.

5. For reviews, see: (a) Rao, Y. S. *Chem. Rev.* 1976, *76*, 625–694; (b) Knight, D. W. *Contemp. Org. Synth.* 1994, *1*, 287–315; (c) Collins, I. *J. Chem. Soc. Perkin Trans. 1,* 1999, 1377–1395; (d) Brückner, R. *Curr. Org. Chem.* 2001, *5*, 679–718.

6. Rauter, A. P.; Ferreira, M. J.; Font, J.; Virgili, A.; Figueredo, M.; Figueiredo, J. A.; Ismael, M. I.; Canda, T. L. *J. Carbohydr. Chem.* 1995, *14*, 929–948

7. Justino, J.; Rauter, A. P.; Canda, T.; Wilkins, R.; Matthews, E. *Pest. Manag. Sci.* 2005, *61*, 985–990.

8. Xavier, N. M.; Rauter, A. P. *Carbohydr. Res.* 2008, *343*, 1523–1539.

9. (a) Bennet, M.; Gill, G. B.; Pattenden, G.; Shuker, A. J.; Stapleton, A. *J. Chem. Soc. Perkin Trans. 1* 1991, *1991*, 929–937; (b) Rychlik, M.; Schieberle, P. *J. Agric. Food Chem.* 1998, *46*, 5163–5169.

10. Liu, H.-M.; Zhang, F.; Zhang, J.; Shi, L. *Carbohydr. Res.* 2003, *338*, 1737–1743.

11. (a) Rauter, A.; Ferreira, M.; Duarte, T.; Piedade, F.; Silva, M.; Santos, H. *Carbohydr. Res.* 2000, *325*, 1–15. (b) Rauter, A. P.; Oliveira, O.; Canda, T.; Leroi, E.; Ferreira, H.; Ferreira, M. J.; Ascenso, J. A. *J. Carbohydr. Chem.* 2002, *21*, 257–274.

12. Rauter, A. P.; Figueiredo, J. A.; Ismael, M. I.; Pais, M. S.; Gonzalez, A. G.; Dias, J.; Barrera, J. B. *J. Carbohydr. Chem.* 1987, *6*, 259–272.

13. (a) Tronchet, J. M. J.; Gentile, B. *Carbohydr. Res.* 1975, *44*, 23–35. (b) Tadano, K.; Idogaki, Y.; Yamada, H.; Suami, T. *J. Org. Chem.* 1987, *52*, 1201–1210.

14. (a) Parr, I. B.; Horenstein, B. A. *J. Org. Chem.* 1997, *62*, 7489–7494; (b) Lu, Y.; Just, G. *Tetrahedron* 2001, *57*, 1677–1687.

15. (a) Robins, M. J.; Doboszewski, B.; Timoshchuk, V. A.; Peterson, M. A. *J. Org. Chem.* 2000, *65*, 2939–2945. (b) Martinková, M.; Gonda, J.; Raschmanová, J. *Molecules* 2006, *11*, 564–573.

16 Glycal Dimerization with High Diastereoselectivity

Andreas H. Franz, Paul H. Gross,
and Katja Michael†*

CONTENTS

Experimental Methods 160
  General Methods 160
    General Method for the Dimerization of Glycals 161
    1,3,4,6-Tetra-*O*-Acetyl-2-*C*-(4,6-Di-*O*-Acetyl-2,3-
    Dideoxy-α-D-*Erythro*-Hex-2-Enopyranosyl)-2-Deoxy-α/β-D-
    Glucopyranose (**2a, 2b**) 162
Acknowledgments 164
References 166

Boron trifluoride-catalyzed dimerization of 3,4,6-tri-*O*-acetyl-1,5-anhydro-2-deoxy-D-*ara-bino*-hex-1-enitol (tri-*O*-acetyl glucal) in dichloromethane in the presence of acetic anhydride (0°C to rt, 2 h). (From Franz, A.H. and Gross, P.H., *Carbohydr. Lett.*, 2, 371, 1997.)

The importance of dendritic carbohydrates and polyhydroxyl clusters in biochemical processes such as reaction site recognition, anti-gene/antibody reactions, cell-to-cell communication, and regulatory effects in cell growth and protein assimilation is well established.[2–12] Because of their mimetic characteristics, C-glycosyl compounds have gained appreciable consideration as anticancer and anti-inflammatory drugs.[13,14] Glycals have been used in the synthesis of such C-glycosyl compounds. Ever since Emil Fischer and Karl Zach discovered the glycals in 1913 and published on the subject in the following years,[15–18] this class of carbohydrates has attracted

---

* Corresponding author.
† Checker.

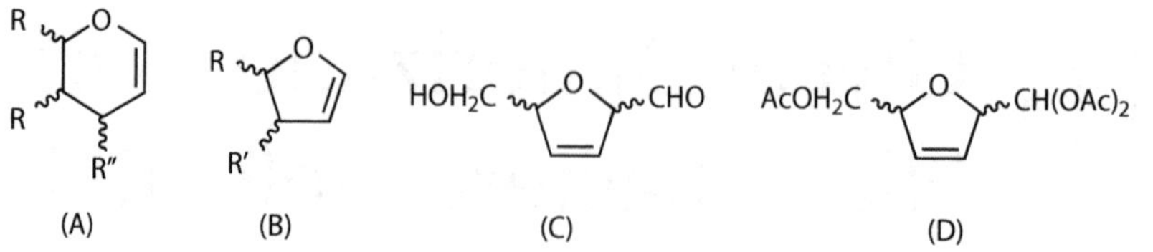

FIGURE 16.1 General structure of glycals (A) and (B). The initial structure proposed for glucal (C) and its per-*O*-acetylated derivative (D) was made tentatively by Emil Fischer based on elemental analysis and a positive Fehling test for (C).

attention of many chemists. Glycals[19] have become very versatile synthons in carbohydrate chemistry, as demonstrated by the assembly of complex oligosaccharides and combinatorial libraries thereof.[20–22] Glycals are 1,5-(or 1,4)-anhydro-2-deoxy-1-enitols, structures-type A and B (Figure 16.1); R, R′, and R″ are most often oxygen functions but can also include branches or deoxy side chains.

Most commonly, *O*-acetylated 1,5-anhydro-2-deoxy-hex-1-enitols are obtained by treatment of per-*O*-acetylated glycosyl halides with zinc in AcOH.[23–27] When Fischer discovered glucal, he initially proposed a dihydrofuran-derived structure with aldehyde functionality because of a positive Fehling test (Figure 16.1C), hence "glycal," and a fully acetylated "methylene diacetate" structure (Figure 16.1D). The early literature shows how inconclusive the structure of glycals remained during Fischer's lifetime.[15–18,23]

By the time it became clear that the positive Fehling test was due to a rearrangement of the double bond with concomitant loss of a molecule of acetic acid and the formation of a reducing hemiacetal, the term "glycal" had already become well established. Later investigations revealed a true aldehyde by-product from ring-opening and subsequent photoisomerization.[28] While working on compound **1**, Ferrier et al.[29–32] found that treatment of this compound with only 0.1 mol% of BF₃·Et₂O in toluene resulted in epimerization at C-3 (Scheme 16.1). The product was a mixture of starting material and 3,4,6-tri-*O*-acetyl-1,5-anhydro-2-deoxy-D-*ribo*-hex-1-enitol. Analogously, 3,4,6-tri-*O*-acetyl-1,5-anhydro-2-deoxy-*lyxo*-hex-1-enitol epimerized partially to 3,4,6-tri-*O*-acetyl-1,5-anhydro-2-deoxy-*xylo*-hex-1-enitol. Acetylated glycals are both vinyl ethers and allylic esters, and can take part in allylic rearrangement reactions (Ferrier rearrangement).[29–34] The resonance-stabilized allylic oxonium electrophile has been used extensively to synthesize O- and S-glycosides, and N- and C-glycosyl compounds. In 1969, Ferrier et al.[32] treated compound **1** in benzene with boron trifluoride and obtained a crystalline dimerization product in 10% yield (Scheme 16.1). Here, we describe an optimized protocol starting from tri-*O*-acetyl-D-glucal, which gives diastereoselectively two (α and β) dimers in the improved, combined yield of 52%–55%. The same procedure has been applied to glycals obtained from D-galactose, L-fucose, D-cellobiose, and D-lactose.[1,35,36]

EXPERIMENTAL METHODS

General Methods

Chemicals, including compound **1**, were purchased from Acros Organics, Part of Thermo Fisher Scientific (Pittsburgh, PA), Aldrich (Milwaukee, WI), Sigma

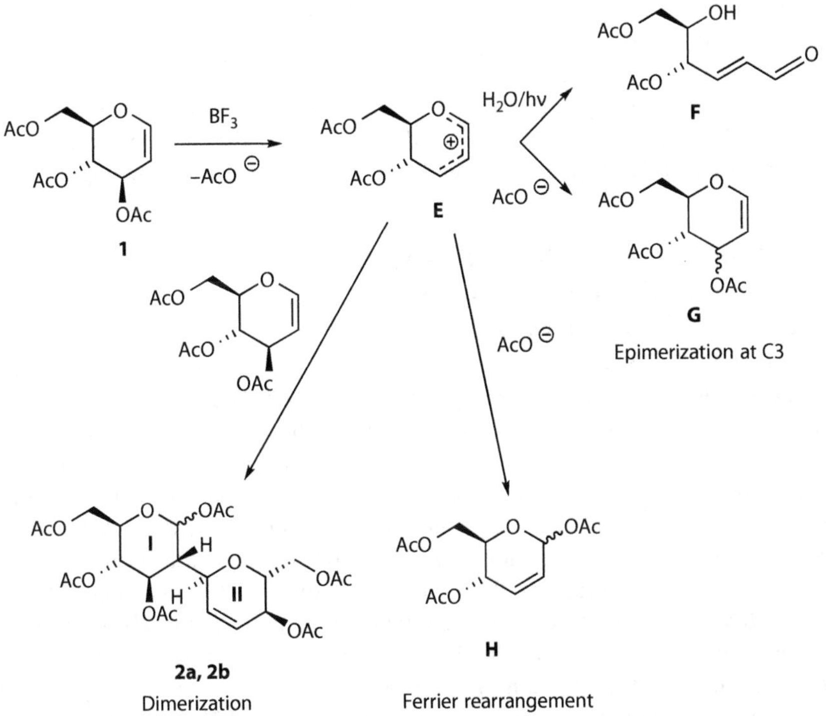

SCHEME 16.1 Chemical transformations of **1**. The resonantly stabilized electrophile (**E**) can lead to ring-opening (**F**), epimerization at C3 (**G**), Ferrier rearrangement (**H**), and dimerization.

(St. Louis, MO), Pfanstiehl (Waukegan, IL), and Lancaster Synthesis, Inc. (Windham, NH) and were used without further purification. Flash chromatography was performed on silica gel from J. T. Baker (40 mm, $r = 0.5$ g/cm^3), or from Natland Int. Corporation (230–400 mesh). Solvents of HPLC grade were used without further purification, unless stated otherwise. TLC was performed on SiO$_2$-coated glass plates (Analtech, Newark, DE) or on SiO$_2$-coated aluminum (EMD Merck). ^{1}H-NMR and ^{13}C-NMR data were acquired with a Varian (Palo Alto, CA) Mercury system at 300 and 75 MHz, respectively. Signals were assigned based on coupling constants and ^{1}H-^{1}H and ^{1}H-^{13}C-COSY (HETCOR) correlations. ^{1}H-NMR data were acquired by the checker with a JEOL ECA-600 NMR spectrometer at 600 MHz. Melting points are uncorrected. Mass spectral data were obtained with an infusion pump in positive and negative atmospheric pressure chemical ionization mode on an LCmate JEOL (Peabody, MD) mass spectrometer, and with electrospray ionization (positive mode) JEOL AccuTOF mass spectrometer (Peabody, MD). Solutions of $c = 100$ nM in MeCN were prepared. A 250 μL syringe was used for continuous injection at a rate of 0.3 mL/h. N$_2$ was used as desolvating gas at a pressure of 700 psi.

General Method for the Dimerization of Glycals

A solution of the glycal (1.0 g) in CH$_2$Cl$_2$ (5 mL) was added to a freshly prepared solution of Ac$_2$O (1.0 equiv.) and BF$_3$·0.5 Et$_2$O (0.1 equiv.) in CH$_2$Cl$_2$ (5 mL), and the mixture was stirred at 0°C for 15 min. The cooling was removed and stirring was continued for 2 h. During this period, the solution reached RT and turned from light yellow to deep purple. Saturated aq. NaHCO$_3$ (2 equiv.) was added to the solution, followed by vigorous stirring for 0.5 h with concomitant change of color to light yellow. Additional CH$_2$Cl$_2$ (20 mL) was added, and the separated organic phase was dried (Na$_2$SO$_4$), concentrated, and the residue was chromatographed as specified.

1,3,4,6-Tetra-O-Acetyl-2-C-(4,6-Di-O-Acetyl-2,3-Dideoxy-α-D-*Erythro*-Hex-2-Enopyranosyl)-2-Deoxy-α/β-D-Glucopyranose (2a, 2b)

Compound **1** (5 g, 18.4 mmol) was treated according to the general procedure to give **2a** and **2b** in an α/β mixture ranging from 1:1 to 1:4. The α/β ratio varies due to small differences of the reaction conditions. When the α/β anomers formed in a 1:1 ratio, the crude reaction mixture was recrystallized from anhydrous methanol, to furnish 1.69 g of a clean 1:1 mixture of **2a** and **2b**. The mother liquor still contained 0.89 g of **2a** and **2b**, which were separated from by-products by flash chromatography on silica (3:5 EtOAc–hexane). The same solvent system was used to separate **2a** and **2b** from each other by flash chromatography. In this reaction, 2.58 g of **2a** and **2b** were obtained (52% yield). When compounds **2a** and **2b** were formed in an α/β ratio of 1:4, some of the β anomer could be recrystallized from anhydrous methanol, and the remaining material was purified by chromatography on silica (3:5 EtOAc–hexane). In this reaction, 2.75 g of **2a** and **2b** were obtained (55% yield). The β-*anomer* (**2b**): Yield, 2.2 g (44%), mp 203°C–204°C (from MeOH); [α]$_D^{20}$ +82.3 (*c* 2, CHCl$_3$). R$_f$ 0.32 (3:5 EtOAc-hexane); R$_f$ 0.13 (1:2:2 EtOAc-hexane-diethyl ether). IR (KBr pellet) [cm^{-1}] 1052, 1220, 1251, 1376, 1438, 1718, 1749, 2958, 2964. ^{13}C-NMR (CDCl$_3$) 20.6, 20.7, 21.0, 47.9, 59.8, 61.8, 63.5, 63.8, 69.5, 69.9, 71.9, 73.7, 91.0, 119.1, 135.7, 168.2, 170.2, 170.4, 170.9, 171.0, 171.2; MALDI-TOF-MS: [M + Na]$^+$ calcd for C$_{24}$H$_{32}$O$_{14}$Na, 567.23; found: 567.24; ESI-TOF-MS: [M + Na]$^+$ calcd 567.1690; found: 567.1728; calcd for [M + K]$^+$ 583.1429; found: 583.1503. Anal. calcd for C$_{24}$H$_{32}$O$_{14}$: C, 52.94%, H 5.92%. Found: C, 52.46%, H 5.96%. *The α-anomer* (**2a**): Yield, 0.55 g (11%), mp 162°C–164°C (from MeOH); [α]$_D^{20}$ +100 (*c* 2, CHCl$_3$). R$_f$ 0.26 (3:5 EtOAc-hexane) R$_f$ 0.10 (1:2:2 EtOAc-hexane-diethyl ether). IR (KBr pellet) [cm^{-1}] 968, 1046, 1078, 1222, 1367, 1432, 1751, 2963. ^{1}H-NMR (CDCl$_3$) δ 1.9–2.0 (6 s, 18H, COCH$_3$), 2.45 (ddd, 1H, $J_{2,1}$ 3.3 Hz, $J_{2,3}$ 11.1 Hz, $J_{2,III}$ 7.5 Hz, H-2^I), ~4.0 (subm, 4H, H-5^I, H-6b^I, H-5^{II}, H-6b^{II}), 4.13 (dd, 1H, $J_{6a,6b}$ 11.7 Hz, $J_{6a,5}$ 7.8 Hz, H-6a^{II}), ~4.3 (subm, 2H, H-6a^I, H-1^{II}), 5.01 (dt ~ s, 1H, $J_{4,3}$ <2 Hz, $J_{4,5}$ <2 Hz, H-4^{II}), 5.04 (t, 1H, $J_{4,3}$ 9.9 Hz, $J_{4,5}$ 9.9 Hz, H-4^I), 5.48 (t, 1H, $J_{3,2}$ 9.6 Hz, $J_{3,4}$ 9.6 Hz, H-3^I), 5.77 (AB-mixing, 1H, H-3^{II}), 5.83 (AB-mixing, 1H, H-2^{II}), 6.34 (d, 1H, $J_{1,2}$ 2.4 Hz, H-1^I); ^{13}C-NMR (CDCl$_3$) 20.5, 20.6, 20.9, 46.1, 61.7, 62.3, 64.4, 68.9, 69.3, 69.4, 70.8, 90.4, 124.6, 130.9, 168.5, 170.0, 170.4, 170.4, 170.8, 171.1; MALDI-TOF-MS: [M + Na]$^+$ calcd for C$_{24}$H$_{32}$O$_{14}$Na, 567.23; found: 567.18; ESI-TOF-MS: [M + Na]$^+$ calcd 567.1690; found: 567.1685; calcd for [M + K]$^+$ 583.1429; found: 583.1549. Anal. calcd for C$_{24}$H$_{32}$O$_{14}$: C, 52.94%, H, 5.92%. Found: C, 52.61%, H, 5.88% (Table 16.1).

TABLE 16.1

Chemical Shifts and Coupling Constants in Different Solvents for Compound 2b (ref. TMS)

	^3J	CDCl$_3$ δ/ppm	CDCl$_3$ ^3J/Hz	[^{2}H$_6$]Acetone δ/ppm	[^{2}H$_6$]Acetone ^3J/Hz	[^{2}H$_5$]Pyridine δ/ppm	[^{2}H$_5$]Pyridine ^3J/Hz	[^{2}H$_6$] DMSO δ/ppm	[^{2}H$_6$] DMSO ^3J/Hz
H-1^I	1^I-2^I	5.85	9.0	5.73	9.0	6.32	9.0	5.82	9.0
H-2^I	2^I-1^I	2.14	9.0	2.09	9.6	2.45	9.0	2.30	9.6
	2^I-3^I		11.1		11.1		10.5		10.5
	2^I-1^{II}		1.8		1.8		1.2		0.9
H-3^I	3^I-2^I	5.38	11.1	5.26	11.4	5.83	10.8	5.30	11.1
	3^I-4^I		9.3		9.0		9.0		9.3
H-4^I	4^I-3^I	4.93	9.9	4.77	9.3	5.37	9.6	4.81	9.9
	4^I-5^I		9.9		9.3		9.6		9.9
H-5^I	5^I-4^I	3.74	10.2	~3.9	—[a]	4.11	10.2	—[a]	—[a]
	5^I-6^I		3.6		—[a]		4.2		—[a]
	5^I-6b^I		2.1		1.5		2.1		—[a]
H-6a^I	6a^I-5^I	4.28	4.2	4.13	6.0	4.56	4.2	—[a]	—[a]
	6a^I-6b^I		12.3		13.0		12.3		—[a]
H-6b^I	6b^I-5^I	3.99	1.8	3.84	2.1	4.31	2.4		—[a]
	6b^I-6a^I		12.6		12.0		12.3		—[a]
H-1^{II}	1^{II}-2^{II}	4.25	<1	4.23	1.8	~4.4	—[a]	—[a]	—[a]
	1^{II}-3^{II}		<1		<1		—[a]		—[a]
	1^{II}-2^I		2.1		1.8		1.2		—[a]
H-2^{II}	2^{II}-1^{II}	5.95	<1	6.00	1.8	6.07	1.2	—[a]	—[a]
	2^{II}-3^{II}		10.5		10.5		10.5		—[a]
	2^{II}-4^{II}		1.5		<1		<1		—[a]
H-3^{II}	3^{II}-1^{II}	~5.8	—[a]	5.76	2.4	5.93	2.4	—[a]	—[a]
	3^{II}-2^{II}		—[a]		9.9		10.5		—[a]
	3^{II}-4^{II}		4.8		5.4		5.7		—[a]
H-4^{II}	4^{II}-2^{II}	4.71	<1	4.66	1.2	4.98	<1	—[a]	—[a]
	4^{II}-3^{II}		5.4		6.0		5.4		—[a]
	4^{II}-5^{II}		<1		1.2		0.9		—[a]
H-5^{II}	5^{II}-4^{II}	4.14	<1	3.99	1.8	—[a]	[a]	—[a]	—[a]
	5^{II}-6a^{II}		9.9		10.5		[a]		—[a]
	5^{II}-6b^{II}		3.6		3.9		[a]		—[a]
H-6a^{II}	6a^{II}-5^{II}	4.43	9.6	4.30	9.6	4.66	9.9	4.31	9.9
	6a^{II}-6b^{II}		12.0		12.0		12.0		12.3
H-6b^{II}	6b^{II}-5^{II}	3.72	3.6	3.75	3.6	3.98	3.6	3.89	3.6
	6b^{II}-6a^{II}		12.0		12.0		12.3		12.3
COCH$_3$		2.0–2.1		1.9–2.1		1.9–2.2		1.9–2.1	

[a] Overlapped.

ACKNOWLEDGMENTS

The authors thank Dr. Vyacheslav V. Samoshin for helpful discussions. This chapter is partially based upon work supported by the National Science Foundation under Grant No. CHE-0840525.

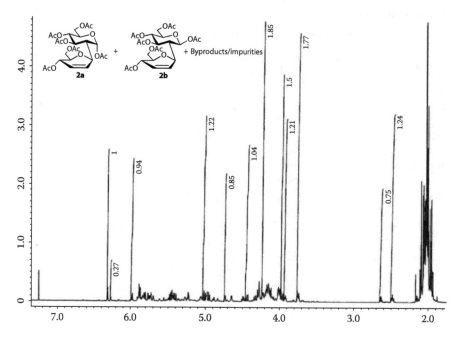

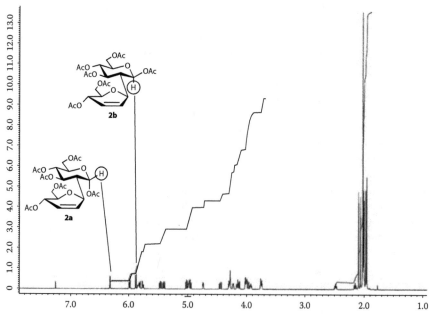

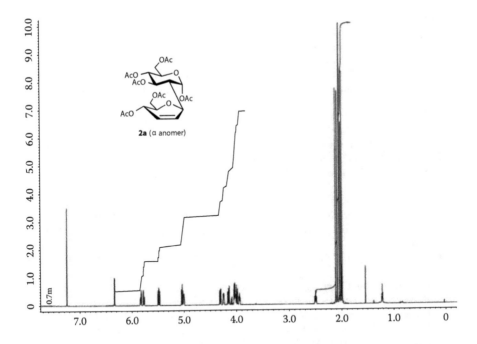

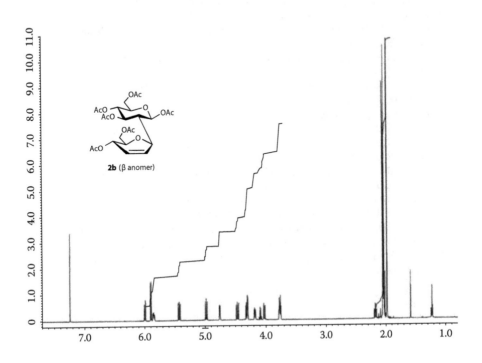

REFERENCES

1. Franz, A. H.; Gross, P. H. *Carbohydr. Lett.*, 1997, *2*, 371–376.
2. Dwek, R. A. *Chem. Rev. (Washington, DC)*, 1996, *96*, 683–720.
3. Mammen, M.; Chio, S.-K.; Whitesides, G. M. *Angew. Chem. Int. Ed.*, 1998, *37*, 2755–2794.
4. Gross, P. H.; Franz, A. H.; Samoshin, V. V. *Recent Res. Dev. Org. Chem.*, 2004, *8*, 255–280.
5. Timmer, M. S. M.; Verhelst, S. H. L.; Grotenbreg, G. M.; Overhand, M.; Overkleeft, H. S. *Pure Appl. Chem.*, 2005, *77*, 1173–1181.
6. Nishida, Y.; Dohi, H.; Kobayashi, K. *Trends Glycosci. Glycotechnol.*, 2005, *17*, 59–69.
7. Murphy, P. V. *Eur. J. Org. Chem.*, 2007, *25*, 4177–4187.
8. Niederhafner, P.; Sebestik, J.; Jezek, J. *J. Pept. Sci.*, 2008, *14*, 2–43.
9. Niederhafner, P.; Sebestik, J.; Jezek, J. *J. Pept. Sci.*, 2008, *14*, 44–65.
10. Niederhafner, P.; Reinis, M.; Sebestik, J.; Jezek, J. *J. Pept. Sci.*, 2008, *14*, 556–587.
11. Imberty, A.; Chabre, Y. M.; Roy, R. *Chem. Eur. J.*, 2008, *14*, 7490–7499.
12. Franz, A. H.; Gross, P. H.; Samoshin, V. V. *ARKIVOC (Gainesville, FL)*, 2008, *1*, 271–308.
13. Levy, D. E.; Tang, C.; Eds. *The Chemistry of C-Glycosides*, Elsevier Science: Oxford, U.K., 1995.
14. Levy, D. E. *Org. Chem. Sugars*, 2006, 269–348.
15. Fischer, E. *Ber. Dtsch. Chem. Ges.*, 1914, *47*, 196–210.
16. Fischer, E.; von Fodor, K. *Ber. Dtsch. Chem. Ges.*, 1914, *47*, 2057–2063.
17. Fischer, E.; Curme, G. O., Jr. *Ber. Dtsch. Chem. Ges.*, 1914, *47*, 2047–2057.
18. Fischer, E.; Bergmann, M.; Schotte, H. *Ber. Dtsch. Chem. Ges.*, 1920, *53B*, 509–547.
19. Roth, W.; Pigman, W. *Methods Carbohydr. Chem.*, 1963, *2*, 405–408.
20. Danishefsky, S. J.; Bilodeau, M. T. *Angew. Chem. Int. Ed. Engl.*, 1996, *35*, 1380–1419.
21. Seeberger, P. H.; Bilodeau, M. T.; Danishefsky, S. J. *Aldrichim. Acta*, 1997, *30*, 75–92.
22. Cirillo, P. F.; Danishefsky, S. J. *Solid Support Oligosaccharide Synth. Comb. Carbohydr. Libr.*, 2001, 15–40.
23. Fischer, E.; Zach, C. *Sitzb. Kgl. Preuss. Akad.*, 1913, *16*, 311–317.
24. Fischer, E. *Ber. Dtsch. Chem. Ges.*, 1916, *49*, 584–585.
25. Lemieux, R. U. *Methods Carbohydr. Chem.*, 1963, *2*, 224–225.
26. Lemieux, R. U. *Methods Carbohydr. Chem.*, 1963, *2*, 223–224.
27. Lemieux, R. U. *Methods Carbohydr. Chem.*, 1963, *2*, 221–222.
28. Fraser-Reid, B.; Radatus, B. *J. Am. Chem. Soc.*, 1970, *92*, 5288–5290.
29. Ferrier, R. J.; Sankey, G. H. *J. Chem. Soc. C*, 1966, 2345–2349.
30. Ferrier, R. J.; Prasad, N. *Chem. Commun.*, 1968, 476–477.
31. Ferrier, R. J.; Prasad, N.; Sankey, G. H. *J. Chem. Soc. C*, 1968, 974–977.
32. Ferrier, R. J.; Prasad, N. *J. Chem. Soc. C*, 1969, 581–586.
33. Ciment, D. M.; Ferrier, R. J. *J. Chem. Soc. Org.*, 1966, 441–445.
34. Ferrier, R. J. *Carbohydr. Chem. Biochem.*, 1980, *1B*, 843–879.
35. Franz, A. H. Dissertation, Oligosaccharide mimics: Synthesis, characterization, and biological properties, University of the Pacific, Stockton, CA, 2000.
36. Franz, A. H.; Wei, Y. Q.; Samoshin, V. V.; Gross, P. H. *J. Org. Chem.*, 2002, *67*, 7662–7669.

17 Regioselective Debenzylation of C-Glycosylpropene

Laura Cipolla, Barbara La Ferla, Amélia Pilar Rauter,[†] and Francesco Nicotra*

CONTENTS

Experimental Methods 168
General Methods 168
General Procedure for Iodocyclization 169
β-Elimination 169
3-*C*-(3,4,6-Tri-*O*-Benzyl-α-D-Glucopyranosyl)Prop-1-Ene (**3**) 169
3-*C*-(3,4,6-Tri-*O*-Benzyl-α-D-Fructofuranosyl)Prop-1-Ene (**6**) 170
Acknowledgment 171
References 173

Reagents and conditions: (a) I_2, dry THF (yield: 81% of **2**, 98% of **5**); (b) Zn, AcOH, 1:1 Et_2O/EtOH (quantitative yield of **3**, 80% of **6**).

---

* Corresponding author.
[†] Checker.

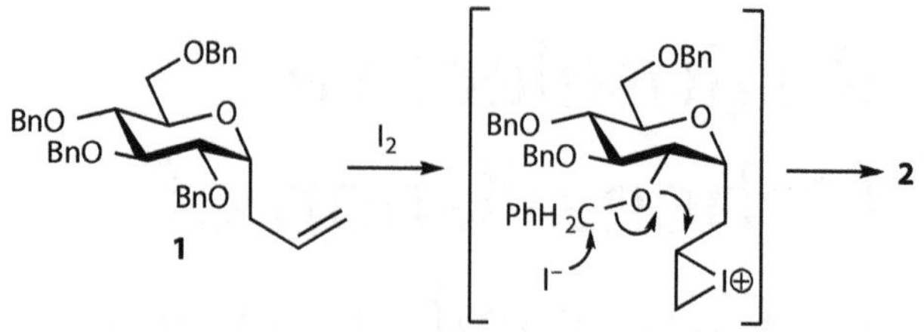

SCHEME 17.1 Mechanism for the iodocyclization/debenzylation reaction.

Analogues of cell surface–associated carbohydrates or inhibitors of carbohydrate-processing enzymes are of great pharmaceutical interest. Therefore, many synthetic efforts have been devoted to mimetics of this class of molecules, such as *C*-glycosyl compounds, which mimic glycosides by replacement of their exocyclic acetalic oxygen with a methylene group. The C–C linkage provides hydrolytic stability without greatly affecting the carbohydrate structure. The *C*-glycosyl scaffolds should be suitably functionalized in order to mimic their natural counterpart. Toward this aim, regioselective deprotection can be useful for the introduction of the required functional groups. Here, we present an easy procedure for the regioselective deprotection of 3-*C*-(2,3,4,6-tetra-*O*-benzyl-α-D-glucopyranosyl)prop-1-ene (**1**)[1] at glycon position 2 and of 3-*C*-(1,3,4,6-tetra-*O*-benzyl-α-D-fructofuranosyl)prop-1-ene (**4**)[2] at glycon position 1, respectively. Reaction of the fully benzylated *C*-glycosylpropene with molecular iodine affords a cyclic iodoether (**2** or **5**), which upon reductive elimination restores the double bond and a free hydroxyl group. The overall process results in regioselective debenzylation, giving products **3** and **6**, respectively. The iodocyclization reaction first involves formation of the iodonium ion, on which the oxygen of the neighboring benzyl ether can act as a nucleophile in a 5-*exo*-type cyclization, with subsequent loss of the benzyl group as benzyl iodide, in an intramolecular process (Scheme 17.1). This regioselective deprotection has been successfully used for the synthesis of a variety of biologically relevant carbohydrate mimetics, such as *C*-glycosyl derivatives of glucosamine and mannosamine,[3] mimics of α- and β-*N*-acetyllactosamine,[4] *N*-acetylgalactosamine,[5] *C*-glycosyl nojirimycins,[6–8] sugar azido acids,[9] fructose-derived scaffolds,[10] and rigid benzodiazepine chimeric scaffolds.[11]

EXPERIMENTAL METHODS

GENERAL METHODS

All solvents were dried over molecular sieves for at least 24 h prior to use. When dry conditions were required, the reaction was performed under Ar atmosphere. Thin-layer chromatography (TLC) was performed on silica gel 60F$_{254}$-coated glass plates (Merck) with UV detection when possible or by charring with 5:45:45 conc. H$_2$SO$_4$/EtOH/H$_2$O. Flash column chromatography was performed on silica gel 230–400 mesh (Merck). Routine ^{1}H and ^{13}C nuclear magnetic resonance (NMR) spectra were recorded at 400 MHz on a Varian Mercury instrument using CDCl$_3$

as solvent. Chemical shifts are reported in parts per million (ppm) downfield from TMS. Optical rotations were measured at room temperature with a Perkin-Elmer 241 polarimeter. Zinc powder was purchased from Sigma-Aldrich and freshly activated by washing with acid as follows. Zn dust was stirred with 5% HCl for 5 min, filtered, and washed three times with distilled water, two times with 95% EtOH, and finally with absolute Et_2O. The material was then dried under vacuum at room temperature (rt). Solutions in organic solvents were dried over Na_2SO_4 and concentrated at reduced pressure.

General Procedure for Iodocyclization*

C-Glycosyl compound (1 mmol) was dissolved in dry THF, and iodine (3 mmol) was added. The reaction mixture was stirred until TLC showed complete consumption of the starting material. The reaction was diluted with H_2O, and solid $Na_2S_2O_3$ was added until the organic phase turned colorless. The mixture was then extracted with AcOEt; and the organic layer was separated, dried (Na_2SO_4), filtered, and concentrated to dryness. The crude residue was purified by flash chromatography, affording a diastereomeric mixture of unseparated cyclic iodoether.

β-Elimination†

Diastereomeric iodoethers (1 mmol) were dissolved in 1:1 Et_2O/EtOH, and dust Zn (10 mmol) and glacial AcOH (2 mmol) were added. After stirring for 24 h, the suspension was filtered through a Celite pad, and the solvent was evaporated. A solution of the residue in CH_2Cl_2 was washed with 5% aqueous HCl, the organic layer was dried, concentrated, and the crude product was chromatographed.

3-C-(3,4,6-Tri-O-Benzyl-α-D-Glucopyranosyl)Prop-1-Ene (3)

To a solution of 1^1 (1.00 g, 1.77 mmol) in dry THF (4 mL) was added iodine (1.3 g, 5.31 mmol) at 0°C, under Ar atmosphere. After 1 h 30 min, when TLC (8:2 petroleum ether–EtOAc) showed that the reaction was complete, workup and chromatography (9:1, petroleum ether–EtOAc) afforded 2 (876 mg, 81%) as a colorless oil (mixture of diastereomers). Yield, 876 mg (81%).

Product 2 (102 mg, 0.17 mmol) was dissolved in a 1:1 mixture of Et_2O–EtOH (2 mL), and powdered zinc (109 mg, 1.66 mmol) was added, followed by glacial acetic acid (19 μL, 0.34 mmol). The suspension was stirred overnight (TLC, 8:2 petroleum ether–EtOAc) and worked up as described previously. Chromatography (8:2 petroleum ether–EtOAc) afforded 3 in theoretical yield, mp 69°C–71°C (Et_2O–petroleum ether); $[\alpha]_D$ +33.3 (c 1, $CHCl_3$); ^1H NMR ($CDCl_3$) δ 7.42–7.28 (m, 15H, Ph-H), 5.95–5.78 (m, 1H, H-2), 5.15 (broad dd, 1H, $J_{2,3a}$ 16.0 Hz, $J_{3a,3b}$ 3.2 Hz, H-3),

---

* Solvents and temperature for the iodocyclization reaction may be changed depending on the substrates. For example 3-C-(2,3,4,6-tetra-O-benzyl-α-D-glucopyranosyl)prop-1-ene (1) gives iodocyclization at room temperature, while the α-anomer reacts at 0°C.

† Zinc powder, freshly activated before use, should be used. The use of old reagent (especially when kept for more than 1 year after activation) results in severely diminished yield.

5.07 (broad dd, 1H, $J_{2,3b}$ 9.6 Hz, $J_{3a,3b}$ 3.2 Hz, H-3b), 4.68–4.46 (m, 6H, OCH_2Ph), 4.11–4.04 (m, 1H, H-5'), 3.93 (ddd, 1H, $J_{1',1a}$ 8.0 Hz, $J_{1',1b}$ 5.8 Hz, $J_{1',2'}$ 3.5 Hz, H-1'), 3.82 (t, 1H, $J_{3',4'}=J_{4',5'}$ 9.3 Hz, H-4'), 3.79 (t, 1H, $J_{3',4'}=J_{2',4'}$ 9.3 Hz, H-3'), 3.76–3.62 (m, 3H, H-2', H-6'), 2.93 (d, 1H, $J_{2,OH}$ 8.0 Hz, OH), 2.53–2.35 (m, 2H, H-1); ^{13}C NMR (CDCl$_3$) δ 139.00, 138.89, 138.15 (3s, C quat. arom.), 135.38 (d, C-2), 129.12–128.23 (m, C arom.), 117.53 (t, C-3), 78.20, 75.47, 74.24, 71.70, 69.75 (5d, C-1', C-2', C-3', C-4', C-5'), 73.90, 73.90, 73.40 (3 t, OCH_2Ph), 68.80 (t, C-6'), 33.92 (t, C-1). Anal. Calcd for C$_{30}$H$_{34}$O$_5$: C, 75.92; H, 7.22. Found: C, 76.08; H, 7.08.

3-C-(3,4,6-Tri-O-Benzyl-α-ᴅ-Fructofuranosyl)Prop-1-Ene (6)

Compound **4**[2] (4.90 g, 8.68 mmol) was dissolved in dry THF (250 mL), and iodine (6.60 g, 26.0 mmol) was added. The mixture was stirred at room temperature and after 1 h (TLC, 9:1 petroleum ether–EtOAc) the reaction was quenched and worked up as described above. The crude residue was chromatographed (8.5:1.5, petroleum ether–EtOAc) to afford the cyclic iodoethers (2'R)-**5** (0.160 g, 0.266 mmol, 56%,) and (2'S)-**5** (0.106 g, 0.177 mmol, 37%,) as clear oils. The isomers were characterized as follows:

(2'R)-5: MS (MALDI-TOF): m/z 623 [M + Na]⁺, 639 [M + K]⁺. C$_{30}$H$_{33}$O$_5$I requires 600.5. $[\alpha]_D^{20}$ = +36.9 (c 1.6, CHCl$_3$). ^{1}H-NMR (400 MHz, CDCl$_3$): δ (ppm) 7.34–7.26 (m, 15H, OCH$_2$*Ph*), 4.59–4.48 (m, 5H, OCH_2Ph), 4.40 (d, 1H, J = 11.6 Hz, OCH_2Ph), 4.25 (d, 1H, J = 10.3, Hz H-1a), 4.18–4.16 (m, 1H, H-5), 4.12–4.06 (m, 1H, H-2'), 3.94 (dd, 1H, J = 3.3, 1.7 Hz, H-4), 3.92 (d, 1H, J = 1.7 Hz, H-3), 3.88 (d, 1H, J = 10.3 Hz, H-1b), 3.58 (dd, 1H, J = 9.9, 5.5 Hz, H-6a), 3.50 (dd, 1H, J = 9.9, 6.6 Hz, H-6b), 3.30–3.18 (m, 2H, H-3'), 2.34 (dd, 1H, J = 12.8, 5.1 Hz, H-1'a), 1.64 (dd, 1H, J = 12.8, 9.9 Hz, H-1'b). ^{13}C-NMR (100.57 MHz, CDCl$_3$): δ (ppm) 92.94 (C-2), 86.80, 83.84, 82.00, 78.31 (C-3, C-4, C-5, C-2'), 74.46, 73.67, 72.06, 71.99, 70.83 (OCH_2Ph, C-1, C-6), 43.68 (C-1'), 10.31 (C-3'). C$_{30}$H$_{33}$IO$_5$: C, 60.00; H, 5.54; found: C, 60.12; H, 5.58.

(2'S)-5: MS (MALDI-TOF): m/z 623 [M + Na]⁺, 639 [M + K]⁺. C$_{30}$H$_{33}$O$_5$I requires 600.5. $[\alpha]_D^{20}$ = +24.7 (c 1.2, CHCl$_3$). ^{1}H-NMR (400 MHz, CDCl$_3$): δ (ppm) 7.34–7.26 (m, 15H, OCH$_2$*Ph*), 4.68-4.47 (m, 5H, OCH_2Ph), 4.38 (d, 1H, J = 12.1 Hz, OCH_2Ph), 4.23–4.12 (m, 2H, H-5, H-2'), 4.11 (d, 1H, J = 10.3 Hz, H-1a), 4.03 (d, 1H, J = 10.3 Hz, H-1b), 3.96 (dd, 1H, J = 3.4, 1.5 Hz, H-4), 3.84 (d, 1H, J = 1.5 Hz, H-3), 3.58 (dd, 1H, J = 10.0, 5.4 Hz, H-6a), 3.48 (dd, 1H, J = 10.0, 6.5 Hz, H-6b), 3.34–3.22 (m, 2H, H-3'), 2.25 (dd, 1H, J = 9.9, 7.4 Hz, H-1'a), 2.06 (dd, 1H, J = 9.9, 5.1 Hz, H-1'b). ^{13}C-NMR (100.57 MHz, CDCl$_3$): δ (ppm) 91.96 (C-2), 86.59, 83.82, 81.91, 79.54 (C-3, C-4, C-5, C-2'), 73.46, 73.37, 71.75, 71.58, 70.30 (OCH_2Ph, C-1, C-6), 41.99 (C-1'), 9.33 (C-3'). C$_{30}$H$_{33}$IO$_5$: C, 60.00; H, 5.54; found: C, 60.14; H, 5.55.

A mixture of the iodoethers **5** (1.48 g, 2.62 mmol) was dissolved in 1:1 Et$_2$O–EtOH (30 mL), and dust Zn (1.49 g, 22.8 mmol) and AcOH (0.26 mL) were added. The suspension was stirred overnight (TLC, 8:2 petroleum ether–EtOAc) and treated as described above in the General Procedure. The crude product was chromatographed (8:2, petroleum ether–EtOAc) to afford alcohol **6** (0.90 g, 80%) as colorless oil. Yield, 0.90 g (80%). MS (MALDI-TOF): m/z 498 [M + Na]⁺, 514

$[M + K]^+$. $C_{30}H_{34}O_5$ requires 474.6. $[\alpha]_D$ +12.9 (*c* 1.6, $CHCl_3$); ^1H NMR ($CDCl_3$) δ 7.38–7.20 (m, 15H, Ph-H), 5.83–5.71 (m, 1H, H-2), 5.09 (d1 H, 10.3 Hz, H-3a), 4.97 (dd, 1H; $J_{2,3b}$ 17.2, H-3b), 4.72–4.46 (m, 6H; PhC*H*$_2$O), 4.45 (t, 1H, $J_{3',4'}=J_{4',5'}$ 7.3 Hz, H-4′), 4.12 (d, 1H; $J_{3',4'}$ 7.3 Hz, H-3′), 3.92 (td, 1H, $J_{5',6'a}=J_{4',5'}$ 7.3 Hz, $J_{5',6'b}$ 3.2 Hz, H-5′), 3.72–3.64 (m, 2H, H-1′a, H-6′a), 3.52–3.46 (m, 2H, H-1′b, H-6′b), 2.30 (dd, 1H, $J_{1a,1b}$ 13.9 Hz, $J_{1a,2}$ 6.2 Hz, H-1a), 2.18 (dd, $J_{1a,1b}$ 13.9 Hz, $J_{1b,2}$ 8.0 Hz, 1H; H-1b), 1.60 (br s, 1H; OH); ^{13}C NMR ($CDCl_3$) δ 138.21, 138.08, 137.63 (3s, C quat. arom.), 132.98 (d, C-2), 128.80–127.00 (m, C arom.), 119.12 (t, C-3), 84.33 (s, C-2′), 86.71, 83.56, 79.40 (3d, C-3′, C-4′, C-5′), 73.70, 73.23, 73.21, 69.71, 66.43 (5 t; C-1′, C-6′, PhC*H*$_2$O), 40.41 (t; C-1); Anal. Calcd for $C_{30}H_{34}O_5$: C 75.92, H 7.22. Found: C 76.03, H 7.25.

ACKNOWLEDGMENT

We gratefully acknowledge Consorzio Interuniversitario Nazionale "Metodologie E Processi Innovativi Di Sintesi" (CINMPIS) for the financial support.

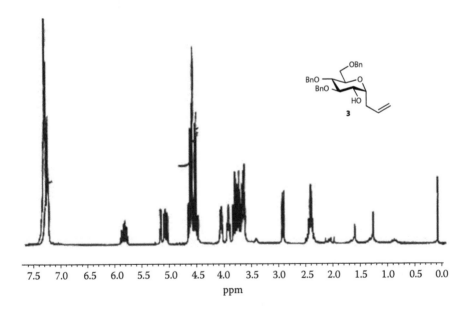

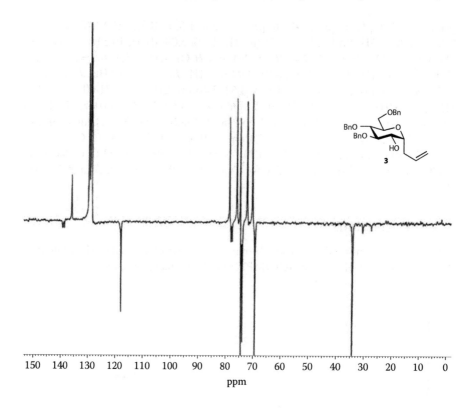

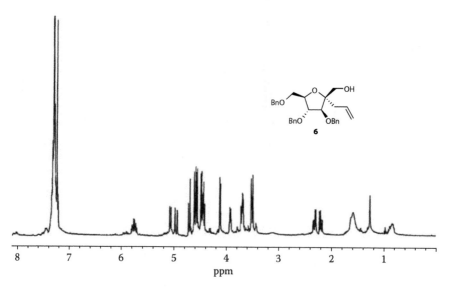

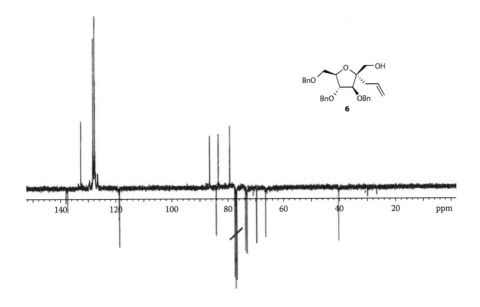

REFERENCES

1. Lewis, M. D.; Kun Cha, J.; Kishi, Y. *J. Am. Chem. Soc.*, 1982, *104*, 4976–4978.
2. Nicotra, F.; Panza, L.; Russo, G. *J. Org. Chem.*, 1987, *52*, 5627–5629.
3. Cipolla, L.; Lay, L.; Nicotra, F. *J. Org. Chem.*, 1997, *62*, 6678–6681.
4. Lay, L.; Cipolla, L.; La Ferla, B.; Peri, F.; Nicotra, F. *Eur. J. Org. Chem.*, 1999, 3437–3440.
5. Cipolla, L.; La Ferla, B.; Lay, L.; Peri, F.; Nicotra, F. *Tetrahedron Asymm.*, 2000, *11*, 295–303.
6. Cipolla, L.; La Ferla, B.; Peri, F.; Nicotra, F. *Chem. Commun.*, 2000, 1289–1290.
7. Cipolla, L.; Palma, A.; La Ferla, B.; Nicotra, F. *J. Chem. Soc. Perkin Trans.*, *1*, 2002, 2161–2165.
8. Cipolla, L.; Reis Fernandes, M.; Gregori, M.; Airoldi, C.; Nicotra, F. *Carbohydr. Res.*, 2007, 342, 1813–1830.
9. Peri, F.; Cipolla, L.; La Ferla, B.; Nicotra, F. *Chem. Commun.*, 2000, 2303–2304.
10. Cipolla, L.; Forni, E.; Jiménez-Barbero, J.; Nicotra, F. *Chem. Eur. J.*, 2002, *8*, 3976–3983.
11. Araújo, A. C.; Nicotra, F.; Airoldi, C.; Costa, B.; Giagnoni, G.; Fumagalli, P.; Cipolla, L. *Eur. J. Org. Chem.*, 2008, 635–639.

18 Synthesis of Azido-Functionalized Carbohydrates for the Design of Glycoconjugates

Samy Cecioni, Mehdi Almant,[†]
Jean-Pierre Praly, and Sébastien Vidal*

CONTENTS

Experimental Methods 176
  General Methods 176
    General Procedure for Glycosylation 177
    1-Azido-3,6-Dioxaoct-8-yl 2,3,4,6-Tetra-*O*-Acetyl-β-D-
    Galactopyranoside **2** 177
    1-Azido-3,6-Dioxaoct-8-yl 2,3,6,2′,3′,4′,6′-Hepta-*O*-Acetyl-β-
    Lactoside **4** 178
Acknowledgments 178
References 180

Reagents and conditions: (a) SnCl$_4$, CF$_3$CO$_2$Ag, H(OCH$_2$CH$_2$)$_3$Cl, CH$_2$Cl$_2$, rt, 2–3 h; (b) NaN$_3$, *n*Bu$_4$NI, DMF, 70°C, 16 h.

---

* Corresponding author.
[†] Checker.

Carbohydrate–protein interactions are among the most important biological processes taking place in Nature and are involved in numerous normal and pathological phenomena such as cell–cell communication, viral infection, cancer metastasis, or even fecundation.[1] While the interaction of a monovalent saccharide is typically weak, with K_d values in the millimolar range, highly specific and strong avidities are reached when multiple carbohydrate epitopes on the surface of a glycoprotein are not localized randomly but are presented for a multivalent interaction with a lectin in the form of clusters, hence the so-called "cluster effect."[2] Over the past decades, to better understand the function(s) of carbohydrate–lectin interactions or as putative therapeutic alternatives, chemists have developed several approaches for the design of multivalent neoglycoconjugates, such as glycoclusters,[3] glycodendrimers,[4] glycopolymers,[5] or glyconanoparticles.[6]

1,3-Dipolar cycloaddition of an alkyne and an azide catalyzed by Cu(I) has recently emerged as a powerful technique[7] for the chemical ligation of carbohydrate probes to synthetic multivalent scaffolds.[8] This conjugation requires the synthesis of azido-functionalized carbohydrate derivatives with the azido moiety attached either directly at the anomeric center providing N-glycosyl-heterocycles or connected through a linker to the saccharide. We have developed a powerful methodology for the synthesis of multivalent glycoconjugates using ω-azido-triethyleneglycol glycosides, such as **2** or **4**, which can be readily prepared in a two-step procedure from the corresponding peracetylated carbohydrates.

Diethylene and triethylene glycol glycosides were first prepared by Szurmai et al.[9] by Hg(CN)$_2$-promoted Koenigs–Knorr glycosylation from the corresponding acetobromo-glycoses. A similar approach was reported later by Wang et al.[10,11] but using BF$_3$·Et$_2$O as a promoter. However, we were not able to reproduce the high yields of the desired compounds reported and have always obtained mixtures of anomers with the concomitant orthoester when Koenigs–Knorr conditions were applied. We have recently applied the glycosylation protocol involving peracetylated carbohydrates in combination with SnCl$_4$ and silver trifluoroacetate (CF$_3$CO$_2$Ag) for the large-scale synthesis (typically 5 g and up to 20 g) of ω-azido-triethyleneglycol glycosides and obtained reproducibly the desired 1,2-trans glycosides in short reaction times (typically 2–3 h) and high yields.

EXPERIMENTAL METHODS

GENERAL METHODS

All reagents were from commercial sources and were used without further purification. Dichloromethane was distilled over CaH$_2$. DMF was purchased from Fluka. All reactions were performed under argon. Thin-layer chromatography (TLC) was carried out on aluminum sheets coated with silica gel 60 F$_{254}$ (Merck). Spots were visualized by UV light ($\lambda = 254$ nm) and by charring with 10% H$_2$SO$_4$ in EtOH/H$_2$O (9:1 v/v). Preparative chromatography was performed with Geduran® silica gel Si 60 (40–63 μm) purchased from Merck (Darmstadt, Germany). 2-[2-(2-Chloroethoxy)ethoxy]ethanol was purchased from Aldrich; SnCl$_4$ (1M solution in CH$_2$Cl$_2$) and silver trifluoroacetate were purchased from Acros Organics. ^{1}H and ^{13}C nuclear magnetic resonance (NMR) spectra were recorded at 298 K using a Bruker Avance DRX300 spectrometer at 300 MHz with the residual solvent as the internal standard (CHCl$_3$ at 7.26 ppm for ^{1}H and 77.0 for ^{13}C). 1,2,3,4,6-Penta-O-acetyl-β-D-galactopyranose was purchased from Carbosynth. With 1,2,3,6,2′,3′,4′,6′-octa-O-acetyl-lactose, the best results were obtained with the per-O-acetate containing the β-anomer as the major isomer, as it is often the case with the product of acetylation with acetic anhydride and anhydrous AcONa.[12,13] Solutions in organic solvents were dried with anhydrous Na$_2$SO$_4$ and concentrated at reduced pressure at 30°C–35°C.

General Procedure for Glycosylation

SnCl$_4$ (1 M in CH$_2$Cl$_2$, 38.4 mL, 38.4 mmol) was added dropwise (within 30 min) at room temperature (rt) to a stirred solution of **1** (5 g, 12.8 mmol), silver trifluoroacetate (4.24 g, 19.2 mmol), and 2-[2-(2-chloroethoxy)ethoxy]ethanol (2.80 mL, 19.2 mmol) in freshly distilled dichloromethane (120 mL). Disappearance of the starting material was observed within 1–3 h, occasionally with the mixture becoming pale pink. Saturated aqueous NaHCO$_3$ (100 mL) was added to adjust pH to >8, and the solution was vigorously stirred for 20 min. A biphasic system formed upon addition of aqueous NaHCO$_3$ with a white suspension in the aqueous layer above the clear CH$_2$Cl$_2$ phase. The biphasic solution was diluted with 500 mL of water and the aqueous layer was extracted with CH$_2$Cl$_2$ (3 × 150 mL).* The organic layers were combined, washed successively with saturated aqueous NaHCO$_3$ (150 mL), water (3 × 150 mL), and brine (2 × 150 mL), and dried (Na$_2$SO$_4$). After concentration, a solution of the crude product (pale yellow gum) was dissolved in anhydrous DMF (150 mL), sodium azide[†] (4.16 g, 64.0 mmol) and tetra-n-butyl ammonium iodide (4.73 g, 12.8 mmol) was added, and the mixture was stirred at 70°C under argon for 16 h.[‡] The mixture was cooled to rt, filtered, and the solid was washed with EtOAc (3 × 100 mL). The filtrate was diluted with EtOAc to reach a total volume of 1 L. The organic layer was washed with aq. NaHCO$_3$ (3 × 300 mL), water (3 × 500 mL), and brine (400 mL) and dried. After concentration, the residue (yellow to orange gum) was chromatographed (internal diameter = 45 mm; length = 250–300 mm) to afford the corresponding azido-functionalized glycosides as colorless gums.

1-Azido-3,6-Dioxaoct-8-yl 2,3,4,6-Tetra-O-Acetyl-β-D-Galactopyranoside 2[9]

Obtained from 1,2,3,4,6-tetra-O-acetyl-β-D-galactopyranose **1** (5 g) according to the general procedure and purified by silica gel column chromatography (isocratic: PE/EtOAc 1:1 v/v).

---

* The solid present in the suspension may be filtered through a bed of Celite for small scale syntheses (>1 g).

† *CAUTION: Sodium azide*, when inhaled, is highly toxic and may cause *death* (MSDS J.T. Baker). Precautions must be taken when weighing the material such as using a powder mask and a *teflon spatula* (metallic spatula may cause explosion). The azidation reaction was performed behind a plastic shield due to the potential explosion. DMF is used as a polar solvent favoring the reaction but also to maintain a basic pH (>8) of the solution. In acidic pH, *hydrazoic acid* (HN$_3$) may be formed, which may explode and/or, when inhaled, may cause intoxication, damage of the central nervous system, and blood pressure effects.

‡ TLC analyses did not show a significant difference between the polarities of the chlorinated precursors and the azido compounds.

Yield, 3.88 g (60%). R_f=0.34 (1:1 PE–EtOAc). ^{1}H NMR (CDCl$_3$) δ 1.99, 2.04, 2.07, 2.15 (4s, 4×3H, 4×CH_3CO), 3.40 (t, 2H, J=5.0 Hz, CH_2N$_3$), 3.60–3.82 (m, 9H, OCH_2), 3.88–4.02 (m, 2H, OCH_2, H-5), 4.08–4.20 (m, 1H, H-6, H-6′), 4.59 (d, 1H, $J_{1,2}$=7.9 Hz, H-1), 5.02 (dd, 1H, $J_{3,4}$=3.4 Hz, $J_{3,2}$=10.5 Hz, H-3), 5.21 (dd, 1H, $J_{2,1}$=7.9 Hz, $J_{2,3}$=10.5 Hz, H-2), 5.39 (dd, 1H, $J_{4,5}$=0.7 Hz, $J_{4,3}$=3.4 Hz, H-4). ^{13}C NMR (CDCl$_3$) δ 20.3, 20.4, 20.4, 20.5 (4s, 4×CH$_3$CO), 50.4 (CH$_2$N$_3$), 61.0 (C-6), 66.8 (C-4), 68.5 (C-2), 68.8, 69.8, 70.1 (3s, 3×CH$_2$O), 70.4 (C-3), 70.4, 70.5 (2s, 2×CH$_2$O), 70.6 (C-5), 101.1 (C-1), 169.2, 169.9, 170.0, 170.1 (4s, 4×CH$_3$CO).

1-Azido-3,6-Dioxaoct-8-yl 2,3,6,2′,3′,4′,6′-Hepta-O-Acetyl-β-Lactoside 4[11]

Obtained from 1,2,3,6,2′,3′,4′,6′-octa-O-acetyl-β-lactose **3** (5 g) according to the general procedure and purified by silica gel column chromatography (Gradient: 7:3 → 2:3 PE–EtOAc with 10% increase every 400 mL).

Yield, 3.73 g (62%). R_f=0.26 (1:1 PE–EtOAc). ^{1}H NMR (CDCl$_3$) δ 1.94, 2.02, 2.04, 2.10, 2.13 (5s, 21H, CH_3CO), 3.37 (t, 2H, J=6.0 Hz, CH_2N$_3$), 3.57–4.15 (m, 16H), 4.42–4.48 (m, 2H), 4.59 (d, 1H, J=7.9 Hz), 4.87 (dd, 1H, J=8.7 Hz, J=8.9 Hz), 4.93 (dd, 1H, J=2.8 Hz, J=8.7 Hz), 5.09 (dd, 1H, J=8.0 Hz, J=11.5 Hz), 5.17 (t, 1H, J=11.5 Hz), 5.31–5.33 (m, 1H).

ACKNOWLEDGMENTS

The authors thank the University Claude Bernard Lyon 1 and the CNRS for financial support. S.C. thanks the Région Rhône-Alpes (Cluster de Recherche Chimie) and the CNRS (Programme Interdisciplinaire: Chimie pour le Développement Durable) for additional funding.

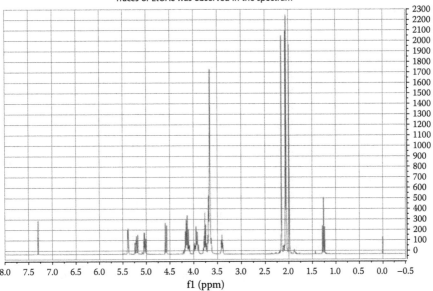

¹H NMR (CDCl₃, 300 MHz, 298 K)

2

Traces of EtOAc was observed in the spectrum

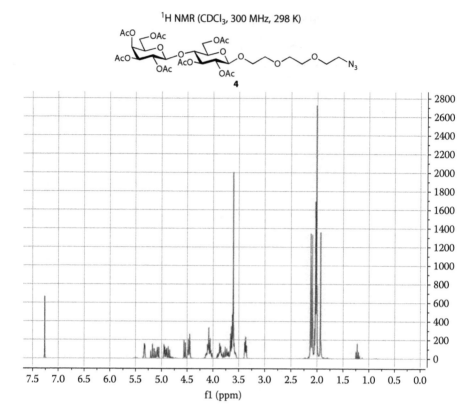

^{1}H NMR (CDCl$_3$, 300 MHz, 298 K)

REFERENCES

1. (a) Dwek, R. A. *Chem. Rev.* 1996, *96*, 683–720. (b) Varki, A.; Cummings, R.; Esko, J.; Freeze, H.; Hart, G. W.; Marth, J. *Essentials of Glycobiology*; Cold Spring Harbor Laboratory Press: New York, 1999.
2. (a) Lundquist, J. J.; Toone, E. J. *Chem. Rev.* 2002, *102*, 555–578. (b) Mammen, M.; Choi, S.-K.; Whitesides, G. M. *Angew. Chem. Int. Ed.* 1998, *37*, 2754–2794.
3. Imberty, A.; Chabre, Y. M.; Roy, R. *Chem. Eur. J.* 2008, *14*, 7490–7499.
4. Cloninger, M. J. *Curr. Opin. Chem. Biol.* 2002, *6*, 742–748.
5. Flitsch, S. L. *Curr. Opin. Chem. Biol.* 2000, *4*, 619–625.
6. de la Fuente, J. M.; Penadés, S. *Biochim. Biophys. Acta* 2006, *1760*, 636–651.
7. (a) Rostovtsev, V. V.; Green, L. G.; Fokin, V. V.; Sharpless, K. B. *Angew. Chem. Int. Ed.* 2002, *41*, 2596–2599. (b) Meldal, M.; Tornoe, C. W. *Chem. Rev.* 2008, *108*, 2952–3015.
8. Dondoni, A. *Chem. Asian J.* 2007, *2*, 700–708.
9. Szurmai, Z.; Szabó, L.; Lipták, A. *Acta Chim. Hung.* 1989, *126*, 259–269.
10. Wang, J.; Zhang, B.; Fang, J.; Sujino, K.; Li, H.; Otter, A.; Hindsgaul, O.; Palcic, M. M.; Wang, P. G. *J. Carbohydr. Chem.* 2003, *22*, 347–376.
11. Li, J.; Zacharek, S.; Chen, X.; Wang, J.; Zhang, W.; Janczuk, A.; Wang, P. G. *Bioorg. Med. Chem.* 1999, *7*, 1549–1558.
12. Wolfrom, M. L.; Thompson, A. *Methods Carbohydr. Chem.* 1963, *1*, 211–215.
13. Hou, S-j.; Kováč, P. *Eur. J. Org. Chem.* 2008, 1947–1952.

19 Synthesis of Thioglycosides and Thioimidates from Glycosyl Halides

Archana R. Parameswar, Daniel Mueller, Lin Liu,[†]
Cristina De Meo, and Alexei V. Demchenko*

CONTENTS

Experimental Methods 182
    1,3-Benzoxazol-2-yl 2,3,4,6-Tetra-*O*-Acetyl-1-Thio-β-D-
    Glucopyranoside (**3**) 182
    Methyl (Phenyl 5-Acetamido-4,7,8,9-Tetra-*O*-Acetyl-3,5-Dideoxy-2-Thio-
    D-*Glycero*-α-D-*Galacto*-Non-2-Ulopyranosid)onate (**6**) 183
Acknowledgments 183
References 185

* Corresponding author.
[†] Checker.

Thioglycosides[1–4] and thioimidates[5] are common glycosyl donors used in chemical glycosylation[6] and important building blocks used for oligosaccharide synthesis.[7]

This contribution describes syntheses of 1,3-benzoxazol-2-yl 2,3,4,6-tetra-O-acetyl-1-thio-β-D-glucopyranoside (**3**) from 1,2,3,4,6-penta-O-acetyl-β-D-glucopyranose (**1**) via 2,3,4,6-tetra-O-acetyl-β-D-glucopyranosyl bromide (**2**) in the presence of potassium carbonate[8] and methyl (phenyl 5-acetamido-4,7,8,9-tetra-O-acetyl-3,5-dideoxy-2-thio-D-*glycero*-α-D-*galacto*-non-2-ulopyranosid)onate (methyl thiosialoside, **6**) from methyl (5-acetamido-2,4,7,8,9-penta-O-acetyl-3,5-dideoxy-D-*glycero*-D-*galacto*-non-2-ulopyranos)onate (sialic acid peracetate, **4**) via methyl (5-acetamido-4,7,8,9-tetra-O-acetyl-3,5-dideoxy-D-*glycero*-β-D-*galacto*-non-2-ulopyranosyl)onate (sialyl chloride, **5**) in the presence of diisopropylethylamine (DIPEA).[9,10]

EXPERIMENTAL METHODS

For **General methods**, see the succeeding contribution Chapter 20 from this laboratory. 2-sulfanylbenzoxazole was purchased from Aldrich and used without further purification.

1,3-Benzoxazol-2-yl 2,3,4,6-Tetra-O-Acetyl-1-Thio-β-D-Glucopyranoside (3)

HBr (30% v/v) in glacial AcOH (5.0 mL) was added to a stirred solution of glucose pentaacetate **1** (5.0 g, 12.6 mmol) in anhydrous CH_2Cl_2 (8 mL). When the reaction was complete (thin-layer chromatography [TLC], ~2 h), the mixture was diluted with CH_2Cl_2 (50 mL) and was washed successively with ice-cold water (20 mL), ice-cold sat. aq. $NaHCO_3$ (2 × 20 mL), and ice-cold water (3 × 20 mL).* The organic layer was separated, dried, filtered, and concentrated at room temperature (rt), and crystallization from dry ether-hexanes afforded 2,3,4,6-tetra-O-acetyl-α-D-glucopyranosyl bromide **2**[11] (3.56 g, 68%), mp 90°C–91°C (ether-hexanes); Ref. [12] mp 89°C–91°C.

A mixture of 2-sulfanylbenzoxazole (0.22 g, 1.5 mmol) and K_2CO_3 (0.2 g, 1.5 mmol) in dry acetone (7 mL) was stirred at 60°C for 4 h. The heating was removed, and a solution of freshly prepared bromide **2** (0.5 g, 1.2 mmol) in dry toluene (5 mL) was added dropwise. The resulting reaction mixture was stirred at rt for ~5 h (TLC). Toluene (30 mL) was added and the mixture was washed successively with 1% aq. NaOH (2 × 15 mL), sat. aq. $NaHCO_3$ (15 mL), and water (3 × 15 mL). The organic layer was separated, dried, filtered, and concentrated; and chromatography (hexane–EtOAc, gradient, starting with 10% EtOAc) gave the title compound **3** (0.55 g, 94%). Analytical data for **3**: $R_f = 0.33$ (2:3 ethyl acetate–hexanes); mp 98°C–100°C (Et_2O–hexanes); $[\alpha]_D^{25}$ −0.43° (*c* 1, $CHCl_3$); ^1H NMR ($CDCl_3$): δ, 2.00, 2.01, 2.02,

---

* Caution! Remaining acid can react violently with $NaHCO_3$ and the separatory funnel must be frequently depressurized.

2.02 (4 s, 12H, 4×–COCH$_3$), 3.88 (m, 1H, $J_{5,6a}$ 4.8 Hz, $J_{5,6b}$ 2.2 Hz, H-5), 4.07 (dd, 1H, H-6b), 4.22 (dd, 1H, $J_{6a,6b}$ 12.5 Hz, H-6a), 5.11 (dd, 1H, $J_{4,5}$ 9.2 Hz, H-4), 5.18 (dd, 1H, $J_{2,3}$ 9.2 Hz, H-2), 5.30 (dd, 1H, $J_{3,4}$ 9.2 Hz, H-3), 5.63 (d, 1H, $J_{1,2}$ 10.3 Hz, H-1), 7.21–7.63 (m, 4H, aromatic) ppm; ^{13}C NMR (CDCl$_3$): δ, 20.7 (×3), 20.8, 61.8, 68.1, 69.8, 73.8, 76.5, 83.6, 110.3, 119.1 (×2), 124.7, 124.8, 141.7, 152.1, 161.0, 169.5, 169.6, 170.2, 170.7 ppm; HR-FAB MS [M+H]$^+$ calcd for C$_{21}$H$_{24}$NO$_{10}$S 482.1121; found: 482.1117. Anal. calcd for C$_{21}$H$_{24}$NO$_{10}$S: C, 52.39; H, 4.81; N, 2.91. Found: C, 52.23; H, 4.74; N, 2.92.

METHYL (PHENYL 5-ACETAMIDO-4,7,8,9-TETRA-*O*-ACETYL-3,5-DIDEOXY-2-THIO-D-*GLYCERO*-α-D-*GALACTO*-NON-2-ULOPYRANOSID)ONATE (6)

Methyl   (5-acetamido-2,4,7,8,9-penta-*O*-acetyl-3,5-dideoxy-D-*glycero*-D-*galacto*-non-2-ulopyranos)onate 4^{13} (100 mg, 0.188 mmol) was dissolved in acetyl chloride (1.2 mL) under argon. The solution was cooled to 0°C, methanol (0.06 mL) was added dropwise and the mixture was stirred at rt until TLC showed that the reaction was complete (~2 h). The mixture was concentrated and dried at rt in vacuo for 1 h. The residue containing crude methyl (5-acetamido-4,7,8,9-tetra-*O*-acetyl-3,5-dideoxy-D-glycero-D-galacto-2-nonulopyranosyl chloride)onate 5 (~90 mg) was dissolved in anhydrous CH$_2$Cl$_2$ (0.94 mL) and thiophenol (29 μL, 0.28 mmol) was added with stirring under argon at rt, followed by the dropwise addition of *N,N*-diisopropylethylamine (DIPEA, 46 μL, 0.28 mmol). The mixture was stirred at rt overnight until TLC showed that the reaction was complete. After concentration, chromatography (hexane–EtOAc, gradient, starting with 10% EtOAc) afforded the title compound 6 (86 mg, 79%). Analytical data for 6: R_f = 0.32 (2:3 acetone–toluene); mp 142°C–144°C (toluene-hexanes); Ref. [9] mp 139°C–140°C (from benzene-hexanes); $[\alpha]_D^{24}$ +19° (*c* 1, CHCl$_3$); Ref. [9] $[\alpha]_D$ +21° (*c* 0.9, CHCl$_3$); ^{1}H NMR (CDCl$_3$): δ 1.78, 1.94, 1.97, 1.98 (4 s, 12H, 4×–COCH$_3$), 2.06 (s, 1H, H-3a). 2.73 (ddd, $J_{3e,4}$ 4.6 Hz, H-3e), 3.49 (s, 3H, –OCH$_3$), 3.89 (dd, $J_{6,7}$ 4.6 Hz, H-6), 3.97 (dd, $J_{5,6}$ 10.2 Hz, H-5), 4.14 (ddd, $J_{8,9b}$ 5.6 Hz, H-9b), 4.32 (ddd, $J_{9a,9b}$ 10.2 Hz, H-9a), 4.81 (ddd, 1H, $J_{4,5}$ 10.3 Hz, H-4), 5.16–5.25 (m, 2H, H-7.8), 5.49 (d, 1H, $J_{5,NH}$ 9.8 Hz, –NH), 7.20–7.45 (m, 5H, aromatic) ppm; ^{13}C NMR (CDCl$_3$): δ, 20.8, 20.9 (×2), 21.1, 23.2, 38.2, 49.2, 52.8, 62.2, 67.9, 69.8, 70.2, 74.9, 87.6, 128.7, 128.9 (×2), 130.0, 136.6 (×2), 168.0, 170.1, 170.2, 170.3, 170.8, 171.0 ppm; HR-FAB MS [M+Na]$^+$ calcd for C$_{26}$H$_{33}$NO$_{12}$SNa 606.1621; found: 606.1622. Anal. calcd for C$_{26}$H$_{33}$NO$_{12}$S: C, 53.51; H, 5.70; N, 2.40. Found: C, 53.59; H, 5.68; N, 2.36.

ACKNOWLEDGMENTS

The chapter was supported by NSF-CAREER Award (CHE-0547566) awarded to A.V.D., Research Corporation-Cottrell College Science Award (CC6776) and SIUE Summer Research Fellowship awarded to C.D.M.

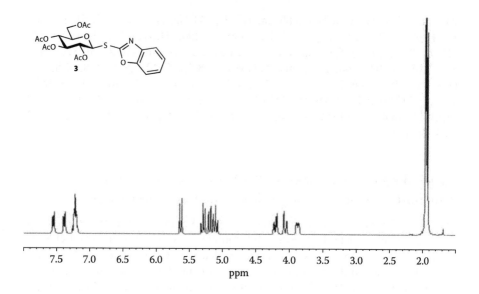

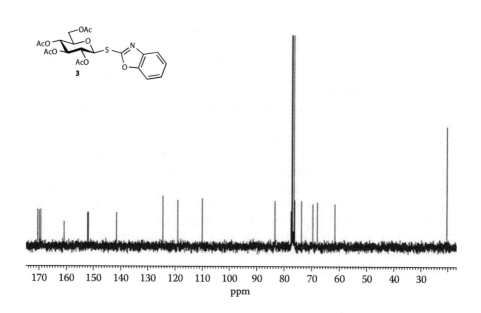

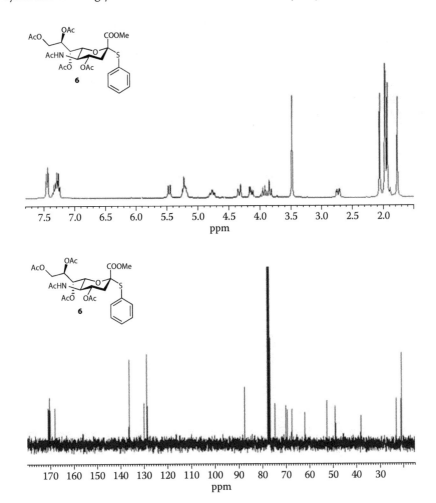

REFERENCES

1. Garegg, P. J. *Adv. Carbohydr. Chem. Biochem.* 1997, *52*, 179–205.
2. Nicolaou, K. C.; Ueno, H. In *Preparative Carbohydrate Chemistry*; Hanessian, S., Ed.; Marcel Dekker, Inc.: New York, 1997, pp. 313–338.
3. Oscarson, S. In *Carbohydrates in Chemistry and Biology*; Ernst, B., Hart, G. W., Sinay, P., Eds.; Wiley-VCH: Weinheim, Germany, 2000; Vol. 1, pp. 93–116.
4. Codee, J. D. C.; Litjens, R. E. J. N.; van den Bos, L. J.; Overkleeft, H. S.; van der Marel, G. A. *Chem. Soc. Rev.* 2005, *34*, 769–782.
5. Pornsuriyasak, P.; Kamat, M. N.; Demchenko, A. V. *ACS Symp. Ser.* 2007, *960*, 165–189.
6. Demchenko, A. V., Ed.; *Handbook of Chemical Glycosylation: Advances in Stereoselectivity and Therapeutic Relevance*; Wiley-VCH: Weinheim, Germany, 2008.
7. Smoot, J. T.; Demchenko, A. V. *Adv. Carbohydr. Chem. Biochem.* 2009, *62*, 161–250.
8. Kamat, M. N.; Rath, N. P.; Demchenko, A. V. *J. Org. Chem.* 2007, *72*, 6938–6946.
9. Marra, A.; Sinay, P. *Carbohydr. Res.* 1989, *187*, 35–42.

10. Cao, S.; Meunier, S. J.; Andersson, F. O.; Letellier, M.; Roy, R. *Tetrahedron: Asymm.* 1994, *5*, 2303–2312.
11. Lemieux, R. U. In *Methods in Carbohydrate Chemistry*; Whistler, R. L., Wolform, M. L., Eds.; Academic Press Inc.: New York, 1963; Vol. 2, pp. 226–228.
12. Latham, H. G.; May, E. L.; Mosrttig, E. *J. Org. Chem.* 1950, *15*, 884–889.
13. Baggett, N.; Mardsen, B. J. *Carbohydr. Res.* 1982, *110*, 11–18.

20 Synthesis of Thioglycosides and Thioimidates from Peracetates

Archana R. Parameswar, Akihiro Imamura,[†] and Alexei V. Demchenko*

CONTENTS

Experimental Methods 189
    General Methods 189
        Phenyl 2,3,4,6-Tetra-*O*-Acetyl-1-Thio-β-D-Glucopyranoside (**2**) 189
        4,5-Dihydro-1,3-Thiazol-2-yl 2,3,4,6-Tetra-O-Acetyl-1-Thio-β-D-
        Glucopyranoside (**3**) 190
        Ethyl 2,3,4,6-Tetra-*O*-Acetyl-1-Thio-β-D-Glucopyranoside (**4**) 190
        p-Tolyl 2,3,4,6-Tetra-*O*-Acetyl-1-Thio-β-D-Glucopyranoside (**5**) 191
Acknowledgment 191
References 195

---

* Corresponding author.
[†] Checker.

Alkyl/aryl thioglycosides. Thioglycosides are the most versatile glycosyl donors for oligosaccharide synthesis.[1-4] They survive many conventional reaction conditions that are often employed in carbohydrate chemistry and can be readily activated with mild electrophilic promoters. Moreover, thioglycosides can be transformed into other common glycosyl donors such as glycosyl halides, sulfoxides, and imidates (via hemiacetals). First attempts to activate 1-thioderivatives employed rather harsh reaction conditions and resulted in only modest yields and stereoselectivities.[5-7] Subsequently introduced milder promoters have been in common use for the past 2 decades.[3] Many successful strategies for expeditious oligosaccharide synthesis have been developed based on thioglycosides.[4,8]

Thioimidates. 2-Thiopyridyl derivatives were among the first thioimidates to be investigated as glycosyl donors.[9] Hanessian based his concept of "remote activation"[10] on 2-pyridyl glycosides and the scope of this technique was expanded by Mereyala who investigated MeI-promoted glycosylation conditions.[11] Demchenko and coworkers have recently introduced *S*-benzoxazolyl (SBox) and *S*-thiazolinyl (IUPAC preferred name: 4,5-dihydro-1,3-thiazolyl) (STaz) glycosides as novel efficient glycosyl donors for stereoselective glycosylation and expeditious oligosaccharide synthesis.[12,13] High anomeric selectivity and yields were achieved for a variety of systems in the presence of stoichiometric amounts of promoters, such as MeOTf or AgOTf. Both armed and disarmed glycosyl thioimidates can be selectively activated in the presence of other common glycosyl donors such as S-alkyl/aryl and O-pentenyl glycosides, as well as fit into a variety of expeditious strategies for oligosaccharide synthesis based on selective or chemoselective activations.[8,9]

This contribution describes transformation of 1,2,3,4,6-tetra-O-acetyl-β-D-glucopyranose (**1**) into phenyl 2,3,4,6-tetra-O-acetyl-1-thio-β-D-glucopyranoside (**2**)[14] and 4,5-dihydro-1,3-thiazol-2-yl 2,3,4,6-tetra-O-acetyl-1-thio-β-D-glucopyranoside (**3**)[15] in the presence of BF_3-etherate, as well as into ethyl 2,3,4,6-tetra-O-acetyl-1-thio-β-D-glucopyranoside (**4**)[16] and tolyl 2,3,4,6-tetra-O-acetyl-1-thio-β-D-glucopyranoside (**5**)[17] in the presence of zirconium(IV) chloride.

EXPERIMENTAL METHODS

GENERAL METHODS

Column chromatography was performed on silica gel 60 (70-230 mesh). Reactions were monitored by TLC on Kieselgel 60 F_{254} and the compounds were detected by UV light and by charring with 10% sulfuric acid in methanol. Solvents were removed under reduced pressure at <40°C. CH_2Cl_2 was distilled from CaH_2 prior to use. Optical rotations were measured at Jasco P-1020 polarimeter. Melting points were measured at Thomas Hoover capillary melting point apparatus. NMR spectra were recorded for solutions in $CDCl_3$ at 300 and 75 MHz, for 1H- and ^{13}C-NMR respectively. HRMS were measured with JEOL MStation (JMS-700) Mass Spectrometer. Thiophenol, 4,5-dihydro-2-sulfanyl-1,3-thiazole, and p-methylthiophenol were purchased from Aldrich and used without further purification. 1,2,3,4,6-Tetra-O-acetyl-β-D-glucopyranose was purchased from TCI.

Phenyl 2,3,4,6-Tetra-O-Acetyl-1-Thio-β-D-Glucopyranoside (2)

Thiophenol (3.1 mL, 30.7 mmol) was added under argon to a stirred solution of pentaacetate **1** (10 g, 25.6 mmol) in anhydrous CH_2Cl_2 (50 mL), followed by the dropwise addition of BF_3-OEt_2 (16.2 mL, 128.2 mmol). When the reaction was complete (TLC, ~4 h), the mixture was diluted with CH_2Cl_2 (250 mL), washed with water (70 mL) followed by sat. aq. $NaHCO_3$ (70 mL) and water (3 × 70 mL). The organic layer was dried, filtered, and concentrated under reduced pressure. Chromatography (hexane–EtOAc, gradient, starting with 10% EtOAc) gave the title compound **2** (8.9–10.4 g, 79%–92%, reported 75%).[18] Analytical data for **2**: R_f = 0.41 (2:3 EtOAc–hexanes); mp 119°C–121°C (Et_2O–hexanes), reported mp 121°C–122°C (EtOH)[18]; $[\alpha]_D^{25}$ −18.5 (c 1, $CHCl_3$), reported $[\alpha]_D^{22}$ −18.1 (c 2.3)[18]; ^{1}H NMR ($CDCl_3$): δ 1.96, 1.98, 2.04, 2.05 (4 s, 12H, 4×–COCH3), 3.68–3.73 (m, 1H, H-5), 4.15 (dd, 1H, $J_{5,6a}$ 5.1 Hz, H-6a), 4.21 (dd, 1H, $J_{6a,6b}$ 12.1 Hz, H-6b), 4.68 (d, 1H, $J_{1,2}$ 10.1 Hz, H-1), 4.92 (dd, 1H, $J_{2,3}$ 9.2 Hz, H-2), 5.04 (dd, 1H, $J_{4,5}$ 9.9 Hz, H-4), 5.23 (dd, 1H, $J_{3,4}$ 9.3 Hz, H-3), 7.26–7.49 (m, 5H, aromatic) ppm; ^{13}C NMR ($CDCl_3$): δ, 20.8 (× 2), 20.9 (× 2), 62.3, 68.4, 70.1, 74.1, 75.9, 85.9, 128.6, 129.1 (× 2), 131.8, 133.3 (× 2), 169.4, 169.6, 170.3, 170.7 ppm; HR-FAB MS $[M+Na]^+$ calcd for $C_{20}H_{24}O_9SNa$ 463.1039; found: 463.1038. Anal. calcd for $C_{20}H_{24}O_9S$: C, 54.54; H, 5.49. Found: C, 54.59; H, 5.44.

4,5-Dihydro-1,3-Thiazol-2-yl 2,3,4,6-Tetra-O-Acetyl-1-Thio-β-D-Glucopyranoside (3)

A mixture of pentaacetate **1** (0.2 g, 0.513 mmol), 4,5-dihydro-2-sulfanyl-1,3-thiazole (0.06 g, 0.513 mmol), and activated molecular sieves (3 Å, 0.4 g) in CH_2Cl_2 (5.0 mL) was stirred for 30 min at room temperature (rt) under argon. BF_3-Et_2O (0.065 mL, 0.513 mmol) was added dropwise, and the mixture was stirred for 45 min at rt. Fresh portions of 4,5-dihydro-2-sulfanyl-1,3-thiazole (0.513 mmol) and BF_3-Et_2O (0.513 mmol) were added and the mixture was refluxed. When TLC (1:1 EtOAc–toluene) indicated that the reaction was complete (~5–6 h),* the mixture was diluted with toluene (20 mL), the solid was filtered off, and the residue was washed with toluene. The combined filtrate (~40 mL) was washed with 1% aq. NaOH (2 × 15 mL), $NaHCO_3$ (15 mL), and water (2 × 15 mL); the organic layer was separated, dried, and concentrated; and chromatography (hexane–EtOAc, gradient, starting with 5% EtOAc) afforded the title compound **3** (0.19–0.21 g, 80%–91%). Analytical data for **3**: R_f=0.28 (1:1 EtOAc–toluene); mp 127°C–128°C (Et_2O–hexanes); $[\alpha]_D^{28}$ +2.0 (c 1, $CHCl_3$); ^{1}H NMR ($CDCl_3$): δ, 2.02, 2.03, 2.06, 2.09 (4s, 12H, 4×$COCH_3$), 3.33 (t, 2H, CH_2N), 3.75 (m, 1H, $J_{5,6a}$ 2.3 Hz, $J_{5,6b}$ 4.5 Hz, H-5), 4.05–4.25 (m, 4H, J_{CH_2S,CH_2N} 8.1 Hz, H-6a, 6b, CH_2S), 5.08 (dd, 1H, $J_{4,5}$ 9.5 Hz, H-4), 5.09 (dd, 1H, $J_{2,3}$ 8.3 Hz, H-2), 5.17 (dd, 1H, $J_{3,4}$ 8.3 Hz, H-3), 5.38 (d, 1H, $J_{1,2}$ 10.4 Hz, H-1) ppm; ^{13}C NMR ($CDCl_3$): δ, 20.7 (× 2), 20.8, 20.9, 35.5, 61.9, 64.4, 68.1, 69.5, 74.0, 76.3, 83.1, 162.7, 169.5, 170.3, 170.8 ppm; HR-FAB MS $[M+H]^+$ calcd for $C_{17}H_{24}NO_9S_2$ 450.0892; found: 450.0891. Anal. calcd for $C_{17}H_{24}NO_9S_2$: C, 45.42; H, 5.16; N, 3.12. Found: C, 45.37; H, 5.07; N, 3.14.

Ethyl 2,3,4,6-Tetra-O-Acetyl-1-Thio-β-D-Glucopyranoside (4)

Ethane thiol (0.96 mL, 12.8 mmol) was added, under argon at 0°C, to a stirred penta-O-acetate **1** (5.0 g, 12.8 mmol) in anhydrous CH_2Cl_2 (100 mL), followed by addition of zirconium(IV) chloride (3.17 g, 13.6 mmol), and stirring at 0°C was continued for 30 min. A second portion of the thiol (0.96 mL, 12.8 mmol) was added, the cooling was removed, and the mixture was allowed to warm to rt. When TLC showed that the reaction was complete (~1 h after second addition of the reagent), the mixture was diluted with CH_2Cl_2 (100 mL), and washed successively with water (50 mL), sat. aq. $NaHCO_3$ (50 mL) and water (2 × 50 mL). The organic layer was separated, dried, filtered, and concentrated under reduced pressure. Chromatography (hexane–EtOAc, gradient, starting with 10% EtOAc) gave the title compound **4** (4.25–4.66 g, 85%–93%, reported 74%).[16] Analytical data for **4**: R_f=0.38 (2:3 ethyl acetate–hexanes); mp 82°C–83°C (Et_2O–hexanes), reported mp 82°C–83°C (EtOH)[16]; $[\alpha]_D^{25}$ −45 (c 1, $CHCl_3$), reported $[\alpha]_D^{20}$ −26.7 (c 1.05)[16]; ^{1}H NMR ($CDCl_3$): δ 1.19 (t, 3H, CH_3), 1.93, 1.95, 1.98, 1.99 (4s, 12H, 4×−COCH3), 2.54–2.72 (m, 2H, CH_2), 3.62–3.67 (m, 1H, H-5), 4.05 (dd, 1H, $J_{5,6a}$ 5.0 Hz, H-6a), 4.16 (dd, 1H, $J_{6a,6b}$ 12.3 Hz, H-6b), 4.42 (d, 1H,

---

* Monitoring this reaction by TLC can be difficult as it often shows a streak below the starting material and a major spot on the baseline. After workup, TLC shows a single spot corresponding to the desired product.

$J_{1,2}$ 10.0 Hz, H-1), 4.95 (dd, 1H, $J_{2,3}$ 9.9 Hz, H-2), 5.00 (dd, 1H, $J_{4,5}$ 9.6 Hz, H-4), 5.16 (dd, 1H, $J_{3,4}$ 8.9 Hz, H-3); ^{13}C NMR (CDCl$_3$): δ, 14.9, 20.6, 20.7, 20.8, 24.2, 62.2, 68.4, 69.9, 73.9, 75.9, 76.8, 83.5, 169.4, 169.5, 170.2, 170.7 ppm; HR-FAB MS [M+Na]$^+$ calcd for C$_{16}$H$_{24}$O$_9$SNa 415.1039; found: 415.1057. Anal. calcd for C$_{16}$H$_{24}$O$_9$S: C, 48.97; H, 6.16. Found: C, 49.20; H, 6.32.

p-Tolyl 2,3,4,6-Tetra-*O*-Acetyl-1-Thio-β-D-Glucopyranoside (5)

p-Methylthiophenol (0.095 g, 0.8 mmol) was added to a solution of pentaacetate **1** (0.5 g, 1.3 mmol) in anhydrous CH$_2$Cl$_2$ (5 mL) followed by zirconium(IV) chloride (0.24 g, 1.0 mmol), and the mixture was stirred for 1 h. Another portion of the thiol (0.064 g, 0.5 mmol) and ZrCl$_4$ (0.12 g, 0.5 mmol) were added, and when the reaction was complete (TLC, ~1 h after the second addition of reagents), the mixture was diluted with CH$_2$Cl$_2$ (25 mL), washed successively with water (15 mL), sat. aq. NaHCO$_3$ (15 mL), and water (2×15 mL). The organic layer was dried, filtered, and concentrated; and chromatography (hexane–EtOAc; gradient, starting with 10% EtOAc) afforded the title compound **5** (0.48–0.51 g, 83%–88%, reported 87%).[17] Analytical data for **5**: R_f=0.42 (2:3 EtOAc–hexanes); mp 114°C–115°C (from ether–hexanes), reported mp 115°C[17]; $[\alpha]_D^{25}$ −18.6 (*c* 1, CHCl$_3$), reported $[\alpha]_D$ −19.05 (*c* 0.21)[17]; ^{1}H NMR (CDCl$_3$): δ 1.96, 1.98, 2.05, 2.06 (4 s, 12H, 4×−COCH3), 2.32 (s, 3H, −CH3), 3.63–3.69 (m, 1H, H-5), 4.16 (dd, 1H, $J_{5,6a}$ 5.2 Hz, H-6a), 4.20 (dd, 1H, $J_{6a,6b}$ 12.0 Hz, H-6b), 4.60 (d, 1H, $J_{1,2}$ 10.1 Hz, H-1), 4.91 (dd, 1H, $J_{2,3}$ 9.3 Hz, H-2), 5.03 (dd, 1H, $J_{4,5}$ 9.6 Hz, H-4), 5.22 (dd, 1H, $J_{3,4}$ 9.3 Hz, H-3), 7.08–7.41 (m, 4H, aromatic) ppm; ^{13}C NMR (CDCl$_3$): δ, 20.6, 20.7 (× 2), 20.8, 21.2, 62.1, 68.3, 69.9, 74.1, 75.8, 85.8, 127.6, 129.7, 133.9, 138.8, 169.3, 169.4, 170.2, 170.6 ppm; HR-FAB MS [M+Na]$^+$ calcd for C$_{21}$H$_{26}$O$_9$SNa 477.1195; found: 477.1211. Anal. calcd for C$_{21}$H$_{26}$O$_9$S: C, 55.50; H, 5.77. Found: C, 55.65; H, 5.72.

ACKNOWLEDGMENT

The chapter was supported by NSF-CAREER award (CHE-0547566).

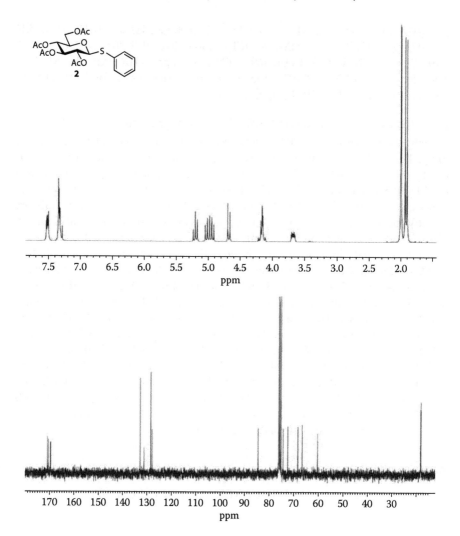

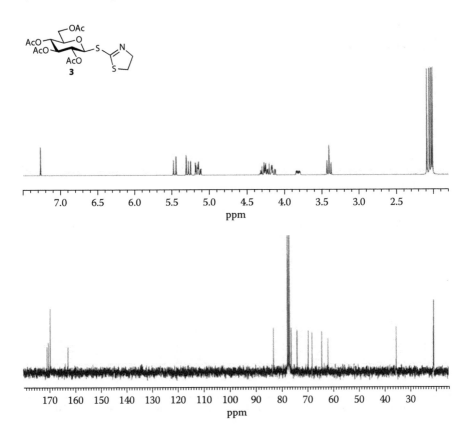

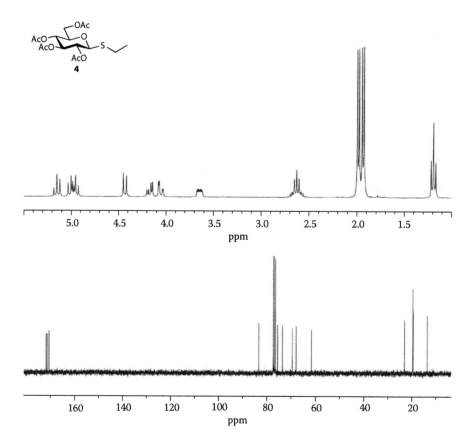

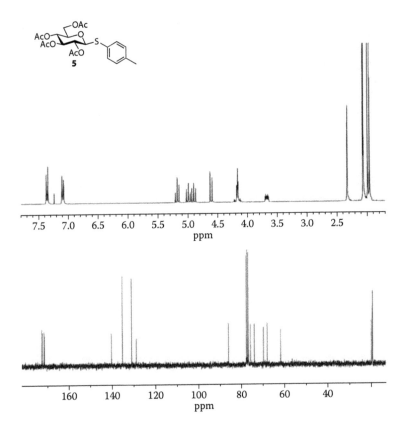

REFERENCES

1. Garegg, P. J. *Adv. Carbohydr. Chem. Biochem.* 1997, *52*, 179–205.
2. Nicolaou, K. C.; Ueno, H. In *Preparative Carbohydrate Chemistry*; Hanessian, S., Ed.; Marcel Dekker, Inc.: New York, 1997, pp. 313–338.
3. Oscarson, S. In *Carbohydrates in Chemistry and Biology*; Ernst, B., Hart, G. W., Sinay, P., Eds.; Wiley-VCH: Weinheim, New York, 2000; Vol. 1, pp. 93–116.
4. Codee, J. D. C.; Litjens, R. E. J. N.; van den Bos, L. J.; Overkleeft, H. S.; van der Marel, G. A. *Chem. Soc. Rev.* 2005, *34*, 769–782.
5. Ferrier, R. J.; Hay, R. W.; Vethaviyasar, N. *Carbohydr. Res.* 1973, *27*, 55–61.
6. Nicolaou, K. C.; Seitz, S. P.; Papahatjis, D. P. *J. Am. Chem. Soc.* 1983, *105*, 2430–2434.
7. Garegg, P. J.; Henrichson, C.; Norberg, T. *Carbohydr. Res.* 1983, *116*, 162–165.
8. Smoot, J. T.; Demchenko, A. V. *Adv. Carbohydr. Chem. Biochem.* 2009, *62*, 161–250.
9. Pornsuriyasak, P.; Kamat, M. N.; Demchenko, A. V. *ACS Symp. Ser.* 2007, *960*, 165–189.
10. Hanessian, S.; Bacquet, C.; Lehong, N. *Carbohydr. Res.* 1980, *80*, c17–c22.
11. Reddy, G. V.; Kulkarni, V. R.; Mereyala, H. B. *Tetrahedron Lett.* 1989, *30*, 4283–4286.
12. Demchenko, A. V.; Malysheva, N. N.; De Meo, C. *Org. Lett.* 2003, *5*, 455–458.
13. Demchenko, A. V.; Pornsuriyasak, P.; De Meo, C.; Malysheva, N. N. *Angew. Chem. Int. Ed.* 2004, *43*, 3069–3072.

14. Janczuk, A. J.; Zhang, W.; Andreana, P. R.; Warrick, J.; Wang, P. G. *Carbohydr. Res.* 2002, *337*, 1247–1259.
15. Pornsuriyasak, P.; Demchenko, A. V. *Chem. Eur. J.* 2006, *12*, 6630–6646.
16. Contour, M. O.; Defaye, J.; Little, M.; Wong, E. *Carbohydr. Res.* 1989, *193*, 283–287.
17. Ding, Y. *Syn. Commun.* 1999, *29*, 3541–3546.
18. Dasgupta, F.; Garegg, P. J. *Acta Chem. Scand.* 1989, *43*, 471–475.

Part II

Synthetic Intermediates

21 2-Acetamido-4,6-O-Benzylidene-2-Deoxy-D-Glucopyranose

Sergey S. Pertel,* Sergey A. Gunchak, Elena S. Kakayan, Vasily Ya. Chirva, and Sébastien Vidal[†]

CONTENTS

Experimental Methods 200
  General Methods 200
    2-Acetamido-4,6-O-Benzylidene-2-Deoxy-D-Glucopyranose (**2**) 200
Acknowledgment 202
References 203

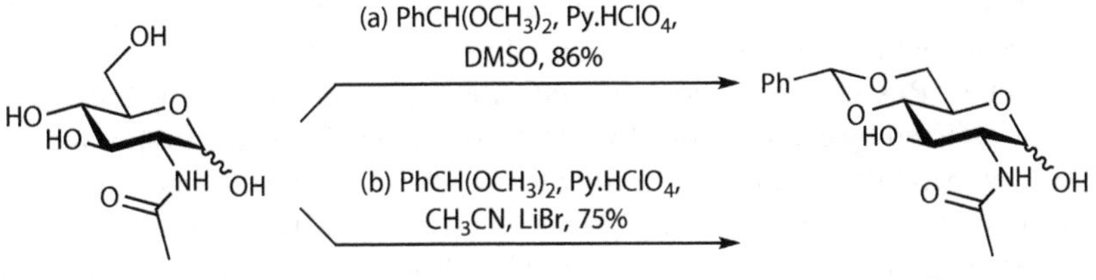

The title compound is used in carbohydrate chemistry as intermediate toward partially O-alkylated[1,2] or O-acylated[3] derivatives of N-acetyl-D-glucosamine, for syntheses of O-glycosaminides,[1,2] 4,6-O-benzylidenated oxazoline derivatives of D-glucosamine,[4,5] glycosyl acceptors,[6,7] C-glycosides,[8–13] and also as an intermediate in the synthesis of neuraminic acid derivatives.[14,15] Compound **2** could also be used for glycoside synthesis via anomeric O-alkylation and trichloroacetimidate method.[16]

Benzylidene derivative **2** was first prepared by classical method, using benzaldehyde and anhydrous zinc chloride as reagents.[1,2,7,17] However, the large excess of reagents used in the absence of additional solvent complicates the workup of the

---

* Corresponding author.
† Checker.

199

reaction mixture, and isolation and purification of the product. The high yield (92%) originally reported[2] could not be reproduced although the reaction was conducted with the aid of sonication.[7] In our laboratory, the yield obtained was the same as that reported recently[7] (58%). The yield of **2** does not improve when external solvents are used during $ZnCl_2$-mediated benzylidenation because of low solubility of both the starting N-acetyl-D-glucosamine and product **2**. N-Acetyl-D-glucosamine is known to be soluble in some organic solvents in the presence of lithium salts, for example, LiBr.[18] Another suitable medium for benzylidenation of N-acetyl-D-glucosamine seems to be DMSO. When more reactive benzylidenating agents are used, such as benzaldehyde dimethyl acetal, the reaction can be conducted with a smaller amount of a less acidic catalyst. We have developed two new, high-yielding methods for preparation of 4,6-O-benzylidene derivative of N-acetyl-D-glucosamine under mild conditions, using polar aprotic solvents and benzaldehyde dimethyl acetal in the presence of pyridinium perchlorate.

EXPERIMENTAL METHODS

GENERAL METHODS

Reagents (Reagent Grade) were purchased from Aldrich or Fluka. DMSO was distilled *in vacuo* over CaH_2. Benzaldehyde dimethyl acetal was distilled in vacuo over NaH. Pyridinium perchlorate was synthesized as described[19] and stored over P_2O_5. LiBr (white crystalline powder) was used as supplied, without further drying. Thin-layer chromatography was performed on silica gel STH-1A-coated aluminum foil (Sorbpolimer, Russian Federation). Visualization of spots of carbohydrate derivatives was effected by exposure of TLC plates to chlorosulfonic acid vapor for 5 min at room temperature followed by heating to ~200°C. Column chromatography was carried out on Silica Gel 60 (Fluka 220-448 mesh). ^{1}H NMR spectra were recorded on a Varian Mercury 400 spectrometer (400.49 MHz). The chemical shifts are referred to the signal of TMS (δ_H 0.0). Assignments of the signals in the NMR spectrum were performed using 2D spectroscopy (COSY) experiment. Optical rotation was measured with a Carl-Zeiss Polamat-S polarimeter.

2-Acetamido-4,6-O-Benzylidene-2-Deoxy-D-Glucopyranose (2)

Method A

To a solution of N-acetyl-D-glucosamine (3.000 g, 13.56 mmol) in DMSO (18 mL), benzaldehyde dimethyl acetal (2.53 mL, 16.92 mmol) and pyridinium perchlorate (360 mg, 2.16 mmol) were added. The reaction mixture was stirred at room temperature (~24°C) for 10 h and periodically evacuated at ~5 Torr* (Six times during 15 min with 1.5 h interval). The stirring was continued and a fresh portion of

---

* The pressure range of 2–7 Torr may be applied; when the pressure during evacuation periods was kept at ~15 Torr (the vacuum normally achieved with a water aspirator) the yield of **2** decreased to 63%.

benzaldehyde dimethyl acetal (5.08 mL, 33.84 mmol) was added after a total 24 h of reaction time. The stirred reaction mixture was evacuated another six times during the following 10 h with 1.5 h interval (15 min at ~5 Torr each time). The progress of the conversion was monitored by TLC (10:1 $CHCl_3$-MeOH). When the reaction was complete, benzene (360 mL) was added and the mixture was kept for 12 h at room temperature. The precipitate was filtered off and washed with benzene. Aqueous sodium hydrocarbonate (5%, 60 mL) was added to the precipitate, the mixture was then stirred for 2 h, filtered, the solids were washed with water, to give, after drying at 25°C for to a constant weight (~5 h), pure (TLC, NMR) **2** (3.32 g). The benzene filtrate and washings were collected, concentrated under reduced pressure, and coevaporated with xylene to remove DMSO and the residual benzaldehyde dimethyl acetal. The dry residue was chromatographed on a column of silica gel (gradient $CHCl_3 \rightarrow$ 100:8 $CHCl_3$-EtOH) to give another crop of **2** (270 mg). Total yield 3.59 g (86%),* $[\alpha]_{546}^{25}$ +55.9° (*c* 2, Py, final 48 h), lit.[2] $[\alpha]_D$ +38.2° (*c* 1, Py, final, 24 h).†

^{1}H NMR (DMSO-d_6), α-anomer: δ 1.87 (s, 3H, CH_3CO), 3.36–3.46 (m, 1H, H-6a), 3.65–3.81 (m, 3H, H-6b,H-3,H-2), 3.88 (ddd, 1H, $J_{5,6a}$ 9.5 Hz, $J_{5,6b}$ 9.5 Hz, $J_{5,4}$ 5 Hz, H-5), 4.12 (dd, 1H, $J_{4,3}$ 10 Hz, H-4), 4.87 (bd, 1H, $J_{OH,3}$ 5 Hz, OH-3), 4.98 (bt, 1H, $J_{1,2}$ 3 Hz, H-1), 5.54 (s, 1H, PhC*H*), 6.59 (bd, 1-H, $J_{OH,1}$ 4 Hz, OH-1), 7.31–7.54 (m, 5H, Ph), 7.61 (d, 1H, $J_{NH,2}$ 8 Hz, NH);

β-anomer: δ 1.87 (s, 3H, CH_3CO), 3.32 (ddd, 1H, $J_{5,6a}$ 9 Hz, $J_{5,6b}$ 9 Hz, $J_{5,4}$ 5 Hz, H-5), 3.36–3.46 (m, 2H, H-2 + H-6a), 3.60 (ddd, 1H, $J_{3,2}$ 9 Hz, $J_{3,OH}$ 5 Hz, H-3), 3.65–3.81 (m, 1H, H-6b), 4.19 (dd, 1H, $J_{4,3}$ 10 Hz, H-4), 4.60 (dd, 1H, $J_{1,2}$ 8 Hz, H-1), 5.06 (bd, 1H, OH-3), 5.54 (s, 1H, PhC*H*), 6.57 (bd, 1-H, $J_{OH,1}$ 7 Hz, OH-1), 7.31–7.54 (m, 5H, Ph), 7.81 (d, 1H, $J_{NH,2}$ 8 Hz, NH).

NMR data for compound **2** also are published by Santhanam et al.[7]

Method B

A mixture of *N*-acetyl-D-glucosamine (1.000 g, 4.50 mmol), benzaldehyde dimethyl acetal (1.36 mL, 9.10 mmol), pyridinium perchlorate (150 mg, 0.90 mmol), LiBr (1.000 g, 11.51 mmol), and acetonitrile (15 mL) was boiled under reflux. When the solids dissolved (~30 min), TLC (10:1 $CHCl_3$-MeOH) showed that the reaction was complete. The mixture was concentrated to dryness at reduced pressure and the residue was chromatographed ($CHCl_3 \rightarrow$ 100:8 $CHCl_3$-EtOH), to give **2** (1.018–1.08 g, 73%–77%). Similar yields could be obtained without chromatography: when the reaction was complete, the mixture was concentrated, the residue was coevaporated with toluene (3 × 25 mL), and the residue was triturated with MeOH (25 mL).

The resulting white powder was filtered off and washed with MeOH (2 × 5 mL) and dried at reduced pressure.

---

* Compound **2** can be crystallized from different solvents (water,[2] methanol,[1] DMSO-H_2O mixture), anomeric ratio of the product and constants substantially depend on crystallization method.

† Because of most products of benzylidenation of **1** are anomeric mixtures, literature data reported for mp and $[\alpha]_D$ for **2** vary.

ACKNOWLEDGMENT

This chapter was funded by Ministry of Education of Ukraine; registration number of financing 0109U001355.

2-Acetamido-4,6-O-benzylidene-2-deoxy-D-glucopyranose (2) (mixture of anomers, 2:3 (α : β) ratio) ^{1}H (400 MHz) in DMSO-d_6

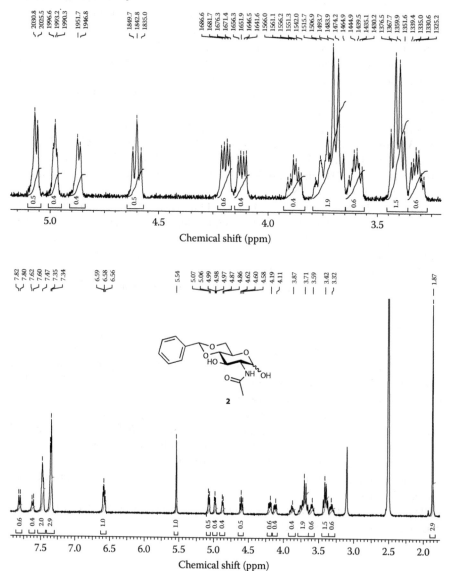

REFERENCES

1. Masamune, H.; Okuyama, T.; Sinohara H. *Tohoku J. Exp. Med.*, 1958, *68*, 181–184.
2. Roth, W., Pigman, W. *J. Am. Chem. Soc.*, 1960, *82*, 4608–4611.
3. Hung, S.-C.; Thopate, S.R.; Wang, C.-C. *Carbohydr. Res.*, 2001, *330*, 177–182.
4. Abdel-Malik, M.M.; Perlin, A.S. *Carbohydr. Res.*, 1989, *189*, 123–133.
5. Yonehara, K.; Hashizume, T.; Mori, K.; Ohe, K.; Uemura, S. *J. Org. Chem.*, 1999, *64*, 9374–9380.
6. Dasgupta, F.; Anderson, L. *Carbohydr. Res.*, 1990, *202*, 239–255.
7. Santhanam, B.; Wolfert, M.A.; Moore, J.N.; Boons, G.-J. *Chem. Eur. J.*, 2004, *10*, 4798–4807.
8. Vyplel, H.; Scholz, D.; Macher, I.; Schindlmaier, K.; Schuetze, E. *J. Med. Chem.*, 1991, *34*, 2759–2767.
9. Mbongo, A.; Frechou, C.; Beaupere, D.; Uzan, R.; Demailly, G. *Carbohydr. Res.*, 1993, *246*, 361–370.
10. Nicotra, F.; Russo, G.; Ronchetti, F.; Toma, L. *Carbohydr. Res.*, 1983, *124*, C5-C7.
11. Beer, D.; Bieri, J.H.; Macher, I.; Prewo, R.; Vasella, A. *Helv. Chim. Acta.*, 1986, *69*, 1172–1190.
12. Werner, R.M.; Williams, L.M.; Davis, J.T. *Tetrahedron Lett.*, 1998, *39*, 9135–9138.
13. Wen, X.; Hultin, P.G. *Tetrahedron Lett.*, 2004, *45*, 1773–1775.
14. Kuhn, R.; Baschang, G. *Liebigs Ann. Chem.*, 1962, *659*, 156–163.
15. Wesemann, W.; Zilliken, F. *Liebigs Ann. Chem.*, 1966, *695*, 209–216.
16. Schmidt, R.R. The anomeric *O*-alkylation and the trichloroacetimidate method—Versatile strategies for glycoside bond formation. In *Modern Methods in Carbohydrate Chemistry*; Khan, S.H., O'Neill, R.A., Eds.; Harwood, Amsterdam, the Netherlands, 1996; pp. 20–54.
17. Holmquist, L. *Acta Chem. Scand.*, 1970, *24*, 173–178.
18. Vauzeilles, B.; Dausse, B.; Palmier, S.; Beau, J.-M. *Tetrahedron Lett.*, 2001, *42*, 7567–7570.
19. Wong, C.L.; Klingler, R.J.; Kochi, J.K. *Inorg. Chem.*, 1980, *19*, 423–430.

22 Synthesis of 1,3,4,6-Tetra-O-Acetyl-2-Azido-2-Deoxy-α,β-D-Glucopyranose and 2-Azido-4,6-O-Benzylidene-2-Deoxy-α,β-D-Glucopyranose

Rafael Ojeda, José Luis de Paz,
Ricardo Lucas, Niels Reichardt, Lin Liu,[†]
and Manuel Martín-Lomas*

CONTENTS

Experimental Methods 206
   General Methods 206
      Preparation of Trifluoromethanesulfonyl Azide (TfN₃) Solution 207
      1,3,4,6-Tetra-O-Acetyl-2-Azido-2-Deoxy-α,β-D-Glucopyranose (**2**) 207
      2-Azido-4,6-O-Benzylidene-2-Deoxy-α,β-D-Glucopyranose (**3**) 208
References 211

---

* Corresponding author.
[†] Checker.

The presence of an azide function at C-2 of sugars has been shown to be of great value in the preparation of complex aminosugars.[1] The reasons for the importance of the azide function as a masking agent for the amine function are twofold: (i) the nonparticipating nature of the azide group enables, depending on the glycosylation conditions and the protecting groups in the glycon, the formation of α- or β-linkages; (ii) the azide group can be smoothly converted under reductive conditions into the free amine function. These azides have been usually prepared by azidonitration of glycals,[2] by addition of halogeno azides to glycals,[3] and from 1,6-anhydroglycoses either by opening of epoxides[4] or by substitution of 2-O-triflates.[5] However, some of these procedures can be problematic because of low selectivity or a large number of steps involved.

Diazo transfer from trifluoromethanesulfonyl azide (TfN_3)[6] to 2-amino-2-deoxy-glycoses constitutes a high-yielding, simple procedure for the preparation of partially protected or unprotected 2-azido-2-deoxy-glycoses.[7] According to this method, glucosamine, an inexpensive starting material, can be transformed into the corresponding azide by diazo transfer from trifluoromethanesulfonyl azide in good yield.[7]

Compounds 2 and 3 are important to differentiate positions in the monosaccharide for latter transformations and to simplify purification of the 2-azidoglucopyranoses. They are important intermediates in the synthesis of complex oligosaccharides. For instance, compound 3 was converted in four steps into the corresponding 3-O-benzyl-1-O- trichloroacetimidate, which was employed in the preparation of heparin-like oligosaccharides.[8]

This methodology has been successfully applied for the preparation of 2-azido-2-deoxy- allo-, manno- and galacto-derivatives.[7]

EXPERIMENTAL METHODS

GENERAL METHODS

Thin layer chromatography (TLC) was performed on silica gel 60 F_{254} precoated on aluminum plates (Merck). Compounds were detected by charring with sulfuric acid/ethanol (1:9) or with anisaldehyde solution [anisaldehyde (25 mL) in a mixture of sulfuric acid (25 mL), ethanol (450 mL), and acetic acid (1 mL)]. Column chromatography was carried out on silica gel 60 (0.2–0.5 mm, 0.2–0.063 mm, or 0.040–0.015 mm; Merck). Optical rotations were determined with a Perkin-Elmer 341 polarimeter. ^{1}H- and ^{13}C-NMR spectra were acquired on Bruker DRX-400 spectrometer and chemical shifts are given in ppm (δ). Signal nuclei assignments were made by 2 D ^{1}H-^{1}H and ^{1}H-^{13}C HSQC experiments. Combustion analyses were performed with a Leco CHNS-932 apparatus, after drying analytical samples over phosphorous pentoxide for 24 h. Melting point was measured using Mel-Temp Capillary Melting Point Apparatus and was not corrected. All chemicals were purchased from Aldrich Chemical Company.

Preparation of Trifluoromethanesulfonyl Azide (TfN₃) Solution*,†

In a 1 L three-neck round-bottom flask, equipped with a dropping funnel, an internal thermometer and an argon balloon, NaN$_3$ (62.22 g, 0.96 mol) was dissolved at room temperature in H$_2$O (150 mL). CH$_2$Cl$_2$ (200 mL) was added, the mixture was cooled to 0°C (internal temperature), and Tf$_2$O (32 mL, 0.190 mol) was added within 1 h 30 min to the vigorously stirred solution, while keeping the temperature unchanged. After the addition was complete, the mixture was stirred for 2 h at 0°C, the organic layer was separated and the aqueous layer was extracted with CH$_2$Cl$_2$ (2×75 mL). The combined organic layers were washed successively with saturated aq NaHCO$_3$ (150 mL) and H$_2$O (150 mL), dried over MgSO$_4$ and filtered, to obtain a 0.4M TfN$_3$ solution (350 mL). The concentration of the TfN$_3$ solution was determined by IR spectroscopy (intensity of the band at 2150 cm^{-1}) to be 0.40 M, using the easily available TsN$_3$ as standard.[7] This solution was prepared immediately before use for the diazo transfer reaction.

1,3,4,6-Tetra-O-Acetyl-2-Azido-2-Deoxy-α,β-D-Glucopyranose (2)

In a 2 L three-neck round-bottom flask, equipped with a dropping funnel and an argon balloon attached through a septum, a suspension of D-glucosamine hydrochloride (10 g, 46.4 mmol) in dry MeOH (200 mL) was treated with a 0.5 M solution NaOMe in MeOH (110 mL, 55 mmol).* After stirring for 30 min at room temperature, the mixture was diluted with MeOH (500 mL) and treated with 4-(dimethylamino)pyridine (6 g, 49.2 mmol) to afford a clear and colorless solution, to which the 0.4M TfN$_3$ solution (350 mL, 140 mmol) was added dropwise at room temperature within 2 h. After stirring for 48 h at room temperature under Ar, solvent was evaporated at 30°C in vacuo to furnish an oily residue that was dissolved in anhydrous pyridine (300 mL) and treated at 0°C with acetic anhydride (200 mL). After stirring for 24 h at 0°C, the mixture was diluted with CH$_2$Cl$_2$ (1.25 L) and washed with 1 N HCl solution (2×1 L). The combined aqueous layers were extracted with CH$_2$Cl$_2$ (3×300 mL) and the combined organic layers were washed with saturated aqueous

---

* Trifluoromethanesulfonyl azide is presumed to be toxic and potentially explosive. Although we have carried out these reactions numerous times and have never had problems, all operations and reactions involving TfN$_3$ should be carried out with caution, behind explosion-proof shield, in a well-ventilated fume hood.

† An alternative diazo transfer reagent, to which the safety considerations (see above) also apply, has recently been described.[9]

NaHCO$_3$ solution (1.25 L), brine (1.25 L), dried (MgSO$_4$) and concentrated in vacuo. The residue was chromatographed (3:1 hexane-ethyl acetate) to yield **2** (12.1 g, 10 g scale, 70%, or 1.04 g, 1 g scale, 61%) as a colorless oil. TLC (3:1 hexane-ethyl acetate) R_f 0.20; Crystallization (EtOH) gives the β anomer, mp 95°C–96°C; lit.[5b] 96°C–97°C. IR (film, CHCl$_3$): 2118, 1755, 1432, 1370, 1220, 1143, 1110, 1075, 1050; ^{1}H-NMR (400 MHz, CDCl$_3$) δ 5.54 (d, 1H, $J_{1,2}$ 8.4 Hz, H-1), 5.05 (t, 1H, J 9.6 Hz, H-3), 5.02 (t, 1H, J 9.6 Hz, H-4), 4.28 (dd, 1H, $J_{5,6a}$ 4.4 Hz, $J_{6a,6b}$ 12.5 Hz, H-6a), 4.05 (dd, 1H, $J_{5,6b}$ 2.2 Hz, 12.5 Hz, H-6b), 3.78 (ddd, 1H, $J_{5,6b}$ 2.2 Hz, $J_{5,6a}$ 4.4 Hz, $J_{4,5}$ 9.7 Hz, H-5), 3.67 (t, 1H, J 8.8 Hz, H-2), 2.17 (s, 3H, –COCH$_3$), 2.08 (s, 3H, –COCH$_3$), 2.06 (s, 3H, –COCH$_3$), 2.00 (s, 3H, –COCH$_3$).^{13}C-NMR (100 MHz, CDCl$_3$) δ 170.56 (C=O), 169.81 (C=O), 169.65 (C=O), 168.59 (C=O), 92.58 (C-1), 72.73 (C-5), 72.69 (C-3), 67.77 (C-4), 62.57 (C-2), 61.40 (C-6), 20.91, 20.71, 20.65, 20.57 (4 *CH$_3$*CO).

2-Azido-4,6-*O*-Benzylidene-2-Deoxy-α,β-D-Glucopyranose (3)

In a 2 L three-neck round-bottom flask, equipped with a dropping funnel, a septum and an argon balloon, a suspension of D-glucosamine hydrochloride (10 g, 46.4 mmol) in dry MeOH (200 mL) was treated with a 0.5 M solution of NaOMe in MeOH (110 mL, 55 mmol).* After stirring for 30 min at room temperature, the mixture was diluted with MeOH (500 mL) and treated with 4-(dimethylamino)pyridine (6 g, 49.2 mmol). A clear and colorless solution was formed, to which 0.4 M TfN$_3$ solution (350 mL, 140 mmol, prepared as described above) was added dropwise at room temperature within 2 h. After stirring for 48 h at room temperature under Ar, solvent was evaporated at 30°C in vacuo to furnish an oily residue which was dissolved in MeOH, treated with NH$_4$Cl to adjust pH to 7, the solution was concentrated and a solution of the residue in 4:1 dichloromethane–methanol was filtered through a short silica gel column. After concentration, a mixture of the residue, benzaldehyde dimethyl acetal (10.4 mL, 69.6 mmol) and a catalytic amount of *p*-toluenesulfonic acid (~10 mg) in 60 mL of dry DMF was stirred for 48 h at 40°C. After neutralization with solid NaHCO$_3$ and concentration, chromatography (6:1 toluene-acetone or 1:1 hexanes–EtOAc) afforded compound **3** as a white solid (8.85 g, 65%). TLC (4:1 toluene–acetone), R_f 0.41; ^{1}H-NMR (400 MHz, CD$_3$OD) δ 7.45 (m, 2H, Ph), 7.31 (m, 3H, Ph), 5.57 (m, 1H, PhC*H*), 5.17 (d, 0.4H, $J_{1,2}$ 3.6 Hz, H-1α), 4.61 (d, 0.6H, $J_{1,2}$ 8.8 Hz, H-1β), 4.23 (dd, 0.6H, $J_{5,6a}$ 5.2 Hz, $J_{6a,6b}$ 10 Hz, H-6aβ), 4.15 (dd, 0.4H, $J_{5,6a}$ 5.2 Hz, $J_{6a,6b}$ 10 Hz, H-6aα), 4.06 (t,0.4H, $J_{2,3}$9.6 Hz, H-3α), 4.01–3.87 (m,0.6H, H-5α), 3.78–3.66 (m,1H, H-6bα, H-6bβ), 3.57 (t,0.6H, $J_{2,3}$9.2 Hz, H-3β), 3.46 (t,1H, $J_{3,4}$ 9.2 Hz, H-4α, H-4β), 3.42 (m,0.6H, H-5β), 3.20–3.15 (m,1H, H-2α, H-2β).^{13}C-NMR(100 MHz, CD$_3$OD) δ137.68 (Ph), 128.59(Ph), 127.67 (Ph), 126.14 (Ph), 101.75 (PhCH), 101.60 (PhCH), 96.48 (C-1β), 92.74 (C-1α), 82.12 (C-4), 80.99 (C-4), 71.81 (C-3β), 68.97 (C-2), 68.70 (C-3α), 68.23 (C-6), 68.19 (C-6), 66.32 (C-5β), 64.40 (C-2), 62.35 (C-5α). Anal. Calcd for C$_{13}$H$_{15}$N$_3$O$_5$: C, 53.24; H, 5.16; N, 14.33. Found: C, 53.02; H, 5.05; N, 13.85.

---

* The concentration of the solution of sodium methoxide in Methanol should be approximately 0.5 M to reproduce the given reaction time.

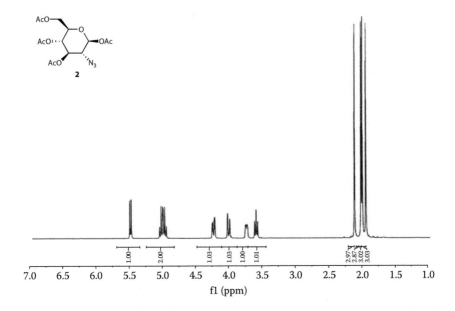

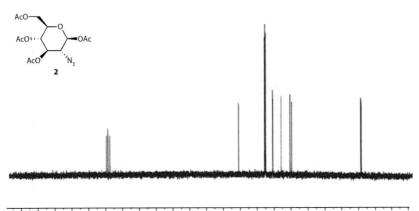

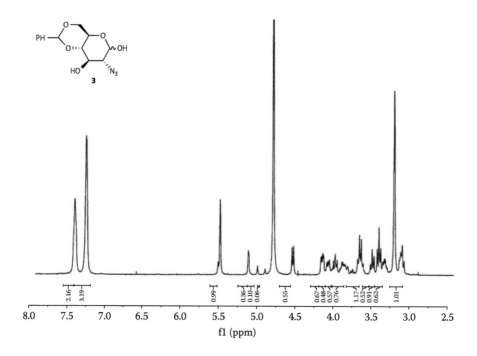

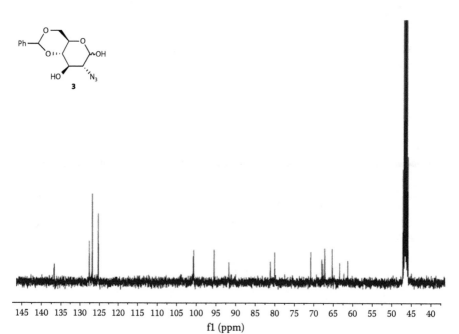

REFERENCES

1. (a) H. Paulsen, *Angew. Chem.* 1982, *94*, 184; (b) R. R. Schmidt, *Angew. Chem.* 1986, *98*, 213; (c) H. Paulsen, *Angew. Chem.* 1990, *102*, 213; (d) H. Kunz, W. Günther, *Angew. Chem.* 1986, *102*, 1068.
2. R. U. Lemieux, R. M. Ratcliffe, *Can. J. Chem.* 1979, *57*, 1244.
3. N. V. Bovin, S. E. Surabyan, A. Y. Khorlin, *Carbohydr. Res.* 1981, *98*, 25.
4. H. Paulsen, W. Stenzel, *Chem. Ber.* 1978, *111*, 2334.
5. (a) M. Kloosterman, M. P. de Nijs, H. van Boom, *J. Carbohydr. Chem.* 1986, *5*, 215; (b) V. Pavliak, P. Kováč, *Carbohydr. Res.* 1991, *210*, 333.
6. (a) C. J. Caveander, V. J. Shiner, *J. Org. Chem.* 1972, *37*, 3567–3569; (b) J. Zaloom, D. C. Roberts, *J. Org. Chem.* 1981, *46*, 5173–5176.
7. (a) A. Vasella, C. Witzig, J. L. Chiara, M. Martín-Lomas, *Helv. Chim. Acta* 1991, *74*, 2073; (b) P. B. Alper, S.-C.Hung, C.-H. Wong, *Tetrahedron Lett.* 1996, *37*, 6092.
8. (a) J. L. de Paz, J. Angulo, J. M. Lassaletta, P. M. Nieto, M. Redondo-Horcajo, R. M. Lozano, G. Giménez-Gallego, M. Martín-Lomas, *ChemBioChem.* 2001, *2*, 673; (b) R. Ojeda, J. Angulo, P. M. Nieto, M. Martín-Lomas, *Can. J. Chem.* 2002, *80*, 917–936; (c) R. Lucas, J. Angulo, P. M. Nieto, M. Martín-Lomas, *Org. Biomol. Chem.* 2003, *1*, 2253–2266; (d) R. Ojeda, J. L. de Paz, M. Martín-Lomas, *Chem. Commun.* 2003, 2486–2487.
9. E. D. Goddard-Borger, R. V. Stick, *Org. Lett.* 2007, *9*, 3797–3800.

REFERENCES

(text illegible — mirrored and faded)

23 An Easy Access to 2,3,4,6-Tetra-*O*-Benzyl-D-Galactopyranose and 2,3,6-Tri-*O*-Benzyl-D-Glucopyranose

Ian Cumpstey, Riccardo Cribiu,
and Lorenzo Guazzelli* [†]

CONTENTS

Experimental Methods 214
General Methods 214
Benzyl 2,3,4,6-Tetra-*O*-Benzyl-β-D-Galactopyranosyl-(1 → 4)-2,3,6-Tri-
O-Benzyl-β-D-Glucopyranoside (**II**) 215
2,3,4,6-Tetra-*O*-Benzyl-D-Galactopyranose (**IV**), 2,3,6-Tri-*O*-Benzyl-
D-Glucopyranose (**V**) and 1-*O*-Acetyl-2,3,4,6-Tetra-*O*-Benzyl-β-D-
Galactopyranose (**III**) 216
References 220

Reagents and conditions. (i) BnBr, NaH, DMF, 0°C, RT, 34%–46%; (ii) H$_2$SO$_{4(aq)}$, AcOH, 85°C; **V**, 26%–29%; (iii) Ac$_2$O, Et$_3$N, 47%–62% from **II**; (iv) NaOMe, MeOH, 97%.

---

* Corresponding author.
[†] Checker.

Protected carbohydrate hemiacetals may be converted into glycosyl donors (e.g., tri-chloroacetimidates)[1] or used as donors directly.[2] Alternatively, they may be used as substrates for nucleophilic addition reactions.[3] The galactose hemiacetal **IV** may be prepared from galactose via a glycoside[4] or a thioglycoside[5] to protect the anomeric position during the introduction of benzyl ethers. Here, we describe a short route[6] to multigram quantities of 2,3,4,6-tetra-*O*-benzyl-D-galactopyranose **IV** and also the *gluco* hemiacetal **V** starting from lactose.

Perbenzylation of reducing monosaccharides will often give the β-pyranosides as major reaction products, but for galactose, the α-furanoside is the major product[7] so a direct benzylation–hydrolysis route from galactose to the *galacto* hemiacetal **IV** is impractical. When a pyranoside is benzylated, an acetal locks the anomeric position, preserving the pyranose ring. A readily available galactopyranoside is present in lactose **I**; O-4 of the reducing *gluco* residue is blocked, preventing *gluco*furanoside formation. Consequently, purification of a possible mixture of perbenzylated products should be simplified.

Perbenzylation of lactose **I** with benzyl bromide and sodium hydride in DMF gave a major perbenzylated β-disaccharide **II** after chromatography and crystallization. The β configuration at the glucose anomeric position is consistent with Schmidt's thesis that the β-hemiacetal anomer is more nucleophilic than its α counterpart; it reacts more quickly to give the β-glycoside under kinetic control.[8] Acidic hydrolysis of disaccharide **II** cleaved both glycosidic bonds in **II**, and gave the two hemiacetals **IV** and **V**, which were easily separable by chromatography. The two hemiacetals may be pure enough for some applications, but traces of inseparable by-products could be detected by ^{1}H nuclear magnetic resonance (NMR) spectroscopy. The *gluco* compound (α/β) was crystallized to give pure **V** (mostly α). The *galacto* compound was converted into the crystalline β anomeric acetate **III** following Gervay–Hague's procedure.[9] This β-acetate was easily purified by crystallization, and then deacetylated to give the pure *galacto* hemiacetal **IV**.

EXPERIMENTAL METHODS

GENERAL METHODS

Melting points were recorded on a Gallenkamp melting point apparatus and are uncorrected. Proton NMR (^{1}H) spectra were recorded on a Bruker Avance II 400 spectrometer; multiplicities are quoted as singlet (s), broad singlet (br s), doublet (d), doublet of doublets (dd), triplet (t), apparent triplet (at), doublet of apparent triplets (dat), AB quartet (ABq) or multiplet (m). Carbon NMR (^{13}C) spectra were recorded on Bruker Avance II 500. Spectra were assigned using COSY, HSQC, and DEPT experiments. All chemical shifts are quoted on the δ-scale in parts per million (ppm). Residual solvent signals ($CHCl_3$, $δ_H$ 7.26, $δ_C$ 77.16) were used as an internal reference. Low- and high-resolution (HRMS) electrospray (ES+) mass spectra were recorded using a Bruker Microtof instrument. Optical rotations were measured on a Perkin–Elmer 241 polarimeter with a path length of 1 dm; concentrations are given in g/100 mL. Thin layer chromatography (TLC) was carried out on Merck Kieselgel sheets, precoated with $60F_{254}$ silica. Plates were visualized with UV light and 10%

sulfuric acid, or a solution of ammonium molybdate (10% w/v) and cerium (IV) sulfate (2% w/v) in 10% sulfuric acid. Flash column chromatography was carried out on silica gel (35–70 micron, Grace). Solutions were dried with anhydrous Na_2SO_4 and concentrated at reduced pressure.

Benzyl 2,3,4,6-Tetra-O-Benzyl-β-D-Galactopyranosyl-(1 → 4)-2,3,6-Tri-O-Benzyl-β-D-Glucopyranoside (II)

Lactose monohydrate **I** (10.0 g, 27.8 mmol) was suspended in benzyl bromide (50 mL, 420 mmol) and DMF (250 mL), and cooled to 0°C under N_2. Sodium hydride (60% in oil, 18.9 g, 473 mmol) was added in portions over 15 min, and the well-stirred reaction mixture was left in the cooling bath and allowed to warm to RT as the ice melted.* After 44 h, TLC (4:1 pentane–EtOAc) showed the presence of a major product (R_f 0.2). The reaction mixture was cooled to 0°C, quenched with MeOH (50 mL), and stirred for 30 min at RT. The solvent was then removed under reduced pressure, and the residue partitioned between EtOAc (2×200 mL) and water (200 mL). The organic phase was washed with brine (200 mL), dried, and concentrated. The residue was partially purified by dry flash column chromatography (10 cm diameter sintered filter funnel, 15:1 pentane–EtOAc, 1 L → 10:1 pentane–EtOAc, 500 mL → 4:1 pentane–EtOAc, 1.5 L – product elutes here) to give, after concentration, pale yellow oil (19 g). Crystallization was effected by addition of pentane (80 mL) to a solution of the partially purified material in EtOAc (25 mL), to give perbenzylated β-lactoside **II**, 10–13 g (34%–46%) as white crystals, mp 83°C–86°C, lit. mp 74°C–76°C[10]†; $[\alpha]_D^{25}$ +0.9 (c, 1.0 in $CHCl_3$), lit. $[\alpha]_D$ +1.5 (c, 1.4 in $CHCl_3$)[11]; ^1H NMR (400 MHz, $CDCl_3$) δ 7.41–7.13 (m, 40H, Ar-CH), 5.05 (d, 1H, J 10.7 Hz, PhCHH'), 4.98 (d, 1H, J 11.3 Hz, PhCHH'), 4.96 (d, 1H, J 11.9 Hz, PhCHH'), 4.93 (d, 1H, J 10.8 Hz, PhCHH'), 4.83 (d, 1H, J 11.1 Hz, PhCHH'), 4.80–4.72 (m, 5H, PhCH_2, 3×PhCHH'), 4.68 (d, 1H, J 12.0 Hz, PhCHH'), 4.60–4.57 (m, 2H, PhCHH', PhCHH'), 4.51 (d, 1H, $J_{1,2}$ 7.7 Hz, H-1^I), 4.47 (d, 1H, $J_{1,2}$ 7.7 Hz, H-1^{II}), 4.43 (d, 1H, J 12.1 Hz, PhCHH'), 4.37, 4.27 (ABq, 2H, J_{AB} 11.8 Hz, PhCH_2), 3.99 (dd, 1H, J 8.9 Hz, J 9.8 Hz, H-4^I), 3.94 (d, 1H, $J_{3,4}$ 3.0 Hz, H-4^{II}), 3.84 (dd, 1H, $J_{5,6'}$ 4.5 Hz, $J_{6,6'}$ 11.0 Hz, H-6'), 3.81–3.76 (m, 2H, H-2^{II}, H-6), 3.60–3.56 (m, 2H, H-3^I, H-6'), 3.51 (dd, 1H, $J_{1,2}$ 7.7 Hz, $J_{2,3}$ 9.2 Hz, H-2^I), 3.44 (dd, 1H, $J_{2,3}$ 9.8 Hz $J_{3,4}$ 3.0 Hz, H-3^{II}), 3.41–3.37 (m, 3H, H-5^I, H-5^{II}, H-6); ^{13}C NMR (125 MHz, $CDCl_3$) δ 139.0, 138.8, 138.7, 138.6, 138.2, 137.7 (Ar-C), 128.5, 128.5, 128.5,128.5, 128.4, 128.4, 128.3, 128.3, 128.3, 128.2, 128.2, 128.1, 128.0, 128.0, 128.0, 127.9, 127.9, 127.8, 127.8, 127.7, 127.7, 127.6, 127.6, 127.5, 127.2 (Ar-CH), 102.9 (C-1^{II}), 102.7 (C-1^I), 83.2 (C-3^I), 82.7 (C-3^{II}), 81.9 (C-2^I), 80.1 (C-2^{II}), 76.9 (C-4^I), 75.5, 75.4, 75.2, 74.8, 73.5, 73.2, 72.7, 71.1 (8×PhCH_2), 75.3, 73.1 (C-5^I, C-5^{II}), 73.8 (C-4^{II}), 68.4, 68.2 (C-6^I, C-6^{II}).

The mother liquor contains (NMR) **II** as the major component, along with another disaccharide likely to be the perbenzylated α-lactoside, with anomeric carbon resonances at δ_C 96.0 and 102.9 ppm.

---

* The reaction mixture should not be removed from the cooling bath until after the reaction has neared completion. Failure to follow this may result in rapid exothermic reaction.
† This melting point is significantly higher than the literature value (for which no crystallization solvent was reported). We did not observe any change in the mp upon recrystallization from EtOAc/pentane.

2,3,4,6-Tetra-*O*-Benzyl-D-Galactopyranose (IV), 2,3,6-Tri-*O*-Benzyl-D-Glucopyranose (V) and 1-*O*-Acetyl-2,3,4,6-Tetra-*O*-Benzyl-β-D-Galactopyranose (III)

Benzyl lactoside **II** (6.84 g, 6.4 mmol) was suspended in a mixture of acetic acid (75 mL) and H_2SO_4 (1 M, 10 mL), and the mixture stirred at 85°C. After 5 h, TLC (3:1 pentane–EtOAc) showed complete conversion of the starting material (R_f 0.5) into three products (R_f 0.4, 0.2 (**IV**), 0.1 (**V**)). The mixture was allowed to cool to RT, and quenched by addition to water (250 mL), extracted with toluene (2 × 250 mL), and the combined organic extracts were washed with $NaHCO_3$ (satd. aq., 250 mL), dried, filtered, and concentrated. The residue was chromatographed (2:1 → 5:4 pentane–EtOAc) to give impure galactose hemiacetal **IV** (3.0–3.2 g), and impure glucose hemiacetal **V** (α:β, 1:1; 1.3–1.6 g). The glucose hemiacetal **V** crystallized from EtOAc–pentane to give white crystals **V**, 750–830 mg (α:β, 7:1; 26%–29%); ^1H NMR (400 MHz, CDCl$_3$)^{12} Data for **Vα**: δ 7.37–7.27 (m, 15H, Ar-H), 5.23 (br s, 1H, H-1), 4.98, 4.76 (ABq, 2H, J_{AB} 12.3 Hz, PhC<u>H</u>$_2$), 4.76, 4.69 (ABq, 2H, J_{AB} 11.7 Hz, PhC<u>H</u>$_2$), 4.59, 4.54 (ABq, 2H, J_{AB} 12.3 Hz, PhC<u>H</u>$_2$), 4.00 (dat, 1H, J 4.5 Hz, J 9.3 Hz, H-5), 3.79 (at, 1H, J 9.2 Hz, H-3 or H-4), 3.68–3.67 (m, 2H, H-6, H-6′), 3.60 (at, 1H, J 9.4 Hz, H-3 or H-4), 3.55 (dd, 1H, $J_{1,2}$ 3.5 Hz, $J_{2,3}$ 9.3 Hz, H-2), 3.03 (br s, 1H, OH), 2.40 (br s, 1H, OH).

Impure galactose hemiacetal **IV** (3.24 g) was dissolved in CH_2Cl_2 (70 mL), and triethylamine (21 mL) and acetic anhydride (4.2 mL) were added. After 2 h, TLC (3:1 pentane–EtOAc) indicated complete conversion of starting material (R_f 0.2) into a major product (R_f 0.4). The reaction mixture was cooled to 0°C, and MeOH (30 mL) was slowly added, after which the mixture was concentrated in vacuo. The residue was dissolved in EtOAc (100 mL) and washed with HCl (1 M, 100 mL). The aqueous phase was reextracted with EtOAc (100 mL), and the combined extracts were dried, filtered, and concentrated. Crystallization from EtOAc–pentane gave the β-acetate **III** (1.8–2.3 g, 47%–62% from **II**), mp 98°C–101°C, lit. mp 102°C–103°C (from ether–hexane)^{13}; $[α]_D^{28}$ +2.5 (c, 1.0 in CHCl$_3$, lit. +3.8 (c, 2.0 in CHCl$_3$).^{13}

The acetate **III** (2.30 g, 4.0 mmol) was suspended in MeOH (50 mL), and a solution of sodium methoxide (prepared from sodium (17 mg) and MeOH (5 mL)) was added. After 3 h, all the starting material had dissolved, and TLC (3:1 pentane–EtOAc) showed a complete conversion of starting material (R_f 0.4) into a single product (R_f 0.2). Dowex 50×8 (H$^+$) ion-exchange resin (2 mL) was added, then the mixture was filtered, and concentrated. The residue was passed through a pad of silica eluting with 1:1 pentane–EtOAc to give the galactose hemiacetal **IV**, 2.06 g (97%) as a colorless oil that crystallized on standing^{14}*; Selected data, ^1H NMR (400 MHz, CDCl$_3$) δ 5.28 (d, 1H, $J_{1,2}$ 3.5 Hz, H-1α), 4.15 (at, 1H, J 6.4 Hz, α), 4.03 (dd, 1H, J 3.6 Hz, J 9.8 Hz, α), 3.97 (dd, 1H, J 1.1 Hz, J 2.8 Hz, H-4α), 3.76 (dd, 1H, J 7.4 Hz, J 9.6 Hz, β), 3.14 (d, 1H, $J_{OH,1}$ 6.4 Hz, OH-1β), 2.93 (br s, 1H, OH-1α).

---

* Crystallization from a suitable solvent was not attempted, to avoid losses due to preferential crystallization of one anomer. The trace impurities present after hydrolysis of **II** were absent: only the α and β anomers of **IV** could be seen in the ^1H NMR spectra.

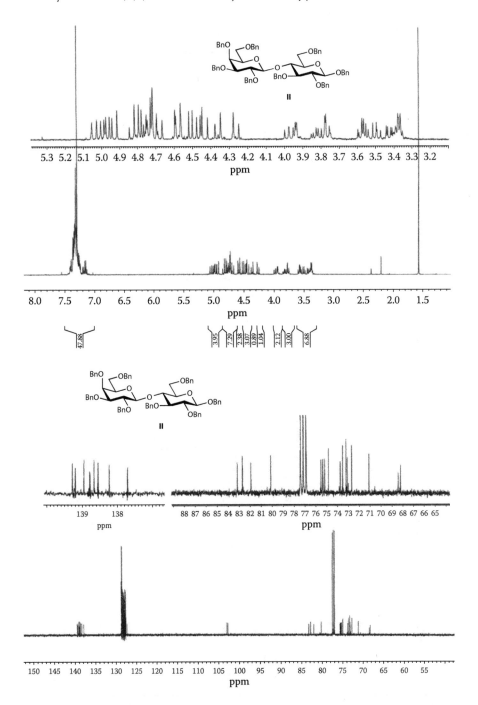

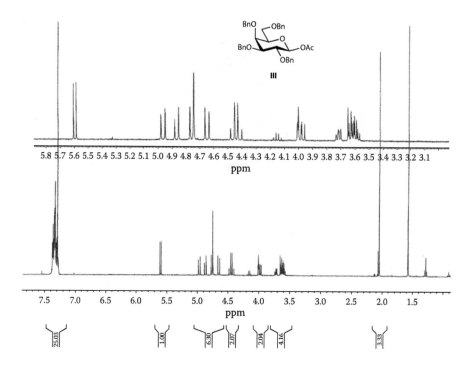

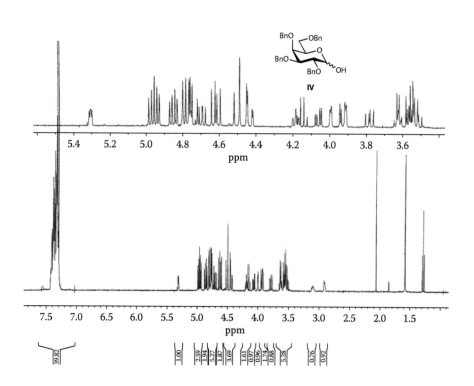

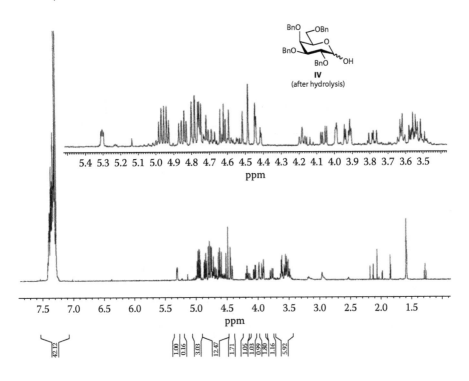

IV
(after hydrolysis)

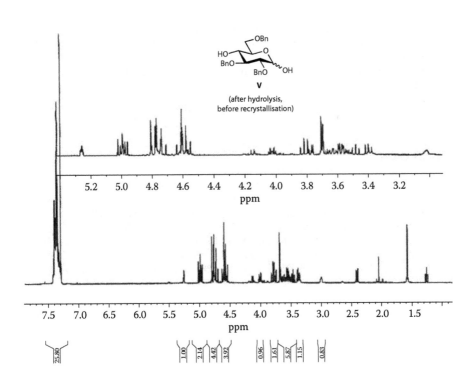

V
(after hydrolysis,
before recrystallisation)

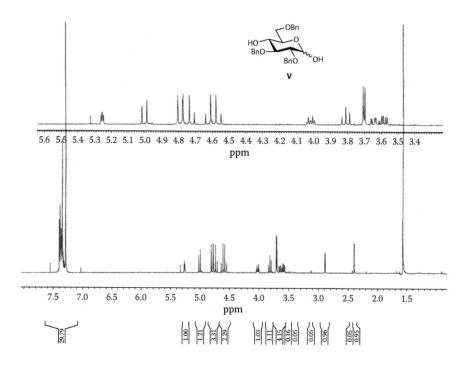

REFERENCES

1. Schmidt, R.R.; Michel, J., *Tetrahedron Lett.* 1984, *25*, 821–824.
2. Nguyen, H.M.; Chen, Y.; Duron, S.G.; Gin, D.Y., *J. Am. Chem. Soc.* 2001, *123*, 8766–8772.
3. Marco-Contelles, J.; de Opazo, E.; Arroyo, N., *Tetrahedron* 2001, *57*, 4729–4739.
4. Beaton, S.A.; Huestis, M.P.; Sadeghi-Khomami, A.; Thomas, N.R.; Jakeman, D.L., *Chem. Commun.* 2009, 238–240.
5. Garegg, P.J.; Hultberg, H.; Lindberg, C., *Carbohydr. Res.* 1980, *83*, 157–162.
6. Cribiu, R.; Borbas, K.E.; Cumpstey, I., *Tetrahedron* 2009, *65*, 2022–2031.
7. Decoster, E.; Lacombe, J.-M.; Strebler, J.-L.; Ferrari, B.; Pavia, A.A., *J. Carbohydr. Chem.* 1983, *2*, 329–341.
8. Schmidt, R.R.; Klotz, W., *Synlett* 1991, 168–170.
9. Kulkarni, S.S.; Gervay-Hague, J., *Org. Lett.* 2006, *8*, 5765–5768.
10. Bieg, T.; Szeja, W., *Carbohydr. Res.* 1990, *205*, C10–C11.
11. Sato, S.; Mori, M.; Ito, Y.; Ogawa, T. *Carbohydr. Res.* 1986, *155*, C6–C10.
12. Sato, T.; Nakamura, H.; Ohno, Y.; Endo, T., *Carbohydr. Res.* 1990, *199*, 31–35.
13. Zinin, A.I.; Eneyskaya, E.V.; Shabalin, K.A.; Kulminskaya, A.A.; Shishlyannikov, S.M.; Neustroev, K.N., *Carbohydr. Res.* 2002, *337*, 635–642.
14. Motawia, M.S.; Olsen, C.E.; Denyer, K.; Smith, A.M.; Møller, B.L., *Carbohydr. Res.* 2001, *330*, 309–318.

24 Benzyl 2,3,6,2',3',6'-Hexa-O-Benzyl-β-Cellobioside

Deepak Sail, Paula Correia da Silva,[†] and Pavol Kováč[*]

CONTENTS

Experimental Methods 222
    General Methods 222
        Benzyl 2,3,6,2',3'-Penta-O-Benzyl-4',6'-O-Benzylidene-α-Cellobioside
        (**2A**) and Benzyl 2,3,6,2',3'-Penta-O-Benzyl-4',6'-O-Benzylidene-β-
        Cellobioside (**2B**) 223
        Benzyl 2,3,6,2',3',6'-Hexa-O-Benzyl-β-Cellobioside (**3**) and Benzyl
        2,3,6,2',3',4'-Hexa-O-Benzyl-β-Cellobioside (**9**) 224
Acknowledgment 225
References 230

(a) BnBr, NaH, DMF, 18 h, 90%; (b) NaBH$_3$CN, HCl in ether, THF, 30 min, 86%.

---

[*] Corresponding author.
[†] Checker.

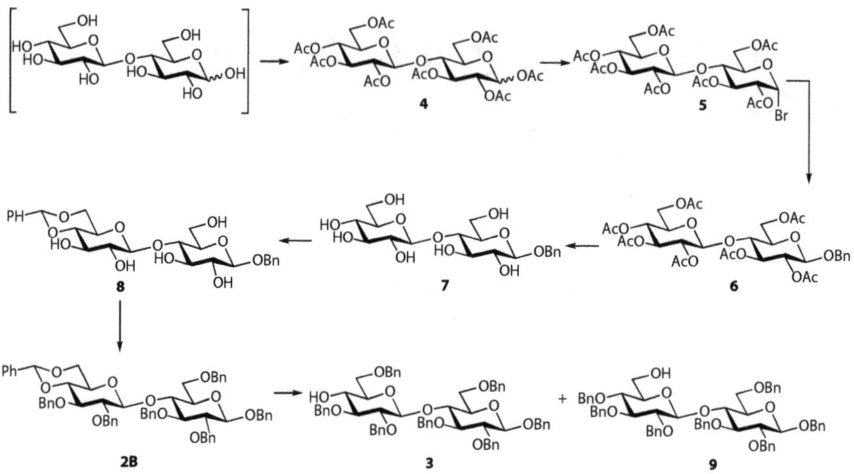

SCHEME 24.1 The original, 7-step route to the synthesis[1] of **3**.

The title compound **3** (see opening scheme of this chapter) is an important intermediate in the preparation of C-4′ modified derivatives of lactose and cellobiose. The
previously reported synthesis[1] of **3** (Scheme 24.1) involved a sequence of reactions,
developed originally by Hess et al.[2] and Lipták et al.[3] which started from cellobiose and
led to benzyl glycoside **8**. After per-*O*-benzylation (**8**→**2B**), reductive opening of the
benzylidene ring in **2B** gave **3** in an overall yield of ~20%. Taking into consideration
improvements made later by Edwards et al.[4] and Twaddle et al.[5] on various aspects of
the sequence from **5** to **8**, the overall yield of **3** could theoretically increase to ~28%.

Here we report a more efficient route to **3** featuring fewer synthetic steps (*cf.* the
opening scheme of this chapter and Scheme 24.1) and an overall yield comparable to
that described previously. Thus, cellobiose was converted into the known[6,7] benzylidene derivative **1** and this product was per-*O*-benzylated, to give a mixture of α and
β benzyl glycosides (**2A** and **2B**). After column chromatography, **2B** was obtained in
~64% yield from **1**, together with the hitherto unknown, crystalline α-anomer **2A**.
Employing the protocol described by Takeo et al.,[1] compound **3** was obtained from
2B in ~85% yield, together with a small amount of the 6′-hydroxy derivative **9**.

EXPERIMENTAL METHODS

GENERAL METHODS

Optical rotations were measured at ambient temperature with a Jasco P-2000 digital
polarimer. All reactions were monitored by thin-layer chromatography (TLC) on
silica gel 60-coated glass slides. For column chromatography, SuperFlash SI 35 pre-
packed columns (Analogix) were used.* The solvents used were as follows: A, hexane; B, 2:1 toluene–EtOAc; C, toluene; and D, 15:1 toluene–acetone. Best resolution

---

* When self-packed columns are used, the size of the sample/column may have to be adjusted accordingly.

of a low-concentration sample of **2** by TLC could be achieved with 4:1 hexane–EtOAc. The purpose of adding toluene to the elution solvent was to minimize tailing of poorly soluble solutes (for details, see below). Nuclear magnetic resonance (NMR) spectra were measured at 600 MHz (^{1}H) and 150 MHz (^{13}C) with a Bruker Avance spectrometer. Assignments of NMR signals were made by homonuclear and heteronuclear two-dimensional correlation spectroscopy, using the software supplied with the spectrometers. When reporting NMR assignments, p.o. denotes signals that were partially overlapped. Atmospheric pressure chemical ionization (APCI) high resolution mass spectrometry (HRMS) was performed with a Waters LCT Premier spectrometer. Solutions in organic solvents were dried with anhydrous Na_2SO_4 and concentrated at 40°C/2 kPa.

Benzyl 2,3,6,2′,3′-Penta-O-Benzyl-4′,6′-O-Benzylidene-α-Cellobioside (2A) and Benzyl 2,3,6,2′,3′-Penta-O-Benzyl-4′,6′-O-Benzylidene-β-Cellobioside (2B)

Sodium hydride (0.72 g, 18.0 mmol, 60% in mineral oil; 3 eq./OH) was added, portionwise at 0°C (ice-water bath) over 15 min, to a solution of 4′,6′-O-benzylidene cellobiose[6,7] (0.430 g, 1 mmol) in DMF (10.0 mL), and the mixture was stirred under argon at the same temperature for 10 min. With continued cooling, benzyl bromide (1.43 mL, 12.0 mmol, 2.0 eq/OH) was added and the mixture was stirred under argon for 30 min. The ice-water cooling was then replaced with tap-water bath, and the mixture was stirred overnight, when TLC (3:1 A–B) showed that all starting material was consumed. Two major products were formed (R_f 0.3 and 0.2; solvent, 2:1 A–B), the one with faster mobility largely predominating, along with very minor by-products. The mixture was cooled in an ice-bath and the reaction was quenched by slow addition of MeOH (10.0 mL). After the mixture had been stirred at 0°C for 15 min, it was allowed to warm up to room temperature (RT). The solvents were evaporated under reduced pressure and the residue was partitioned between CH_2Cl_2 and water. The organic phase was separated, dried, and concentrated. ^{1}H NMR spectrum of the crude mixture showed that the α:β ratio was ~3:7. With the aid of toluene* (3 mL + 2 × 1 mL to rinse the flask), the crude product was applied on top of a column of silica gel (115 g). Isocratic elution with 2 column volumes of 8:1 A–B was followed by a gradient of 10 column volumes of 8:1 A:B → 2.5:1 A–B, and continued isocratically with 2.5:1 A–B. Baseline resolution of the anomers was achieved.

Eluted first was benzyl 2,3,6,2′,3′-penta-O-benzyl-4′,6′-O-benzylidene-β-cellobioside (**2B**, 0.62 g, 64%); mp 165°C–167°C (acetone); $[\alpha]_D = -12.3°$ (c 1.0, CHCl$_3$); lit.[3] mp 170°C–174°C (acetone); $[\alpha]_D = -13.5°$ (c 1.72, chloroform); APCI HRMS: m/z for $[M+NH_4]^+$ Calcd 988.4636; found: 988.4662; ^{1}H NMR (CDCl$_3$): δ 7.49–7.23 (m, 35H, aromatic protons), 5.49 (s, 1H, PhC*H*), 4.96–4.39 (m, 12H, 6 PhC*H*$_2$), 4.54 (d, 1H, $J_{1',2'}$ = 7.8 Hz, H-1′), 4.48 (d, 1H, $J_{1,2}$ = 7.4 Hz, H-1), 4.18 (dd, 1H, $J_{6a',6b'}$ = 10.5 Hz, $J_{5',6a'}$ = 4.9 Hz, H-6a′), 4.00 (bt, 1H, J = 9.2 Hz, H-4), 3.85 (dd, 1H, $J_{6a,6b}$ = 11.0 Hz, $J_{5,6a}$ = 4.0 Hz, H-6a), 3.69 (dd, 1H, $J_{5,6b}$ = 1.7 Hz, H-6b), 3.61 (t, p.o., 1H, J = ~9.2 Hz, H-3′), 3.58 (t, p.o., 1H, J = ~9.1 Hz, H-4′), 3.53 (t, p.o., 1H, J = ~8.9 Hz, H-3), 3.50 (dd, 1H, $J_{2',3'}$ = 9.0 Hz, H-2), 3.47 (t, p.o., J = ~10.5 Hz,

---

* Slight warming may be necessary to form a clear solution.

H-6b′), 3.36 (t, 1H, $J=8.0$ Hz, H-2′), 3.32 (ddd, 1H, $J_{4,5}=9.8$ Hz, H-5), 3.15 (ddd, 1H, $J4′,5′=14.1$ Hz, H-5′). ^{13}C NMR (CDCl$_3$) δ ppm: 139.0, 138.52, 138.50, 138.32, 138.2, 137.5, 137.4, 128.9, 128.4, 128.29, 128.27, 128.26, 128.22, 128.1, 127.9, 127.82, 127.79, 126.03, 102.8 (C-1′), 102.5 (C-1), 101.1 (PhCH), 82.9 (C-3), 82.5 (C-2′), 81.8 (C-4′), 81.7 (C-2), 81.1 (C-3′), 76.8 (C-4), 75.42 (PhCH$_2$), 75.41 (PhCH$_2$), 75.1 (C-5), 75.0 (PhCH$_2$), 74.95 (PhCH$_2$), 73.2 (PhCH$_2$), 70.9 (PhCH$_2$), 68.8 (C-6′), 67.9 (C-6), 65.8 (C-5′).

Eluted next was benzyl 2,3,6,2′,3′-penta-O-benzyl-4′,6′-O-benzylidene-α-cellobioside (**2A**, 0.188 g, 19%); mp 163°C–165°C (CH$_2$Cl$_2$-MeOH); [α]$_D$=+24.6° (*c* 1.0, chloroform); APCI HRMS *m/z*: for [M+NH$_4$]$^+$ Calcd 988.4636; found: 988.4655. ^{1}H NMR (CDCl$_3$): δ 7.49–7.23 (m, 35H, aromatic protons), 5.49 (s, 1H, PhCH), 4.93–4.29 (m, 12H, 6 PhCH$_2$), 4.81 (d, 1H, $J_{1,2}=3.6$ Hz, H-1), 4.37 (d, 1H, $J_{1′,2′}=7.7$ Hz, H-1′), 4.18 (dd, 1H, $J_{6a′,6b′}=10.5$ Hz, $J_{5′,6a′}=4.9$ Hz, H-6a′), 3.95 (t, 1H, $J=9.1$ Hz, H-4), 3.88 (t, 1H, $J=9.1$ Hz, H-3), 3.82 (dd, 1H, $J_{6a,6b}=10.9$ Hz, $J_{5,6a}=2.9$ Hz, H-6a), 3.65 (m, 1H, H-5), 3.56 (t, p.o., 1H, $J=~9.2$ Hz, H-4′), 3.52 (t, p.o., 1H, $J=~8.6$ Hz, H-3′), 3.51 (dd, 1H, $J_{2,3}=9.5$ Hz, H-2), 3.46 (t, 1H, $J=10.5$ Hz, H-6b′), 3.36 (dd, p.o., 1H, $J_{5,6b}=~1.7$ Hz, H-6b), 3.33 (t, p.o., 1H, $J=~8.3$ Hz, H-2′), 3.09 (m, 1H, H-5′). ^{13}C NMR (CDCl$_3$) δ ppm: 139.4, 138.6, 138.4, 137.9, 137.5, 137.3, 128.9, 128.44, 128.39, 128.29, 128.1, 127.8, 127.3, 126.1, 102.9 (C-1′), 101.1 (PhCH), 95.9 (C-1), 82.5 (C-2′), 81.7 (C-4′), 81.0 (C-3′), 80.2 (C-3), 79.0 (C-2), 76.9 (C-4), 75.44 (PhCH$_2$), 75.39 (PhCH$_2$), 74.9 (PhCH$_2$), 73.3 (2 PhCH$_2$), 70.3 (C-5), 69.3 (PhCH$_2$), 68.8 (C-6′), 67.6 (C-6), 65.7 (C-5′). Anal. Calcd for C$_{61}$H$_{62}$O$_{11}$: C, 75.44; H, 6.43. Found: C, 75.38; H, 6.32.

Benzyl 2,3,6,2′,3′,6′-Hexa-*O*-Benzyl-β-Cellobioside (3) and
Benzyl 2,3,6,2′,3′,4′-Hexa-*O*-Benzyl-β-Cellobioside (9)

Sodium cyanoborohydride (0.41 g, 6.5 mmol) was added to a mixture of benzylidene derivative **2B** (0.486 g, 0.5 mmol) and molecular sieves 4 Å (0.5 g) in THF (~5.0 mL), which had been stirred for 5 min under argon. When the reagent dissolved, the mixture was cooled in an ice-bath and 2 M solution of HCl in ether was added slowly until evolution of gas ceased (~2.5 mL). The cooling was removed and stirring at RT was continued until TLC (solvent D) showed that the starting material was consumed (~5 min). Two products were formed (R_f 0.4 and 0.25), the one showing faster mobility largely predominating, together with a very minor product moving close to the baseline. The mixture was diluted with EtOAc (20.0 mL) and transferred to a separatory funnel with the aid of EtOAc (10.0 mL). The mixture was then washed successively with aq. NaHCO$_3$ and NaCl solutions. The aqueous phases were combined and washed once with 20.0 mL of CH$_2$Cl$_2$. The combined organic phases were dried, concentrated, and a solution of the residue in toluene (3 mL plus 3 rinses, 2 mL each) was applied on top of a column of 60 g of silica gel. The first elution with solvent C (one column volume) was followed successively with a gradient of C→D (10 CV) and isocratic elution with solvent D.

Eluted first was the 4′-OH product (**3**, 0.419 g, 86%), mp 83°C–87°C (isopropyl ether); [α]$_D$=−7.2° (*c* 1.0, CHCl$_3$); lit.[1] mp 82°C–83°C (hexane); [α]$_D$=−7.5° (*c* 1.3, CHCl$_3$); APCI HRMS *m/z*: for [M+NH$_4$]$^+$ Calcd 990.4792; found: 990.4778. ^{1}H NMR (CDCl$_3$) δ ppm: 7.37–7.2 (m, 35H, aromatic protons), 4.95–4.37 (m, 14H, 7 PhCH$_2$), 4.48 (d, p.o., 1H, $J_{1′,2′}=~7.7$ Hz, H-1′), 4.47 (d, p.o., 1H, $J_{1,2}=~7.7$ Hz, H-1),

3.99 (t, 1H, $J=9.3\,Hz$, H-4), 3.83 (dd, 1H, $J_{6a,6b}=11.0\,Hz$, $J_{5,6a}=4.0\,Hz$, H-6a), 3.70 (dd, 1H, $J_{5,6b}=1.7\,Hz$, H-6b), 3.62 (t, 1H, $J=9.1\,Hz$, H-4′), 3.54 (m, 3H, H-3, H-6a′, H-6b′), 3.48 (dd,1H, $J_{2,3}=9.1\,Hz$, H-2), 3.33 (m, 3H, H-3′, H-5, H-2′), 3.25 (m, 1H, H-5′), 2.91 (s, 1H, -OH); ^{13}C NMR (CDCl$_3$): δ 139.1, 138.7, 138.5, 138.4, 138.1, 137.7, 137.5, 128.4, 128.37, 128.34, 128.33, 128.25, 128.2, 128.05, 127.9, 127.83, 127.82, 127.78, 127.74, 127.72, 127.66, 127.64, 127.59, 127.54, 102.4 (C-1), 102.3 (C-1′), 84.3 (C-3′), 82.8 (C-3), 82.0 (C-2′), 81.7 (C-2), 76.5 (C-4), 75.2 (PhCH$_2$), 75.1 (PhCH$_2$), 75.0 (C-5), 74.94 (PhCH$_2$), 74.87 (PhCH$_2$), 73.6 (PhCH$_2$), 73.4 (C-4′), 73.2 (PhCH$_2$), 73.0 (C-5′), 71.1 (C-6′), 70.9 (PhCH$_2$), 68.0 (C-6).

Eluted next was a small amount of benzyl 2,3,6,2′,3′,4′-hexa-O-benzyl-β-cellobioside (**9**). For characterization, products from several experiments were combined, mp 136°C–138°C (CH$_2$Cl$_2$–MeOH); $[\alpha]_D=+7.6°$ (c 1.0, chloroform); lit.[3] mp 96°C–98°C; $[\alpha]_D=+7.5°$ (c 1.06, chloroform); APCI HRMS m/z for $[M+NH_4]^+$ Calcd 990.4792; found: 990.4753; ^{1}H NMR (600 MHz, CDCl$_3$) δ ppm: 7.38–7.23 (m, 35H, aromatic protons), 4.96–4.44 (m, 14H, 7 PhCH$_2$), 4.49 (d, 1H, $J_{1,2}=7.5\,Hz$, H-1), 4.45 (d, p.o., 1H, $J_{1',2'}=7.9\,Hz$, H-1′), 3.94 (t, 1H, $J=9.2\,Hz$, H-4), 3.81 (dd, 1H, $J_{6a,6b}=10.9\,Hz$, $J_{5,6a}=4.0\,Hz$, H-6a), 3.70 (dd, 1H, $J_{5,6b}=1.7\,Hz$, H-6b), 3.62 (ddd, 1H, $J_{6a',6b'}=11.9\,Hz$, $J_{6a',OH}=7.0\,Hz$, $J_{5',6a'}=2.5\,Hz$, H-6a′), 3.53 (t, p.o., 1H, $J=\sim9.0\,Hz$, H-3), 3.52 (t, p.o., 1H, $J=\sim9.0\,Hz$, H-3′), 3.49 (dd, p.o., 1H, $J_{2,3}=\sim9.2\,Hz$, H-2), 3.43 (t, 1H, $J=9.4\,Hz$, H-4′), 3.36–3.30 (m, p.o., 3H, H-5, H-6b′, H-2′), 3.14 (ddd, 1H, $J_{4',5'}=9.4\,Hz$, $J_{5',6b'}=5.1\,Hz$, H-5′), 1.57 (t, 1H, $J=7.0\,Hz$, -OH); ^{13}C NMR (151 MHz, CDCl$_3$) δ ppm: 139.0, 1238.4, 138.3, 137.5, 128.4, 128.37, 128.37, 128.35, 128.29, 128.25, 128.11, 127.8, 127.2, 102.45 (C-1), 102.38 (C-1′), 84.7 (C-3′), 82.74 (C-3), 82.71 (C-2′), 77.9 (C-4′), 76.8 (C-4), 75.7 (PhCH$_2$), 75.2 (PhCH$_2$), 74.97 (C-5), 74.93 (2 PhCH$_2$), 74.85 (C-5′), 74.81 (PhCH$_2$), 73.3 (PhCH$_2$), 70.9 (PhCH$_2$), 67.8 (C-6), 61.7 (C-6′).

Anal. Calcd for C$_{61}$H$_{64}$O$_{11}$: C, 75.29; H, 6.63. Found: C, 75.07; H, 6.85.

ACKNOWLEDGMENT

This research was supported by the Intramural Research Program of the NIH, NIDDK.

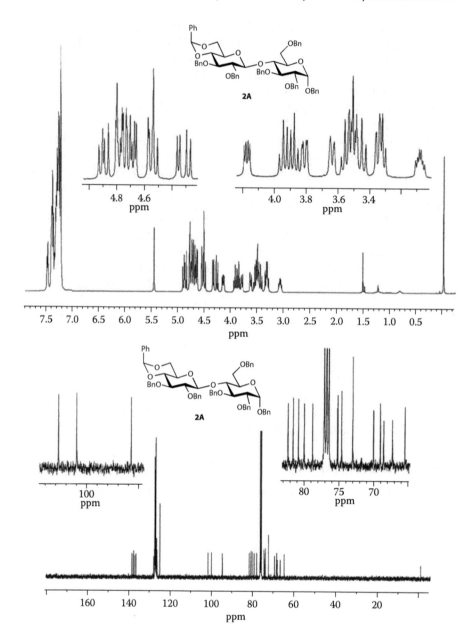

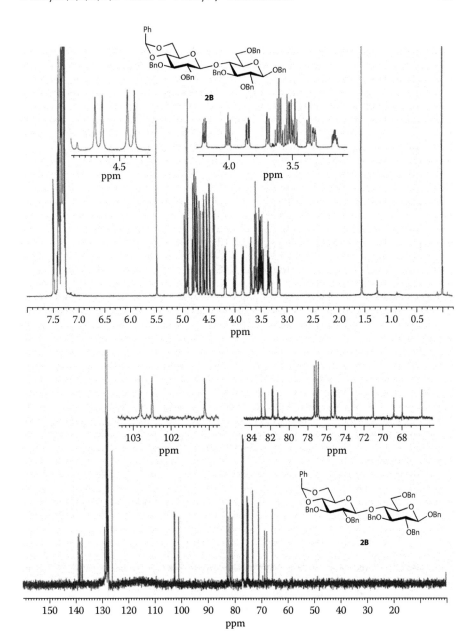

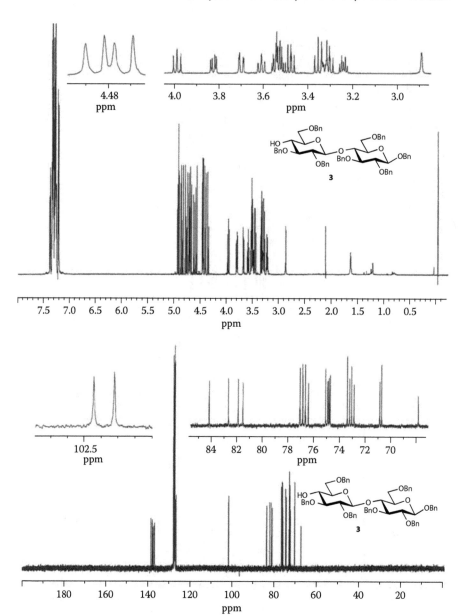

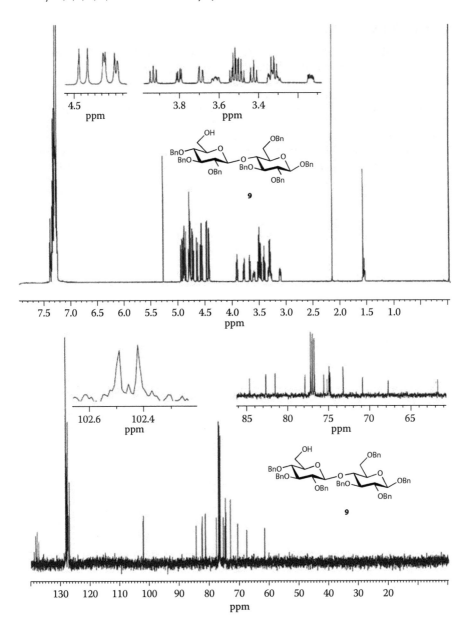

REFERENCES

1. Takeo, K.; Okushio, K.; Fukuyama, K.; Kuge, T. *Carbohydr. Res.* 1983, *121*, 163–173.
2. Hess, K.; Hammerstein, H.; Gramberg, W. *Ber.* 1937, *70*, 1134–1138.
3. Liptak, A.; Jodal, I.; Nanasi, P. *Carbohydr. Res.* 1976, *52*, 17–22.
4. Edwards, R. G.; Hough, L.; Richardson, A. C. *Carbohydr. Res.* 1977, *57*, 129–148.
5. Twaddle, G. W. J.; Yashunsky, D. V.; Nikolaev, A. V. *Org. Biomol. Chem.* 2003, *1* 623–628.
6. Mani, N. S. *Indian J. Chem.* 1989, *28B*, 602–603.
7. Day, D.; Du, M.; Mendez, R.; Maunder, D. *Preparation of Non-Animal Based Lactose from Cellobiose via Epimerization Reaction*, US 2008/0004438 A1, Jan. 3, 2008.

25 One-Step Syntheses of 1,2,3,5,6-Penta-O-Benzoyl-α,β-D-Galactofuranose and 1,2,3,5-Tetra-O-Benzoyl-α,β-D-Arabinofuranose

*Carla Marino, Lucía Gandolfi-Donadío,
Carola Gallo Rodriguez, Yu Bai,[†]
and Rosa M. de Lederkremer**

CONTENTS

Experimental Methods 233
   General Methods 233
      1,2,3,5,6-Penta-*O*-Benzoyl-α,β-D-Galactofuranose (**1α** and **1β**) 233
      1,2,3,5-Tetra-*O*-Benzoyl-α,β-D-Arabinofuranose (**2αβ**), 1,2,3,5-Tetra-
      O-Benzoyl-α-D-Arabinofuranose (**2α**) and 1,2,3,4-Tetra-*O*-Benzoyl-α-
      D-Arabinopyranose (**3**) 234
Acknowledgments 235
References 237

* Corresponding author.
[†] Checker.

D-Arabinofuranose (Ara$f$) and D-galactofuranose (Gal$f$) are found in the arabinoga-lactan of the cell wall of mycobacteria.[1,2] D-Gal$f$ is also present in glycoconjugates of infectious protozoa like *Trypanosoma cruzi* and Leishmania,[3,4] and of fungi.[5,6] The chemistry and biology of arabinofuranosyl and galactofuranosyl containing polysac-charides has been reviewed.[7] The furanose form of arabinose and galactose is absent in mammals, hence the interest of several groups in the synthesis of the oligosac-charides containing these sugars for metabolic and immunological studies. Per-O-acylated monosaccharides are important synthons for the synthesis of glycosides, in particular oligosaccharides.[8] We have used galactofuranose per-O-benzoate for the first synthesis of α-D-Gal$f$ phosphate[9] and 1-thio-β-D-galactofuranosides.[10] Also, Ara$f$ and Gal$f$ were introduced as the terminal quasinonreducing (upstream) unit in oligosaccharides using the tin(IV) chloride–promoted condensation.[11,12] The perben-zoate **1** was also used as precursor of the trichloroacetimidate derivative employed in oligosaccharide syntheses.[13,14] These per-O-benzoates are obtained as a crystal-line, anomeric mixture of the α,β-furanoses, and it can be used, without separation, for the glycosylation reactions. The method is based on the tautomerization of the monosaccharide in hot pyridine that yields a considerable proportion of the furano-syl forms, which are then benzoylated. We have optimized the original method for the preparation of 1,2,3,5,6-penta-O-benzoyl-α,β-D-Gal$f$,[15] and extended the reaction to D-arabinose.

Peracetylated galactofuranose and arabinofuranose were previously most often synthesized from glycosides obtained by Fisher glycosidation of free sugars. The mixture of pyranose and furanose glycosides thus obtained was then acetylated and the peracetates were acetolysed to obtain furanose peracetates. In this way, crystal-line penta-O-acetyl-β-D-galactofuranose was obtained in 37%–41% yield (in three steps).[16,17] Difficulties to separate the mixture of glycosides have been reported.[18] When octyl galactofuranosides were used for the acetolysis reaction,[19] the yield of penta-O-acetyl-β-D-galactofuranose was ~40% but the protocol, in addition to the three synthetic steps, involved repeated chromatography.

The tetra-O-acetyl-α,β-D-arabinofuranose was obtained by the Fisher glyco-sidation as a syrup, after column chromatography.[20] Earlier, tetra-O-benzoyl-α-D-arabinofuranose was prepared in three steps in a low yield,[21] starting from the methyl glycoside.

A different approach comprised acetolysis of D-galactose diethyl dithioacetal, obtained from D-galactose in 47% yield.[22] It afforded 1,2,3,5,6-penta-*O*-acetyl-β-D-galactofuranose in a yield of 30% (from galactose).[23] This method has the disadvantage of employing the odorous ethanethiol for preparation of the starting material.

By the present procedure, the yields of the crystalline furanose perbenzoates are also moderate (26%–33%) but the easy one step synthesis from inexpensive reagents makes it an attractive approach.

EXPERIMENTAL METHODS

GENERAL METHODS

Thin layer chromatography (TLC) was performed on Silica Gel $60 F_{254}$ (Merck) aluminum-supported plates. Detection was effected by UV light and by charring with 10% (v/v) H_2SO_4 in EtOH. Column chromatography was performed on Silica Gel 60 (230–400 mesh, Merck). NMR spectra were recorded with a Bruker AM 500 spectrometer at 500 MHz (^{1}H) and 125.8 MHz (^{13}C). Melting points were determined with a Fisher–Johns apparatus and are uncorrected. Optical rotations were measured with a Perkin-Elmer 343 polarimeter, with a path length of 1 dm at 25°C.

1,2,3,5,6-Penta-*O*-Benzoyl-α,β-D-Galactofuranose (1α and 1β)

The reaction setup consists of a 250 mL, three-neck round bottom flask with a magnetic stirring bar. One neck is connected to an addition funnel and the other equipped with a thermometer. A reflux condenser with a calcium chloride drying tube is attached to the third neck. The flask is charged with D-galactose (5.0 g, 0.028 mol) and anhydrous pyridine (70 mL),* and the suspension is stirred in a gently boiling water bath for 2 h, while the bath and the flask are covered with aluminum foil. In this way, any water condenses under the foil. The flask is then removed from the bath, vigorous stirring is continued, and the mixture is allowed to cool to 60°C–65°C. BzCl (20 mL, 0.17 mol) is added in portions (within approx. 5 min), while the content of the flask is stirred manually and the internal temperature is kept at 60°C, by cooling with an ice-water bath, if necessary.[†] When the addition of BzCl is complete, the solution is stirred in a water bath kept at 60°C.[2] After 1.5 h, water (10 mL) is slowly added, and vigorous stirring is continued for 0.5 h at room temperature. The solution is poured slowly with stirring (glass rod) into ice-water (500 mL) affording an amorphous solid. Immediately after the ice had melted, the liquid is decanted and the remaining solid is thoroughly washed with ice-water (5 × 500 mL), rubbing the solid with the rod. The solid is filtered,[‡] rapidly washed with cold water, transferred into an Erlenmeyer flask, and dissolved in boiling ethanol (800 mL). The solution is kept at room temperature (covered loosely with an aluminum foil) with occasional

---

* D-Galactose or D-arabinose is dried under vacuum (P_2O_5, toluene reflux); pyridine is distilled from NaOH pellets and stored over NaOH under nitrogen.
[†] The reaction mixture turns brown if the temperature rises above 70°C.
[‡] If the product cannot be filtered it is transferred to the Erlenmeyer flask with the aid of hot ethanol and finally dissolved in a total of 800 mL ethanol.

scratching the walls of the flask with the rod, to induce crystallization, and after 2 days, a crop of crystals of 1,2,3,5,6-penta-*O*-benzoyl-α,β-D-galactofuranose (**1α,β**) is obtained. After three crops of the crystals are collected (2, 4, and 8 days), the total yield of **1α,β** is 5.0–6.4 g (26%–33%), R_f 0.60 and 0.54 (9:1 toluene–EtOAc). If TLC analysis of the crystals shows presence of the β-pyranose benzoate, with mobility (R_f 0.57) between that of the furanose forms, it can be removed by recrystallization from EtOH. ^{1}H NMR (CDCl$_3$) β-anomer: δ 8.12-7.13 (H-aromatic), 6.84 (s, $J <$ 0.5 Hz, 1H, H-1), 5.14 (m, 1H, H-5), 5.78 (d, J=4,1 Hz, 1H, H-3), 5.77 (s, 1H, H-2), 4.87 (apparent t, J=4.0 Hz, 1H, H-4), 4.78 (m, 2H, H-6,6′); α-anomer: δ 8.13-7.10 (H-aromatic), 6.84 (d, J=4.7 Hz, 1H, H-1), 6.39 (apparent t, J=7.2 Hz, 1H, H-3), 5.90 (dd, J=7.5, 4.7 Hz, 1H, H-2), 5.88 (m, 2H, H-5), 4.79 (m, 2H, H-4,6), 4.70 (dd, J=6.3, 11.9 Hz, 1H, H-6′).

1,2,3,5-Tetra-*O*-Benzoyl-α,β-D-Arabinofuranose (2αβ),
1,2,3,5-Tetra-*O*-Benzoyl-α-D-Arabinofuranose (2α) and
1,2,3,4-Tetra-*O*-Benzoyl-α-D-Arabinopyranose (3)

D-Arabinose (3.05 g, 20.3 mmol), in dry pyridine (63.9 mL) is heated, for 45 min with the exclusion of moisture, in a boiling water bath, as described for galactose, The bath is rapidly cooled to 60°C–65°C and freshly distilled benzoyl chloride (11.3 mL, 97.4 mmol) is slowly added to the reaction mixture (approx. 3 min), keeping the internal temperature at 60°C. After stirring at 60°C for 1.5 h, water (6 mL) is slowly added to the orange mixture, and the stirring is continued for 30 min at room temperature. With continuous stirring with a glass rod, the solution is poured slowly into ice-water (400 mL), affording an amorphous solid. After decantation, the remaining solid is washed five times with cold water (5×300 mL). ^{1}H NMR spectrum (CDCl$_3$) of the solid shows the anomeric signals with the following integrations: δ 6.88 (d, 0.30H, J=4.4 Hz, H-1β furanoside), 6.76 (s, 0.27H, H-1α furanoside), 6.26 (d, 0.43H, J=5.6 Hz, H-1α pyranoside). The solid is dissolved in boiling EtOH (400 mL) and the flask is loosely closed with aluminum foil to allow slow evaporation of the solvent. Occasional scratching the walls of the flask with a glass rod causes slow crystallization and, after 2 days, 1,2,3,4-tetra-*O*-benzoyl-α-D-arabinopyranose (**3**) is filtered and washed twice with 5 mL of cold ethanol (yield: 3.02 g, 26%,* R_f 0.46, 3:1 hexane–EtOAc, double development); mp 161°C–162°C; [α]$_D$ −113.8 (*c* 1, CHCl$_3$) [lit.^{24} mp 164°C–165°C; [α]$_D$ −114.4 (*c* 0.8, CHCl$_3$)]; ^{1}H NMR (CDCl$_3$) δ 8.08–7.33 (m, 20H), 6.26 (d, 1H, J=5.6 Hz, H-1), 5.95 (dd, 1H, J=5.6, 7.3 Hz, H-2), 5.80 (ddd, 1H, J=2.9, 3.6, 5.2 Hz, H-4), 5.78 (dd, 1H, J=3.6, 7.3 Hz, H-3), 4.43 (dd, 1H, J=5.2, 12.6 Hz, H-5a), 4.14 (dd, 1H, J=2.9, 12.6 Hz, H-5b); ^{13}C NMR (CDCl$_3$) δ 164.5–164.7 (COPh), 133.7–128.5 (aromatic), 92.4 (C-1), 69.9 (C-3), 68.9 (C-2), 67.5 (C-4), 62.7 (C-5).

The mother liquors combined with the washings are kept at room temperature (20°C–23°C). Crystallization is induced by scratching the walls of the flask with

---

* These yields and periods for crystallization may slightly vary. Shorter standardized periods of crystallization are obtained by seeding the solution with the benzoates **3** and **2αβ**, respectively, obtained in a previous preparation.

a rod.* After 2 days at room temperature, the crystals are filtered and washed as described above giving 3.34 g of 1,2,3,5-tetra-*O*-benzoyl-α,β-D-arabinofuranose (**2αβ**) (29%, R_f 0.53 and 0.49, 3:1 hexane–EtOAc, double development) in a ~7:3 α:β ratio; ^{1}H NMR (CDCl$_3$) δ 8.13–7.24 (m, 20H), 6.87 (d, 0.3H, J=4.7 Hz, H-1 β anomer), 6.76 (s, 0.7H, H-1 α anomer), 6.11 (dd, 0.3H, J=5.2, 7.0 Hz, H-3), 5.94 (dd, 0.3H, J=4.7, 7.0 Hz, H-2), 5.82 (d, 0.7H, J=0.8 Hz, H-2), 5.68 (dd, 0.7H, J=3.7, 0.8 Hz, H-3), 4.83 (dd, 0.7H, J=3.9, 12.7 Hz, H-5a), 4.82 (m, 0.7H, H-4), 4.81 (dd, 0.3H, J=6.7, 14.1 Hz, H-5a), 4.73 (dd, 0.7H, J=6.4, 12.7 Hz, H-5b), 4.67 (m, 0.3H, H-4), 4.66 (dd, 0.3H, J=6.1, 14.1 Hz, H-5b); ^{13}C NMR (CDCl$_3$) δ 166.2–164.6 (*C*OPh), 133.7–128.2 (aromatic), 99.8 (C-1 α anomer), 94.5 (C-1 β anomer), 83.9 (C-4 α anomer), 80.9 (C-2 α anomer), 79.8, 77.5, 76.2, 75.5, 64.7, 63.7.

The pure α-anomer (**2α**), obtained by recrystallization, showed mp 100°C–101°C (EtOH); [α]$_D$ +26.7 (*c* 1, CHCl$_3$) [lit.[21] mp 117°C–121°C (EtOH), [α]$_D$ +27.9 (*c* 2.13, CHCl$_3$)]; ^{1}H NMR (CDCl$_3$) δ 8.14–7.26 (m, 20H), 6.76 (s, 1H, H-1), 5.82 (d, 1H, J=0.8 Hz, H-2), 5.68 (dd, 1H, J=3.7, 0.8 Hz, H-3), 4.83 (dd, 1H, J=3.9, 12.7 Hz, H-5a), 4.82 (m, 1H, H-4), 4.73 (dd, 1H, J=6.4, 12.7 Hz, H-5b); ^{13}C NMR (CDCl$_3$) δ 166.2–164.6 (*C*OPh), 133.8–128.3 (aromatic), 99.8 (C-1), 83.9 (C-4), 80.9 (C-2), 77.5 (C-3), 63.7 (C-5). These assignments were supported by HETCOR experiments.

ACKNOWLEDGMENTS

We are indebted to Agencia Nacional de Promoción Científica y Tecnológica and Universidad de Buenos Aires for financial support. C. Marino, C. Gallo-Rodriguez, and R. M. de Lederkremer are research members of CONICET.

---

* Crystals for seeding (**2**, α,β mixture) can be obtained after chromatography of a small portion of the mother liquor.

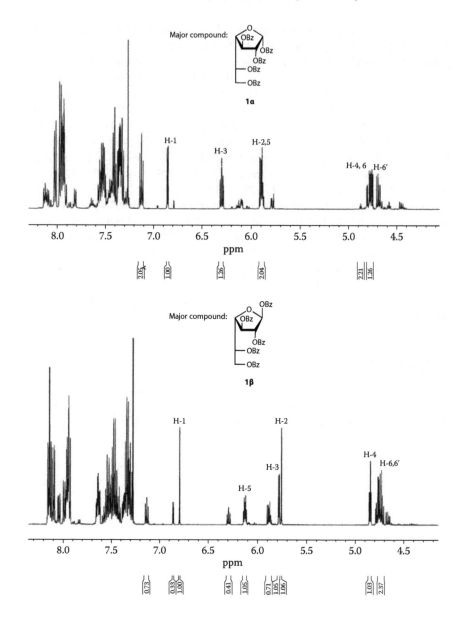

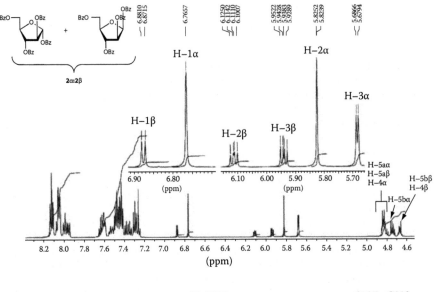

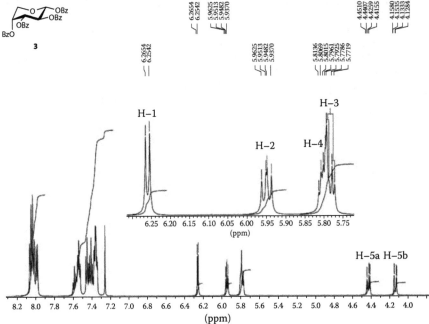

REFERENCES

1. Crick, D. C.; Mahaprata, S.; Brennan, P. J. *Glycobiology* 2001, *11*, 107–118.
2. Pan, F.; Jackson, M.; Ma, Y.; McNeil, M. *J. Bacteriol.* 2001, *183*, 3991–3998.
3. Lederkremer, R. M.; Colli, W. *Glycobiology* 1995, *5*, 547–552.
4. Pedersen, L. L.; Turco, S. J. *Cell Mol. Life Sci.* 2003, *60*, 259–266.

5. Latge, J. P. *Med. Mycol.* 2008, *5*, 1–6.
6. Levery, S. B.; Toledo, M. S.; Straus, A. H.; Takahashi, H. K. *Biochemistry* 1998, *37*, 8764–8775.
7. Houseknecht, J. B.; Lowary, T. L. *Curr. Opin. Chem. Biol.* 2001, *5*, 677–682.
8. Schmidt, R. R. *Angew. Chem. Int. Ed.* 1986, *25*, 212–235.
9. Lederkremer, R. M.; Nahmad, V. B.; Varela, O. *J. Org. Chem.* 1994, *59*, 690–692.
10. Marino, C.; Mariño, K.; Miletti, L.; Manso Alves, M. J.; Colli, W.; Lederkremer, R. M. *Glycobiology* 1998, *8*, 901–904.
11. Gallo-Rodriguez, C.; Varela, O.; Lederkremer, R. M. *Carbohydr. Res.* 1998, *305*, 163–170.
12. Gandolfi-Donadio, L.; Gallo-Rodríguez, C.; Lederkremer, R. M. *Can. J. Chem.* 2006, *84*, 486–491.
13. Gallo-Rodriguez, C.; Gandolfi, L.; de Lederkremer, R. M. *Org. Lett.* 1999, *1*, 245–247.
14. Gandolfi-Donadio, L.; Gallo-Rodriguez, C.; de Lederkremer, R. M. *J. Org. Chem.* 2003, *68*, 6928–6934.
15. D'Accorso, N. B.; Thiel, I. M. E.; Schüller, M. *Carbohydr. Res.* 1983, *124*, 177–184.
16. Chittenden, G. J. F. *Carbohydr. Res.* 1972, *25*, 35–41.
17. Owen, D. J.; Davis, C. B.; Hartnell, R. D.; Madge, P. D.; Thomson, R. J.; Chong, A. K. J.; Coppel, R. L.; von Itzstein, M. *Bioorg. Med. Chem. Lett.* 2007, *17*, 2274–2277.
18. Completo, G. C.; Lowary, T. L. *J. Org. Chem.* 2008, *73*, 4513–4525.
19. Ferrières, V.; Gelin, M.; Boulch, R.; Toupet, L.; Plusquellec, D. *Carbohydr. Res.* 1998, *314*, 79–83.
20. Kam, B. L.; Barascut, J.-L.; Imbach, J.-L. *Carbohydr. Res.* 1979, *69*, 135–142.
21. Ness, R. K.; Fletcher, H.G. *J. Am. Chem. Soc.* 1958, *80*, 2007–2010.
22. Horton, D.; Norris, P. In *Preparative Carbohydrate Chemistry*; Hanessian, S. Ed; Marcel Dekker, Inc, New York, 1997, pp. 35–52.
23. Lerner, L. M. *Carbohydr. Res.* 1996, *282*, 189–192.
24. Fetcher, H. G., Jr.; Hudson, C. S. *J. Am. Chem. Soc.* 1947, *69*, 1145–1147.

26 Stereoselective Synthesis of α-C-Sialyl Compounds

Jin-Hwan Kim, Fei Huang, Sayaka Masuko,
Deepak Sail,[†] and Robert J. Linhardt*

CONTENTS

Introduction 239
Experimental Methods 240
  General Methods 240
    SmI$_2$-Mediated *C*-Sialylation: 4,4-Dimethyl-1-[Methyl (5-Acetamido-
    4,7,8,9-Tetra-*O*-Acetyl-3,5-Dideoxy-D-*Glycero*-α-D-*Galacto*-Non-2-
    Ulopyranosyl)onate]cyclohexanol (**3**) 240
References 242

INTRODUCTION

Sialic acids (or neuraminic acids) are often found at the outmost ends of the oligosaccharide components of cell-surface glycoproteins and glycolipids. They are involved in a number of important biological events including cell recognition and interaction, neuronal transmission, ion transport, reproduction, differentiation, epitope masking, and protection. They are also involved in pathological processes including infection, inflammation, cancer, neurological, cardiovascular, endocrine, and autoimmune diseases.[1-4] Cell surfaces containing sialic acids interact with receptors, hormones, enzymes, toxins, and viruses and other pathogens that use them to localize on the surface of cells they infect.[5] The linkage of sialic acid to oligosaccharide is among the most labile glycosidic linkages and is cleaved in vitro under mildly acidic conditions.[6] In vivo, sialic acid–containing glycoconjugates are catabolized through the removal of the terminal sialic acid residue by the action of hydrolase-type enzymes called neuraminidases.[7] A nonhydrolyzable glycosidic linkage to sialic acid is an attractive approach to design reagents for glycobiology and immunology. The replacement of the interglycosidic oxygen atom with a hydroxymethylene group using SmI$_2$ chemistry affords hydrolytically and metabolically inert α-*C*-sialyl analogues of natural glycoconjugates. This stable linkage is being studied to improve our understanding of biological recognition and to enhance or suppress biological events at the molecular level.

---

* Corresponding author.
[†] Checker.

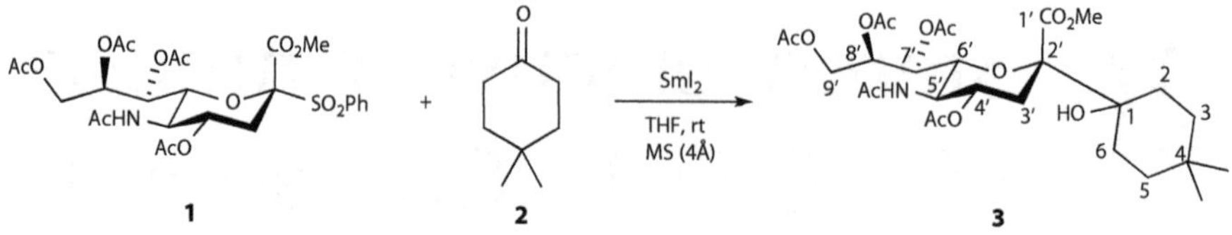

SCHEME 26.1　Stereoselective synthesis of 4,4-dimethyl-1-α-C-sialylcyclohexanol.

A method for the stereoselective preparation of α-C-sialyl compounds was pioneered in our laboratory.[8a] Since 1997, this method has been applied for the diastereocontrolled synthesis of α-C-sialyl compounds, using samarium iodide under Barbier conditions,[8] a method that had been previously used to prepare C-glycosyl compounds.[9–11] This approach is tolerant of a wide variety of protecting groups.[8–11] The reducing potential of SmI_2 is exploited through the in situ generation of a neuraminyl samarium (III) species and its coupling to carbonyl compounds. Through a simple, high-yielding reaction, this same chemistry could be used to couple different ketones or aldehydes with peracetylated sialic acid sulfone and form α-C-sialyl compounds (Scheme 26.1).

EXPERIMENTAL METHODS

GENERAL METHODS

All chemicals were purchased from commercial suppliers and used without further purification, unless otherwise noted. Column chromatography was performed on silica gel 60 (EM Science, 70-230 mesh). Reaction was monitored by TLC on Kieselgel $60 F_{254}$ (EM Science) and the compounds were detected by UV light and visualized by dipping the plates in a cerium sulfate-ammonium molybdate solution followed by heating. Solutions in organic solvents were concentrated by rotary evaporation below 40°C under reduced pressure. ¹H NMR and ¹³C NMR spectra were recorded with a Bruker, 600 MHz instrument. When reporting NMR data, nuclei associated with the sugar are denoted with a prime ('). Chemical shifts are reported in parts per million (ppm) downfield from tetramethylsilane. Data are presented as follows: Chemical shift, multiplicity (s = singlet, d = doublet, t = triplet, dd = double of doublet, ddd = doublet of doublet of doublet, dt = double of triplet, m = multiplet and/or multiple resonances), integration, and coupling constant in Hertz (Hz). High-resolution mass spectra were run in a JMS SX/SX102A tandem mass spectrometer, equipped with FAB source. The matrix used was DHB and the internal standards ultramark 1621 and PEG. SmI_2 solution was purchased from Aldrich.

SmI₂-Mediated C-Sialylation: 4,4-Dimethyl-1-[Methyl (5-Acetamido-4,7,8,9-Tetra-O-Acetyl-3,5-Dideoxy-D-*Glycero*-α-D-*Galacto*-Non-2-Ulopyranosyl)onate]cyclohexanol (3)

To a solution of sulfone donor 1[12] (308 mg, 0.5 mmol) and 4,4-dimethylcyclohexanone 2 (94 mg, 0.75 mmol) in anhydrous THF (7.5 mL) was added molecular sieves (4 Å,

500 mg).* After stirring for 2 h at room temperature under a positive pressure of Argon, SmI$_2$ solution (30.0 mL, 0.1 M in THF, 3.0 mmol)† was added to the reaction mixture and stirring was continued for 1 h under argon. During initial addition of the SmI$_2$, the solution decolorized and the mixture turned yellow but when the addition was complete the reaction mixture turned dark green and maintained that color for ~1 h.‡ TLC (3:2 hexane-acetone) then showed reaction to be complete.§ The mixture was diluted with Et$_2$O (50 mL), and washed successively with aqueous 1 N HCl (50 mL), aqueous 0.1 M Na$_2$S$_2$O$_3$ (50 mL), and saturated aqueous NaHCO$_3$ (50 mL). The organic phase was dried over anhydrous MgSO$_4$, filtered, the filtrate was concentrated, and chromatography (2:1 hexane–acetone) afforded **3** (219 mg, 73%): R_f=0.4 (3:2 hexane–acetone), c.f. R_f=0.3 for the starting material; $[α]_D$=−19° (c=0.7, CHCl$_3$); ^{1}H NMR (600 MHz, CDCl$_3$) δ 5.41 (ddd, 1H, J=8.8, 6.5, 2.7 Hz, H-8′), 5.35–5.24 (m, 2H, H-7′, NH), 4.78–4.73 (m, 1H, H-4′), 4.35 (dd, 1H, H-9′a, J=12.4, 2.7 Hz), 4.07 (dd, 1H, J=12.4, 6.4 Hz, H-9′b), 4.03–3.98 (m, 2H, H-5′, H-6′), 3.79 (s, 3H, CO$_2$$CH_3$), 2.56 (s, 1H, OH), 2.48 (dd, 1H, J=12.8, 4.6 Hz, H-3′eq), 2.17 (s, 3H, Ac), 2.12 (s, 3H, Ac), 2.05 (s, 3H, Ac), 2.03 (s, 3H, Ac), 1.97 (t, 1H, J=12.4 Hz, H-3′ax), 1.88 (s, 3H, NAc), 1.68–1.16 (m, 8H, 4×CH$_2$), 0.92 (s, 3H, CH$_3$), 0.84 (s, 3H, CH$_3$); ^{13}C NMR (151 MHz, CDCl$_3$) δ 171.1, 170.70, 170.68, 170.35, 170.18, 170.02, 86.0 (C-2′), 74.9 (C-1), 73.2 (C-6′), 70.4 (C-4′), 68.7 (C-8′), 67.8 (C-7′), 62.6 (C-9′), 52.3 (CO$_2$$CH_3$), 49.5 (C-5′), 34.1, 33.9 (C-3, 5), 32.9 (C-3′), 32.5 (CH$_3$), 29.3 (C-4), 27.6, 27.3 (C-2, 6), 23.2 (CH$_3$), 23.1 (NAc), 21.2 (Ac), 20.9 (Ac), 20.74 (Ac), 20.72 (Ac); HR MALDI-TOF MS: m/z: calcd for C$_{28}$H$_{43}$NNaO$_{13}$ [M + Na]$^+$: 624.2627; found: 624.2624. Anal. Calcd for C$_{28}$H$_{43}$NO$_{13}$: C, 55.90; H, 7.20; N, 2.33; O, 34.57. Found: C, 56.07; H, 7.23; N, 2.42.

---

* Molecular sieves (4 Å) were crushed and activated in vacuo >160°C for 5 h before use.
† Commercial 0.1 M samarium iodide solution in THF should be clear blue with only small amount of solid samarium present, which is used as stabilizer.
‡ Blue, instead of green color was observed when the reaction was carried out on much smaller scale.
§ Frequent monitoring of progress of the reaction by TLC is not recommended, to prevent the mixture from exposure to atmospheric air and moisture.

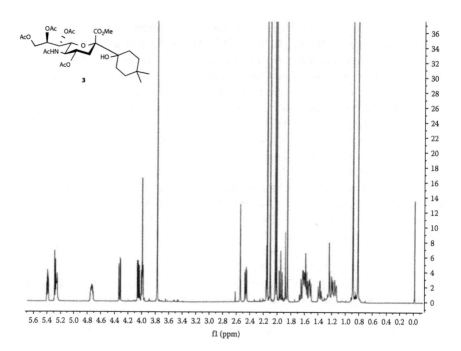

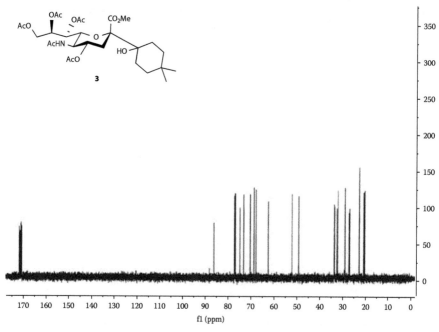

REFERENCES

1. Schauer, R. *Glycoconj. J.* 2000, *17*, 485–499.
2. Angata, T.; Varki, A. *Chem. Rev.* 2002, *102*, 439–469.

3. Varki, A. *Nature* 2007, *446*, 1023–1029.
4. Varki, A. *Trands Mol. Med.* 2008, *14*, 351–360.
5. Swartley, J. S.; Marfin, A. A.; Edupugantis, D.; Liu, L. J.; Cieslak, P.; Perkins, B.; Wenger, J. D.; Stephans, D. S. *Proc. Nat. Acad. Sci. U.S.A.* 1997, *94*, 271–276.
6. Sharon, N.; Lis, H. *Science* 1989, *246*, 227–234.
7. Air, G. M.; Laver, W. *Proteins Struct. Funct. Genet.* 1989, *6*, 341–356, and references therein.
8. (a) Vlahov, I. R.; Vlahova, P. I.; Linhardt, R. J. *J. Am. Chem. Soc.* 1997, *119*, 1480–1481. (b) Du, Y.; Linhardt, R. J. *Carbohydr. Res.* 1998, *308*, 161–164. (c) Du, Y.; Polat, T.; Linhardt, R. J. *Tetrahedron Lett.* 1998, *39*, 5007–5010. (d) Polat, T.; Du, Y.; Linhardt, R. J. *Synlett* 1998, *11*, 1195–1196. (e) Bazin, H. G.; Du, Y.; Polat, T.; Linhardt, R. J. *J. Org. Chem.* 1999, *64*, 7254–7259. (f) Wang, Q.; Linhardt, R. J. *J. Org. Chem.* 2003, *68*, 2668–2672. (g) Kuberan, B.; Sikkander, S. A.; Tomiyama, H.; Linhardt, R. J. *Angew. Chem. Int. Ed. Engl.* 2003, *42*, 2073–2075. (h) Ress, D. K.; Baytas, S. N.; Wang, Q.; Munoz, E. M.; Tokuzoki, K.; Tomiyama, H.; Linhardt, R. J. *J. Org. Chem.* 2005, *70*, 8197–8200. (i) Yuan, X.; Ress, D. K.; Linhardt, R. J. *J. Org. Chem.* 2007, *72*, 3085–3088. (j) Kim, J. –H.; Huang, F.; Ly, M.; Linhardt, R. J. *J. Org. Chem.* 2008, *73*, 9497–9500.
9. Mazeas, D.; Skrydstrup, T.; Beau, J. M. *Angew. Chem. Int. Ed. Engl.* 1995, *34*, 909–9012.
10. Hung, S.-C.; Wong. C.-H. *Angew. Chem. Int. Ed. Engl.* 1996, *35*, 2671–2674.
11. Depouilly, P.; Chenede, A.; Mallet, J. M.; Sinaÿ, P. *Bull. Soc. Chim. Fr.* 1993, *130*, 256–265.
12. Marra, A.; Sinay, P. *Carbohydr. Res.* 1989, *187*, 35–42.

27 Synthesis of O-Acetylated N-Acetylneuraminic Acid Glycal

Nadezhda Y. Kulikova, Anna M. Shpirt,
A. Chinarev,[†] and Leonid O. Kononov*

CONTENTS

Experimental Methods...246
    General Methods...246
        Methyl (5-Acetamido-4,7,8,9-Tetra-*O*-Acetyl-3,5-Dideoxy-β-D-
        Glycero-D-*Galacto*-Non-2-Ulopyranosyl)onate Chloride (2).....................246
        Methyl (5-Acetamido-4,7,8,9-Tetra-*O*-Acetyl-3,5-Dideoxy-2,6-
        Anhydro-D-*Glycero*-D-*Galacto*-Non-2-Enopyranos)onate (3)....................249
Acknowledgment...250
References..250

Reagents and conditions: (a) HCl (generated in situ by reaction of AcCl with MeOH), AcCl, CH$_2$Cl$_2$, +4°C; (b) Na$_2$HPO$_4$, MeCN, reflux.

O-Acetylated *N*-acetylneuraminic acid (Neu5Ac) glycal (**3**) is the key intermediate for preparation of the corresponding glycosyl donors with an auxiliary stereocontrolling group at the C-3, which have been glycosyl donors of choice for the synthesis of complex sialooligosaccharides.[1] Compound **3** has also found application in synthesis of an anti-influenza drug (Zanamivir), which has recently been commercialized.[2] Although several methods for the preparation of this important intermediate

---

* Corresponding author.
[†] Checker.

have been developed,[3] all of them have their own disadvantages (for more detailed discussion see Ref. [4]).

The synthesis of Neu5Ac glycal **3** described here[4] is experimentally simple, high yielding, and devoid of drawbacks inherent to the known approaches. Neu5Ac glycosyl chloride **2**,[5] readily accessible from the corresponding glycosyl acetate **1**,[5,6] was found to react smoothly with anhydrous Na_2HPO_4 in refluxing acetonitrile to give the target Neu5Ac glycal **3** in high yield (one-product conversion **2 → 3**, thin-layer chromatography [TLC]). The product of substantial purity (see Figures 27.1 through 27.3 for copies of nuclear magnetic resonance [NMR] spectra), suitable for most applications, can be isolated from the reaction mixture by simple filtration and subsequent concentration of the filtrate. As chromatography or crystallization is often not required, the protocol is applicable to large-scale preparation of **3**.

EXPERIMENTAL METHODS

GENERAL METHODS

The reactions were performed using commercial reagents (Aldrich and Fluka) and solvents purified according to standard procedures. Dichloromethane was distilled over P_2O_5. Acetonitrile used for small-scale preparation of **3** was distilled over CaH_2 under argon. Acetonitrile used for large-scale preparation was used as supplied (HPLC grade, $H_2O < 0.02\%$, Biosolve, the Netherlands). Fully acetylated methyl ester of Neu5Ac **1** was synthesized as described before.[5,6] TLC was carried out on silica gel 60 F_{254}-coated aluminum foil (Merck). Spots were visualized under UV light (254 nm) and by heating the plates after immersion in a 1:10 (v/v) mixture of 85% aqueous H_3PO_4 and 95% EtOH. The ^{1}H and ^{13}C NMR spectra were recorded for solutions in $CDCl_3$ with a Bruker Avance 800 (800 and 200 MHz, respectively) or Bruker AC-200 instruments (200.13 and 50.32 MHz, respectively). The ^{1}H and ^{13}C chemical shifts are referred to the signal of the residual $CHCl_3$ (δ 7.27) and $CDCl_3$ (δ 77.0), respectively. The signal assignment was made by ^{1}H,^{1}H-COSY 2D NMR, and APT (JMODXH) experiments. Electrospray ionization mass spectra (ESI-MS) were recorded with a Finnigan LCQ mass spectrometer and MALDI-TOF mass spectra (MALDI-MS) with a Vision-2000 MALDI-TOF spectrometer. The specific optical rotation ($[\alpha]_D$) of **3** was measured with a JASCO DIP-360 polarimeter.

Methyl (5-Acetamido-4,7,8,9-Tetra-O-Acetyl-3,5-Dideoxy-β-D-Glycero-D-Galacto-Non-2-Ulopyranosyl)onate Chloride (2)

Small Scale

Anhydrous MeOH (1.8 mL, 0.04 mol) was slowly added dropwise, with cooling in an ice–water bath, to AcCl (4.5 mL, 0.06 mol). The resulting solution was added to a cold solution of acetate **1** (102 mg, 0.19 mmol) in a mixture of anhydrous CH_2Cl_2 (4.5 mL) and AcCl (4.5 mL, 0.06 mol), and the reaction mixture was kept at +4°C for 12 h (TLC: R_f 0.50 (**2**), R_f 0.30 (**1**), AcOEt). Volatile components were evaporated, and a solution of the residue in CCl_4 (5 mL) was concentrated five times. Drying in vacuum gave glycosyl chloride **2** as a white foam (114 mg), which was used without additional purification.

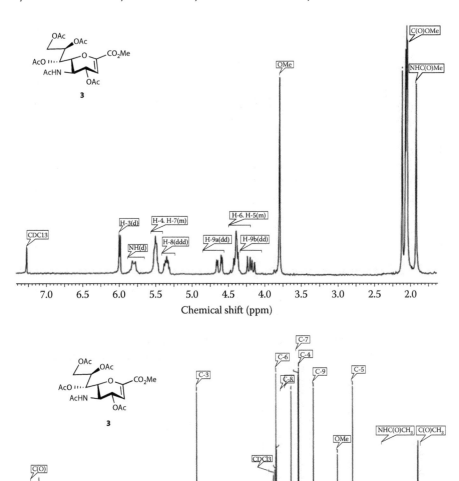

FIGURE 27.1 ^{1}H and ^{13}C NMR spectra (obtained at 200.13 and 50.32 MHz, respectively) of Neu5Ac glycal **3**, which was obtained by small-scale procedures without purification by chromatography.

Large Scale

AcCl (110 mL, 1.54 mol) was added to a solution of acetate **1** (15 g, 28.1 mmol) in CH$_2$Cl$_2$ (480 mL) placed in 1 L round-bottom flask equipped with magnetic stirrer, and the solution was cooled to ~−20°C. Cold MeOH (30 mL, 0.74 mol) was added to

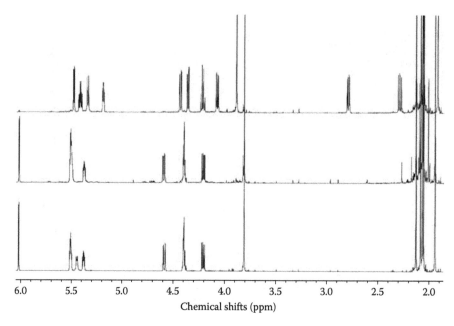

FIGURE 27.2 ¹H NMR spectra (obtained at 800 MHz) of Neu5Ac chloride **2** (top) and Neu5Ac glycal **3** before (middle) and after chromatography (bottom), which were prepared by large-scale procedures.

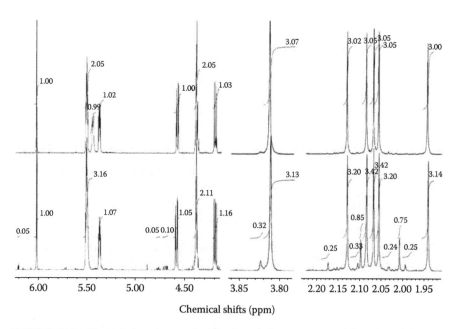

FIGURE 27.3 Expanded regions of ¹H NMR spectra (obtained at 800 MHz) of Neu5Ac glycal **3** before (bottom) and after chromatography (top), which were prepared by large-scale procedures.

the stirred solution in one portion, which made the concentration of HCl in the reaction mixture ~1.2 M. The stirring and cooling were discontinued, the flask was tightly closed, and a stopper was secured. The reaction mixture was kept at room temperature for 72 h and then concentrated. The residue was dried in vacuum, affording glycosyl chloride **2** as colorless foam in virtually theoretical yield; the product obtained was used for further synthesis without purification. $[\alpha]_D^{20}$ −62.3 (*c* 1.0, CHCl$_3$), lit.: $[\alpha]_D^{20}$ −63.0 (*c* 1, CHCl$_3$)^{5a}; TLC: R_f 0.50 (**2**), R_f 0.32 (**1-β**), R_f 0.30, (**1-α**) (AcOEt). ^{1}H NMR (800 MHz): δ 1.92 (s, 3H, NC(O)CH$_3$), 2.06, 2.07, 2.09, 2.13 (4 s, 4 × 3H, 4 × OC(O)CH$_3$), 2.30 (dd, 1H, $J_{3ax,3eq}$ 13.9 Hz, $J_{3ax,4}$ 11.2 Hz, H-3$_{ax}$), 2.80 (dd, 1H, $J_{3eq,4}$ 4.9 Hz, H-3$_{eq}$), 3.89 (s, 3H, OMe), 4.08 (dd, 1H, $J_{9a,9b}$ 12.7 Hz, $J_{9b,8}$ 5.9 Hz, H-9$_b$), 4.22 (ddd, 1H, H-5), 4.36 (dd, 1H, $J_{6,5}$ 10.5 Hz, $J_{7,6}$ 2.4 Hz, H-6), 4.43 (dd, 1H, $J_{9a,8}$ 2.7 Hz, H-9$_a$), 5.20 (ddd, 1H, H-8), 5.34 (d, 1H, $J_{5,NH}$ 10.2 Hz, NH), 5.42 (ddd, 1H, $J_{5,4}$ 10.4 Hz, H-4), 5.48 (dd, 1H, $J_{8,7}$ 10.4 Hz, H-7). MALDI-MS: 510 [M]$^+$, 533 [M + Na]$^+$, 549 [M + K]$^+$; Anal. calcd for C$_{20}$H$_{28}$ClNO$_{12}$: C, 47.11; H, 5.54; N, 2.75. Found: C, 47.00; H, 5.65; N, 2.70.

Methyl (5-Acetamido-4,7,8,9-Tetra-*O*-Acetyl-3,5-Dideoxy-2,6-Anhydro-D-*Glycero*-D-*Galacto*-Non-2-Enopyranos)onate (3)

Small Scale

Na$_2$HPO$_4$ (33 mg, 0.23 mmol) was added to a solution of glycosyl chloride **2** [prepared from **1** (103.6 mg, 0.194 mmol)] in MeCN (4 mL), and the suspension was heated under reflux.* The course of the reaction was monitored by TLC (AcOEt). After 3 h, when TLC (AcOEt) showed that the conversion **2 → 3** was complete (**3**, R_f 0.48; **2**, R_f 0.50), the colorless mixture was cooled to room temperature, filtered through Celite pad, the volatiles were evaporated, and the residue was dried in vacuo (~0.1 Torr) to give glycal **3** (87.1 mg) (for purity, see Figure 27.1). The product was chromatographed (gradient, AcOEt–hexanes 1:1 → AcOEt) to give pure **3** (87.1 mg, 95% from **1** over two steps), R_f 0.48 (AcOEt). $[\alpha]_D^{20}$ +56.6 (*c* 1.3, CHCl$_3$), lit.: $[\alpha]_D^{20}$ +56.0 (*c* 1.3, CHCl$_3$)^{3g}, $[\alpha]_D^{20}$ +79.9 (*c* 1.3, CHCl$_3$)^{3b}. ESI-MS: [M + Na]$^+$ calcd for C$_{20}$H$_{27}$NNaO$_{12}$, 496.1; found: 496.0. ^{1}H NMR (200 MHz): δ 1.92 (s, 3H, NC(O)CH$_3$), 2.04, 2.05, 2.07, 2.11 (4 s, 3H each, OC(O)CH$_3$), 3.79 (s, 3H, OMe), 4.18 (dd, 1H, $J_{9a,9b}$ 12.4 Hz, $J_{8,9b}$ 7.1 Hz, H-9b), 4.34–4.45 (m, 2H, H-5, H-6), 4.63 (dd, 1H, $J_{9a,8}$ 3.0 Hz, H-9a), 5.28–5.39 (m, 1H, H-8), 5.45–5.54 (m, 2H, H-4, H-7), 5.92 (d, 1H, $J_{NH,5}$ 8.7 Hz, NH), 5.98 (d, 1H, $J_{3,4}$ 2.9 Hz, H-3). ^{13}C NMR (CDCl$_3$): δ 20.7, 20.8 (OC(O)CH$_3$), 23.1 (NC(O)CH$_3$), 46.4 (C-5), 52.5 (OMe), 61.9 (C-9), 67.6 (C-4), 67.9 (C-7), 70.7 (C-8), 76.4 (C-6), 107.9 (C-3), 145.0 (C-2), 161.6 (C-1), 170.2, 170.6, 170.8 (C=O).

Large Scale

Na$_2$HPO$_4$ (5 g, 35.2 mmol) was added to a solution of the glycosyl chloride **2** (14.4 g, 28.1 mmol) in 600 mL of MeCN. The mixture was heated in a tightly closed flask for 3 h at 80°C, cooled to room temperature, the solids were filtered off, and the filtrate was concentrated to dryness. The residue was dried in vacuum to give glycal **3** (for purity, see Figures 27.2 and 27.3), which was chromatographed on silica gel (*i*-PrOH

---

* No glycal formation was observed at *ambient* temperature even after prolonged treatment with Na$_2$HPO$_4$.

5%→15% gradient in hexane–CHCl$_3$, 2:1) to give glycal **3** (10.1 g, 76%) identical to that obtained by small-scale procedure.

ACKNOWLEDGMENT

This chapter was financially supported by the Russian Foundation for Basic Research (Project No. 04-03-32854).

REFERENCES

1. Boons, G.-J.; Demchenko, A. V. *Chem. Rev.*, 2000, *100*, 4539–4565.
2. von Itzstein, M. *Nat. Rev. Drug Discov.*, 2007, *6*, 967–974.
3. (a) Meindl, P.; Tuppy, H. *Monatsh. Chem.*, 1969, *100*, 1295–1306; (b) Okamoto, K.; Kondo, T.; Goto, T. *Bull. Chem. Soc. Jpn.*, 1987, *60*, 631–636; (c) Claesson, A.; Luthman, K. *Acta Chem. Scand., Ser. B*, 1982, *B36*, 719–720; (d) Schmid, W.; Christian, R.; Zbiral, E. *Tetrahedron Lett.*, 1988, *29*, 3643–3646; (e) Ercegovic, T.; Magnusson, G. *J. Chem. Soc. Chem. Comm.*, 1994, 831–832; (f) Kok, G. B.; Mackey, B. L.; von Itzstein, M. *Carbohydr. Res.*, 1996, *289*, 67–75; (g) Ikeda, K.; Konishi, K.; Sano, K.; Tanaka, K. *Chem. Pharm. Bull.*, 2000, *48*, 163–165; (h) Kononov, L. O.; Komarova, B. S.; Nifantiev, N. E. *Russ. Chem. Bull.*, 2002, *51*, 698–702.
4. Kulikova, N. Yu.; Shpirt, A. M.; Kononov, L. O. *Synthesis.*, 2006, *24*, 4113–4114.
5. (a) Kuhn, R.; Lutz, P.; MacDonald, D. L. *Chem. Ber.*, 1966, *99*, 611–617; (b) Sharma, M. N.; Eby, R. *Carbohydr. Res.*, 1984, *127*, 201–210; (c) Byramova, N. E.; Tuzikov, A. B.; Bovin, N. V. *Carbohydr. Res.*, 1992, *237*, 161–175; (d) Kononov, L. O.; Magnusson, G. *Acta. Chem. Scand.*, 1998, *52*, 141–144; (e) Shpirt, A. M.; Kononov, L. O.; Torgov, V. I.; Shibaev, V. N. *Russ. Chem. Bull.*, 2004, *53*, 717–719.
6. Marra, A.; Sinaÿ, P. *Carbohydr. Res.*, 1989, *190*, 317–322.

28 Substituted Benzyl Glycosides of N-Acetylneuraminic Acid

A. Chinarev, A.B. Tuzikov,
A.I. Zinin,† and N.V. Bovin*

CONTENTS

Experimental Methods 253
  General Methods 253
    Methyl {4-[(*Tert*-Butyloxycarbonyl)glycylamido]benzyl 5-Acetamido-
    4,7,8,9-Tetra-*O*-Acetyl-3,5-Dideoxy-D-*Glycero*-D-*Galacto*-Non-2-
    Ulopyranosid}onate (**3**) 253
    4-[(*Tert*-Butyloxycarbonyl)glycylamido]benzyl 5-Acetamido-3,5-
    Dideoxy-D-*Glycero*-D-*Galacto*-Non-2-Ulopyranosidonic Acid (**5**) 256
    4-(Glycylamido)benzyl 5-Acetamido-3,5-Dideoxy-D-*Glycero*-D-
    Galacto-Non-2-Ulopyranosidonic Acid (**6**) 256
    4-[(4-Nitrophenoxy)adipoylglycylamido]benzyl 5-Acetamido-3,5-
    Dideoxy-D-*Glycero*-D-*Galacto*-Non-2-Ulopyranosidonic Acid (**8**) 257
Acknowledgment 257
References 257

---

* Corresponding author.
† Checker.

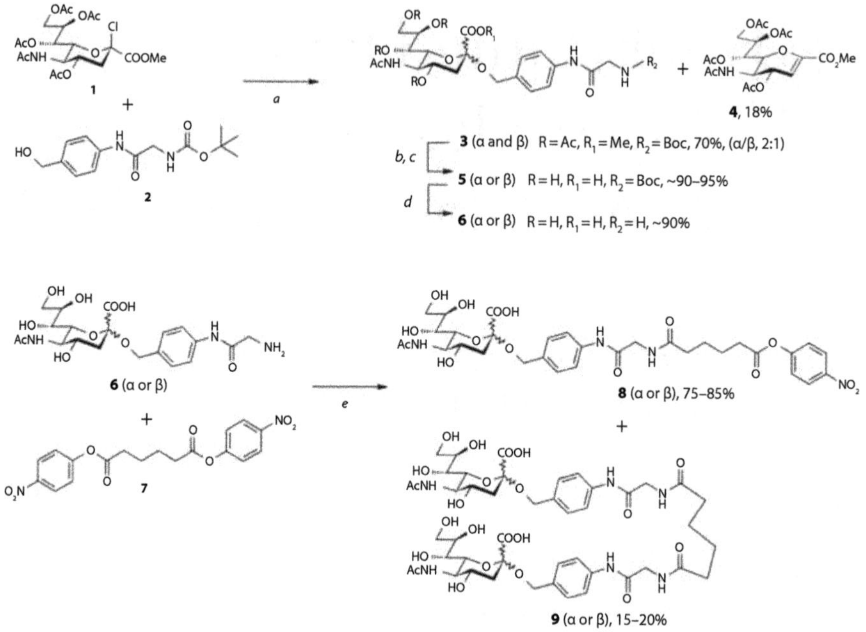

4, 18%

3 (α and β) R = Ac, R$_1$ = Me, R$_2$ = Boc, 70%, (α/β, 2:1)

5 (α or β) R = H, R$_1$ = H, R$_2$ = Boc, ~90–95%

6 (α or β) R = H, R$_1$ = H, R$_2$ = H, ~90%

6 (α or β)

8 (α or β), 75–85%

9 (α or β), 15–20%

Reagents and conditions: a. Ag$_2$CO$_3$/AgOTf, 2.5:1, MS 4 Å, CH$_2$Cl$_2$, 72 h, room temperature; separation of anomers; *b.* 0.1 M MeONa in absolute MeOH, 1 h, room temperature; *c.* 0.05 M NaOH in MeOH/H$_2$O, 1:1, 12 h, room temperature; *d.* TFA, 2 h, room temperature; *e.* DMSO/DMF 1:1, 24 h, room temperature.

Benzyl and substituted benzyl glycosides of α-*N*-acetylneuraminic acid (Neu5Ac) are important tools in glycobiology because their binding affinity toward proteins that recognize sialic acid, including H1 and H3 subtypes of human influenza virus hemagglutinin, siglecs, and anti-glycan antibodies, can be finely tuned.[1–3]

Here, we describe the synthesis of 4-(glycylamido)benzyl glycoside of Neu5Ac **6** having a free amino group, which can be used for direct coupling with a variety of labels, tags, and also with macromolecules or supports (ELISA plates, microchips, affinity matrices, beads) that carry an activated carboxylic group. By additional derivatization, glycoside **6** can be converted into a compound with an activated carboxyl group in the aglycon part, namely, into [4-(4-nitrophenoxy)adipoylglycylamido]benzyl glycoside **8**, followed by coupling with various entities, including peptides and proteins, which have a free amino group. UV absorbance of 4-(glycylamido)benzyl residue (λ_{max} 247 nm, ε = 17,000) allows performing a quantitative monitoring of reactions of **6** or **8**.[4] Finally, it should be noted that although α-glycosides **6** and **8** are the objects of primary interest, the correspondent β-glycosides are important as the negative control counterparts in studies of carbohydrate–protein interactions. Thus, the glycosides **6** and **8** were used for syntheses of different carbohydrate multimerics, sialoglycopolymers, sialoglycoclusters, and self-assembling sialoglycopeptides, to study influenza viruses binding to host cells.[4–6]

Earlier, a small-scale preparation of 4-[(*tert*-butyloxycarbonyl)glycylamido)]ben-zyl glycoside of peracetylated methyl ester of Neu5Ac **3** was described, which was based on Helferich reaction of the readily accessible glycosyl chloride **1** with the cor-responding alcohol **2** in acetonitrile–dichloromethane mixture using $HgBr_2/Hg(CN)_2$ as a catalyst. The yield of **3** was ~60% (anomeric α/β mixture,~3/2, as revealed by ^1H nuclear magnetic resonance [NMR]).[1c] We have developed an improved proce-dure where coupling of chloride **1** with alcohol **2** is performed in dichloromethane in the presence of $Ag_2CO_3/AgOTf$.[7] Individual anomers of **3** are obtained by chro-matography of the reaction mixture on silica gel in ~70% yield, α/β ~2:1. Stepwise deprotection of **3** (α or β), involving sequential Zemplén deacetylation (MeONa/MeOH), hydrolysis of the methyl ester group (0.05 M NaOH), and N-deprotection (TFA), gives glycoside **6** (α or β) with 80%–85% yield (over three steps). A treatment of glycoside **6** (α or β) with a fivefold excess of bis(4-nitrophenyl) adipate **7** in DMF/DMSO mixture gives two products, the monosialoside **8** (major, α or β, 75%–85%) and the disialoside **9** (minor, α or β, 15%–20%). The products can be purified by gel-permeation chromatography on Sephadex LH-20. The prepared glycoside **8** is stable for several months when stored at –20°C.

EXPERIMENTAL METHODS

GENERAL METHODS

The reactions were performed using commercial reagents (Aldrich, Merck, and Fluka) and solvents were purified according to standard procedures. The glycosyl chloride **1**, 4-[(*tert*-butyloxicarbonyl)glycylamido)]]benzyl alcohol **2**, and bis-(4-nitrophenyl) adipate **7** were synthesized as described before.[1c,6–8] Thin-layer chro-matography (TLC) was carried out on silica gel $60F_{254}$-coated aluminum sheets (Merck). Spots were visualized by dipping the plates in 10% aqueous H_3PO_4 or in a solution of ninhydrin (2.5 g in a mixture of 95:4:1 $Me_2CO–H_2O–AcOH$, 500 mL) and heating. The presence of compounds bearing the 4-nitrophenyl ester group was revealed by exposing the plates to NH_3 atmosphere. The ^1H NMR spectra were recorded in $CDCl_3$ or D_2O with a Bruker WM-500 (500 MHz) (Figure 28.1). Chemical shifts are referenced to the signal of the residual $CHCl_3$ (δ 7.27) and H_2O (δ 4.75), respectively; the data obtained are summarized in the Table 28.1. MALDI-TOF mass spectra (MALDI-MS) were recorded with a Vision-2000 MALDI-TOF spectrometer. The specific optical rotation ($[α]_D$) was measured with a PerkinElmer 341LC polarimeter.

Methyl {4-[(*Tert*-Butyloxycarbonyl)glycylamido]benzyl 5-Acetamido-4,7,8,9-Tetra-*O*-Acetyl-3,5-Dideoxy-D-*Glycero*-D-*Galacto*-Non-2-Ulopyranosid}onate (3)

A mixture of alcohol **2** (1.23 g, 4.41 mmol), Ag_2CO_3 (1.08 g, 5.88 mmol), AgOTf (600 mg, 2.34 mmol), freshly activated molecular sieves 4 Å (4.0 g), and absolute CH_2Cl_2 (30 mL) was stirred for 1 h at room temperature, and a solution of chloride **1** (1.5 g, 2.94 mmol) in absolute CH_2Cl_2 (30 mL) was added. The formed suspension was stirred in the dark at room temperature, while the reaction was periodically

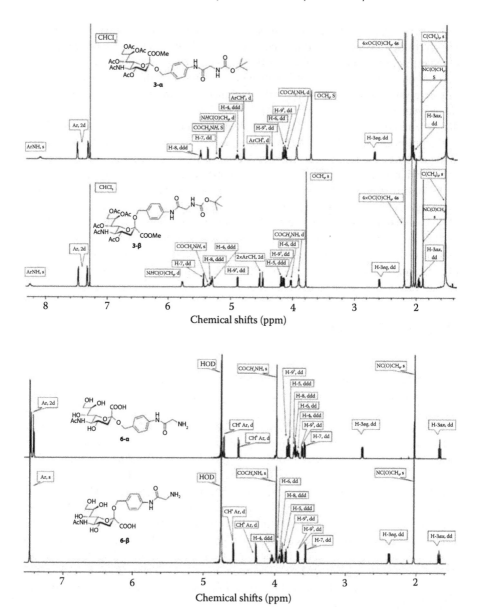

FIGURE 28.1 ¹H NMR spectra (obtained at 500 MHz in CHCl₃ and D₂O) of the substituted benzyl glycosides Neu5Ac.

checked by TLC: R_f 0.51 (**2**), R_f 0.38 (**1**), R_f 0.30 (**4**), R_f 0.19 (**3-α + β**) (AcOEt). After 3–5 days, when chloride **1** was consumed, the mixture was filtered, the solids were washed with CHCl₃ (2 × 50 mL) and 1:1 CHCl₃–MeOH (2 × 50 mL), and the combined filtrates were concentrated to dryness. The residue was dissolved in CHCl₃ (150 mL), the chloroform solution was washed with 10% Na₂S₂O₃ (30 mL) and H₂O (30 mL), kept for 12 h over anhydrous Na₂SO₄ (20 g), filtered, and then concentrated

TABLE 28.1

Proton Chemical Shifts (δ, ppm; 500 MHz) and Coupling Constants (J, Hz) for the Substituted Benzyl Glycosides of Neu5Ac[a]

	H-3ax	H-3eq	H-4	H-5	H-6	H-7	H-8	H-9	H-9	ArCH	ArCH	NC(O) CH$_3$	COCH$_2$NH
3-α (CDCl$_3$)	2.03, dd, $J_{4,3ax}$ 12.5	2.65, dd, $J_{3ax,3eq}$ 12.5, $J_{4,3eq}$ 4.5	4.88, ddd, $J_{5,4}$ 10.0	4.10, ddd	4.15, dd, $J_{6,5}$ 11.0	5.35, dd, $J_{7,6}$ 8.0	5.46, ddd	4.33, dd, $J_{9a,8}$ 3.0	4.11, dd, $J_{9a,9b}$ 12.5, $J_{9b,8}$ 6.0	4.78, d	4.40, d, J_{hem} 12.0	1.90, s	3.92, d, J 6.0
3-β (CDCl$_3$)	1.93, dd, $J_{4,3ax}$ 12.0	2.57, dd, $J_{3ax,3eq}$ 13.0, $J_{4,3eq}$ 5.0	5.30, ddd, $J_{5,4}$ 10.0	4.17, ddd	4.03, dd, $J_{6,5}$ 10.5	5.42, dd, $J_{7,6}$ 3.0	5.27, ddd	4.87, dd, $J_{9a,8}$ 2.5	4.13, dd, $J_{9a,9b}$ 12.5, $J_{9b,8}$ 7.5	4.52, d	4.46, d, J_{hem} 11.5	1.87, s	3.87, d, J 6.0
5, 6, 8-α (D$_2$O)	1.67, dd, $J_{4,3ax}$ 12.5	2.76, dd, $J_{3ax,3eq}$ 12.5, $J_{4,3eq}$ 4.5	3.68, ddd, $J_{5,4}$ 10.0	3.80, ddd	3.72, dd, $J_{6,5}$ 10.0	3.58, dd, $J_{8,7}$ 9.2, $J_{7,6}$ 1.3	3.73, ddd	3.82, dd, $J_{9a,8}$ 2.5	3.62, dd, $J_{9a,9b}$ 12.5, $J_{9b,8}$ 6.0	4.72, d	4.51, d, J_{hem} 11.0	2.02, s	3.97, s
5, 6, 8-β (D$_2$O)	1.68, dd, $J_{4,3ax}$ 12.0	2.38, dd, $J_{3ax,3eq}$ 13.0, $J_{4,3eq}$ 5.0	4.04, ddd, $J_{5,4}$ 10.0	3.89, ddd	3.97, dd, $J_{6,5}$ 10.7	3.57, dd, $J_{8,7}$ 9.6, $J_{7,6}$ <1.0	3.93, ddd	3.85, dd, $J_{9a,8}$ 2.5	3.67, dd, $J_{9a,9b}$ 12.0, $J_{9b,8}$ 5.7	4.58, d	4.26, d, J_{hem} 10.5	2.04, s	3.98, s

Additional signals. **3-α:** 1.49 (s, 9H, C(CH$_3$)$_3$), 2.04, 2.06, 2.16, 2.18 (4s, 4×3H, 4×OC(O)CH$_3$), 3.68 (s, 3H, OCH$_3$), 5.16 (d, 1H, $J_{NH,5}$ 10.0 Hz, N*H*C(O)CH$_3$), 5.21 (br. s, 1H, COCH$_2$N*H*), 7.30, 7.48 (2d, 2×2H, J 8.5 Hz, Ar), 8.16 (s, 1H, ArN*H*); **3-β:** 1.50 (s, 9H, C(CH$_3$)$_3$), 1.99, 2.02, 2.06, 2.17 (4s, 4×3H, 4×OC(O)CH$_3$), 3.78 (s, 3H, OCH$_3$), 5.41 (br. s, 1H, COCH$_2$N*H*), 5.96 (d, 1H, $J_{NH,5}$ 10.0 Hz, N*H*C(O)CH$_3$), 7.30, 7.45 (2d, 2×2H, J 8.1 Hz, Ar), 8.31 (s, 1H, ArN*H*); **5-α:** 1.45 (s, 9H, C(CH$_3$)$_3$), 7.48, 7.44 (2d, 2×2H, J 8.5 Hz, Ar); **5-β:** 1.50 (s, 9H, C(CH$_3$)$_3$), 7.50 (br. s, 4H, Ar); **6-β:** 7.50 (br. s, 4H, Ar); **8-α:** 2.01–1.96 (m, 4H, 2×CH$_2$CH$_2$CO), 2.66, 2.87 (2t, 2×3H, J 6.8 Hz, 2×CH$_2$CO), 7.47, 7.71 (2d, 2×2H, J 8.3 Hz, Ar), 7.56, 8.47 (2d, 2×2H, J 8.8 Hz, ArNO$_2$); **8-β:** 1.83–1.76 (m, 4H, CH$_2$CH$_2$CO), 2.44–2.41 (m, 2H, CH$_2$COArNO$_2$), 2.72 (t, 2H, J 6.8 Hz, CH$_2$CO), 7.38 (br. s, 4H, Ar), 7.31, 8.27 (2d, 2×2H, J 9.1 Hz, ArNO$_2$).

[a] The spectra of **8** (α or β) were recorded at a concentration 5 mg/mL; at higher concentrations of **8** in D$_2$O, considerable peak broadening is observed, apparently due to micellization of **8** in aqueous solutions, caused by the hydrophobic aglycon.

to dryness. The residue was dissolved in 1:1 toluene–AcOEt (40 mL), chromato-graphed on a column of silica gel (250 g) packed in toluene, and eluted with a gra-dient of 1:1 toluene–AcOEt→AcOEt, to give, in the order of elution: recovered **2** (260 mg, 43%), **4** (252 mg, 18%), and **3** (**α + β**) (1.55 g, 70%). The mixture of the anomers was dissolved in $CHCl_3$ (20 mL), applied on a column of silica gel (250 g) packed in $CHCl_3$, and eluted with a gradient of 2%→5% i-PrOH–$CHCl_3$ to give **3-α** (1.0 g, 45%) and **3-β** (492 mg, 22%) as colorless foams. **3-α**: $[\alpha]_D^{20}$ +1.0 (c 0.7, $CHCl_3$); TLC: R_f 0.27 (15:1CH_3Cl–i-PrOH); MALDI-MS: 754 [M]$^+$, 777 [M + Na]$^+$, 793 [M + K]$^+$; Anal. Calcd for $C_{34}H_{47}N_3O_{16}$: C 54.18; H 6.29; N 5.57. Found: C 54.08; H 6.42; N 5.49.

3-β: $[\alpha]_D^{20}$ −10.5 (c 1.5, $CHCl_3$); TLC: R_f 0.20 (15:1 $CHCl_3$–i-PrOH,); MALDI-MS: 754 [M]$^+$, 777 [M + Na]$^+$, 793 [M + K]$^+$; Anal. Calcd for $C_{34}H_{47}N_3O_{16}$: C 54.18; H 6.29; N 5.57. Found: C 54.10; H 6.37; N 5.46.

4-[(*Tert*-Butyloxycarbonyl)glycylamido]benzyl 5-Acetamido-3,5-Dideoxy-D-*Glycero*-D-*Galacto*-Non-2-Ulopyranosidonic Acid (5)

To a solution of **3** (**α** or **β**) (500 mg, 0.66 mmol) in dry MeOH (40 mL), 2M MeONa in MeOH (2.0 mL) was added. The mixture was kept for 2 h at room temperature and for a further 12 h following the addition of H_2O (40 mL). After acidification with AcOH (300 μL), the mixture was concentrated, the residue was dissolved in H_2O (2 mL) and chromatographed on a column (2 × 15 cm) of Dowex 50X4-400 (Py-form in H_2O), using H_2O as eluent to give **5** (**α** or **β**) as a colorless foam, (340–360 mg, 90%–95%).

5-α: $[\alpha]_D^{20}$ −24.7 (c 0.5, H_2O), lit.: $[\alpha]_D^{20}$ −24.5 (c 0.4, H_2O);[1c] TLC: R_f 0.6 (4:3:2 i-PrOH–MeCN–H_2O); MALDI-MS: 572 [M]$^+$, 596 [M + Na]$^+$, 611 [M + K]$^+$; Anal. Calcd for $C_{25}H_{37}N_3O_{12}$: C 52.53; H 6.52; N 7.35. Found: C 52.43; H 6.64; N 7.33.

5-β: $[\alpha]_D^{20}$ +12.5 (c 0.5, H_2O), lit.: $[\alpha]_D^{20}$ +12.6 (c 0.47, H_2O);[1c] TLC: R_f 0.5 (4:3:2 i-PrOH–MeCN–H_2O); MALDI-MS: 572 [M]$^+$, 596 [M + Na]$^+$, 611 [M + K]$^+$; Anal. Calcd for $C_{25}H_{37}N_3O_{12}$: C 52.53; H 6.52; N 7.35. Found: C 52.45; H 6.60; N 7.29.

4-(Glycylamido)benzyl 5-Acetamido-3,5-Dideoxy-D-*Glycero*-D-*Galacto*-Non-2-Ulopyranosidonic Acid (6)

TFA (5 mL) was added to **5** (**α** or **β**, 200 mg, 0.35 mmol), the mixture was kept for 2 h at room temperature and concentrated to dryness below 30°C using a high vacuum pump.* Without any delay, the residue was dissolved in H_2O (1 mL) and chromato-graphed on a column (1.5 × 10 cm) of Dowex 50X4-400 (H$^+$-form in H_2O) using as eluent H_2O (10 mL) followed by 2M aqueous Py. Fractions containing the product were combined and concentrated, the residue was dried in vacuum, suspended in dry MeOH (10 mL), and the suspension was stirred 12 h at room temperature to remove small amounts of MeOH-soluble impurities and filtered to give **6** (**α** or **β**) as a color-less solid (150 mg, 90%). **6-α**: $[\alpha]_D^{20}$ −27.0 (c 0.3, 1:1 MeOH–H_2O); TLC: R_f 0.34 (4:3:2

---

* The residue should be kept under high vacuum with slow rotation at room temperature for 15–30 min, to insure complete removal of TFA.

i-PrOH–MeCN–H$_2$O); MALDI-MS: 472 [M]$^+$, 493 [M+Na]$^+$, 511 [M+K]$^+$; Anal. Calcd for C$_{20}$H$_{29}$N$_3$O$_{10}$: C 50.95; H 6.20; N 8.91. Found: C 50.78; H 6.32; N 8.83.

6-β: [α]$_D^{20}$ +5.6 (*c* 0.6, 1:1 MeOH–H$_2$O); TLC: R_f 0.13 (4:3:2 *i*-PrOH–MeCN–H$_2$O); MALDI-MS: 472 [M]$^+$, 493 [M+Na]$^+$, 511 [M+K]$^+$; Anal. Calcd for C$_{20}$H$_{29}$N$_3$O$_{10}$: C 50.95; H 6.20; N 8.91. Found: C 50.80; H 6.34; N 8.81.

4-[(4-Nitrophenoxy)adipoylglycylamido]benzyl 5-Acetamido-3,5-Dideoxy-D-*Glycero*-D-*Galacto*-Non-2-Ulopyranosidonic Acid (8)

A solution of **7** (400 mg, 1.03 mmol) in DMF (2.5 mL) was added to a solution of **6** (α or β, 100 mg, 0.21 mmol) in DMSO (0.7 mL). The mixture was stirred 24 h at room temperature, diluted with 1% AcOH$_{(aq)}$ (15 mL) to precipitate excess of **7**, and filtered. The filtrate was concentrated in vacuum to ~3.5 mL, the residue was chromatographed on a column (2×30 cm) of Sephadex LH-20 with 0.2% AcOH in 1:1 MeCN–H$_2$O as eluent to give, in the order of elution, **9** (α or β) and crude **8** (α or β) in a mixture with DMSO. To remove residual DMSO, the fractions containing **8** (α or β) were concentrated to dryness, and the residues were subjected to reversed-phase chromatography on a Supelco Supelclean™ LC-18 SPE tube (bed weight 0.5 g, volume 6 mL) eluting with a stepwise gradient 0 → 50 vol. % MeCN in H$_2$O, containing 0.2% of AcOH (in 10% increments, 6 mL per step). The fractions containing the products were combined, concentrated to dryness, and solutions of the residues in 0.5% AcOH$_{(aq)}$ (1–2 mL) were freeze-dried giving **8** (α or β, 115–130 mg, 75%–80%) and **9** (α or β, 33–45 mg, 15%–20%) as a colorless solid. **8-α**: [α]$_D^{20}$ −12.1 (*c* 0.5, DMSO); TLC: R_f 0.95 (**7**); R_f 0.66 (**8-α**), R_f 0.20 (**9-α**), R_f 0 (**6-α**) (4:3:2 *i*-PrOH–AcOEt–H$_2$O); MALDI-MS: 721 [M]$^+$, 746 [M+Na]$^+$, 760 [M+K]$^+$; Anal. Calcd for C$_{32}$H$_{40}$N$_4$O$_{15}$: C 53.33; H 5.59; N 7.77. Found: C 53.23; H 5.72; N 7.63.

8-β: [α]$_D^{20}$ −10.1 (*c* 1.0, DMSO); TLC: R_f 0.95 (**7**); R_f 0.59 (**8-β**), R_f 0.10 (**9-β**), R_f 0 (**6-β**) (4:3:2 *i*-PrOH–AcOEt–H$_2$O); MALDI-MS: 721 [M]$^+$, 746 [M+Na]$^+$, 760 [M+K]$^+$; Anal. Calcd for C$_{32}$H$_{40}$N$_4$O$_{15}$: C 53.33; H 5.59; N 7.77. Found: C 53.25; H 5.78; N 7.61.

ACKNOWLEDGMENT

This chapter was supported by the RAS Presidium program "Molecular and Cell Biology."

REFERENCES

1. (a) Pritchett, T.J.; Brossmer, R.; Rose, U.; Paulson, J.C. *Virology*, 1987, *160*, 502–506; (b) Matrosovich, M.N.; Mochalova, L.V.; Marinina, V.P.; Byramova, N.E.; Bovin, N.V. *FEBS Lett.*, 1990, *272*, 209–212; (c) Byramova, N.E.; Mochalova, L.V.; Belyanchikov, I.M.; Matrosovich, M.N.; Bovin, N.V.; *J. Carbohydr. Chem.*, 1991, *10*, 691–700.

2. Rapoport, E.M.; Sapot'ko, Yu.B.; Pazynina, G.V.; Bojenko, V.K.; Bovin, N.V. *Biochemistry(Moscow)*, 2005, *70*, 330–338.

3. Huflejt, M.E.; Vuscovic, M.; Vasiliu, D.; Xu, H.; Obukhova, P.; Shilova, N.; Tuzikov, A.; Galanina, O.; Arun, B.; Lu, K.; Bovin, N. *Mol. Immunol.*, 2009, *46*, 3037–3049.

4. Bovin, N.V.; Korchagina, E.Yu.; Zemlyanukhina, T.V.; Byramova, N.E.; Galanina, O.E.; Zemlyakov, A.E.; Ivanov, A.E.; Zubov, V.P.; Mochalova, L.V. *Glycoconj. J.*, 1993, *10*, 142–151.
5. Chinarev, A.; Tuzikov, A.; Gambaryan, A.; Matrosovich, M.; Imberty, A.; Bovin, N. In: *Sialobilolgy and Other Novel Forms of Glycosylation*; Innoue, Y., Lee Y., Troy F., (eds.); Gakushin Publishing Company, Osaka, Japan, 1999; pp. 135–143.
6. Tuzikov, A.B.; Chinarev, A.A.; Gambaryan, A.S.; Oleinikov, V.A.; Klinov, D.V.; Matsko, N. B.; Kadykov, V.A.; Ermishov, M.A.; Demin, I.V.; Demin, V.V.; Rye, P.D.; Bovin, N.V. *ChemBioChem*, 2003, *4*, 147–154.
7. Byramova, N.E.; Tuzikov, A.B.; Bovin, N.V. *Carbohydr. Res.*, 1992, *237*, 161–175.
8. Kulikova, N.Y.; Shpirt, A.M.; Chinarev, A.; Kononov, L.O. In: *Carbohydrate Chemistry: Proven Methods;* Vol. 1., Kováč, P., (ed.); CRC Press/Taylor & Francis, Boca Raton, FL, 2011.

29 Synthesis of 1,5-Di-C-Alkyl 1,5-Iminoxylitols Related to 1-Deoxynojirimycin

Vincent Chagnault, Philippe Compain, Olivier R. Martin,* and Jean-Bernard Behr†

CONTENTS

Introduction 259
Experimental Methods 261
  General Methods 261
    1,5-Di-(1/2-Benzotriazolyl)-*N*-Benzyl-1,5-Dideoxy-1,5-Iminoxylitol (**4**) ... 261
    2,3,4-Tri-*O*-Acetyl-1,5-Di-*C*-Allyl-*N*-Benzyl-1,5-Dideoxy-1,5-
    Iminoxylitol (**5**) 262
    Meso-(1*R*,5*S*)-, *Meso*-(1*S*,5*R*)-, and *Rac*-(1*R*,5*R*)-2,3,4-Tri-*O*-Acetyl-
    1,5-Di-*C*-Allyl-1,5-Dideoxy-1,5-Iminoxylitol (**6a**, **6b**, and **6c**) 262
Acknowledgment 263
References 267

INTRODUCTION

Iminosugars form a class of carbohydrate mimics of increasing importance.[1] Historically known as potent glycosidase inhibitors,[2] the scope of their biological activity has been extended recently to a diversity of enzymes such as glycosyltransferases,[3] glycogen phosphorylases,[4] and nucleoside-processing enzymes.[5] As a consequence, iminosugars are now lead compounds for the treatment of a variety of diseases including diabetes,[6] cancers,[7] viral infections,[8] and rare genetic diseases (lysosomal storage disorders[9] and cystic fibrosis[10]). The recent approval of *Zavesca*™ as the first oral treatment for Gaucher disease, a rare glycosphingolipidose, is a remarkable demonstration of the importance of iminosugars as medicines

---

* Corresponding author.
† Checker.

for unmet medical needs.[9] In this context, the development of rapid and general access to original iminosugars is highly needed.

We have recently developed a convenient access to polyhydroxylated 10-azabicyclo[4.3.1]decanes as new calystegine analogs, using bis(benzotriazolyl) intermediate **4** as a key intermediate.[11] This compound, originally reported by Shankar et al.,[12] is readily available from diacetone-D-glucose and constitutes a convenient entry into a diversity of piperidine derivatives related to DNJ (1-deoxynojirimycin) carrying various substituents at C-2 and C-6.

The conditions for the synthesis of **4** have been optimized, and the condensation of **4** with various organometallic nucleophiles has been considerably improved. Here, we report detailed conditions for a reliable preparation of **4** on a multigram scale (45% overall) by a four-step process without any purification by chromatography, conversion of **4** into the 2,6-bis(C-allyl) piperidine **5** by addition of an organozinc species, and the subsequent acetylation and N-debenzylation reactions, which give a mixture of three stereoisomers (**6a–6c**) that can be separated at that stage (Scheme 29.1).

The double benzotriazolyl/carbon nucleophile exchange was first investigated with alkyl, allyl- or vinylmagnesium bromide with little success. With or without additives, such as $ZnBr_2$ or $MgBr_2$, the expected 2,6-dialkyl piperidines were obtained in poor and unreproducible yields. The best results were finally obtained with 5 equiv of allyl zinc bromide, generated by treatment of allyl bromide with activated Zn dust according to Knochel's procedure.[13] Following these conditions, 2,6-diallyl piperidines **5** were obtained as a mixture of stereoisomers in 57% yield after protection of the hydroxyl groups. Subsequent acetylation of the crude product was necessary for the next step of the synthesis and for the separation of the desired products from benzotriazole. The chemoselective removal of the N-benzyl group using CAN[14] and the separation of the stereoisomers were performed in the same step (Scheme 29.1), thus providing the two *meso* 2,6-*cis* piperidines **6a** and **6b** in a

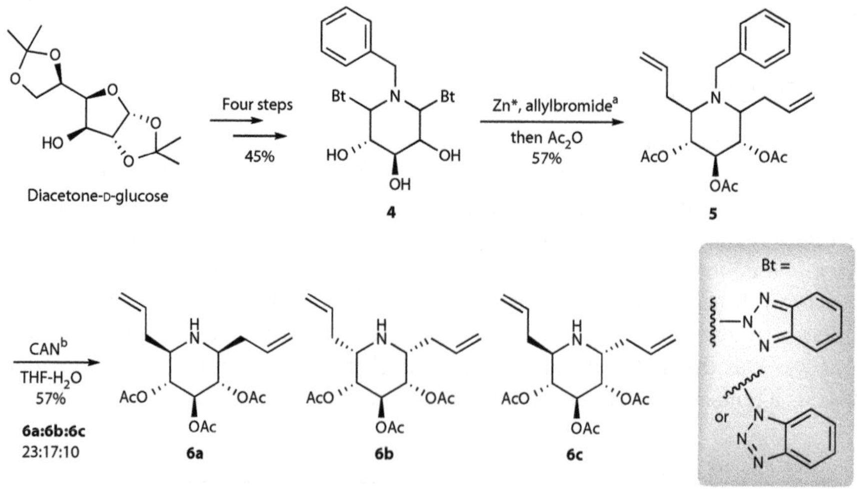

SCHEME 29.1   Synthetic scheme for **6a–6c**. (a) (i) Zn, allyl bromide, THF; (ii) Ac$_2$O, DMAP, CH$_2$Cl$_2$; (b) CAN, 5:1 THF–H$_2$O. The ratio found by Jean-Bernard Behr, **6a:6b:6c** = 36:13:7.

ratio of about 4:3 (2,3-*trans*:2,3-*cis*), the racemic 2,6-*trans* diallylated piperidine in a ratio of 4:1 with respect to the *cis* isomers (2,6-*cis*:2,6-*trans*), and an overall yield of 57%. The 2,6-*cis* stereoisomers have been used as substrates for a ring-closing metathesis, thus affording the skeleton of calystegin analogs.

EXPERIMENTAL METHODS

GENERAL METHODS

Solvents were evaporated under reduced pressure below 40°C. Solvents were dried using standard procedures, and reactions requiring anhydrous conditions were performed under argon. All reactions were monitored by thin-layer chromatography (TLC) on aluminum sheets precoated with 60 F-254 silica gel; spots were visualized by UV light (254 nm) or by spraying with aqueous $KMnO_4$ solution or with Hanessian's stain (prepared by dissolving ammonium molybdate [5 g] and cerium sulfate [1 g] in water, followed by the careful addition of concentrated sulfuric acid [10 mL]. Cerium sulfate can be replaced with cerium ammonium sulfate, which is significantly cheaper. Staining with Hanessian's stain requires spraying and heating until permanent spots are visible). Flash chromatography was performed under slight pressure using silica gel 60 (230–400 mesh).[15] Diacetone-D-glucose was obtained from Acros Organics. Zinc dust (98+%, particle size <10 μ) was obtained from Aldrich Chemical Co.

1,5-Di-(1/2-Benzotriazolyl)-N-Benzyl-1,5-Dideoxy-1,5-Iminoxylitol (4)

Using a 250 mL round-bottom flask, diacetone-D-glucofuranose (12 g, 46.1 mmol) was dissolved in 60% aqueous acetic acid (180 mL), and the reaction mixture was stirred at room temperature for 21 h (TLC, Et_2O). Solvents were evaporated and residual acetic acid was removed by coevaporation with H_2O (about 50 mL) to give 1,2-O-isopropylidene-α-D-glucofuranose (1)[16,17] (Scheme 29.2) as a white solid, which was used without further purification in the next step. The residue thus obtained (10.15 g, 46.1 mmol) was dissolved in water (180 mL), and sodium periodate (11.07 g, 51.8 mmol) was added portionwise over 10 min at room temperature. After stirring overnight (16 h), the precipitated white solids were removed by filtration over cotton wool and the filtrate was extracted with EtOAc (4×200 mL). The organic phases were combined, dried over magnesium sulfate, and concentrated to provide crude 1,2-O-isopropylidene-α-D-*xylo*-pentodialdo-1,4-furanose (2, 8.67 g, 46.1 mmol).[18] The crude aldehyde 2 was redissolved in water (115 mL) and the solution was treated with cation exchange resin (Dowex® 50WX8-100, H⁺ form, 14.75 g) at 70°C overnight

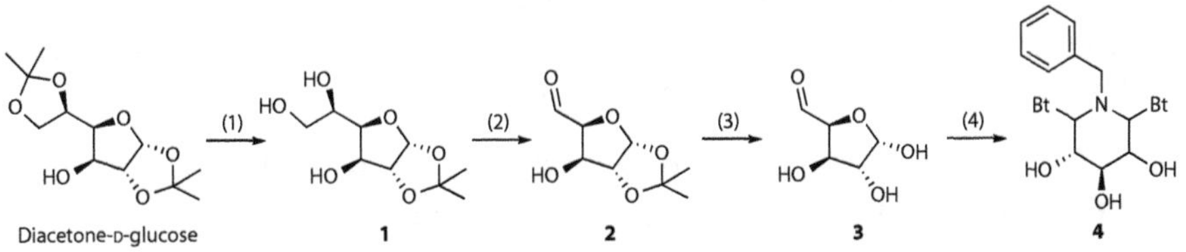

Diacetone-D-glucose   1   2   3   4

SCHEME 29.2   Synthetic scheme for compound **4**.

(16 h). The resin was removed by filtration and the slightly orange filtrate containing *xylo*-pentodialdose (**3**)[19] (6.82 g, 46.0 mmol) was cooled down to room temperature and was added to a vigorously stirred mixture of commercial benzotriazole (10.97 g, 92 mmol) and benzylamine (5 mL, 46.0 mmol) in water (360 mL). The mixture immediately turned cloudy and a gummy solid formed over a period of ~6 h, causing the stirring to stop. The product was extracted into EtOAc (5 × 200 mL) and the organic phases were combined, dried (MgSO$_4$), and concentrated. Reduction of the volume to 200 mL under reduced pressure resulted in crystallization of **4**. After standing for 1–2 h at room temperature, the product was collected by filtration as a white solid and rinsed with cold AcOEt; additional product crystallized from the mother liquors upon standing overnight at room temperature. The combined overall yield of **4** from diacetone-D-glucose was 9.4 g (45%). Attempts to obtain a third crop of **4** from the mother liquors failed. Anal. calcd for C$_{24}$H$_{23}$N$_7$O$_3$·2H$_2$O: C, 58.41; H, 5.51; N, 19.87. Found: C, 58.23; H, 5.56; N, 19.65; mp$_{(dec.)}$ 102°C (from AcOEt); R_F=0.4 (9:1 AcOEt–petroleum ether).

2,3,4-Tri-*O*-Acetyl-1,5-Di-*C*-Allyl-*N*-Benzyl-1,5-Dideoxy-1,5-Iminoxylitol (5)

A three-neck round-bottom flask (500 mL) containing Zinc dust (5.15 g, 79 mmol) and a magnetic stirring bar was dried in an oven (120°C) for 12 h. A condenser was attached, and a solution of 1,2-dibromoethane (0.34 mL, 3.93 mmol) in anhydrous THF (60 mL) was added under argon. The mixture was vigorously stirred and heated to 65°C for 15 min. The mixture was allowed to reach room temperature and chlorotrimethylsilane (0.1 mL, 0.787 mmol) was added. After the mixture had been vigorously stirred for 15 min, a solution of allyl bromide (2.8 mL, 32.8 mmol) in anhydrous THF (30 mL) was added slowly, and the mixture was stirred for another 30 min. A solution of compound **4** (3 g, 6.56 mmol) in anhydrous THF (350 mL) was added slowly at room temperature and the reaction mixture was stirred overnight (20 h). Water (100 mL) was added, and the solids were removed by filtration over Celite. Satd. aq. Na$_2$CO$_3$ (100 mL) was added and another filtration over Celite was carried out to remove zinc salts. EtOAc (200 mL) was added to the filtrate, the organic phase was separated, and the remaining aqueous phase was extracted with fresh EtOAc (2 × 200 mL); the organic phases were combined, dried (MgSO$_4$), and concentrated to give 1.99 g (6.56 mmol) of crude **5**. 4-(N,N-Dimethylamino)pyridine (DMAP, 0.401 g, 3.28 mmol) was added to a solution of the aforementioned material (1.99 g) in dry CH$_2$Cl$_2$ (100 mL). Acetic anhydride (6.19 mL, 65.6 mmol) was then added dropwise, and the reaction mixture was stirred overnight at room temperature. Water (20 mL) was added and the mixture was stirred for 30 min, followed by addition of solid Na$_2$CO$_3$ until a basic pH (9–10) was reached. The organic phase was separated and the aqueous phase was extracted with CH$_2$Cl$_2$ (3 × 100 mL); the organic phases were combined, dried over MgSO$_4$, and concentrated. The residue was chromatographed (1:4 EtOAc–PE), which afforded piperidine derivatives **5** as a mixture of stereoisomers (1.611 g, 3.75 mmol, 57% yield).

Meso-(1R,5S)-, Meso-(1S,5R)-, and Rac-(1R,5R)-2,3,4-Tri-*O*-Acetyl-1,5-Di-C-Allyl-1,5-Dideoxy-1,5-Iminoxylitol (6a, 6b, and 6c)

Cerium ammonium nitrate (7.38 g, 13.47 mmol) was added portionwise to a solution of the foregoing mixture of stereoisomers **5** (1.446 g, 3.37 mmol) in a mixture of

THF (190 mL) and water (37 mL). When the reaction was complete (TLC, <5 h),* sat. aq. $NaHCO_3$ was added until basic pH was reached, and the mixture was extracted with EtOAc (3 × 150 mL). The organic phases were combined, dried ($MgSO_4$), and concentrated. The different isomers were isolated by flash column chromatography (gradient 5:95 → 20:80 EtOAc–PE). **6a**: *meso-1R, 5S* (1,5-*cis*-1,2-*trans*): 331 mg (29%) (R_F 0.25, EtOAc:PE 20:80). **6c**: *rac-1R, 5R* (1,5-*trans*): 149 mg (13%, containing ~50% of **6a**) (R_F 0.20, EtOAc:PE 20:80). **6b**: *meso 1S, 5R* (1,5-*cis*-1,2-*cis*): 149 mg (13%) (R_F 0.05, EtOAc:PE 20:80).

Compound **6a**: ^1H NMR (400 MHz, $CDCl_3$) δ 5.71 (tdd, J=6.0, 8.4, 14.5, 2H, H-8, H-11), 5.15–5.08 (m, 4H, H-9, H-12), 5.04 (t, J=9.4, 1H, H-4), 4.78 (t, J=9.6, 2H, H-3, H-5), 2.71 (td, J=3.4, 9.2, 2H, H-2, H-6), 2.32 (dd, J=5.2, 10.0, 2H, H-10, H-7), 2.07–2.00 (m, 2H, H-10, H-7), 2.02 (s, 6H, CH_3CO), 1.99 (s, 3H, CH_3CO), 1.68 (s, NH). ^{13}C NMR (101 MHz, $CDCl_3$) δ 170.7 (CO), 170.1 (CO), 134.0 (C-11, C-8), 119.0 (C-12, C-9), 75.7 (C-4), 74.0 (C-3, C-5), 56.5 (C-2, C-6), 36.3 (C-10, C-7), 21.0 (2 × CH_3CO), 20.9 (CH_3CO). IR (cm^{-1}) (NaCl; FTIR): 1749.0; 1247.6; 1225.7; 1030.0; HRMS: calcd for $C_{17}H_{26}NO_6$, 340.1760; found: 340.1753. Compound **6b**: ^1H NMR (400 MHz, $CDCl_3$) δ 5.77 (ddt, J=7.1, 10.2, 17.3, 2H, H-11, H-8), 5.20–5.05 (m, 4H, H-9, H-12), 4.99 (t, J=2.6, 1H, H-4), 4.82–4.71 (m, 2H, H-3, H-5), 3.04 (t, J=7.1, 2H, H-2, H-6), 2.21 (t, J=6.9, 4H, H-7, H-10), 2.12 (s, 6H, CH_3COO), 2.11 (s, 3H, CH_3COO). ^{13}C NMR (101 MHz, $CDCl_3$) δ 169.7 (CO), 168.3 (CO), 134.2 (C-8, C-11), 118.1 (C-9, C-12), 68.1 (C-3, C-5), 67.5 (C-4), 54.2 (C-2, C-6), 35.9 (C-7, C-10), 20.9 (CH_3CO). IR (cm^{-1}) (NaCl; FTIR): 1741.0; 1370.2; 1246.0; 1218.8; 1036.9; HRMS: calcd for $C_{17}H_{26}NO_6$, 340.1760; found: 340.1765. Compound **6c**: ^1H NMR (400 MHz, $CDCl_3$) δ 5.75–5.59 (m, 2H, H-8, H-11), 5.24 (t, J=8.0, 1H, H-4), 5.17–5.06 (m, 4H, H-9, H-12), 5.03 (dd, J=5.7, ~10.0, 1H, H-5), 4.73 (t, J=9.4, 1H, H-3), 3.34 (ddd, J=4.2, 5.5, ~10.0, 1H, H-6), 2.90 (td, J=3.4, 9.2, 1H, H-2), 2.40 (ddd, J=8.6, 11.3, 14.2, 1H, H-7), 2.35–2.21 (m, 2H, H-10, H-7), 2.07–1.96 (m, 11H, CH_3CO, H-10). ^{13}C NMR (101 MHz, $CDCl_3$) δ 170.3, 170.0 and 169.9 (COO), 134.6 and 133.9 (C-8, C-11), 118.7 and 118.1 (C-9, C-12), 74.3 (C-4), 72.5 (C-5), 71.6 (C-3), 52.6 (C-6), 50.1 (C-2), 36.4 (C-10), 30.3 (C-7), 20.9, 20.8 and 20.8 (CH_3CO). IR (cm^{-1}) (NaCl; FTIR): 1746.5; 1225.2; 1030.3. HRMS: calcd for $C_{17}H_{26}NO_6$, 340.1760; found: 340.1747.

Numbering scheme for the NMR spectra

ACKNOWLEDGMENT

Financial support from a grant from ANR (Agence Nationale de la Recherche), program MRAR (Maladies Rares) is gratefully acknowledged.

---

* Longer heating than the time indicated results in significantly lower yield.

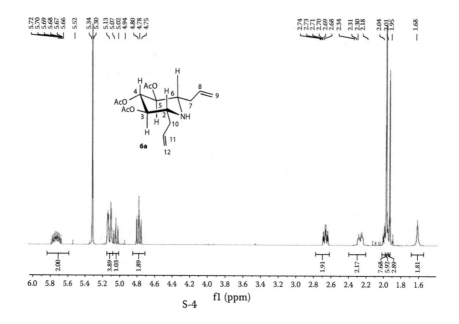

S-4

f1 (ppm)

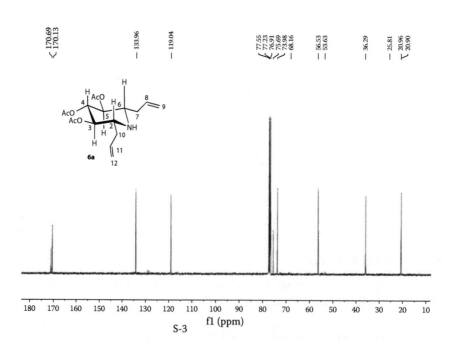

S-3

f1 (ppm)

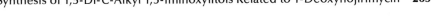

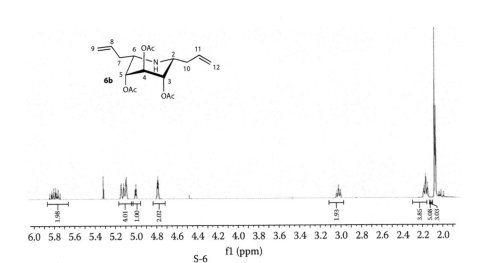

S-6

fl (ppm)

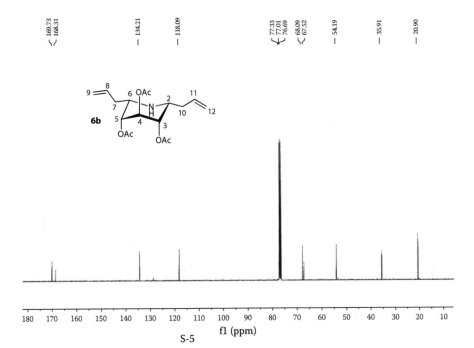

S-5

fl (ppm)

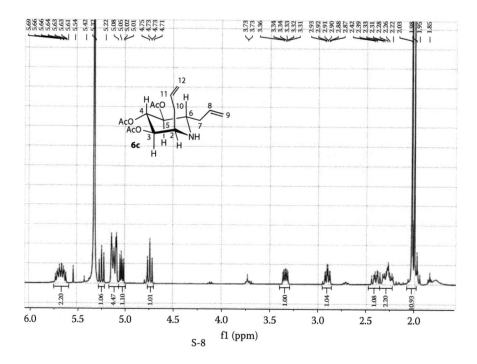

S-8

f1 (ppm)

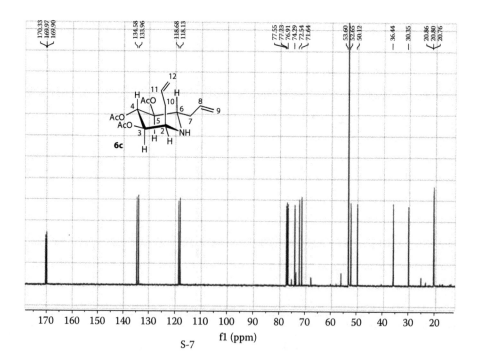

S-7

f1 (ppm)

REFERENCES

1. Compain, P.; Martin, O. R., Eds. *Iminosugars: From Synthesis to Therapeutic Applications*; Wiley-VCH: Weinheim, Germany, 2007.
2. Stütz, A. E., Ed. *Iminosugars as Glycosidase Inhibitors: Nojirimycin and Beyond*; Wiley-VCH, New York, 1999.
3. (a) Compain, P.; Martin, O. R. *Bioorg. Med. Chem.* 2001, *9*, 3077–3092. (b) Whalen, L. J.; Greenberg, W. A.; Mitchell, M. L.; Wong, C.-H. In *Iminosugars: From Synthesis to Therapeutic Applications*; Compain, P., Martin, O. R., Eds.; Wiley-VCH: Weinheim, Germany, 2007, pp. 153–176.
4. (a) Bols, M.; Hazelle, R.; Thomsen, I. B. *Chem. Eur. J.* 1997, *3*, 940–947. (b) Heightman, T. D.; Vasella, A.; Tsitsanou, K. E.; Zographos, S. E.; Skamnaki, V. T.; Oikonomakos, N. G. *Helv. Chim. Acta* 1998, *81*, 853–864.
5. Schramm, V. L.; Tyler, P. C. *Curr. Top. Med. Chem.* 2003, *3*, 525–540.
6. Somsak, L.; Nagy, V.; Hadazy, Z.; Docsa, T.; Gergely, P. *Curr. Pharm. Des.* 2003, *9*, 1177–1189.
7. Nishimura, Y. In *Iminosugars: From Synthesis to Therapeutic Applications*; Compain, P., Martin, O. R., Eds.; Wiley-VCH: Weinheim, Germany, 2007, pp. 269–294.
8. (a) Greimel, P.; Spreitz, J.; Stütz, A. E.; Wrodnigg, T. M. *Curr. Top. Med. Chem.* 2003, *3*, 513–523. (b) Robina, I.; Moreno-Vargas, A. J.; Carmona, A. T.; Vogel, P. *Curr. Drug Met.* 2004, *5*, 329–361. (c) Norton, P. A.; Baohua, G.; Block, T. M. In *Iminosugars: From Synthesis to Therapeutic Applications*; Compain, P., Martin, O. R., Eds.; Wiley-VCH: Weinheim, Germany, 2007, pp. 209–224.
9. (a) Butters, T. D.; Dwek, R. A.; Platt, F. M. *Chem. Rev.* 2000, *100*, 4683–4696. (b) Butters, T. D.; Dwek, R. A.; Platt, F. M. *Glycobiology* 2005, *10*, 43R–52R.
10. Norez, C.; Noel, S.; Wilke, M.; Bijvelds, M.; Jorna, H.; Melin, P.; DeJonge, H.; Becq, F. *FEBS Lett.* 2006, *580*, 2081–2086.
11. Chagnault, V.; Compain, P.; Lewinski, K.; Ikeda, K.; Asano, N.; Martin, O.R. *J. Org. Chem.* 2009, *74*, 3179–3182.
12. Shankar, B. B.; Kirkup, M. P.; McCombie, S. W.; Ganguly, A. K. *Tetrahedron Lett.* 1993, 34, 7171–7174.
13. Knochel, P.; Yeh, M. C. P.; Beck, S. C.; Talbert, J. *J. Org. Chem.* 1988, *53*, 2390–2392.
14. (a) Bull, S. D.; Davies, S. G.; Fenton, G.; Mulvaney, A. W.; Prasad, R. S.; Smith, A. D. *Chem. Commun.* 2000, 337–338. (b) Cipolla, L.; Palma, A.; La Ferla, B.; Nicotra, F. *J. Chem. Soc. Perkin Trans. 1*, 2002, 2161–2165.
15. Still, W.C.; Kahn, M.; Mitra, A. *J. Org. Chem.* 1978, *43*, 2923–2925.
16. Schmidt, O.T. *Methods Carbohydr. Chem.* 1963, *2*, 318–325.
17. Gramera, R.E.; Park, A.; Whistler, R.L. *J. Org. Chem.* 1963, *28*, 3230–3231.
18. (a) Schaffer, R.; Isbell, H. S. *J. Res. Natl. Bur. Stand.* 1956, *56*, 191–195; *J. Am. Chem. Soc.* 1957, *79*, 3864. (b) Youssefyeh, R.D.; Verheyden, J.P.H.; Moffatt, J.G. *J. Org. Chem.* 1979, *44*, 1301–1309.
19. Lichtenthaler, F.W.; Yahya, H.K. *Carbohydr. Res.* 1967, *5*, 485–489.

30 Synthesis of 1,6-Anhydro-2,3,5-Tri-O-Benzoyl-α-D-Galactofuranose

*Sujit K. Sarkar, Ambar K. Choudhury,
Ján Hirsch,† and Nirmolendu Roy**

CONTENTS

Experimental Methods 270
    General Methods 270
        6-O-Benzyl-1,2:3,4-Di-O-Isopropylidene-α-D-Galactopyranose (2) 270
        Methyl 2,3,5-Tri-O-Benzoyl-6-O-Benzyl-β-D-Galactofuranoside (4) 270
        1,6-Anhydro-2,3,5-Tri-O-Benzoyl-α-D-Galactofuranose (5) 271
        1,6-Anhydro-α-D-Galactofuranose (6) 271
        1,6-Anhydro-2,3,5-Tri-O-Acetyl-α-D-Galactofuranose (7) 271
Acknowledgment 271
References 274

* Corresponding author.
† Checker.

6-*O*-Benzyl-1,2:3,4-di-*O*-isopropylidene-α-D-galactopyranose (**2**),[1] prepared from 1,2:3,4-di-*O*-isopropylidene-α-D-galactopyranose (**1**),[2] can be converted to a number of useful synthetic intermediates. *p*-Toluenesulfonic acid-catalyzed methanolysis gives methyl 6-*O*-benzyl-β-D-galactofuranoside (**3**), which can be readily benzoylated. The resulting methyl 2,3,5-tri-*O*-benzoyl-6-*O*-benzyl-β-D-galactofuranoside (**4**),[1] when treated with stannic chloride in dichloromethane, gives 1,6-anhydro-2,3,5-tri-*O*-benzoyl-α-D-galactofuranose (**5**)[3] as the only product. Compound **5** can be further characterized by conversion to triol **6** and the triacetate **7**.

EXPERIMENTAL METHODS

GENERAL METHODS

All reactions were monitored by thin-layer chromatography (TLC) on Silica gel G (E. Merck).

Column chromatography was performed on 100–200 mesh silica gel (SRL, India). All solvents were distilled and/or dried before use and all evaporations were conducted below 40°C under reduced pressure, unless stated otherwise. Optical rotations were measured with a Perkin-Elmer model 241 MC polarimeter. ^{1}H and ^{13}C nuclear magnetic resonance (NMR) spectra were recorded on a Bruker DPX 300 or a Varian-MR spectrometer, respectively.

6-*O*-Benzyl-1,2:3,4-Di-*O*-Isopropylidene-α-D-Galactopyranose (2)

To a solution of (**1**)[4] (8.86 g, 34.1 mmol) in CH_2Cl_2 (80 mL) was added 50% sodium hydroxide (80 mL), benzyl bromide (4.9 mL, 40.9 mmol), and Bu_4NBr (1.1 g, 3.4 mmol). The mixture was stirred vigorously at room temperature for 24 h when TLC (2:1 toluene–EtOAc) showed that the reaction was virtually complete. The organic layer was separated and the aqueous layer was extracted with CH_2Cl_2 (3×20 mL). The combined organic phase was washed with water, dried (Na_2SO_4), and concentrated. Column chromatography (4:1 toluene–EtOAc) gave amorphous **2** (9.55 g, 80%) $[\alpha]_D^{25}$ −60° (*c* 1.2, $CHCl_3$); ^{1}H NMR (300 MHz, $CDCl_3$): δ 7.35–7.25 (m, 5H, aromatic protons), 5.55 (d, 1H, $J_{1,2}$=5 Hz, H-1), 4.63, 4.55 (2 d, 2H, J=12.1 Hz, CH_2Ph), 4.32-4.29 (m, 2H, H-2, H-3), 4.26 (d, 1H, J=1.7 Hz, H-4), 4.01 (m, 1H, H-5), 3.67 (m, 2H, H-6a,b). Anal. Calcd for $C_{19}H_{26}O_6$: C, 65.12; H, 7.48. Found: C, 65.02; H, 7.35.

Methyl 2,3,5-Tri-*O*-Benzoyl-6-*O*-Benzyl-β-D-Galactofuranoside (4)[1]

A solution of **2** (4 g, 11.4 mmol) and *p*-TsOH (1.52 g) in MeOH (80 mL) was refluxed for 6 h. The solution was then neutralized with Et_3N and concentrated. Column chromatography with (12:1 $CHCl_3$–MeOH) gave methyl 6-*O*-benzyl-β-D-galactofuranoside (**3**, 2. g, 61.5%), $[\alpha]_D^{25}$ −76° (*c* 1.4, $CHCl_3$); ^{1}H NMR (300 MHz, $CDCl_3$): δ 7.37–7.19 (m, 5H, aromatic protons), 4.83 (s, 1H, H-1), 4.54, 4.48 (2 d, 2H, J=12.1 Hz, CH_2Ph), 4.12–3.98 (m, 3H, H-2, H-3, H-5), 3.90 (bs, 1H, H-4), 3.62-3.54 (m, 2H, H-6a,b), 3.32 (s, 3H, COOCH_3). Anal. Calcd for $C_{14}H_{20}O_6$: C, 59.14; H, 7.09. Found: C, 59.47; H, 7.07. Benzoylation of **3** (2 g, 7.04 mmol) with benzoyl chloride (4 mL, 34.4 mmol) in pyridine (30 mL) at 0°C for 1 h, followed by column chromatography (10:1 toluene–EtOAc) gave **4** (3.85 g, 91.7%): mp 62–63°C (EtOH); $[\alpha]_D^{25}$ −16° (c 2.6, CHCl$_3$); ^{1}H NMR (300 MHz, CDCl$_3$): δ 8.06-7.20 (m, 20H, aromatic protons), 5.66 (m, 1H, H-5), 5.64 (d, 1H, $J_{3,4}$=5 Hz, H-3), 5.44 (s, 1H, H-2), 5.22 (s, 1H, H-1), 4.55 (dd, 1H, $J_{3,4}$ = 5 Hz, $J_{4,5}$=4 Hz, H-4), 4.50 (s, 2H, CH$_2$Ph), 3.80 (d, 2H, $J_{5,6}$=6 Hz, H-6a,b), 3.42 (s, 3H, OCH$_3$). Anal. Calcd for C$_{35}$H$_{32}$O$_9$: C, 70.46; H, 5.41. Found: C, 70.65; H, 5.60.

1,6-Anhydro-2,3,5-Tri-O-Benzoyl-α-D-Galactofuranose (5)[3]

SnCl$_4$ (70 mL, 0.38 mmol) was added under nitrogen, with vigorous stirring at 25°C, to a solution of **4**[1] (190 mg, 0.32 mmol) in CH$_2$Cl$_2$ (3 mL). The mixture was stirred for 3 h, diluted with CH$_2$Cl$_2$, and stirred with cold aq NaHCO$_3$ (1 mL). After 30 min, the organic layer was washed with water, dried (Na$_2$SO$_4$), filtered, and concentrated. The residue was chromatographed (10:1 toluene–EtOAc) to give **5** (105 mg, 69.5%) mp 141°C (EtOH); $[\alpha]_D^{25}$ +133° (c 0.9, CHCl$_3$); ^{1}H NMR (400 MHz, CDCl$_3$) δ 4.02 (t, 1H, $J_{6a,6b}$ = 11.3 Hz, H-6a), 4.40, (ddd, 1H, $J_{5,6b}$=3.7 Hz, H-6b), 4.72 (d, 1H, $J_{4,5}$ = 4.4 Hz, H-4), 5.42 (ddd, 1H, H-5), 5.59 (dd, 1H, $J_{1,2}$=4.5 Hz, $J_{2,3}$=2.4 Hz, H-2), 5.81 (d, 1H, H-1), 5.95 (d, 1H, H-3), 7.43–8.18 (m, 15H, aromatic protons); ^{13}C NMR (100 MHz, CDCl$_3$) δ 62.82 (C-6), 64.05 (C-5), 75.99 (C-3), 79.06 (C-2), 79.71 (C-4), 96.96 (C-1), 128.11–134.44 (aromatic carbons), and 165.42–165.83 (3 OCOPh). Anal. Calcd for C$_{27}$H$_{22}$O$_8$: C, 68.34; H, 4.67. Found: C, 68.20; H, 4.51.

1,6-Anhydro-α-D-Galactofuranose (6)

Compound **5** (200 mg, 0.42 mmol) was de-O-benzoylated with methanolic 0.1 M NaOMe to give **6** (65 mg, 95%); mp 180°C–182°C (EtOH); $[\alpha]_D^{25}$ +54° (c 1.4, water). Lit.[4] mp 181°C–182°C (EtOH), $[\alpha]_D^{25}$ +55°. ^{1}H NMR (400 MHz, D$_2$O) δ 3.45 (m, 1H, $J_{6a,6b}$= 10.2 Hz, H-6a), 3.89–3.98 (m, 2H, H-5, H-6b), 4.09 (m, 1H, H-3), 4.13–4.16 (m, 2H, H-4, H-2), 5.21 (d, 1H, $J_{1,2}$=4.3 Hz, H-1); ^{13}C NMR (100 MHz, D$_2$O) δ 61.73 (C-5), 64.62 (C-6), 74.55 (C-2), 79.98 (C-4), 84.50 (C-3), and 97.86 (C-1).

1,6-Anhydro-2,3,5-Tri-O-Acetyl-α-D-Galactofuranose (7)

Conventional acetylation of **3** (50 mg, 0.31 mmol) with pyridine (0.5 mL) and Ac$_2$O (0.5 mL) gave, after chromatography (3:1 toluene–EtOAc), the crystalline triacetate **4** (84 mg, 95%) (80 mg; mp 77°C–79°C (EtOH); $[\alpha]_D$ +144° (c 0.5, ethanol); lit.[5] mp 79°C–80°C (EtOH), $[\alpha]_D$ +144.9°. ^{1}H NMR (400 MHz, CDCl$_3$) δ 2.11, 2.12 and 2.15 (3 s, 9H, 3 OCOCH$_3$), 3.72 (t, 1H, $J_{6a,6b}$= 10.9 Hz, H-6a), 4.09 (dd, 1H, $J_{5,6b}$=6.7 Hz, H-6b), 4.41 (dd, 1H, $J_{3,4}$=4.3 Hz, H-4), 5.04 (m, 1H, H-5), 5.11 (dd, 1H, $J_{1,2}$=4.7 Hz, $J_{2,3}$=2.3 Hz, H-2), 5.30 (d, 1H, H-3), 5.52 (d, 1H, H-1). ^{13}C NMR (100 MHz, CDCl$_3$) δ 20.5, 20.7 and 20.8 (3 CH$_3$), 62.2 (C-6), 63.5 (C-5), 75.4 (C-3), 78.4 (C-2), 79.0 (C-4), 96.5 (C-1), 169.8, 169.9 and 170.5 (3 CO). Anal. Calcd for C$_{12}$H$_{16}$O$_8$: C, 50.00; H,5.59. Found: C, 50.36; H, 5.75.

ACKNOWLEDGMENT

The work was supported by the Department of Science and Technology, New Delhi (Project No. SP/S1/G14/95). The checking process was partially supported by the APVV-0366-07 and VEGA 2/0128/08 Grants.

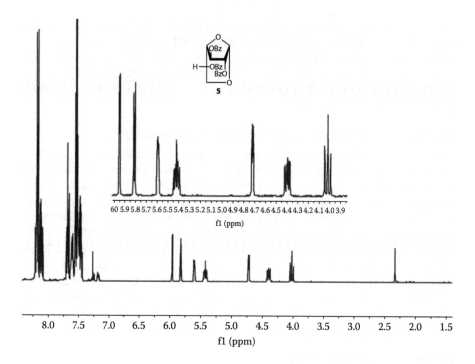

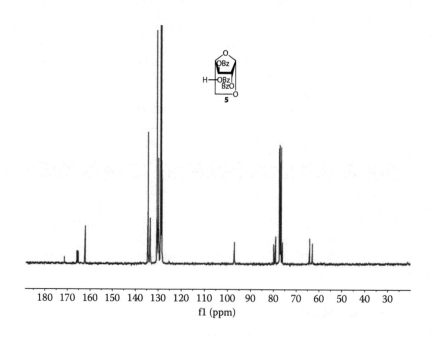

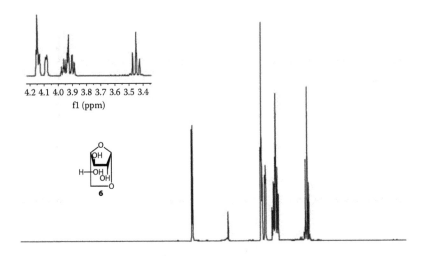

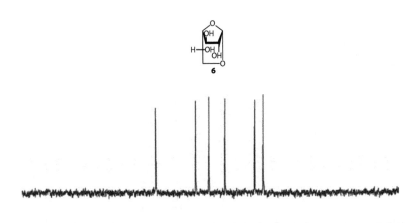

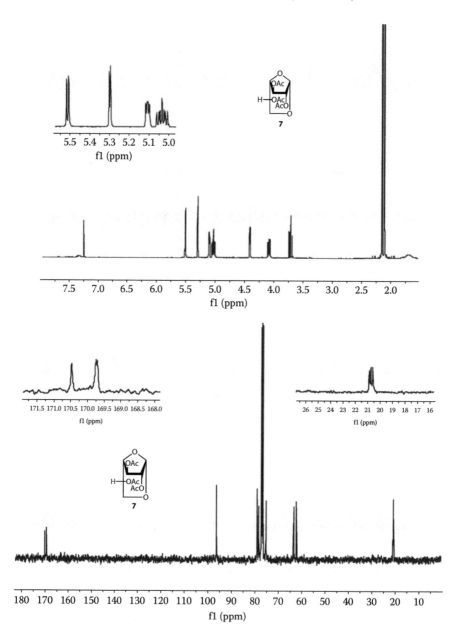

REFERENCES

1. *Choudhury*, A. K. and Roy, N. *Carbohydr. Res.* 1998, *308*, 207–211.
2. Tipson, R. S. *Methods Carbohydr. Chem.* 1963, *2*, 246–250.
3. Sarkar, S. K.; Choudhury, A. K.; Mukhopadhyay, B.; and Roy, N. *J. Carbohydr. Chem.* 1999, *18*, 1121–1130.
4. Richtmyer, N. K. *Methods Carbohydr. Chem.* 1963, *2*, 390.
5. Alexander, B. H.; Dimler, R. J.; and Mehltretter, C. L. *J. Am. Chem. Soc.* 1951, *73*, 4658.

31 Synthesis of Prop-2-Ynyl 2,3,4,6-Tetra-O-Acetyl-α-D-Mannopyranoside

Yoann M. Chabre, Tze Chieh Shiao,
*Sébastien Vidal,† and René Roy**

CONTENTS

Experimental Methods 276
General Methods 276
Prop-2-Ynyl 2,3,4,6-Tetra-*O*-Acetyl-α-D-Mannopyranoside (**2**) 276
Acknowledgments...277
References..278

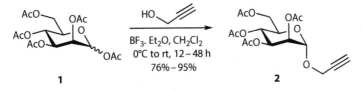

Synthesis of propargyl 2,3,4,6-tetra-*O*-acetyl-α-D-mannopyranoside **2**.

Advances in glycobiology have highlighted the critical role played by complex oligosaccharides and glycoconjugates in various biological processes.[1] Despite recent progress, access of this class of substances in large quantities is still problematic. In order to make such complex materials efficiently, ready access to saccharidic precursors is required. Among the wide variety of suitable derivatives, propargyl glycosides provide the much needed synthetic versatility. Indeed, besides easy introduction and derivatization of the propargyl aglycone, this function has been described as a stable and versatile anomeric protecting group.[2] Propargyl glycosides have also been described as stable glycosyl donors.[3] Consequently, they have been used in the synthesis of glycoconjugates,[4] oligosaccharides,[5] and glycomimetics.[6] More recently, these substances have been used as intermediates toward multivalent

---

* Corresponding author.
† Checker.

neoglycoconjugates through the Cu[I]-catalyzed Huisgen azide-alkyne 1,3-dipolar cycloaddition ("click chemistry"),[7] palladium(0)-catalyzed Sonogashira couplings,[8] or organometallic coupling reactions.[9] Many methods for the preparation of propargyl glycosides have been described: (1) from reducing sugars by classical Fischer glycosidation,[2] (2) from glycosyl donors such as halides[10] and trichloroacetimidates,[11] and (3) from per-acetylated precursors and propargyl alcohol by Lewis acid-catalyzed glycosidation.[12] Here, we describe an improved synthesis of prop-2-ynyl 2,3,4,6-tetra-O-acetyl-α-D-mannopyranoside from D-mannopyranose pentaacetate and propargyl alcohol in the presence of boron trifluoride-diethyl etherate.

EXPERIMENTAL METHODS

GENERAL METHODS

The reaction was carried out in dichloromethane (freshly distilled from P_2O_5) under nitrogen. Solutions in organic solvents were dried over anhydrous Na_2SO_4 and concentrated at reduced pressure. Progress of reactions was monitored by thin-layer chromatography (TLC) using silica gel 60 F_{254} precoated plates (E. Merck). Optical rotations were measured with a JASCO P-1010 polarimeter. Melting points were measured on a Fisher Jones apparatus and are uncorrected. NMR spectra were recorded for solutions in $CDCl_3$ with a Varian Innova AS600 600 MHz spectrometer. Proton and carbon chemical shifts are reported in ppm (δ) relative to the signal of $CDCl_3$ (δ 7.27 and 77.23 ppm for ^{1}H and ^{13}C, respectively). Coupling constants (J) are reported in Hertz (Hz), and the following abbreviations are used for signal multiplicities: singlet (s), doublet (d), doublet of doublets (dd), and multiplet (m). Assignments of nuclear magnetic resonance (NMR) signals were made by COSY, DEPT, and HETCOR experiments. The α-stereochemistry of the O-glycosidic linkage was deduced from $^1J_{C-1,H-1}$ coupling constants.[13] Low- and high-resolution mass spectra (HRMS) were taken by the analytical platform of UQAM (Université du Québec à Montréal, Quebec, Canada).

Prop-2-Ynyl 2,3,4,6-Tetra-O-Acetyl-α-D-Mannopyranoside (2)

To a solution of penta-O-acetyl-α,β-D-mannopyranose **1**[14] (250 mg, 0.64 mmol, 1.00 equiv.) in dry dichloromethane (10 mL), boron trifluoride etherate (150 μL, 1.19 mmol, 1.9 equiv.) was added dropwise at 0°C under nitrogen. The mixture was allowed to warm-up and stirred at room temperature for 4 h. Propargyl alcohol (150 μL, 2.56 mmol, 4.00 equiv.) was added, and the mixture was stirred at room temperature until TLC (1:1 hexane-AcOEt) showed complete disappearance of the starting material (12–48 h). After addition of CH_2Cl_2 (20 mL), the solution was washed successively with 20% aqueous Na_2CO_3 solution (2 × 40 mL) and water (2 × 40 mL). The organic phase was dried, concentrated, and chromatography (2:1 hexane-AcOEt) gave prop-2-ynyl 2,3,4,6-tetra-O-acetyl-α-D-mannopyranoside (**2**, 234 mg, 0.61 mmol, 95%), which crystallized after drying under vacuum. The reaction time and the yield depend on the ratio α/β of the starting material (that can vary over 3:1 to pure α). Best yields and faster reactions are obtained when the configuration is α (ex: α pure, 12h, 95%). Crystallization from CH_2Cl_2–petroleum ether and recrystallization from petroleum ether gave material melting at 99°C–100°C, lit.[15] 99°C–100°C); $[\alpha]_D$ +56 (*c* 2.0, $CHCl_3$) [lit.[9a] $[\alpha]_D$ +56 (*c* 2.0, $CHCl_3$)]; ^{1}H NMR ($CDCl_3$) δ 5.31 (dd, 1H, $J_{2,3}$ 3.4 Hz, $J_{3,4}$ 10.0 Hz, H-3), 5.26 (t, 1 H, $J_{3,4} = J_{4,5}$ 10.0 Hz, H-4), 5.23 (dd, 1H, $J_{1,2}$ 1.7 Hz, $J_{2,3}$ 3.4, H-2), 4.99 (d, 1H, $J_{1,2}$ 1.7 Hz, H-1), 4.24 (dd, 1H, $J_{6a,6b}$ 5.2 Hz, $J_{5,6}$ 12.2 Hz, H-6a), 4.24 (d, 2H, $J_{H-1',H-2'}$ 2.4 Hz, H-1'), 4.07 (dd, 1H, $J_{6a,6b}$ 2.5 Hz, H-6a), 4.00 (ddd, 1H, H-5), 2.44 (t, 1H, $J_{H-1',H-2'}$ 2.4 Hz, H-2'), 2.12, 2.07, 2.01, 1.96 ppm (4×s, 12H, CH_3); ^{13}C NMR ($CDCl_3$) δ 170.5, 169.9, 169.7, 169.6 (CO), 96.1 (C-1, $J_{C-1,H-1}$ 173.4 Hz), 77.8 (C-2'), 75.5 (C-1'), 69.2 (C-5), 68.9 (C-3), 68.8 (C-2), 65.9 (C-4), 62.2 (OCH_2), 54.9 (C-6), 20.8, 20.7, 20.6, 20.6 ppm ($COCH_3$). ESI[+]-HRMS: $[M+Na]^+$ calcd for $C_{17}H_{22}O_{10}Na$, 409.11052; found: 409.11004.

ACKNOWLEDGMENTS

This chapter was supported by Natural Sciences and Engineering Research Council of Canada (NSERC) and a Canadian Research Chair in Therapeutic Chemistry to R.R. Y.M.C. thanks FQRNT (Québec) for a postdoctoral fellowship.

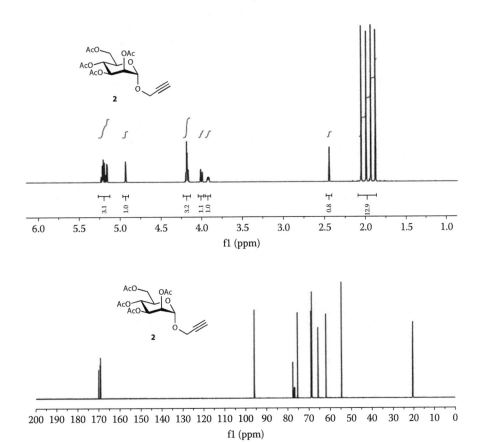

REFERENCES

1. (a) Bertozzi, C. R.; Kiessling, L. *Science*, 2001, *291*, 2357–2364; (b) Varki, A. *Glycobiology*, 1997, *3*, 97–130.
2. (a) Izumi, M.; Fukase, K.; Kusumoto, S. *Biosci. Biotechnol. Biochem.*, 2002, *66*, 211–214; (b) Mereyala, H. B.; Gurrala, S. R. *Carbohydr. Res.*, 1998, *307*, 351–354.
3. Hotha, S.; Kashyap, S. *J. Am. Chem. Soc.*, 2006, *128*, 9620–9621.
4. (a) Pourceau, G.; Meyer, A.; Vasseur, J.-J.; Morvan, F. *J. Org. Chem.*, 2009, *74*, 1218–1222; (b) Wankhede, K. S.; Vaidya, V. V.; Sarang, P. S.; Salunkhe, M. M.; Trivedi, G. K. *Tetrahedron Lett.*, 2008, *49*, 2069–2073; (c) Mandal, S.; Gauniyal, H. M.; Pramanik, K.; Mukhopadhyay, B. *J. Org. Chem.*, 2007, *72*, 9753–9756; (d) Mereyala, H. B.; Pathuri, G. *Synthesis*, 2006, *17*, 2944–2950.
5. (a) Dasgupta, S.; Mukhopadhyay, B. *Eur. J. Org. Chem.*, 2008, 5770–5777; (b) Sureshkumar, G.; Hotha, S. *Chem. Commun.*, 2008, 4282–4284.
6. (a) Giguère, D.; Patnam, R.; Bellefleur, M.-A.; St-Pierre, C.; Sato, S.; Roy, R. *Chem. Commun.*, 2006, *22*, 2379–2381; (b) Béha, S.; Giguère, D.; Patnam, R.; Roy, R. *Synlett*, 2006, *11*, 1739–1743.
7. (a) Touaibia, M.; Roy, R. In *Comprehensive Glycoscience*; Kamerling, J. P. Ed.; Elsevier: Amsterdam, the Netherlands, 2007; Vol. 3, pp. 821–870; (b) Chabre, Y. M.; Roy, R. *Curr. Top. Med. Chem.*, 2008, *8*, 1237–1285; (c) Touaibia, M.; Shiao, T. C.; Papadopoulos, A.; Vaucher, J.; Wang, Q.; Benhamioud, K.; Roy. R. *Chem. Commun.*, 2007, *4*, 380–382; (d) Deguise, I.; Lagnoux, D.; Roy, R. *New J. Chem.*, 2007, *7*, 1321–1331; (e) Fernandez-Megia, E.; Correa, J.; Riguera, R. *Biomacromolecules*, 2006, *7*, 3104–3111; (f) Koumbis, A. E.; Gallos, J. K. *Curr. Org. Chem.*, 2003, *7*, 771–797; (g) Dedola, S.; Nepogodiev, S. A.; Field, R. A. *Org. Biomol. Chem.*, 2007, *5*, 1006–1017; (h) Calvo-Flores, F.; Isac-Garcia, J.; Hernandez-Mateo, F.; Perez-Balderas, F.; Calvo-Asin, J. A.; Sanchez-Vaquero, E.; Santoyo-Gonzalez, F. *Org. Lett.*, 2000, *2*, 2499–2502.
8. (a) Touaibia, M.; Wellens, A.; Shiao, T. C.; Wang, Q.; Sirois, S.; Bouckaert, J.; Roy, R. *Chem. Med. Chem.*, 2007, *2*, 1190–1201; (b) Lowary, T.; Meldal, M.; Helmboldt, A.; Vasella, A.; Bock, K. *J. Org. Chem.*, 1998, *63*, 9657–9668; (c) Sengupta, S.; Sadhukhan, S. K. *Carbohydr. Res.*, 2001, *332*, 215–219.
9. (a) Saito, S.; Yamamoto, Y. *Chem. Rev.*, 2000, *100*, 2901–2916; (b) Roy, R.; Trono, M. C.; Giguère, D. In *Glycomimetics Modern Synthetic Methodologies*, Ed. R. Roy, *ACS Symp. Ser.*, 2005, Vol. 896, pp. 137–150.
10. Horisberger, M.; Lewis, B. A.; Smith, F. *Carbohydr. Res.*, 1972, *23*, 144–147.
11. Megia, E. F.; Correa, J.; Rodriguez-Meizoso, I.; Riguera, R. *Macromolecules*, 2006, *39*, 2113–2120.
12. (a) Kaufman, R. J.; Sidhu, R. S. *J. Org. Chem.*, 1982, *47*, 4941–4947. (b) Roy, R.; Das, S. K.; Hernandez-Mateo, F.; Santoyo-Gonzalez, F.; Gan, Z. *Synthesis*, 2001, *7*, 1049–1052.
13. Bock, K.; Pedersen, C. *J. Chem. Soc. Perkin Trans. 2*, 1974, *3*, 293–297.
14. Levene, P. A. *J. Biol. Chem.*, 1924, *59*, 141–144.
15. Das, S. K.; Trono, C. M.; Roy, R. *Methods Enzymol.*, 2003, *362*, 3–18.

32 Synthesis of 3-C-(2,3,4,6-Tetra-O-Acetyl-β-D-Galactopyranosyl) prop-1-Ene

Subhash Rauthu, Tze Chieh Shiao,
Dominique Lafont,† and René Roy*

CONTENTS

Experimental Methods 280
   General Methods 280
      2,3,4,6-Tetra-O-Acetyl-α-D-Galactopyranosyl Bromide (1) 280
      3-C-(2,3,4,6-Tetra-O-Acetyl-β-D-Galactopyranosyl)Prop-1-Ene (2) 281
Acknowledgments 281
References 282

Synthesis of 3-C-(2,3,4,6-tetra-O-acetyl-β-D-galactopyranosyl)prop-1-ene using allylmagnesium bromide (yields in parentheses refer to the reaction carried out with a solution of AllylMgBr in THF).

C-Glycosyl compounds are important precursors toward stable and biologically active glycomimetics.[1] Among these, 3-C-glycosylprop-1-enes represent powerful and versatile precursors toward other functionalities and as key intermediates in several natural product syntheses. 3-C-Glycosylprop-1-enes can be prepared from glycosyl halides, anomeric acetates, methyl glycosides, and even sugar lactones

---

* Corresponding author.
† Checker.

using a wide range of procedures.[1] Some of the most common and practical methods involve treating sugar lactones with excess allylmagnesium bromide, followed by reduction of the ensuing tertiary alcohol with silanes and a Lewis acid (Kishi's procedure),[2] allylation using allyl trimethylsilane and Lewis acids such as BF_3 etherate or TMSOTf (Sakurai reaction),[3] epoxide opening with organometallic reagents,[4] and radical allylation of glycosyl halides using allyl stannanes or sulfones (Keck allylation).[5] However, most protocols provide anomeric mixtures of the desired 3-C-glycosylprop-1-enes that are not always readily separable. We provide herein a slight modification of the procedure described by Wong and coworkers,[6] which improves the stereoselectivity of the formation of the C-β-glycosyl derivative.

Thus, peracetylated 3-C-(β-D-galactopyranosyl)prop-1-ene (**2**) can be obtained in a stereoselective fashion, in overall 36% yield for the two steps, from tetra-O-acetyl-α-D-galactopyranosyl bromide (**1**) using excess allylmagnesium bromide (10 eq) followed by an aqueous workup and re-O-acetylation. Concomitantly, C-2-allylated anhydro sugar (**3**) was formed as a side product in 15% yield. The stereochemistry of **3**, arising from a 2-keto intermediate has been unambiguously determined by x-ray data.[6]

3-C-Glycopyranosylprop-1-enes can be further transformed into a wide array of useful derivatives, such as C-(β-D-glycopyranosyl)propynes,[7] carboxylic acids,[8] aldehydes, alcohols,[9] azides and amines.[10] Moreover, the terminal double bond can also undergo isomerization[11] and olefin cross metathesis.[12]

EXPERIMENTAL METHODS

GENERAL METHODS

Progress of reactions was monitored by thin-layer chromatography (TLC) using silica gel $60 F_{254}$ precoated plates (E. Merck). Optical rotations were measured with a JASCO P-1010 polarimeter. Melting points were measured on a Fisher Jones apparatus and are uncorrected. Nuclear magnetic resonance (NMR) spectra were recorded for solutions in $CDCl_3$ with a Varian Innova AS600 600 MHz spectrometer. Proton and carbon chemical shifts are reported in parts per million (ppm) (δ) relative to the signal of $CDCl_3$ (δ 7.27 and 77.23 ppm for ^1H and ^{13}C, respectively). Coupling constants (J) are reported in Hertz (Hz), and the following abbreviations are used for signal multiplicities: singlet (s), doublet (d), doublet of doublets (dd), and multiplet (m). Analysis and assignments were made by COSY, DEPT, and HETCOR experiments. Low- and high-resolution mass spectra (HRMS) were carried out by the analytical platform of UQAM (Université du Québec à Montréal, Quebec, Canada). The 1 M solution of allylmagnesium bromide in Et_2O was purchased from Aldrich Chemical Company.

2,3,4,6-Tetra-O-Acetyl-α-D-Galactopyranosyl Bromide (1)

A 33% solution of HBr in AcOH (11.0 equiv.) was added dropwise to a solution of β-D-galactose pentaacetate (500 mg, 1.28 mmol) in dry CH_2Cl_2 (13 mL) at 0°C.[13] The resulting mixture was stirred at 0°C for 30 min and then at room temperature for 1 h. The mixture was diluted with CH_2Cl_2 (13 mL) and washed with cold water, followed by cold $NaHCO_3$ solution. The organic phase was dried (Na_2SO_4) and concentrated under reduced pressure to give **1** (white foam, 516 mg, 1.26 mmol, 98%), which was used for the next step without further purification; $R_f = 0.68$, 1:1 hexane–AcOEt. ^{1}H NMR: δ 6.67 (d, 1H, $J_{1,2}$ 3.9 Hz, H-1), 5.49 (d, 1H, $J_{4,5}$ 2.3 Hz, H-4), 5.37 (dd, 1H, $J_{3,4}$ 3.3 Hz, $J_{2,3}$ 10.6 Hz, H-3), 5.01 (dd, 1H, $J_{1,2}$ 4.0 Hz, $J_{2,3}$ 10.6 Hz, H-2), 4.46 (t, 1H, $J_{5,6}$ 6.3 Hz, H-5), 4.19–4.04 (m, 2H, H-6a,b), 2.12, 2.08, 2.03, 1.98 ppm (4 × s, 12H, 4 × COCH$_3$); ^{13}C NMR: δ 170.2, 170.0, 169.8, 169.6 (*CO*), 88.0 (C-1), 71.0 (C-5), 67.9 (C-3), 66.9 (C-2), 66.8 (C-4), 60.7 (C-6), 20.6, 20.5 ppm (4 × CH$_3$).

3-*C*-(2,3,4,6-Tetra-*O*-Acetyl-β-D-Galactopyranosyl)Prop-1-Ene (2)

Allylmagnesium bromide (1 M in Et$_2$O, 15.9 mL) was added at −78°C to a solution of **1** (690 mg, 1.68 mmol) in THF (7.5 mL). The mixture was slowly (~30 min) allowed to warm-up to room temperature and poured into H$_2$O (45 mL). Glacial acetic acid (3 mL) was added to dissolve the magnesium salts, causing two layers to be formed. The ethereal phase was discarded and the aqueous layer was washed with Et$_2$O. The phases were separated, and the aqueous layer was concentrated to dryness. The residue was stirred overnight at room temperature with 1:1 Ac$_2$O–pyridine (30 mL) and a catalytic amount of DMAP. After excess Ac$_2$O was destroyed with ice (1 h, rt), the mixture was concentrated, and the remaining oil was diluted with EtOAc (80 mL), washed with saturated NaHCO$_3$ solution, brine, and dried over MgSO$_4$. After concentration, the crude product was chromatographed (4:1 → 1:1) (petroleum ether–AcOEt 4:1) to afford compound **2** as a colorless oil (220 mg, 36%),* $R_f = 0.63$, 1:1 petroleum ether–AcOEt; $[α]_D$ +4.82 (*c* 1.0, CH$_2$Cl$_2$); lit.^{5c} $[α]_D$ +6.6 (*c* 0.4, CHCl$_3$); ^{1}H NMR δ 5.86-5.73 (m, 1H, H-2′), 5.39 (dd, 1H, *J* = 1.0, 3.4 Hz, H-4), 5.12–4.95 (m, 3H, H-2, H-3 and H3′), 4.14–3.99 (m, 2H, H-6a,b), 3.83 (td, 1H, *J* = 1.0, 6.7 Hz, H-5), 3.44 (td, 1H, *J* = 5.9, 10.1 Hz, H-1), 2.34–2.22 (2H, m, H-1′), 2.12–1.94 ppm (4 × s, 12H, CH$_3$); ^{13}C NMR δ 170.24, 170.14, 170.04, 169.56 (*CO*), 133.20 (C-2′), 117.26 (C-3′), 77.69 (C-5), 74.05 (C-1), 72.16 (C-3), 69.21 (C-2), 67.70 (C-4), 61.50 (C-6), 35.95 (C-1′), 20.67–20.46 ppm (CH$_3$). ESI$^+$-MS: [M + H]$^+$ calcd for C$_{17}$H$_{25}$O$_9$, 373.1; found: 373.1.

The presence of approximately 15% of compound **3** was determined from the ^{1}H NMR spectrum of the crude reaction mixture.

ACKNOWLEDGMENTS

This chapter was supported from Natural Sciences and Engineering Research Council of Canada (NSERC) and a Canadian Research Chair in Therapeutic Chemistry to R.R.

---

* The yield increases to ~50% when the reaction is carried out in THF with a solution of AllylMgBr in THF (currently not available commercially).

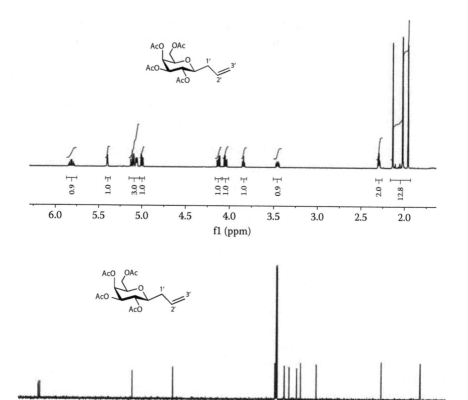

REFERENCES

1. (a) Postema, M. H. D. *Tetrahedron* 1992, *48*, 8545–8599. (b) Leavy, D. E.; Tang, C. *The Chemistry of C-Glycosides*; Pergamon: Oxford, U.K., 1995. (c) Du, Y.; Linhardt, R. J.; Vlahow, I. R. *Tetrahedron* 1998, *54*, 9913–9959. (d) Jaramillo, C.; Kanapp, S. *Synthesis* 1994, 1–20. (e) Postema, M. H. D. *C-Glycosides Synthesis*; CRC: Boca Raton, FL, 1995.
2. (a) Goekjian, P.; Wu, T.-C.; Kang, H. Y.; Kishi, Y. *J. Org. Chem.* 1991, *56*, 6422–6434. (b) Terauchi, M.; Abe, H.; Matsuda, A.; Shuto, S. *Org. Lett.* 2004, *6*, 3751–3754.
3. (a) Hosomi, A.; Sakata, Y.; Sakurai, H. *Tetrahedron Lett.* 1984, *25*, 2383–2386. (b) Giannis, A.; Sandhoff, K. *Tetrahedron Lett.* 1985, *26*, 1479–1482. (c) Hosomi, A.; Sakata, Y.; Sakurai, H. *Carbohydr. Res.* 1987, *171*, 223–232. (d) BeMiller, J. N.; Yadav, MP.; Lalabokis, V. N.; Myers, R. W. *Carbohydr. Res.* 1990, *200*, 111–126. (e) Horton, D.; Miyake, T. *Carbohydr. Res.* 1988, *184*, 221–229. (f) Czechura, P.; Tam, R.; Dimitrijevic, E.; Murphy, A.; Ben, R. *J. Am. Chem. Soc.* 2008, *130*, 2928–2929.
4. (a) Hanessian, S.; Liak, T. J.; Dixit, D. M. *Carbohydr. Res.* 1981, *88*, C14-C19. (b) Rainer, J. D.; Allwein, S. P. *J. Org. Chem.* 1998, *63*, 5310–5311.
5. (a) Pontén, F.; Magnusson, G. *J. Org. Chem.* 1996, *61*, 7463–7466. (b) Roe, B. A.; Boojamra, C. G.; Griggs, J. L.; Bertozzi, C. R. *J. Org. Chem.* 1996, *61*, 6442–6445. (c) Praly, J. P.; Chen, G. R.; Gola, J.; Hetzer, G. *Eur. J. Org. Chem.* 2000, 2831–2838.

6. Uchiyama, T.; Vassilev, V. P.; Kajimoto, T.; Wong, W.; Huang, H.; Lin, C. C.; Wong, C.-H. *J. Am. Chem. Soc.* 1995, *117*, 5395–5396.

7. Giguère, D.; Patnam, R.; Roy, R. *Chem. Commun.* 2006, *22*, 2379–2381.

8. Arya, P.; Barkley, A.; Randell, K. D. *J. Comb. Chem.* 2002, *4*, 193–198.

9. (a) Liu, S.; Ben, R. N. *Org. Lett.* 2005, *7*, 2385–2388. (b) Betancor, C.; Dorta, R. L.; Freire, R.; Prangé, T.; Suárez, E. *J. Org. Chem.* 2000, *65*, 8822–8825. (c) Nolen, E. G.; Watts, M. M.; Fowler, D. J. *Org. Lett.* 2002, *4*, 3963–3965.

10. Podlipnik, C.; Velter, I.; Ferla, B.; Marcou, G.; Belvisi, L.; Nicotra, F.; Bernardi, A. *Carbohydr. Res.* 2007, *342*, 1651–1660.

11. Patnam, R.; Jursez-Ruiz, J.; Roy, R. *Org. Lett.* 2006, *8*, 2691–2694.

12. (a) Roy, R.; Das, S. K. *Chem. Commun.* 2000, 519–529. (b) Meinke, S.; Thiem, J. *Carbohydr. Res.* 2008, *343*, 1824–1829. (c) Dominique, R.; Liu, B.; Das, S. K.; Roy, R. *Synthesis.* 2000, 862–868. (d) Liu, B.; Das, S. K.; Roy, R. *Org. Lett.* 2002, *4*, 2723–2726. (e) Roy, R.; Dominique, R.; Das, S. K. *J. Org. Chem.* 1999, *64*, 5408–5412. (f) Dominique, R.; Das, S. K.; Roy, R.; *Chem. Commun.* 1998, 2437–2438. (g) Hu, Y.-J.; Roy, R. *Tetrahedron Lett.* 1999, *40*, 3305–3308. (h) Plettenburg, O.; Mui, C.; Bodmer-Narkevitch, V.; Wong, C.-H. *Adv. Synth. Catal.* 2002, *344*, 622–626.

13. Bock, K.; Refn, S. *Acta Chem. Scand.* 1987, *B41*, 469–472.

33 Synthesis of (E)-Methyl 4-(2,3,4,6-Tetra-O-Acetyl-β-D-Galactopyranosyl) but-2-Enoate by Cross-Metathesis Reaction

Denis Giguère, Jacques Rodrigue,
David Goyard,† and René Roy*

CONTENTS

Experimental Methods 286
  General Methods 286
    (*E*)-Methyl 4-(2,3,4,6-Tetra-*O*-Acetyl-β-D-Galactopyranosyl)but-2-
    Enoate (**2**) 286
Acknowledgment 287
References...288

Catalytic synthesis of α,β-unsaturated ester **2** from glycosyl-1-propene-3 **1** using Grubbs' catalyst second-generation and methyl acrylate.

---

* Corresponding author.
† Checker.

α,β-Unsaturated esters are abundant in nature and are known to show various biological properties.[1] Indeed, sugars bearing this functionality have become an important class of molecules with respect to their significant versatility.[2] The incorporation of α,β-unsaturated ester motif has been achieved in our laboratory[3] and others,[4] providing galectin inhibitors, insecticides, and conferring antibacterial and antifungal activity. With the aim of generating a wide range and hydrolytically stable carbohydrate mimetics using the versatile α,β-unsaturated ester functionality, the cross-metathesis reaction between a glycosyl-1-propene-3 and an acrylate was explored.

The reaction described herein (see the opening scheme of this chapter) is the cross-metathesis reaction between 3-galactosylprop-1-ene **1**[5] and methyl acrylate catalyzed by Grubbs' second-generation catalyst.[6] This transition-metal-catalyzed cross-coupling reaction has proven to be a powerful tool for mild, highly efficient carbon–carbon bond formations.[6d,7] Product **2**[3] can be obtained in 83% yield, with only the *E*-configuration being produced owing to the conjugated system. Other method for the synthesis of such motif includes olefination reactions starting with the corresponding *C*-aldehyde of **1**, which may give a diastereomeric mixture of the double bond configuration.[8] Furthermore, contrary to the conversion described here, olefination reactions usually require the use of a strong base, which is incompatible with the acetyl protecting groups.

EXPERIMENTAL METHODS

GENERAL METHODS

The reaction was carried out under nitrogen using CH_2Cl_2, which was freshly distilled from P_2O_5. Progress of reactions was monitored by analytical thin-layer chromatography (TLC) using silica gel $60F_{254}$ precoated plates (E. Merck). Optical rotations were measured with a JASCO P-1010 polarimeter. Melting points were measured on a Fisher Jones apparatus and are uncorrected. Nuclear magnetic resonance (NMR) spectra were recorded for solutions in $CDCl_3$ with a Varian Innova AS600 600 MHz spectrometer. Proton and carbon chemical shifts are reported in parts per million (ppm) (δ) relative to $CDCl_3$ (δ 7.27 and 77.23 ppm for 1H- and 13C-NMR, respectively). Coupling constants (J) are reported in Hertz (Hz), and the following abbreviations are used for peak multiplicities: singlet (s), doublet (d), doublet of doublets (dd), and multiplet (m). Analysis and assignments were made by COSY, DEPT, and HETCOR experiments. Low- and high-resolution mass spectra (HRMS) were carried out by the analytical platform of UQAM (Université du Québec à Montréal, Quebec, Canada). Grubbs' second-generation catalyst was obtained from Boehringer Ingelheim Canada Ltd. or Aldrich Chemical Company.

(*E*)-Methyl 4-(2,3,4,6-Tetra-*O*-Acetyl-β-D-Galactopyranosyl)but-2-Enoate (2)

To a solution of 3-(β-D-galactosyl)prop-1-ene **1**[5] (200 mg, 0.537 mmol) in CH_2Cl_2 (13.4 mL, 0.04 M), methyl acrylate (145 μL, 1.611 mmol) and Grubbs' second-generation catalyst (23 mg, 0.027 mmol, 5 mol%) were added. The mixture was stirred under reflux for 3 h, concentrated under reduced pressure, and chromatography of the brown residue on silica gel (30%→45% EtOAc–Hexanes) gave **2** (192 mg, 0.446 mmol, 83%), mp 64°C–65°C (EtOAc–Hexanes); R_f=0.62 (1:1 EtOAc–Hexanes); $[\alpha]_D^{25}$: +9.6 (*c* 1.0, CHCl₃); ¹H NMR δ: 6.91–6.86 (m, 1H, CH₂C$\underline{H}$), 5.85 (d, *J*=15.7 Hz, 1H, C$\underline{H}$CO₂CH₃), 5.36 (dd, *J*=0.9, 3.3 Hz, 1H, H-4), 5.06 (dd, *J*=9.9 Hz, 1H, H-2), 4.97 (dd, *J*=3.4, 10.1 Hz, 1H, H-3), 4.1–4.07 (m, 1H, H-6), 4.01–3.99 (m, 1H, H-6), 3.85–3.82 (m, 1H, H-5), 3.68 (s, 3H, CHCO₂C$\underline{H}_3$), 3.51–3.49 (m, 1H, H-1), 2.41–2.39 (m, 2H, CH₂C$\underline{H}$), 2.10 (s, 3H, CO₂C$\underline{H}_3$), 1.99 (s, 3H, CO₂C$\underline{H}_3$), 1.92 (s, 3H, CO₂C$\underline{H}_3$); ¹³C NMR (150 MHz, CDCl₃, δ ppm): 170.5 ($\underline{C}$OCH₃), 170.2 (2×$\underline{C}$OCH₃), 169.8 ($\underline{C}$OCH₃), 166.6 (CH$\underline{C}$O₂CH₃), 143.6 (CH₂$\underline{C}$H), 123.5 ($\underline{C}$HCO₂CH₃), 76.8 (C-1), 74.2 (C-5), 72.0 (C-3), 69.2 (C-2), 67.6 (C-4), 61.6 (C-6), 51.5 (CHCO₂$\underline{C}$H₃), 34.4 ($\underline{C}$H₂CH), 20.8 (CO$\underline{C}$H₃), 20.7 (2×CO$\underline{C}$H₃), 20.6 (CO$\underline{C}$H₃); ESI-MS *m/z*: 431.3 [M+H]⁺; HRMS *m/z* calcd C₁₉H₂₆O₁₁ [M+H]⁺: 431.1555; found: 431.1538.

ACKNOWLEDGMENT

This chapter was supported by a grant from the Natural Science and Engineering Research Council of Canada (NSERC) to R.R. D.G. is thankful to the FQRNT for a postgraduate fellowship. The authors are thankful to Boehringer Ingelheim Canada Ltd (P. L. Beaulieu) for a generous donation of Grubbs' second-generation catalyst.

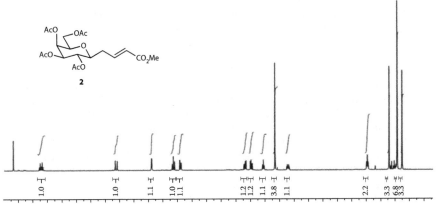

fl (ppm)

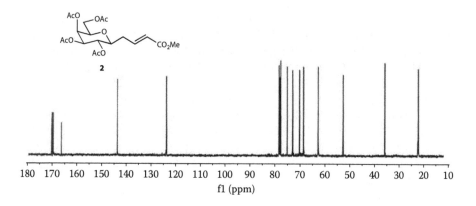

REFERENCES

1. (a) Husain, A.; Hasan, S. M.; Lal, S.; Alam, M. M. *Indian J. Pharm. Sci.* 2006, *68*, 536–538. (b) Li, D.-H.; Zhu, T.-J.; Liu, H. B.; Fang, Y.-C.; Gu, Q.-Q.; Zhu, W.-M. *Arch. Pharm. Res.* 2006, *29*, 624–626. (c) Cateni, F.; Zilic, J.; Zacchigna, M.; Bonivento, P.; Frausin, F.; Scarcia, V. *Eur. J. Med. Chem.* 2006, *41*, 192–200. (d) Ma, S.; Shi, Z.; Yu, Z. *Tetrahedron* 1999, *55*, 12137–12148. (e) Anke, T.; Watson, W.; Gianneti, B.; Steglich, W. *J. Antibiot.* 1981, *34*, 1271–1277.
2. (a) Roy, R.; Das, S. K. *Chem. Commun.* 2000, 519–529. (b) Madsen, R. *Eur. J. Org. Chem.* 2007, *3*, 399–415. (c) Xavier, N. M.; Rauter, A. P. *Carbohydr. Res.* 2008, *343*, 1523–1539.
3. Giguère, D.; Bonin, M.-A.; Cloutier, P.; Patnam, R.; St-Pierre, C.; Sato, S.; Roy, R. *Bioorg. Med. Chem.* 2008, *16*, 7811–7823.
4. (a) Xavier, N. M.; Silva, S.; Madeira, P. J. A.; Florêncio, M. H.; Silva, F. V. M.; Justino, J.; Thiem, J.; Rauter, A. P. *Eur. J. Org. Chem.* 2008, 6134–6136. (b) Rauter, A. P.; Ferreira, M. J.; Font, J.; Virgili, A.; Figueredo, M.; Figueiredo, J. A.; Ismael, M. I.; Canda, T. L. J. *Carbohydr. Chem.* 1995, *14*, 929–948. (c) Justino, J.; Rauter, A. P.; Canda, T.; Wilkins, R.; Matthews, E. *Pest. Manag. Sci.* 2005, *61*, 985–990. (d) Rauter, A. P.; Figueiredo, J. A.; Ismael, M. I.; Pais, M. S.; Gonzalez, A. G.; Dias, J.; Barrera, J. B. *J. Carbohydr. Chem.* 1987, *6*, 259–272.
5. Uchiyama, T.; Vassilev, V. P.; Kajimoto, T.; Wong, W.; Huang, H.; Lin, C. C.; Wong, C.-H. *J. Am. Chem. Soc.* 1995, *117*, 5395–5396.
6. (a) Scholl, M.; Ding, S.; Lee, C. W.; Grubbs, R. H. *Org. Lett.* 1999, *1*, 953–956. (b) Grubbs, R. H.; Chang, S. *Tetrahedron* 1998, *54*, 4413–4450. (c) Schmidt, B. *Angew. Chem. Int. Ed.* 2003, *42*, 4996–4999. (d) Roy, R.; Das, S. K.; Dominique, R.; Trono, M. C.; Hermandez-Mateo, F.; Santoyo-Gonzalez, F. *Pure App. Chem.* 1999, *71*, 565–571.
7. (a) Dominique, R.; Liu, B.; Das, S. K.; Roy, R. *Synthesis* 2000, 862–868. (b) Liu, B.; Das, S. K.; Roy, R. *Org. Lett.* 2002, *4*, 2723–2726. (c) Roy, R.; Dominique, R.; Das, S. K. *J. Org. Chem.* 1999, *64*, 5408–5412. (d) Hu, Y.-J.; Roy, R. *Tetrahedron Lett.* 1999, *40*, 3305–3308. (e) Liu, S.; Ben, R. N. *Org. Lett.* 2005, *7*, 2385–2388.
8. (a) Flynn, A.; Ogilvie, W. W. *Chem. Rev.* 2007, *107*, 4698–4745; (b) Maryanoff, B. E.; Reitz, A. B. *Chem. Rev.* 1989, *89*, 863–927.

34 Preparation of O-β-D-Galactopyranosyl-hydroxylamine

Tze Chieh Shiao, Alex Papadopoulos,
Olivier Renaudet,[†] and René Roy*

CONTENTS

Experimental Methods 290
  General Methods 290
    O-(2,3,4,6-Tetra-O-Acetyl-β-D-Galactopyranosyl)-N-
    Hydroxysuccinimide (**2**) 290
    O-β-D-Galactopyranosylhydroxylamine (**3**) 291
Acknowledgments 291
References 293

Synthesis of O-β-D-galactopyranosylhydroxylamine (**3**) under PTC conditions.

Ligation of aldehydes and ketones with aminooxy, hydrazide, or semicarbazide groups is an important tool toward neoglycoconjugates.[1] In this context, the transformation of the anomeric position into O-oxyamino glycosides and glycopeptide mimetics has been extensively studied.[2,3] Also, inter-glycosidic oxyamino linkages have been observed to occur in some natural products, such as calicheamicin and esperamicin.[4] Efforts toward synthesis of the corresponding oligosaccharides have also been described.[5] The ready formation of oximes from glycosylhydroxylamines has served for the preparation of chemical library of glycomimetic inhibitors for galectins[6] and more recently for construction of glycan microarrays.[7]

---

* Corresponding author.
[†] Checker.

Anomeric hydroxylamines have been stereoselectively synthesized under our original phase transfer catalyzed (PTC) conditions.[2] More recently, other procedures have also been used, albeit with the loss of anomeric stereoselectivity.[8] The complementarity of these procedures expanded the scope and limitation initially observed for 1,2-*trans*-glycosides.[2] Hence, we described herein a simplified and high-yielding stereoselective synthesis of *O*-β-D-galactopyranosylhydroxylamine (see opening scheme of this chapter) from acetobromogalactose (**1**). Thus, treatment of **1** with *N*-hydroxysuccinimide under PTC conditions[2] provided pure *O*-(2,3,4,6-tetra-*O*-acetyl-β-D-galactopyranosyl)-*N*-hydroxysuccinimide (**2**, 88%). Subsequent hydrazinolysis gave pure (NMR) *O*-β-D-galactopyranosylhydroxylamine (**3**), which was isolated by simple precipitation (87%), thus avoiding tedious purification by chromatography.

EXPERIMENTAL METHODS

GENERAL METHODS

The reaction was carried out under nitrogen using CH_2Cl_2, which was freshly distilled from P_2O_5. Progress of reactions was monitored by thin-layer chromatography using silica gel $60 F_{254}$ precoated plates (E. Merck). Spot visualization was performed with ammonium molybdate (50 g ammonium heptamolybdate tetrahydrate, 12. 2 g ceric sulfate, 200 mL concentrated sulfuric acid, and 1.8 L distilled water). Optical rotations were measured with a JASCO P-1010 polarimeter. Melting points were measured on a Fisher Jones apparatus and are uncorrected. Nuclear magnetic resonance (NMR) spectra were recorded at 22°C on Varian Gemini 300 MHz or Innova 600 MHz spectrometers. Proton and carbon chemical shifts are reported in parts per million (ppm) (δ) relative to $CDCl_3$ (δ 7.27 and 77.23 ppm for ${}^1H$- and ${}^{13}C$-NMR, respectively) or relative to the signal of D_2O (δ 4.81 ppm for ${}^1H$) and relative to the signal of MeOH in D_2O (δ 49.50 ppm for ${}^{13}C$). Coupling constants (J) are reported in Hertz (Hz), and the following abbreviations are used for signal multiplicities: singlet (s), doublet (d), doublet of doublets (dd), triplet (t), multiplet (m), and broad (b). Analysis of the spectra and assignments were made by COSY, DEPT, and HETCOR experiments. High-resolution mass spectrometry (HRMS) was carried out in our analytical laboratory.

O-(2,3,4,6-Tetra-*O*-Acetyl-β-D-Galactopyranosyl)-*N*-Hydroxysuccinimide (2)

Acetobromo-galactose (**1**)[9] (1.55 g, 3.76 mmol), *N*-hydroxysuccinimide (1.30 g, 11.10 mmol, 3.0 equiv.), and tetrabutylammonium hydrogen sulfate (TBAHS, 1.89 g, 5.50 mmol, 1.50 equiv.) in CH_2Cl_2 (20 mL) and 1 M Na_2CO_3 (20 mL) were vigorously stirred at room temperature for 6 h. After addition of dichloromethane (20 mL), the organic phase was washed with distilled water (2×) and brine (2 × 40 mL). The organic phase was dried (Na_2SO_4), filtered, and concentrated under reduced pressure, to give a white residue. Crystallization from ethanol gave pure *N*-hydroxysuccinimide **2** (1.36 g, 80%), mp 190°C–191°C [lit.[2] 190.1°C–191.4°C (from AcOEt–hexane)]; [α]$_D$ −52 (*c* 1, $CHCl_3$) [lit.[2] [α]$_D$ −52.1 (*c* 1, $CHCl_3$)]. ${}^1H$ NMR ($CDCl_3$) δ 5.38 (dd, 1H, $J_{2,3}$ = 10.4 Hz,

H-2), 5.36 (dd, 1H, $J_{4,5}$ = 1.0 Hz, H-4), 5.07 (dd, 1H, $J_{3,4}$ = 3.4 Hz, $J_{2,3}$ = 10.4 Hz, H-3), 4.90 (d, 1H, $J_{1,2}$ = 8.2 Hz, H-1), 4.25 (ddd, 1H, $J_{6a,6b}$ = 6.2 Hz, $J_{5,6a}$ = 6.2 Hz, H-6a), 4.11 (ddd, 1H, $J_{5,6b}$ = 7.4 Hz, H-6b), 3.90 (ddd, 1H, H-5), 2.75 (s, 4H, 2×CH$_2$), 2.18, 2.16, 2.03, 2.00 ppm (4×s, 12H, 4×CH$_3$); ^{13}C NMR (CDCl$_3$) δ 170.2, 170.1, 169.9, 169.8, 169.7 (CO), 105.2 (C-1), 71.1 (C-5), 70.3 (C-3), 66.7 (C-2), 66.1 (C-4), 60.6 (C-6), 25.3 (CO$\underline{C}$H$_2$), 20.6, 20.5, 20.4 ppm (4×CH$_3$). ESI$^+$-HRMS: [M+Na]$^+$ calcd for C$_{18}$H$_{23}$NO$_{12}$Na, 468.11125; found: 468.11077.

O-β-D-Galactopyranosylhydroxylamine (3)

To a suspension of exactly 0.1 M O-(2,3,4,6-tetra-O-acetyl-β-D-galactopyranosyl)-N-hydroxysuccinimide (**2**) (445 mg, 1.00 mmol) in methanol (10 mL) was added 97% hydrazine hydrate (267 μL, 5.50 mmol, 5.5 equiv.). The mixture was stirred at room temperature until the solution became clear (2–4 min), indicating completion of the reaction. The reaction mixture was stirred at room temperature in an open flask for 1–3 h, to allow precipitation of butanedioic acid dihydrazide. R_f = 0.15, EtOH–H$_2$O (7:3); ESI$^+$-HRMS: [M+H]$^+$ calcd for C$_4$H$_{11}$N$_4$O$_2$, 147.08765; found: 147.08772. The mixture was filtered* and the filtrate was cooled to –78°C† overnight (6 h minimum) affording pure crystalline piperazine-3,6-dione, which was separated by filtration. R_f = 0.24, 7:3 EtOH–H$_2$O (detection with ammonium molybdate solution); ESI$^+$-HRMS: [M+H]$^+$ calcd for C$_4$H$_7$N$_2$O$_2$, 115.05020; found: 115.05014. The filtrate was concentrated under reduced pressure to afford a residue, which was a mixture of white solid and colorless oil. It was dissolved in a minimum amount of warmed methanol and the resulting solution was added to excess of CH$_2$Cl$_2$ whereupon O-β-D-galactopyranosylhydroxylamine (**3**) precipitated as a white solid (164 mg, 0.87 mmol, 84%) free of N-acetylhydrazide (NMR). R_f = 0.06, EtOH–H$_2$O (7:3), mp 173°C–174°C (from ethanol); [α]$_D$ –7 (*c* 1.0, H$_2$O), [α]$_D$ –6.4 (*c* 3.0, H$_2$O); ^{1}H NMR, 600 MHz (D$_2$O+CH$_3$OH‡): ^{1}H NMR (D$_2$O+CH$_3$OH) δ 4.54 (d, 1H, $J_{1,2}$ = 8.2 Hz, H-1), 3.95 (d, 1H, $J_{3,4}$ = 3.2 Hz, H-4), 3.81 (m, 2H, H-6a, H-6b), 3.74 (m, 1H, H-5), 3.69 (dd, 1H, $J_{2,3}$ = 9.9 Hz, H-3), 3.55 ppm (dd, 1H, H-2); ^{13}C NMR (D$_2$O+CH$_3$OH) δ 106.2 (C-1), 75.7 (C-5), 73.4 (C-3), 70.0 (C-2), 69.2 (C-4), 61.7 ppm (C-6). ESI$^+$-HRMS: [M+H]$^+$ calcd for C$_6$H$_{14}$NO$_6$, 196.08156; found: 196.08156.§,¶

ACKNOWLEDGMENTS

This chapter was supported from Natural Sciences and Engineering Research Council of Canada (NSERC) and a Canadian Research Chair in Therapeutic Chemistry to R. R.

---

* Without further washing with methanol.
$\dagger$ Crystallization does not occur at higher temperature.
$\ddagger$ Acetone cannot be used as internal reference as it rapidly forms the corresponding oxime.
$\S$ Some authors[8a] prefer the use of the more volatile N-methylhydrazine but this reagent is not always readily available. Deviation from the prescribed reaction concentration may complicate the selective crystallization process used herein.
$\P$ Discrepancies exist with the lit. values[3e]: mp 156°C; [α]$_D^{25}$ +68 (*c* 3.0, H$_2$O), but independent preparation (by Olivier Renaudet) confirmed the values reported here.

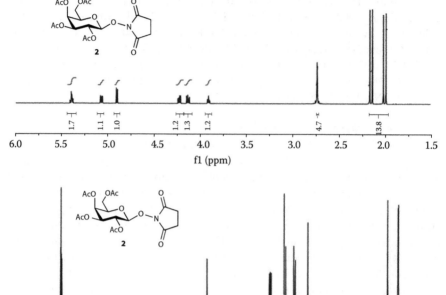

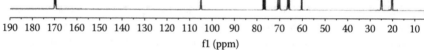

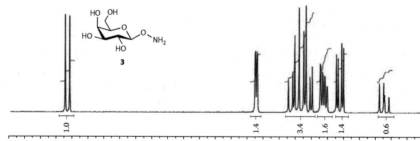

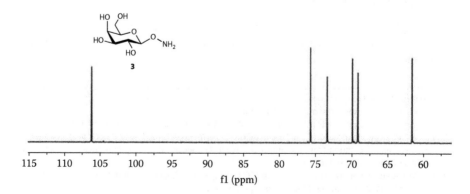

REFERENCES

1. (a) Stowell, C. P.; Lee, Y. C. *Adv. Carbohydr. Chem. Biochem.* 1980, *37*, 225–281. (b) Roy, R. *The Chemistry of Neoglycoconjugates.* In *Carbohydrate Chemistry*, Boons, G.-J. (Ed.). Blackie Academic and Professional, London, U.K., 1998, pp. 243–321.
2. Cao, S.; Tropper, F. D.; Roy, R. *Tetrahedron* 1995, *51*, 6679–6686.
3. (a) Rodriguez, E. C.; Winans, K. A.; King, D. S.; Bertozzi, C. R. *J. Am. Chem. Soc.* 1997, *119*, 9905–9906. (b) Rodriguez, E. C.; Marcaurelle, L. A.; Bertozzi, C. R. *J. Org. Chem.* 1998, *63*, 7134–7135. (c) Marcaurelle, L. A.; Shin, Y.; Goon, S.; Bertozzi, C. R. *Org. Lett.* 2001, *3*, 3691–3694. (d) Renaudet, O.; Dumy, P. *Eur. J. Org. Chem.* 2008, 5383–5386. (e) Brunner, H.; Schönherr, M.; Zabel, M. *Tetrahedron Asymm.* 2001, *12*, 2671–2675. (f) Mitchell, M. B.; Whitcombe, I. W. A. *Tetrahedron Lett.* 2000, *41*, 8829–8834. (g) Andreana, P. R.; Xie, W.; Cheng, H. N.; Qiao, L.; Murphy, D. J.; Gu, Q.-M.; Wang, P. G. *Org. Lett.* 2002, *4*, 1863–1866. (h) Liu, H.; Wang, L.; Brock, A.; Wong, C.-H.; Schultz, P. G. *J. Am. Chem. Soc.* 2003, *125*, 1702–1703.
4. (a) Nicolaou, K. C. *J. Org. Chem.* 2009, *74*, 951–972. (b) Galm, U.; Hager, M. H.; Van Lanen, S. G.; Ju, J.; Thorson, J. S.; Shen, B. *Chem. Rev.* 2005, *105*, 739–758. (c) Van Lanen, S. G.; Shen, B. *Curr. Top. Med. Chem.* 2008, *8*, 448–459.
5. (a) Groneberg, R. D.; Miyazaki, T.; Stylianides, N. A.; Schulze, T. J.; Stahl, W.; Schreiner, E. P.; Suzuki, T.; Iwabuchi, Y.; Smith, A. L.; Nicolaou, K. C. *J. Am. Chem. Soc.* 1993, *115*, 7593–7611. (b) Renaudet, O.; Dumy, P. *Tetrahedron* 2002, *58*, 2127–2135. (c) Johnson, H. D.; Thorson, J. S. *J. Am. Chem. Soc.* 2008, *130*, 17662–17663.
6. Tejler, J.; Leffler, H.; Nilsson, U. J. *Bioorg. Med. Chem. Lett.* 2005, *15*, 2343–2345.
7. (a) Wilczewski, M.; Van der Heyden, A.; Renaudet, O.; Dumy, P.; Coche-Guéerente, L.; Labbé, P. *Org. Biomol. Chem.* 2008, *6*, 1114–1122. (b) Renaudet, O.; Dumy, P. *Org. Biomol. Chem.* 2006, *4*, 2628–2636. (c) Scheibler, L.; Dumy, P.; Stamou, D.; Duschl, C.; Vogel, H.; Mutter, M. *Polym. Bull.* 1998, *40*, 151–157. (d) Park, S.; Lee, M.; Shin, I. *Chem. Commun.* 2008, *37*, 4389–4399.
8. (a) Renaudet, O.; Dumy, P. *Tetrahedron Lett.* 2001, *42*, 7575–7578. (b) Lagnoux, D.; Darbre, T.; Lienhard Schmitz, M.; Reymond, J.-L. *Chem. Eur. J.* 2005, *11*, 3941–3950. (c) Grigalevicius, S.; Chierici, S.; Renaudet, O.; Lo-Man, R.; Dériaud, E.; Leclerc, C.; Dumy, P. *Bioconjugate Chem.* 2005, *16*, 1149–1159. (d) Forget, D.; Renaudet, O.; Boturyn, D.; Defrancq, E.; Dumy, P. *Tetrahedron Lett.* 2001, *42*, 9171–9174. (e) Renaudet, O.; Dumy, P. *Open Glycoscience* 2008, *1*, 1–7.
9. Bock, K.; Refn, S. *Acta Chem. Scand.* 1987, *B41*, 469–472.

35 Synthesis of 2,3,4,6-Tetra-O-Acetyl-1,5-Anhydro-D-*Lyxo*-Hex-1-Enitol and Its Conversion into a Hex-3-Enopyranosid-2-Ulose Analogue of Levoglucosenone

Verónica E. Manzano, Evangelina Repetto, María Laura Uhrig, Marek Baráth,[†] and Oscar Varela[*]

CONTENTS

Experimental Methods 296
General Methods 296
2,3,4,6-Tetra-*O*-Acetyl-1,5-Anhydro-D-*Lyxo*-Hex-1-Enitol (**3**) 297
Benzyl 3,4-Dideoxy-α-D-*Glycero*-Hex-3-Enopyranosid-2-Ulose (**4**) 298
Acknowledgments 298
References 301

[*] Corresponding author.
[†] Checker.

The α,β-unsaturated carbonyl group is found in a large number of natural and synthetic products. This functionality is commonly related to a wide range of biological activities, such as antitumor, antiviral, antimicrobial, and gastric antiulcer activities.[1] Particularly, sugar enones have become important synthetic targets not only due to their bioactivity but also for their use as building blocks in the synthesis of varied targets.[1,2] The usefulness of sugar enones as chiral building blocks relies upon the fact that they posses olefinic and carbonyl unsaturations to which a number of well-established reactions may be applied. In addition, because of the chiral environment generated by the remaining stereocenters, reactions applied to the enone system are usually highly diastereoselective.

Levoglucosenone and isolevoglucosenone are common sugar-derived enuloses that have been employed as dienophiles in Diels–Alder cycloadditions[3] and as Michael acceptors in the synthesis of thiodisaccharides.[4] While levoglucosenone is usually obtained in a very low yield, as one of the products of pyrolysis of cellulose, we have described a mild procedure for the preparation of analogous 3-enopyranosid-2-uloses from hexoses[5] and pentoses,[6] via the corresponding 2-acetoxyglycal derivatives. These compounds undergo a double allylic rearrangement by the tin(IV) chloride-promoted glycosylation to give the enones in good yields. The 3-enopyranosid-2-uloses proved to be convenient dienophiles in Diels–Alder reactions with butadienes and cyclic dienes.[6-10] They have also been employed as Michael acceptors of thiols in the synthesis of glycosides of 3-deoxy-4-thiopyranosid-2-ulose and 3-deoxy-4-thiopyranosides.[11,12] This reaction has been extended to the synthesis of thiodisaccharides as sugar mimetics and enzyme inhibitors. Thus, the conjugate addition of 1-thioaldoses to sugar enones led to 3-deoxy-4-S-(1→4)thiodisaccharides formed by hexopyranose units[13] or their analogues constituted by pentoses and hexoses,[14] or having a furanose as nonreducing end.[15,16] The methodology has also been employed for the synthesis of 4,6′-thioether-linked disaccharides as hydrolytically stable glycomimetics.[17] Reduction of the carbonyl of the 3-en-2-ulopyranoses followed by oxidation of the double bond afforded sugar 3,4-epoxides, that underwent nucleophilic substitution by 1-thioaldoses to give (1→3)- and (1→4)-linked thiodisaccharides.[18] Naturally occurring amino deoxy sugars, constituents of antibiotics, have been synthesized from hex-3-enopyranosid-2-uloses.[19,20]

We describe herein a straightforward and high-yielding synthesis of benzyl 3,4-dideoxy-α-D-*glycero*-hex-3-enopyranosid-2-ulose (**4**) from D-galactose, via the 2,3,4,6-tetra-O-acetyl-1,5-anhydro-D-*lyxo*-hex-1-enitol (**3**). A convenient preparation of this intermediate is also described, as glycal derivatives themselves are useful chiral synthons.[2,21] Glycal **3** has been prepared in low yield a long time ago,[22] and it has been determined that in the crystalline state it adopts the $^4H_5$ half-chair conformation.[23]

EXPERIMENTAL METHODS

GENERAL METHODS

1,2,3,4,6-Penta-O-acetyl-β-D-galactopyranose was purchased from Fluka. Analytical thin layer chromatography (TLC) was performed on Silica Gel 60 F254 (Merck) aluminum-supported plates (layer thickness 0.2 mm) with solvent systems given in the text. Visualization of the spots was effected by exposure to UV light and charring with a solution of 5% (v/v) sulfuric acid in EtOH, containing 0.5% *p*-anisaldehyde. Column chromatography was carried out with Silica Gel 60 (230–400 mesh, Merck). Optical rotations were measured with a Perkin-Elmer 241 polarimeter. Nuclear magnetic resonance (NMR) spectra were recorded with a Bruker AMX 500 instrument. Solutions in organic solvents were dried with anhydrous Na_2SO_4 and concentrated at reduced pressure.

2,3,4,6-Tetra-*O*-Acetyl-1,5-Anhydro-D-*Lyxo*-Hex-1-Enitol (3)

1,2,3,4,6-Penta-*O*-acetyl-β-D-galactopyranose (5.0 g, 0.0128 mol) was placed in a 100 mL round bottom flask* and dissolved in anhydrous CH_2Cl_2 (5.0 mL).† The solution was magnetically stirred and cooled to 0°C in an ice bath. Acetic acid containing 33% HBr (5.1 mL, 0.0287 mol) was added slowly, over a period of 5–10 min. The mixture was stirred for 1 h at 0°C, allowed to reach room temperature, and the stirring was continued for 1 h. Monitoring of the reaction mixture by TLC (1:1 hexane–EtOAc) showed complete conversion of **1** (R_f 0.44) into the faster moving 2,3,4,6-tetra-*O*-acetyl-α-D-galactopyranosyl bromide (**2**, R_f 0.58).

The solution was concentrated and a solution of the residue in toluene was concentrated several times until the acids were removed. The resulting yellowish syrup (5.26 g, quantitative) was dissolved in dry CH_2Cl_2 (9.0 mL) and cooled in an ice-water bath. To this solution was added dropwise and with vigorous magnetic stirring diazabicyclo[5.4.0]-undec-7-ene (DBU, 3.0 mL, 0.0175 mL). The mixture was stirred for 30 min al 0°C and then at room temperature for additional 30 min, when TLC (1:1, hexane–EtOAc) revealed a single spot of **3** (R_f 0.45), slower moving than the glycosyl bromide **2** (R_f 0.58).

The mixture was diluted with CH_2Cl_2 (30 mL) and the solution was successively washed with 1 M aqueous HCl (2 × 15 mL), satd aq NaCl (15 mL), satd aq $NaHCO_3$ (2 × 15 mL), and satd aq NaCl (15 mL). The organic layer was dried (Na_2SO_4), filtered, and concentrated to afford glycal **3** as a yellowish solid. The solid was transferred to a 50 mL Erlenmeyer flask and dissolved in boiling isopropanol (20 mL). When the solution reached room temperature, crystallization was spontaneous or could be induced by occasional scratching of the walls of the flask. Finally, the flask was cooled in an ice bath for 2 h. The crystals were collected by filtration, and washed with cold isopropanol (2 mL). Compound **3** was obtained as white needles. Yield, 3.6–3.8 g (85%–90%), mp 113°C–114°C (from iPrOH), $[\alpha]_D$ −8.4° (*c* 1, CHCl₃), lit.[21] 111°C; $[\alpha]_D$ −3.8 (*c* 1.2, CHCl₃). ¹H NMR (CDCl₃, 500 MHz) δ: 6.63 (d, 1H, $J_{1,3}$ 1.2 Hz, H-1), 5.85 (ddd, 1H, $J_{1,3}$ 1.2, $J_{3,4}$ 4.8, $J_{3,5}$ 0.7 Hz, H-3), 5.49 (dd, 1H, $J_{3,4}$ 4.8, $J_{4,5}$ 2.3 Hz, H-4), 4.39 (ddd, 1H, $J_{3,5}$ 0.7, $J_{5,6}$ 7.6, $J_{5,6'}$ 5.0 Hz, H-5), 4.32 (dd, 1H, $J_{5,6}$ 7.6, $J_{6,6'}$ 11.7 Hz, H-6), 4.24 (dd, 1H, $J_{5,6'}$ 5.0, $J_{6,6'}$ 11.7 Hz, H-6′), 2.14, 2.12, 2.09, 2.05 (CH_3CO); ¹³C NMR (CDCl₃, 125.7 MHz) δ: 170.5, 170.0, 169.9, 169.3 (CH_3CO), 138.8 (C-1), 127.2 (C-2), 73.2 (C-5), 63.9 (× 2, C-3, C-4), 61.4 (C-6), 20.7, 20.6, 20.4 (CH_3CO).

---

* To protect the preparation from light and to avoid the release of bromine, an amber flask was employed. Alternatively, the flask was wrapped up with aluminum foil.

† CH_2Cl_2 was dried by refluxing with P_2O_5 followed by distillation.

Benzyl 3,4-Dideoxy-α-D-*Glycero*-Hex-3-Enopyranosid-2-Ulose (4)

Glycal **3** (3.5 g, 0.0106 mol) was dried in vacuum and dissolved in anhydrous CH_2Cl_2 (40 mL) in a 100 mL round bottom flask. The solution was cooled to approximately −10°C with NaCl–ice bath and benzyl alcohol (2.5 mL, 0.024 mol) was added. The cooled solution (−10°C) was magnetically stirred and $SnCl_4$ (1.5 mL, 0.0125 mol) was slowly added while the temperature was kept at −10°C. The mixture was stirred, keeping the temperature between −5°C and 0°C, for 1.5 h.* Monitoring by TLC (2:1 hexane–EtOAc) showed a main spot of R_f 0.50, higher moving than the starting **3** (R_f 0.27). The reaction mixture was diluted with CH_2Cl_2 (20 mL) and poured into satd aq $NaHCO_3$ (20 mL) in a separatory funnel. The mixture was vigorously shaken and the operation was repeated three times for the complete removal of $SnCl_4$. The organic extract was washed with satd aq NaCl (2 × 20 mL), dried (Na_2SO_4) and concentrated. The residue was purified through a silica gel column, which was eluted with 10:1 hexane–EtOAc (~150 mL) and then 9:1→4:1 hexane–EtOAc, to afford pale yellow, syrupy enone **4**. Yield, 2.5–2.7 g (85%–92%); $[\alpha]_D$ +34.1 (*c* 1, $CHCl_3$). ^1H NMR ($CDCl_3$, 500 MHz) δ: 7.35 (br s, 5H, H-aromatic), 6.94 (dd, 1H, $J_{4,5}$ 1.8, $J_{3,4}$ 10.6 Hz, H-4), 6.18 (dd, $J_{3,4}$ 10.6, $J_{3,5}$ 2.7 Hz, H-3), 4.99 (br s, 1H, H-1), 4.82, 4.74 (2 d, 1 H each, *J* 12.1 Hz, PhCH_2), 4.70 (m, 1H, $J_{3,5}$ 2.7, $J_{4,5}$ 1.8, $J_{5,6}$ 5.4, $J_{5,6'}$ 4.4 Hz, H-5), 4.34 (dd, 1H, $J_{5,6}$ 5.5, $J_{6,6'}$ 11.7 Hz, H-6), 4.22 (dd, 1H, $J_{5,6'}$ 4.4, $J_{6,6'}$ 11.7 Hz, H-6'), 2.10 (s, 3H, CH_3CO); ^{13}C NMR ($CDCl_3$, 125.7 MHz) δ: 188.1 (C-2), 170.6 (CH_3*C*O), 147.0 (C-4), 136.5, 128.5, 128.1 (C-aromatic), 126.3 (C-3), 96.9 (C-1), 71.1 (Ph*C*H$_2$O), 66.9 (C-5), 64.5 (C-6), 20.7 (*C*H$_3$CO).

ACKNOWLEDGMENTS

Support of this chapter by the University of Buenos Aires (Project X227), the National Research Council of Argentina (CONICET, Project PIP 2008-0064), and the National Agency for Promotion of Science and Technology (ANPCyT, PICT 2007-00291) is gratefully acknowledged. O.V. and M.L.U. are Research Members from CONICET, V.E.M. and E.R. are Research Fellows from CONICET.

    The checking process was partially supported by the VEGA 2/0199/09 and CE Glycomed Grants.

---

* The temperature should not be allowed to rise, as higher temperature favors formation of 5-acetoxy-methyl-2-furaldehyde (R_f 0.38) as by-product.

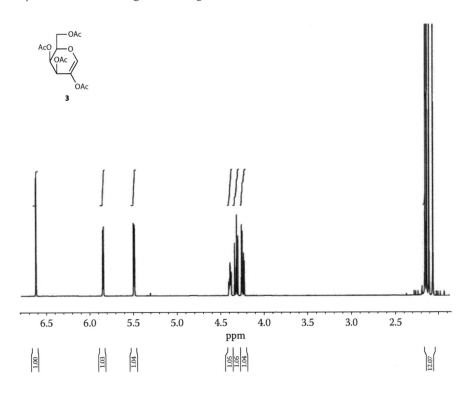

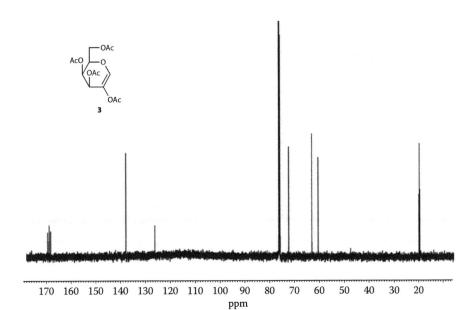

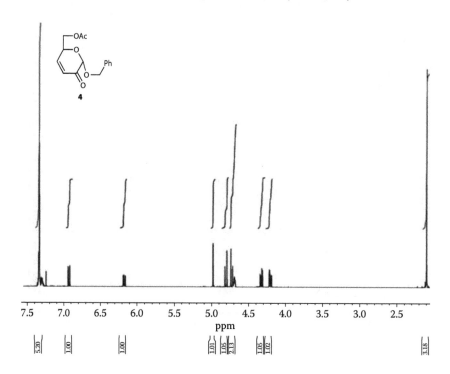

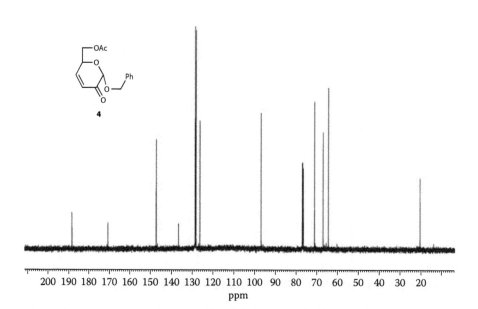

REFERENCES

1. Xavier, N. M.; Reuter, A. P. *Carbohydr. Res.* 2008, *343*, 1523–1539.
2. (a) Ferrier, R. J.; Hoberg, J. O. *Adv. Carbohydr. Chem. Biochem.* 2003, *58*, 55–119; (b) Lichtenthaler, F. W. *Acc. Chem. Res.* 2002, *35*, 728–737; (c) Fraser-Reid, B. *Acc. Chem. Res.* 1996, *29*, 57–66; (d) Lichtenthaler, F. W. In *Natural Product Synthesis*; Atta-ur-Rahman, ed., Springer: New York, 1986, p. 227; (e) Trost, B. M.; King, S. A.; Schmidt, T. *J. Am. Chem. Soc.* 1989, *111*, 5902–5915; (f) Holder, N. L. *Chem. Rev.* 1982, *82*, 287–332.
3. (a) Horton, D.; Roski, J. P.; Norris, P. *J. Org. Chem.* 1996, *61*, 3783–3793; (b) Horton, D.; Roski, J. P. *J. Chem. Soc. Chem. Commun.* 1992, *10*, 759–760; (c) Bhaté, P.; Horton, D. *Carbohydr. Res.* 1983, *122*, 189–199; (d) Ward, D. D.; Shafizadeh, F. *Carbohydr. Res.* 1981, *95*, 155–176.
4. (a) Witczak, Z. J.; Sun, J.; Mielguj, R. *Bioorg. Med. Chem. Soc.* 1995, *5*, 2169–2174; (b) Becker, B.; Thimm, J.; Thiem, J. 1996, *15*, 1179–1181; (c) Witczak, Z. J.; Chhabra, R.; Chen, H.; Xie, X.-Q. *Carbohydr. Res.* 1997, *301*, 167–175; (d) Witczak, Z. J.; Chen, H.; Kaplon, P. *Tetrahedron: Asymm.* 2000, *11*, 519–532; (e) Witczak, Z. J.; Kaplon, P.; Dey, P. M. *Carbohydr. Res.* 2003, *338*, 11–18.
5. De Fina, G. M.; Varela, O.; Lederkremer, R. M. *Synthesis* 1988, 891–893.
6. Iriarte Capaccio, C. A.; Varela, O. *J. Org. Chem.* 2001, *66*, 8859–8866.
7. Iriarte Capaccio, C. A.; Varela, O. *J. Org. Chem.* 2002, *67*, 7839–7846.
8. Iriarte Capaccio, C. A.; Varela, O. *Tetrahedron Lett.* 2003, *44*, 4023–4026.
9. Iriarte Capaccio, C. A.; Varela, O. *Carbohydr. Res.* 2004, *339*, 1207–1213.
10. Iriarte Capaccio, C. A.; Varela, O. *Tetrahedron: Asymm.* 2004, *15*, 3023–3028.
11. Uhrig, M. L.; Varela, O. *Aust. J. Chem.* 2002, *55*, 155–160.
12. Uhrig, M. L.; Varela, O. *Carbohydr. Res.* 2002, *337*, 2069–2076.
13. Uhrig, M. L.; Manzano, V. E.; Varela, O. *Eur. J. Org. Chem.* 2006, *13*, 162–168.
14. Cagnoni, A. J.; Uhrig, M. L.; Varela, O. *Bioorg. Med. Chem.* 2009, *17*, 6203–6212.
15. Repetto, E.; Marino, C.; Uhrig, M. L.; Varela, O. *Eur. J. Org. Chem.* 2008, *3*, 540–547.
16. Repetto, E.; Marino, C.; Uhrig, M. L.; Varela, O. *Bioorg. Med. Chem.* 2009, *17*, 2703–2711.
17. Uhrig, M. L.; Szilágyi, L.; Kövér, K. E.; Varela, O. *Carbohydr. Res.* 2007, *342*, 1841–1849.
18. Manzano, V. E.; Uhrig, M. L.; Varela, O. *J. Org. Chem.* 2008, *73*, 7224–7235.
19. Zunszain, P. A.; Varela, O. *Tetrahedron: Asymm.* 1998, *9*, 1269–1276.
20. Iriarte Capaccio, C. A.; Varela, O. *Tetrahedron: Asymm.* 2000, *11*, 4945–4954.
21. (a) Herscovici, J.; Muleka, K.; Boumaiza, L.; Antonakis, K.; *J. Chem. Soc. Perkin Trans. 1* 1990, 1995–2009; (b) Ferrier, R. J. *Top. Curr. Chem.* 2001, *215*, 153–175; (c) Toshima, K.; Tatsuta, K. *Chem. Rev.* 1993, *93*, 1503–1531.
22. (a) Maurer, M. *Ber.* 1930, *63*, 2069–2073; (b) Blair, M. G. *Adv. Carbohydr. Chem.* 1954, *9*, 97–129.
23. Zhang, Y.; Jia, J.; Pang, L.-N.; Wang, J.-W. *Acta Cryst. E* 2007, *63*, o4321.

36 Efficient Synthesis of Methyl(Allyl 4-O-Acyl-2,3-Di-O-Benzyl-β-D-Galactopyranosid) uronates from D-Galacturonic Acid[‡]

Alice Voss, Navid Nemati, Hmayak Poghosyan, Hans-Ulrich Endress, Andreas Krause,[†] and Christian Vogel[*]

CONTENTS

Experimental Methods 306
   General Methods 306
      1,2,3,4-Tetra-O-Acetyl-α-D-Galactopyranuronic Acid (**11**)........................307
      Methyl 1,2,3,4-Tetra-O-Acetyl-α-D-Galactopyranuronate (**12**) 308
      Methyl 2,3,4-Tri-O-Acetyl-α-D-Galactopyranosyluronate Bromide (**13**)....308
      Methyl (Allyl 2,3,4-Tri-O-Acetyl-β-D-Galactopyranosid)uronate (**14**).......308
      Methyl (Allyl β-D-Galactopyranosid)uronate (**19**).....................................309
      Regioselective Ring Opening in Orthoester Structures **20** and **21** 309
      Methyl (Allyl 4-O-Acetyl-β-D-Galactopyranosid)uronate (**22**) 309
      Methyl (Allyl 4-O-Benzoyl-β-D-Galactopyranosid)uronate (**23**).................310
      Benzylation of Compounds **22** and **23** 310
      Methyl (Allyl 4-O-Acetyl-2,3-Di-O-Benzyl-β-D-Galactopyranosid)
      uronate (**1**) 310

[‡] Presented at *13th European Carbohydrate Symposium*, Bratislava, Slovakia, August, 2005 as Part XVI of the series "Galacturonic Acid Derivatives," for Part XV, see Ref. [5].

[*] Corresponding author.

[†] Checker.

Methyl (Allyl 4-*O*-Benzoyl-2,3-Di-*O*-Benzyl-β-D-Galactopyranosid)
uronate (**2**) 310
Methyl (Allyl 2,3-Di-*O*-Benzyl-β-D-Galactopyranosid)uronate (**5**) 311
References 326

Blockwise buildup of homogalacturonan and rhamnogalacturonan fragments by modular design principle is based on an orthogonal protecting group strategy.[1] Following the present methodology, glycosyl acceptors and donors derived from D-galacturonic acid could be synthesized from monosaccharide modules **1** and **2** (Scheme 36.1) in one and two steps, respectively. Accordingly, deacylation of **1** or **2** with 0.28 M methanolic HCl provided acceptor **5** (90%) having only HO-4 unsubstituted. On the other hand, modules **1** and **2** were deallylated and transformed into α-trichloroacetimidates **3** and **4**, respectively. Trimethylsilyl trifluoromethanesulfonate-mediated glycosylation of the galacturonate acceptor **5** with donor **3** or **4** furnished the corresponding α-linked disaccharides **6** and **7** in 60% and 70% yield, respectively.[2,3] In this strategy, the benzyl group plays an important role as permanent, arming, and nonparticipating protecting group.

For the preparation of disaccharide module **9**, the 4-*O*-benzoyl rhamnose acetate **8** was employed as glycosyl donor, and coupled with the galacturonate acceptor **5** (Scheme 36.1).[4] The analogous disaccharide glycosyl acceptor and glycosyl donor were prepared in a similar way from module **9** either by selective deacetylation at O-2′ or by deallylation and trichloroacetimidation.[5]

We have previously shown preparation of the key modules **1** and **2** directly from commercially available D-galacturonic acid (Scheme 36.2), thus avoiding the oxidation step, required when starting from D-galactose-derived intermediates.[3,6] That synthesis[3,6] started with tetra-*O*-acetyl-D-galactopyranuronic acid **11**, which was earlier reported by Tajima[7] and used by Steglich et al.,[8] but experimental details and characterization of **11** were not included. We have later reported preparation of **11** in 85% yield, and its full characterization.[9] Esterification of the latter was achieved with diazomethane to provide compound **12** in 95% yield. The Helferich glycosylation with bromide **13**, obtained (90%) by treatment of **12** with HBr in acetic acid, led to the allyl glycoside **14** (90%).[6] Enzyme-catalyzed, regioselective deacetylation at optimized conditions gave the 2-*O*-unprotected derivative **15** in 95% yield.[6,10] After acid catalyzed benzylation[6,11] (**16**, 62%), the deacetylation with methanolic 0.28 M HCl provided compound **17** in 90% yield. Since esters of galacturonic acid tend to undergo base-catalyzed β-elimination,[12] most protection and deprotection operations were performed under acidic conditions. One of the exceptions was the regioselective benzylation of **17** via a 3,4-*O*-butylstannyl intermediate,[13,14] which gave the desired glycosyl acceptor **5** in 58% yield, together with benzyl ester **18** (25%), which can also be used as acceptor in glycosylation reactions. Finally, the acylation with acetic anhydride or benzoyl chloride in pyridine provided both modules **1** and **2** in 95% yield.[2,3] In summary, starting from D-galacturonic acid, the desired compounds **1** and **2** were obtained in nine steps in about 18% overall yield.

Here, we report an improved synthesis of **1** and **2** (Scheme 36.3). Accordingly, deacetylation of **14** with 0.28 M methanolic HCl (90% yield)[6] followed by treatment of the product **19** with triethyl orthoacetate or triethyl orthobenzoate and

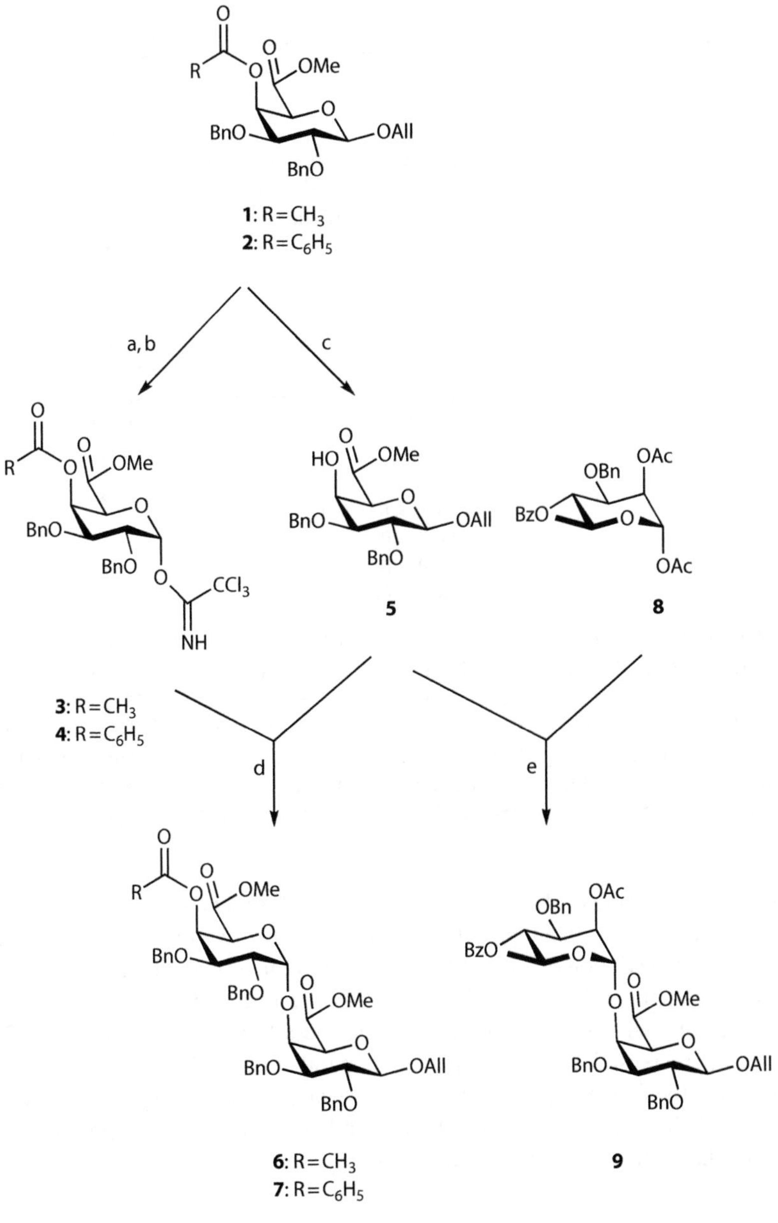

SCHEME 36.1 Reagents and conditions: (a) PdCl$_2$, NaOAc, AcOH–H$_2$O, 40°C–45°C, 4–6 h, (75%–85%); (b) Cl$_3$CCN, DBU, −20°C to 20°C, Ar atmosphere, 3 h, (70%–75%); (c) 0.28 M methanolic HCl, 20°C, Ar atmosphere, 12 h, (90%); (d) (H$_3$C)$_3$SiO$_3$SCF$_3$, CH$_2$Cl$_2$, MS 4 Å, −70°C to 20°C, Ar atmosphere, darkness, 24 h, (60%–70%); (e) (H$_3$C)$_3$SiO$_3$SCF$_3$, CH$_2$Cl$_2$, MS 4 Å, 20°C, Ar atmosphere, darkness, 24 h, (88%).

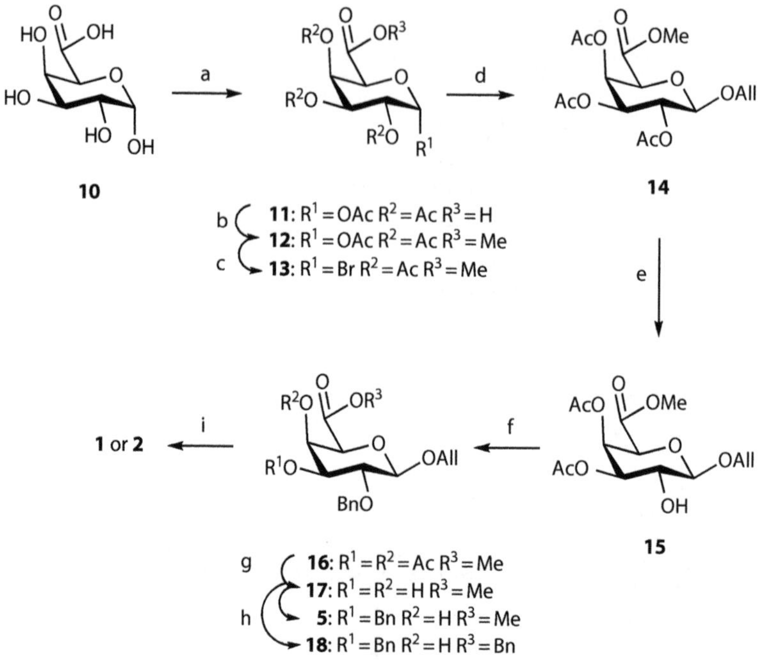

10 → a → **11**: R¹ = OAc R² = Ac R³ = H

10

b ⎰ **11**: R¹ = OAc R² = Ac R³ = H
  ⎱ **12**: R¹ = OAc R² = Ac R³ = Me
c ⤷ **13**: R¹ = Br R² = Ac R³ = Me

14

15

g ⎰ **16**: R¹ = R² = Ac R³ = Me
  ⎱ **17**: R¹ = R² = H R³ = Me
h ⤷ **5**: R¹ = Bn R² = H R³ = Me
  ⤷ **18**: R¹ = Bn R² = H R³ = Bn

1 or 2 ← i

SCHEME 36.2   Reagents and conditions: (a) cat. 70% HClO₄, Ac₂O, 5°C–20°C, 5 h, (85%); (b) ethereal CH₂N₂, CHCl₃, 20°C, 1 h, (95%); (c) HBr–AcOH, 0°C–20°C, 4 h, (90%); (d) Hg(CN)₂, HgBr₂, AllOH, MS 3 Å, 20°C, 12 h (90%); (e) KH₂PO₄–Na₂HPO₄, ethanol–water, Acylase I (from hog kidney), 25°C, 5 h (95%); (f) BnO(HN=)CCl₃, CH₂Cl₂–heptane, cat. F₃CSO₃H, 2 h, 20°C, (62%); (g) 0.28 M methanolic HCl, 20°C, Ar atmosphere, 12 h, (90%); (h) 1. n-Bu₂SnO, toluene, reflux on Dean-Stark apparatus, 2 h, 2. n-Bu₄NBr, BnBr, 60°C–85°C, 4 h, compound **5** (58%) and compound **18** (25%); (i) Ac₂O or PhCOCl, pyridine, –20°C to 20°C, Ar atmosphere 5 h, (90%).

regioselective opening of the orthoester structures[14,15] in **20** and **21**, thus formed, led to the 4-O-acetyl and 4-O-benzoyl derivatives **22** and **23** in 65% and 80% yields, respectively. Benzylation of **22** and **23** according to Madsen and Lauritsen[16] gave the monosaccharide modules **1** and **2** (75% and 70%, respectively).

Thus, compared to the former pathway, the overall yield of modules **1** and **2** was significantly increased (nearly 30%), the total number of synthetic steps was reduced to seven, and the formation of benzyl ester as a side product of one of the conversions was avoided. In addition, every synthetic step lead to a crystalline product, which makes the laboratory work more convenient.

EXPERIMENTAL METHODS

GENERAL METHODS

Melting points were determined with a Boetius micro-heating plate BHMK 05 (Rapido, Dresden) and were not corrected. Optical rotation was measured with an automatic polarimeter GYROMAT (Dr. Kernchen Co.). ¹H NMR Spectra (250.13

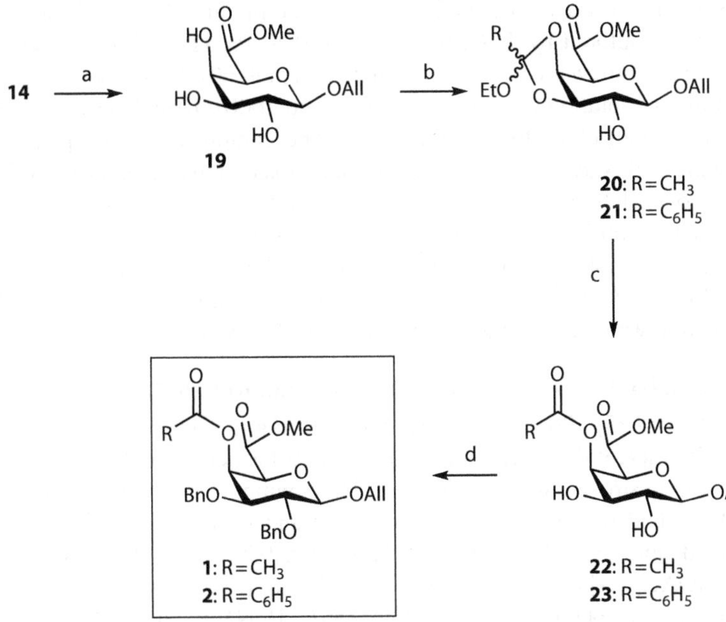

SCHEME 36.3 Reagents and conditions: (a) 0.28 M methanolic HCl, 20°C, 24 h, (90%); (b) $H_3C(OEt)_3$ or $C_6H_5C(OEt)_3$, cat. camphersulfonic acid, CH_2Cl_2, 20°C, Ar atmosphere, 100 min; (c) aq 95% AcOH, 20°C, 10 min, compound **22** (65%) and compound **23** (80%); (d) BnO(HN=)CCl_3, dioxane, F_3CSO_3H, 15–30 min, 0°C, compound **1** (75%) and compound **2** (70%).

and 500.13 MHz) and ^{13}C NMR spectra (62.9 and 125.8 MHz) were recorded with Bruker instruments AV 250 and AV 500, respectively. The chemical shifts are reported relative to solvent signals ($CDCl_3$: δ $^1H = 7.25$, δ $^{13}C = 77.0$; DMSO-d_6: δ $^1H = 2.50$, δ $^{13}C = 39.7$). ^1H and ^{13}C NMR signals were assigned by DEPT, two-dimensional $^1H,^1H$ COSY and NOESY and $^1H,^{13}C$ correlation spectra (HMBC and HSQC). Elemental analysis was performed with a CHNS-Flash-EA-1112 instrument (Thermoquest). Washing solutions were cooled to ∼5°C. The $NaHCO_3$ solution was saturated. Reactions were monitored by thin-layer chromatography (TLC, Silica Gel 60, F_{254}, Merck KGaA). The following solvent systems (v/v) were used: (A) 4:2:2:1 toluene–EtOH–EtOAc–AcOH, (B) 1:2 toluene–EtOAc, (C) 1:1 toluene–EtOAc, (D) 2:1 toluene–EtOAc, (E) 1:2 heptane–EtOAc, (F) 1:1 heptane–EtOAc, (G) 2:1 heptane–EtOAc, (H) 10:1 $CHCl_3$–MeOH, (I) 8:1 EtOAc–MeOH. The spots were visualized by charring with ethanolic 10% H_2SO_4. Flash chromatography was performed by elution from columns of slurry-packed Silica Gel 60 (Merck, 63–200 μm). All solvents and reagents were purified and dried according to standard procedures.[17] Solutions in organic solvents were dried over $MgSO_4$ and concentrated under reduced pressure (rotary evaporator).

1,2,3,4-Tetra-*O*-Acetyl-α-D-Galactopyranuronic Acid (11)[9]

To a stirred solution of 70% perchloric acid (1.5 mL) and acetic anhydride (250 mL), D-galacturonic acid monohydrate **10** (40.32 g, 190 mmol) was added in small portions at 5°C. Stirring was continued for 30 min with cooling and then for 3 h at ambient temperature (monitored by TLC, solvent A; R_f 0.40 for **11**) until one product was formed. The mixture was cooled to 0°C, and methanol (60 mL) was added dropwise. After 30 min, the solution was poured into ice/water (600 mL) and the aqueous phase was extracted with chloroform (3 × 100 mL). The combined organic phases were washed with iced water (3 × 25 mL), dried, and concentrated. Heptane (15–20 mL) was added to a solution of the crude material in EtOAc (100 mL) and the precipitate was collected. A similar precipitation procedure was repeated with the mother liquor (3–4 times) and crystallization from ether gave **11** (58.5 g, 85%); mp 162°C–164°C (from diethyl ether); $[\alpha]_D^{21} = +125$ (c 1.0, chloroform). Melting point and the value of optical rotation were identical with the data in lit.[9] For NMR data, see lit.[9]

Methyl 1,2,3,4-Tetra-*O*-Acetyl-α-D-Galactopyranuronate (12)[6]

Compound **11** (7.25 g, 20.0 mmol) was dissolved in a minimum of chloroform and treated with ethereal diazomethane until yellow color persisted. The excess diazomethane was destroyed with acetic acid. The solution was diluted with heptane (200 mL), washed with aq $NaHCO_3$ (2 × 60 mL) and iced water (2 × 60 mL), dried, concentrated; and crystallization gave **12** (7.15 g, 95%); mp 138°C–140°C (from heptane–EtOAc); $[\alpha]_D^{23} = +159.9$ (c 1.0, chloroform); (R_f 0.35, solvent D); lit.,[18] mp 141°C–142°C; $[\alpha]_D = +136.8$ (c 1.0, chloroform); ¹H NMR (300.13 MHz, $CDCl_3$): δ 6.50 (d, 1H, $^3J_{1,2} = 2.5$ Hz, H-1), 5.80 (m, 1H, $^3J_{4,5} = 1.5$ Hz, H-4), 5.37 (m, 2H, $^3J_{3,4} = 1.1$ Hz, H-3, H-2), 4.73 (d, 1H, H-5), 3.73 (s, 3H, OCH_3), 2.13, 2.10, 2.00 (3s, 12H, $OCOCH_3$, one signal is isochronic); ¹³C NMR (75.5 MHz $CDCl_3$): δ 170.00, 169.66, 168.43, 166.52 (4 × $OCOCH_3$, C-6, one signal is isochronic), 89.54 (C-1), 70.72 (C-5), 68.58 (C-4), 66.96 (C-2), 65.96 (C-3), 51.82 (OCH_3), 20.75, 20.57, 20.47, 20.44 (4 × $OCOCH_3$). Anal. Calcd for $C_{15}H_{20}O_{11}$ (376.31): C, 47.88; H, 5.36. Found: C, 47.64; H, 5.18.

Methyl 2,3,4-Tri-*O*-Acetyl-α-D-Galactopyranosyluronate Bromide (13)[6]

To a stirred solution of tetraacetate **12** (18.37 g, 48.8 mmol), acetic anhydride (6 mL), acetic acid (23.5 mL), and acetyl bromide (32.8 mL, 439.2 mmol) in dry chloroform (49 mL) was added, dropwise at 0°C, a solution of water (7.74 mL, 430 mmol) in acetic acid (26.5 mL). After 15 min, the cooling was removed, and the mixture was stirred for 3 h at ambient temperature (monitored by TLC for absence of **12**, solvent D; R_f 0.35 for **12**; R_f 0.49 for **13**). The solution was poured into iced water (600 mL), the aqueous layer was extracted with chloroform (3 × 150 mL), the combined organic phase was washed successively with iced water (300 mL), cold aq $NaHCO_3$ (2 × 300 mL), iced water (2 × 300 mL), dried, and concentrated, to give **13** (17.4 g, 90%), which was sufficiently pure (NMR) to be used in the next step without further purification. Crystallization gave an analytical sample, mp 128°C–130°C (from dry diethyl ether); $[\alpha]_D^{20} = +240$ (c 1.0, chloroform); lit.[18] mp 130°C, $[\alpha]_D = +242$ (c 1.0, chloroform).

Methyl (Allyl 2,3,4-Tri-*O*-Acetyl-β-D-Galactopyranosid)uronate (14)[6]

A suspension of bromide **13** (18.5 g, 46.6 mmol), mercuric cyanide (5.88 g, 23.3 mmol), mercuric bromide (865 mg, 2.4 mmol), and molecular sieves (3A, 5.0 g) in dry allyl alcohol (100 mL) was stirred overnight at ambient temperature (monitored by TLC for absence of **13**, solvent C; R_f 0.60 for **13**; R_f 0.62 for **14**). The mixture was concentrated, diluted with chloroform (200 mL), and filtered. The filtrate was washed with aq 10% potassium bromide (3 × 50 mL) and water (2 × 50 mL), dried, concentrated; and crystallization gave **14** (13.7 g, 90%); mp 98°C–99°C (from EtOAc–heptane); $[\alpha]_D^{20} = 0$ (c 1.0, chloroform). The physical and NMR data of **14** were fully consistent with those of the product obtained by an alternative synthetic route.[19]

Methyl (Allyl β-D-Galactopyranosid)uronate (19)[6]

To methanolic 0.28 M hydrochloric acid (prepared by adding acetyl chloride [7.3 mL] to ice-cold dry methanol [360 mL]) was added compound **14** (3.74 g, 10 mmol) with stirring and the mixture kept for 24 h at ambient temperature (monitored for absence of **14** by TLC, solvent C; R_f 0.62 for **14**; monitored for presence of **19** by TLC in solvent I; R_f 0.30 for **19**). For neutralization, $PbCO_3 \times Pb(OH)_2$ (30 g) was added, and the reaction mixture was stirred for 2 h at ambient temperature. The salts were then centrifuged off, washed with methanol, the combined supernatants were subjected to another centrifugation to remove salts that were carrier over, and concentrated. The residue was chromatographed (solvent H), to give **19** (2.22 g, 90%); mp 151°C–153°C (from MeOH–EtOAc); $[\alpha]_D^{22} = -62.9$ (c 1.0, acetone). The physical constants were identical with the data in lit.[6] For NMR data, see lit.[6]

Regioselective Ring Opening in Orthoester Structures 20 and 21

Triethyl orthoacetate (5 × 0.74 mL, 20.2 mmol) or triethyl orthobenzoate (5 × 1.0 mL, 20.2 mmol) and anhydrous camphorsulfonic acid (2 × 40 mg, 0.04 mmol) were added in portions, at room temperature under an inert atmosphere, to a stirred solution of compound **19** (1.0 g, 4.02 mmol) in dry CH_2Cl_2 (20 mL). After ~100 min (monitored for absence of **19** by TLC, solvent I; R_f 0.30 for **19**), the reaction was terminated by addition of triethylamine (1.0 mL), and the mixture was diluted with $CHCl_3$ (100 mL). The organic phase was washed with iced water, dried, and concentrated. The residue (**20** or **21**) was immediately dissolved in aq 95% acetic acid (10 mL), in order to inhibit the formation of the regioisomer at C-3 as by-product, and the solution was kept for 10 min at room temperature. After concentration, the residue was co-evaporated with toluene (4 × 25 mL) to remove traces of acetic acid. The crude products **22** and **23** were chromatographed with solvent B as eluent.

Methyl (Allyl 4-O-Acetyl-β-D-Galactopyranosid)uronate (22)

Yield, 757 mg (65%); mp 105°C–107°C (from hot EtOAc); $[\alpha]_D^{23} = +2.2$ (c 1.0, methanol); R_f 0.46 (solvent E); ¹H NMR (500.13 MHz, DMSO-d_6): δ 5.91 (m, 1H, CH₂CH=CH₂), 5.33, 5.15 (2m, 2H, CH₂CH=CH₂), 5.27 (d, 1H, H-4), 5.22 (d, 1H, H-2), 5.19 (d, 1H, H-3), 4.47 (d, 1H, H-5), 4.27 (d, 1H, ³$J_{1,2}$ = 7.8 Hz, H-1), 4.25, 4.05 (2m, 2H, CH₂CH=CH₂), 3.61 (m, 1H, OH-3), 3.59 (s, 3H, OCH₃), 3.25 (m, 1H, OH-2), 1.96 (s, 3H, OCOCH₃); ¹³C NMR (125.8 MHz, DMSO-d_6): δ 169.37 (OCOCH₃), 167.70 (C-6), 134.62 (CH₂CH=CH₂), 116.72 (CH₂CH=CH₂), 102.06 (C-1), 71.77

(C-5), 71.27 (C-4), 70.61 (C-2), 70.30 (C-3), 69.24 ($CH_2CH=CH_2$), 51.85 (OCH_3), 20.59 ($OCOCH_3$). Anal. Calcd for $C_{12}H_{18}O_8$ (290.27): C, 49.65; H, 6.25. Found: C, 49.54; H, 6.18.

Methyl (Allyl 4-O-Benzoyl-β-D-Galactopyranosid)uronate (23)

Yield, 1.13 g (80%); mp 88°C–90°C (from EtOAc–heptane); $[\alpha]_D^{23}$ –12.7 (c 1.0, methanol); R_f 0.40 (solvent E); ^{1}H NMR (250.13 MHz, DMSO-d_6): δ 8.00–7.46 (m, 5H, OCOC_6H_5), 5.93 (m, 1H, CH$_2$CH=CH$_2$), 5.54 (d, 1H, H-4), 5.45–5.27 (m, 3H, CH$_2$CH=CH_2, H-2, H-3), 5.17 (m, 1H, CH$_2$CH=CH_2), 4.62 (d, 1H, H-5), 4.37 (d, 1H, $^3J_{1,2}$=7.8 Hz, H-1), 4.30, 4.10 (2m, 2H, CH_2CH=CH$_2$), 3.75 (m, 1H, OH-3), 3.54 (s, 3H, OCH_3), 3.42 (m, 1H, OH-2); ^{13}C NMR (62.8 MHz, DMSO-d_6): δ 167.79 (OCH$_3$), 164.85 (C-6), 134.61 (CH$_2$CH=CH$_2$), 133.32, 129.64, 129.24, 128.67 (OCOC$_6H_5$, two signals are isochronic), 116.77 (CH$_2$CH=CH_2), 102.13 (C-1), 72.23 (C-5), 71.91 (C-4), 70.77 (C-2), 70.48 (C-3), 69.32 (CH$_2$CH=CH$_2$), 51.90 (OCH$_3$). Anal. Calcd for $C_{17}H_{20}O_8$ (352.34): C, 57.95; H, 5.72. Found: C, 57.75; H, 5.81.

Benzylation of Compounds 22 and 23

Freshly distilled benzyl 2,2,2-trichloroacetimidate (3.36 mL, 18.02 mmol) was added at 0°C to a solution of **22** or **23** (5.0 mmol) in freshly distilled dry dioxane (30 mL) under Ar atmosphere. The mixture was made strongly acidic by addition of trifluoromethanesulfonic acid (~0.30 mL). After stirring for 15–30 min (monitored for absence of **22** or **23** by TLC, solvent E; R_f 0.46 and 0.40, respectively), the reaction mixture was passed through a layer of alkaline alumina and concentrated. The residue was suspended in heptane–Et$_2$O (6:1 v/v, 100 mL), the carbohydrate-free precipitates were filtered off and washed with heptane–Et$_2$O (6:1 v/v, 50 mL). The filtrate and washings were combined, concentrated, and the crude products were chromatographed (solvent G) to give compounds **1** and **2** as colorless crystals.

Methyl (Allyl 4-O-Acetyl-2,3-Di-O-Benzyl-β-D-Galactopyranosid)uronate (1)

Yield, 1.05 g (75%); mp 136°C (from EtOAc–heptane); $[\alpha]_D^{23}$ =+35.8 (c 1.0, chloroform); R_f 0.45 (solvent G). The physical constants were identical with the data in lit.[2] For NMR data, see lit.[2]

Methyl (Allyl 4-O-Benzoyl-2,3-Di-O-Benzyl-β-D-Galactopyranosid)uronate (2)

Yield, 1.94 g (70%); mp 147°C (from EtOAc–heptane); $[\alpha]_D^{25}$ =+4.1 (c 1.0, chloroform); R_f 0.56 (solvent G). ^{1}H NMR (250.13 MHz, CDCl$_3$): δ 3.69 (s, 3H, OCH$_3$), 3.65–3.78 (m, 2H, $^3J_{3,4}$=3.7 Hz, $^3J_{2,3}$=9.5 Hz, H-2, H-3), 4.19, 4.51 (2m, 2H, CH_2CH=CH$_2$), 4.24 (d, 1H, H-5), 4.50 (d, 1H, $^3J_{1,2}$=7.6 Hz, H-1), 4.58, 4.71, 4.83, 4.89 (4d, 4H, ^2J=10.9 Hz, ^2J=11.6 Hz, 2×CH_2C$_6H_5$), 5.22, 5.35 (2m, 2H, CH$_2$CH=CH_2), 5.97 (m, 1H, CH$_2$CH=CH$_2$) 6.01 (dd, 1H, $^3J_{4,5}$=1.2 Hz, H-4), 7.20–8.10 (m, 15H, 2×CH$_2$C$_6H_5$, OCC$_6H_5$); ^{13}C NMR (62.8 MHz, CDCl$_3$): δ 52.63 (OCH$_3$), 68.32 (C-4), 70.73, 72.14 (2×CH$_2$C$_6H_5$), 72.81 (C-5), 75.46 (CH$_2$CH=CH$_2$), 78.36 (C-2), 78.75 (C-3), 102.53 (C-1), 117.75 (CH$_2$CH=CH_2), 127.64, 127.68, 128.02, 128.15, 128.25,

128.29, 128.37, 129.43, 129.94, 130.11, 137.60, 138.37, 147.79, 147.87 ($2 \times CH_2C_6H_5$, OCC_6H_5, four signals are isochronic), 133.25 ($CH_2CH{=}CH_2$), 165.52 (OCC_6H_5) 167.35 (C-6). Anal. Calcd for $C_{31}H_{32}O_8$ (532.58): C, 69.91; H, 6.06. Found: C, 69.82; H, 6.01.

Methyl (Allyl 2,3-Di-*O*-Benzyl-β-ᴅ-Galactopyranosid)uronate (5)

Compound **1** (480 mg, 1.0 mmol) was added with stirring to methanolic 0.28 ᴍ hydrochloric acid (prepared by adding of acetyl chloride [2 mL] to ice-cold dry methanol [100 mL]) and the mixture was stirred at ambient temperature for 24 h under Ar atmosphere (monitored for absence of **1** by TLC, solvent G; R_f 0.45 for **1**). The solution was filtered through a layer of alkaline alumina by elution with $CHCl_3$. The combined eluates (ca. 400 mL) were dried, concentrated, and the crude product was chromatographed (solvent F) to provide acceptor **5** (430 mg, 90%); mp 111°C (from EtOAc–heptane); $[\alpha]_D^{22} = -4.7$ (c 1.0, chloroform); R_f 0.50 (F). The physical constants were identical with the data in lit.[6] For NMR data, see lit.[6]

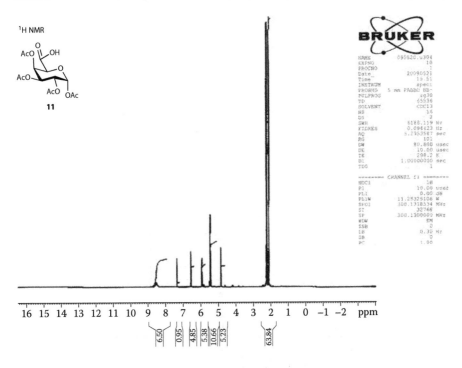

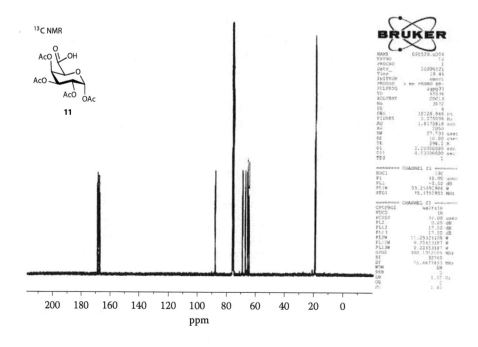

^{13}C NMR

11

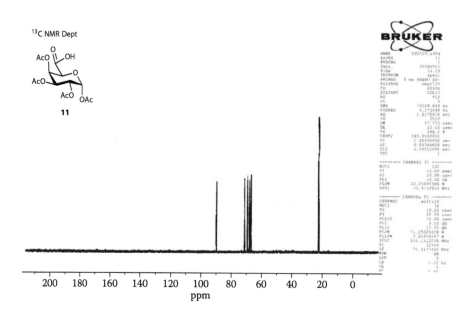

^{13}C NMR Dept

11

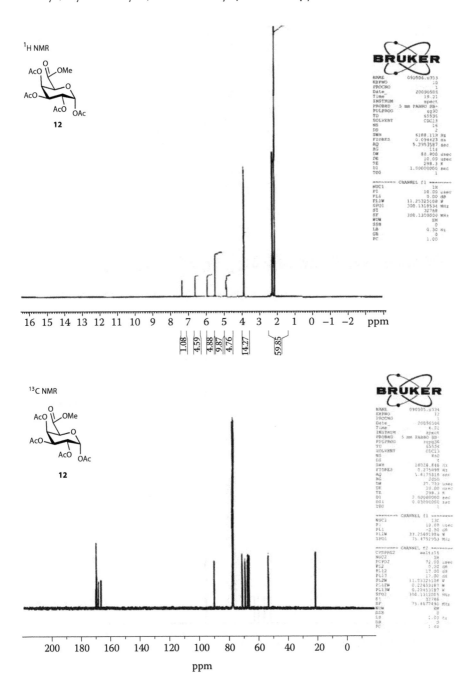

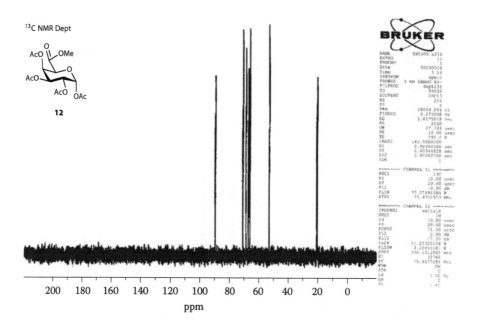

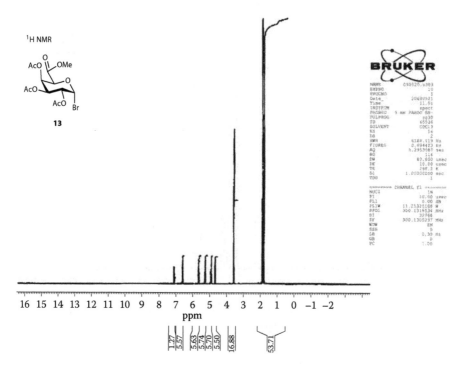

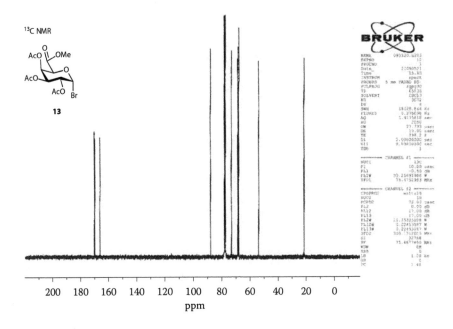

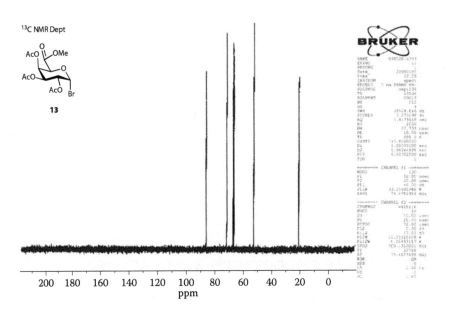

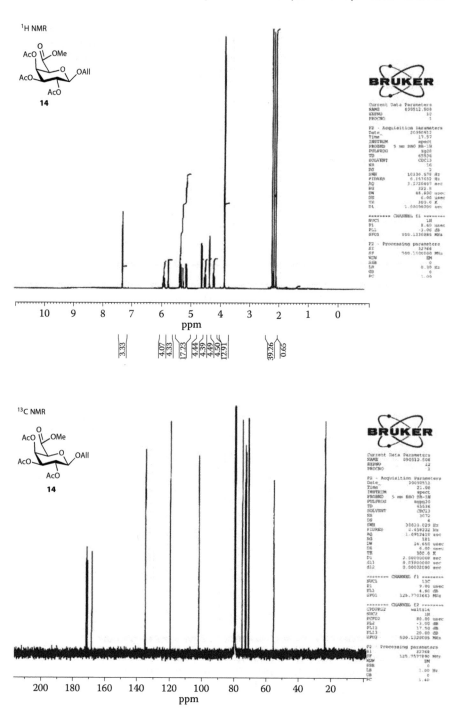

¹H NMR

14

¹³C NMR

14

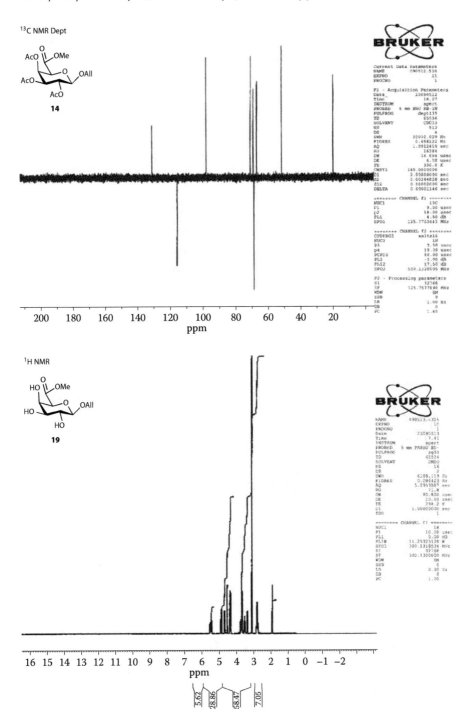

¹³C NMR Dept

14

¹H NMR

19

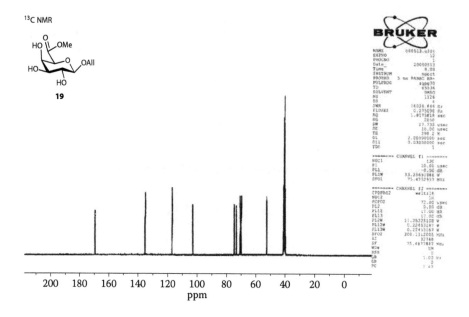

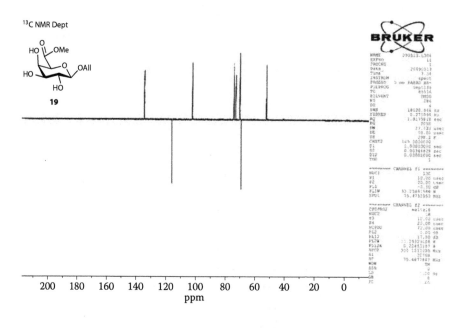

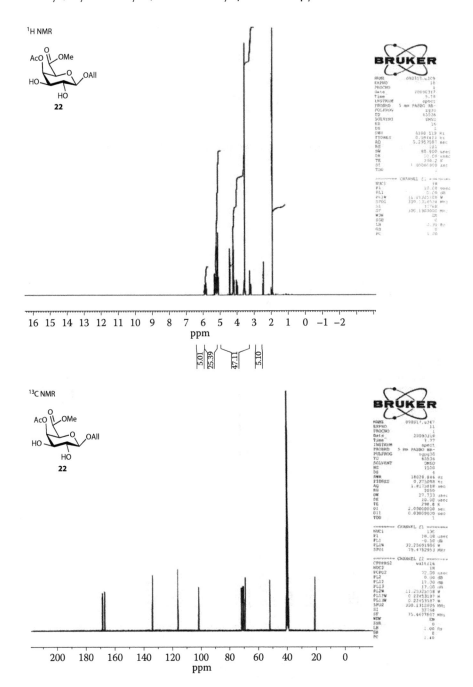

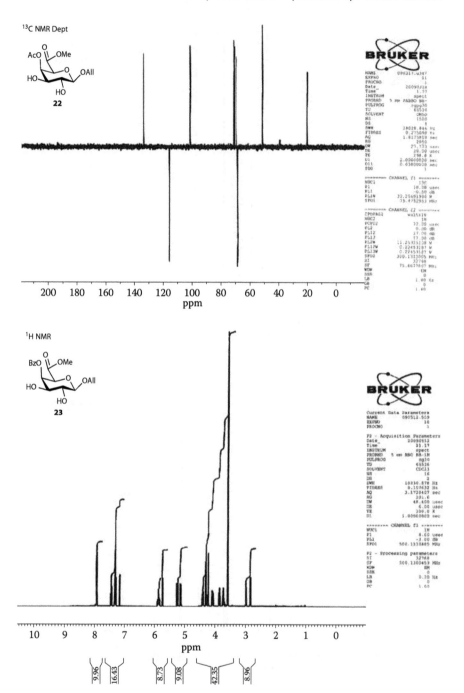

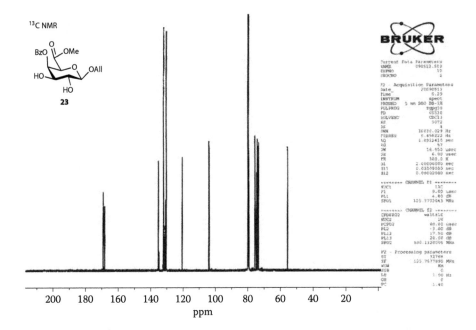

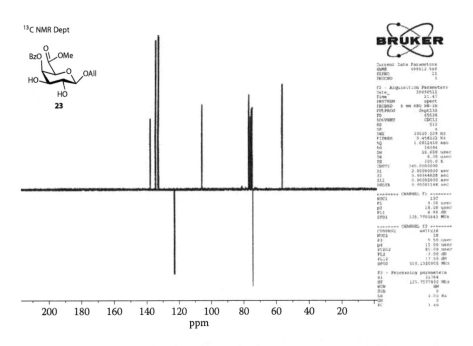

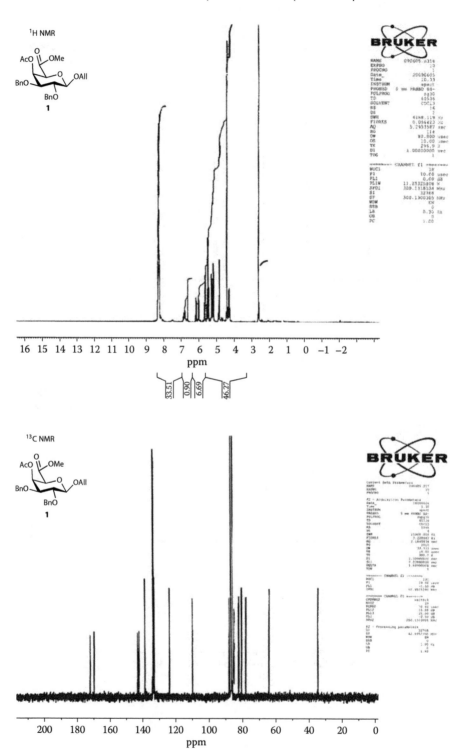

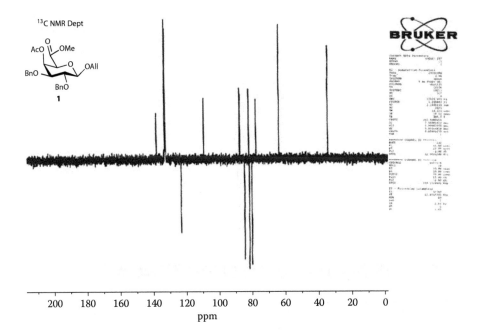

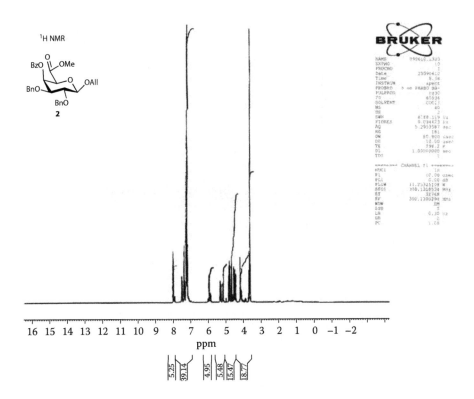

324

324

Carbohydrate Chemistry: Proven Synthetic Methods

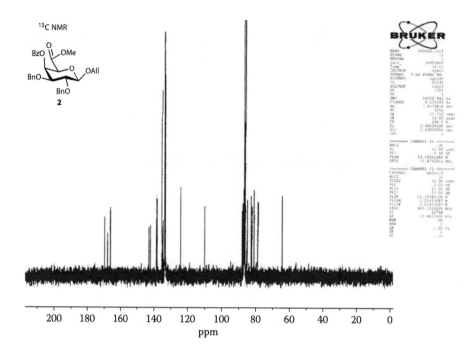

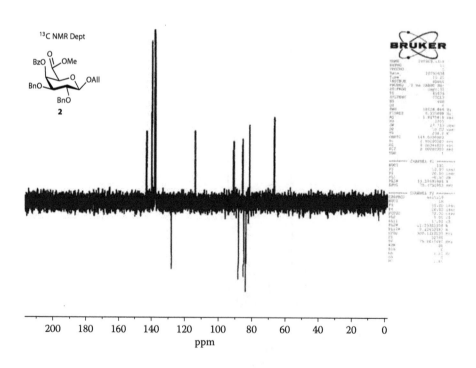

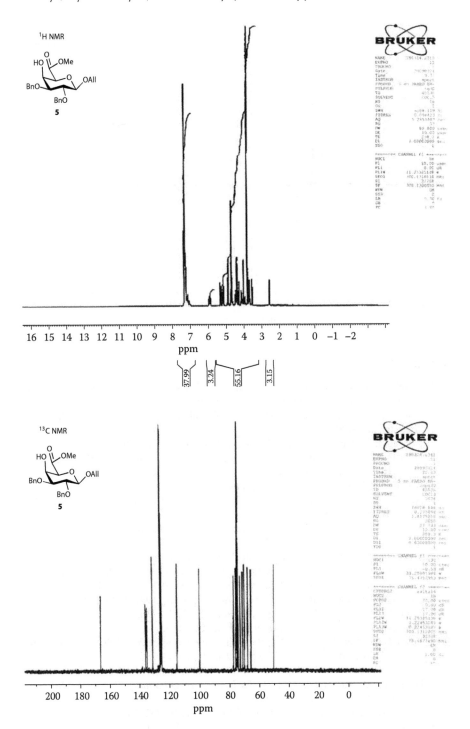

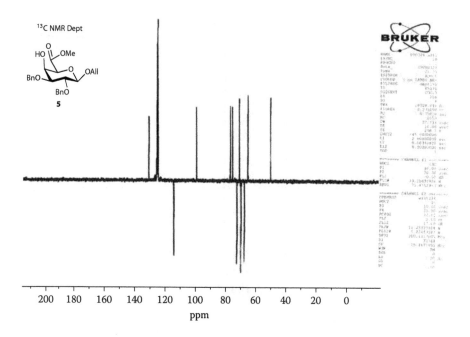

REFERENCES

1. Vogel, C.; Nolting. B.; Kramer, S.; Steffan, W.; Ott, A.-J. Synthesis of pectin fragments by modular design principle. In *Advances in Pectin and Pectinase Research*; Voragen, F., Schols, H., Visser, R., Eds.; Kluwer Academic Publishers: Dordrecht, the Netherlands, 2003; pp. 209–220.
2. Nolting, B.; Boye, H.; Vogel, C. *J. Carbohydr. Chem.* 2001, *20*, 585–610.
3. Nemati, N. Synthesis of ramified rhamnogalacturonan I fragments. PhD dissertation, University of Rostock, Rostock, 2007.
4. Nolting, B.; Boye, H.; Vogel, C. *J. Carbohydr. Chem.* 2000, *19*, 923–938.
5. Nemati, N.; Karapetyan, G.; Nolting, B.; Endress, H.-U.; Vogel, C. *Carbohydr. Res.* 2008, *343*, 1730–1742.
6. Kramer, S.; Nolting, B.; Ott, A.-J.; Vogel, C. *J. Carbohydr. Chem.* 2000, *19*, 891–921.
7. Tajima, K. *Chem. Lett.* 1985, 49–52.
8. Wild, H.; Mohrs, K.; Niewöhner, U.; Steglich, W. *Liebigs Ann. Chem.* 1986, 1548–1567.
9. Vogel, C.; Jeschke, U.; Kramer, S.; Ott, A.-J. *Liebigs Ann./Recueil* 1997, 737–743.
10. Vogel, C.; Kramer, S.; Ott, A.-J. *Liebigs Ann./Recueil* 1997, 1425–1428.
11. Iversen, T.; Bundle, D. R. *J. Chem. Soc. Chem. Commun.* 1981, 1240–1241.
12. Heim, P.; Neukom, H. *Helv. Chim. Acta* 1962, *45*, 1737–1738.
13. David, S.; Hanessian, S. *Tetrahedron* 1985, *41*, 643–663.
14. Vogel, C.; Steffan, W.; Ott, A. Ya.; Betaneli, V. I. *Carbohydr. Res.* 1992, *237*, 115–129.
15. King, J. F.; Allbutt, A. D. *Can. J. Chem.* 1970, *48*, 1754–1769.
16. Madsen, R.; Lauritsen, A. *Org. Biomol. Chem.* 2006, *4*, 2898–2905.
17. Perrin, D. D.; Armarego, W. L. F. *Purification of Laboratory Chemicals*, 3rd edn.; Pergamon Press: Oxford, U.K., 1988.
18. Pippen, E. L., McCready, R. M. *J. Org. Chem.* 1951, *16*, 262–268.
19. Steffan, W.; Vogel, C.; Kristen, H. *Carbohydr. Res.* 1990, *204*, 109–120.

37 Methyl(Ethyl 2,3,5-Tri-O-Benzoyl-1-Thio-α,β-D-Galactofuranosid) uronate

Ambar K. Choudhury, Dirk Michalik, Andreas Gottwald,[†] and Nirmolendu Roy*

CONTENTS

Experimental Methods 329
   General Methods 329
     tert-Butyl 1,2:3,4-Di-*O*-Isopropylidene-α-D-Galactopyranuronate (**2**) 330
     Methyl (Methyl α,β-D-Galactofuranosid)uronate (**3**) 330
     Methyl (Methyl α-D-Galactofuranosid)uronate (**3α**) 330
     Methyl (Methyl β-D-Galactofuranosid)uronate (**3β**) 330
     Methyl (Methyl 2,3,5-Tri-*O*-Benzoyl-α,β-D-Galactofuranosid)uronate (**4**) 330
     Methyl (Methyl 2,3,5-Tri-*O*-Benzoyl-α-D-Galactofuranosid)uronate (**4α**) ... 331
     Methyl (Methyl 2,3,5-Tri-*O*-Benzoyl-β-D-Galactofuranosid)uronate (**4β**) ... 331
     Methyl 1-*O*-Acetyl-2,3,5-Tri-*O*-Benzoyl-α,β-D-Galactofuranuronate (**5**) ... 331
     Methyl 1-*O*-Acetyl-2,3,5-Tri-*O*-Benzoyl-α-D-Galactofuranuronate (**5α**) ... 331
     Methyl 1-*O*-Acetyl-2,3,5-Tri-*O*-Benzoyl-β-D-Galactofuranuronate (**5β**) 332
     Methyl (Ethyl 2,3,5-Tri-*O*-Benzoyl-1-Thio-α,β-D-Galactofuranosid)
     uronate (**6**) 332
     Methyl (Ethyl 2,3,5-Tri-*O*-Benzoyl-1-Thio-α-D-Galactofuranosid)
     uronate (**6α**) 332
     Methyl (Ethyl 2,3,5-Tri-*O*-Benzoyl-1-Thio-β-D-Galactofuranosid)
     uronate (**6β**) 332
References 339

---

* Corresponding author.
† Checker.

(a) Pyr, CrO_3, CH_2Cl_2, DMF, t-BuOH-Ac_2O, 25°C, 16 h, 79%; (b) 0.1 M p-TsOH, MeOH, 6 h, reflux, 60%; (c) BzCl, Pyr, 0°C, 1 h, 90%; (d) AcOH-Ac_2O-H_2SO_4 (4:1:0.1), 25°C, 75%; (e) EtSH, $BF_3 \cdot OEt_2$, CH_2Cl_2, 0°C, 2 h, 60%.

Reexamination of toluene-p-sulfonic acid-catalyzed methanolysis of *tert*-butyl 1,2:3,4-di-O-isopropylidene-α-D-galactopyranuronate (2)[1] prepared from 1,2:3,4-di-O-isopropylidene-α-D-galactopyranose (1)[2] showed that an anomeric mixture (α:β = 28:72) of methyl (methyl D-galactofuranosid)uronate (3)[3,4] was formed. After column chromatography, the NMR spectra showed the material collected as 3 was pyranosides free. Benzoylation of 3 gave the corresponding 4. Acetolysis[3,5] of 4 followed by treatment of the product 5 with ethanethiol and $BF_3 \cdot Et_2O$ afforded methyl (ethyl 2,3,5-tri-O-benzoyl-1-thio-α,β-D-galactofuranosid)uronate 6[3] (α:β = 15:85, see opening scheme of this chapter). This thioglycoside donor has been used for the synthesis of several disaccharides.[3]

The α and β galactofuranosidic structures of compounds 3–6 were confirmed by ^{1}H and ^{13}C NMR spectroscopy. The furanosidic structure was proven at the stage of the synthesis when compound 3 was obtained. The 2D COSY NMR spectrum in DMSO-d_6 showed correlations confirming that in both α and β anomers, one OH group was attached to the carbon atom 5, in contrast to pyranoses having the OH group at C-4. In addition, the 2D NOESY NMR experiment for 4β showed an NOE correlation for the protons H-4 and MeO, which confirmed the β anomeric and also the furanose structure for the compound. In the ^{13}C NMR spectra of compounds 3 through 6, the signals for the anomeric carbon atoms of the β anomers appear at lower field than those of the α anomers. This is in agreement with data published for compound 3 and the corresponding acetyl derivative of 3 in the literature.[4] Furthermore, the vicinal coupling constants $^3J_{1,2}$ for the compounds 3–6 were found to be smaller for the β than for the α anomers.[4] This is caused by the fact that in the case of β anomers the furanose ring adopts a conformation in which the dihedral angle for the protons H-1 and H-2 is closer

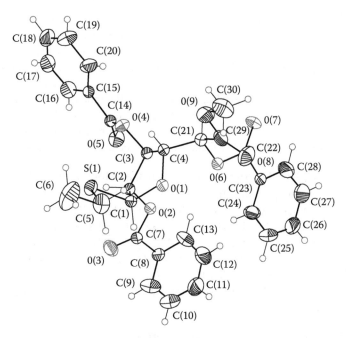

FIGURE 37.1   ORTEP view of the molecular structure of **6β**; 50% probability for the displacement ellipsoids.

to 90°, which corresponds to smallest value for the vicinal couplings according to the Karplus relationship.

Finally, we obtained crystals of compound **6β** suitable for x-ray analysis, which further confirmed the structure (Figure 37.1) previously indicated by NMR.

EXPERIMENTAL METHODS

GENERAL METHODS

All reactions were monitored by TLC on Silica gel 60 F_{254}.

Column chromatography was performed on Silica Gel (chromatography grade, Acros; 0.06–0.2 mm 60 A). HPLC was performed with a KNAUER 364 system on a Nucleosil-100 column; Ø4.5 cm·20 cm. All solvents were distilled and/or dried prior to use and all evaporations were conducted at 40°C under reduced pressure unless stated otherwise. Mass spectra were obtained on an Agilent 6210 Time-of-Flight LC/MS (ESI). All NMR spectra (α/β mixtures of **3**, **4**, **5**, and **6**, as well as for pure **4β**, **6β**, and **6α** that were obtained after chromatography; ^{1}H NMR at 500.13 MHz and ^{13}C NMR spectra at 125.8 MHz) were recorded with a Bruker AVANCE 500 spectrometer. The chemical shifts are referenced to solvent signals (CDCl$_3$: δ ^{1}H=7.26, δ ^{13}C=77.0; DMSO-d_6: δ ^{1}H=2.50, δ ^{13}C=39.7). The NMR signals were assigned by DEPT and two-dimensional ^{1}H,^{1}H COSY, ^{1}H,^{1}H NOESY and ^{1}H,^{13}C correlation spectra (HSQC, HETCOR, HMBC) using standard pulse sequences and software supplied with the spectrometer. For the x-ray structure determination of compound **6β**, an X8Apex system with CCD area detector was used ($\lambda=0.71073\,\text{Å}$, graphite monochromator). The structures were solved by direct methods (Bruker-SHELXTL). The refinement calculations were done by the full-matrix least-squares method of Bruker SHELXTL (Vers.5.10, Copyright 1997, Bruker Analytical x-ray Systems). All non-hydrogen atoms were refined anisotropically. The hydrogen atoms were put into theoretical positions and refined using the riding model. Crystallographic data for the structural analysis has been deposited with the Cambridge Crystallographic Data Centre, CCDC No. 775749. A copy of this information may be obtained free of charge from the Cambridge Crystallographic Data Center via www.ccdc.cam.ac.uk/data_request/cif.

tert-Butyl 1,2:3,4-Di-*O*-Isopropylidene-α-D-Galactopyranuronate (2)

This compound was prepared from **1** in 79% yield as described.[1] TLC (R_f 0.42, 4:1 petroleum ether–EtOAc); ^{1}H NMR (500.13 MHz, CDCl$_3$): $\delta=5.63$ (d, 1H, $^3J_{1,2}=5.0\,\text{Hz}$, H-1); 4.62 (dd, 1H, $^3J_{3,4}=7.6\,\text{Hz}$, $^3J_{2,3}=2.8\,\text{Hz}$, H-3); 4.51 (dd, 1H, $^3J_{3,4}=7.6\,\text{Hz}$, $^3J_{4,5}=2.5\,\text{Hz}$, H-4); 4.35 (dd, 1H, $^3J_{1,2}=5.0\,\text{Hz}$, $^3J_{2,3}=2.8\,\text{Hz}$, H-2); 4.27 (d, 1H, $^3J_{4,5}=2.5\,\text{Hz}$, H-5); 1.52 (s, 3H), 1.43 (s, 3H), 1.32 (s, 6H), 2 C*Me*$_2$); 1.48 (s, 9H, C*Me*$_3$). ^{13}C NMR (125.8 MHz, CDCl$_3$): $\delta=167.0$ (*C*OO); 109.9, 108.8 (2 *C*Me$_2$); 96.5 (C-1); 82.0 (*C*Me$_3$); 72.4 (C-4); 70.8 (C-3); 70.2 (C-2); 68.5 (C-5); 26.0, 25.9, 25.0, 24.8 (2 C*Me*$_2$); 28.0 (C*Me*$_3$).

Methyl (Methyl α,β-D-Galactofuranosid)uronate (3)

A solution of **2** (1.0 g, 3.02 mmol) in 0.1 M methanolic *p*-TsOH (50 mL) was refluxed for 6 h. The solution was neutralized with Et$_3$N and concentrated [^{1}H NMR (500.13 MHz, DMSO-d_6) α:β=28:72, based on intensity of signals at δ 4.59 and 4.60, respectively]. Column chromatography (20:1 EtOAc–MeOH) gave **3α,β** (403 mg, 62%); TLC (R_f 0.53, 8:1 EtOAc–MeOH); HRMS (ESI): calcd for C$_8$H$_{14}$NaO$_7$: 245.0632; found: 245.0634.

Methyl (Methyl α-D-Galactofuranosid)uronate (3α)

^{1}H NMR (500.13 MHz, DMSO-d_6): $\delta=5.20$ (d, 1H, $^3J_{3,OH}=6.3\,\text{Hz}$, OH-3); 5.02 (d, 1H, $^3J_{5,OH}=6.8\,\text{Hz}$, OH-5); 4.92 (d, 1H, $^3J_{2,OH}=7.4\,\text{Hz}$, OH-2); 4.59 (d, 1H, $^3J_{1,2}=4.5\,\text{Hz}$, H-1); 4.06 (dd, 1H, $^3J_{5,OH}=6.8\,\text{Hz}$, $^3J_{4,5}=4.0\,\text{Hz}$, H-5); 4.01 (m, 1H, H-3); 3.80–3.77 (m, 2H, H-2,4); 3.64 (s, 3H, COO*Me*); 3.21 (s, 3H, O*Me*). ^{13}C NMR (125.8 MHz, DMSO-d_6): $\delta=172.6$ (*C*OOMe); 102.0 (C-1); 82.8 (C-4); 77.2 (C-2); 73.3 (C-3); 70.8 (C-5); 55.3 (O*Me*); 51.8 (COO*Me*).

Methyl (Methyl β-D-Galactofuranosid)uronate (3β)

^{1}H NMR (500.13 MHz, DMSO-d_6): $\delta=5.43$ (d, 1H, $^3J_{5,OH}=7.5\,\text{Hz}$, OH-5); 5.35 (d, 1H, $^3J_{2,OH}=5.5\,\text{Hz}$, OH-2); 5.25 (d, 1H, $^3J_{3,OH}=5.5\,\text{Hz}$, OH-3); 4.60 (d, 1H, $^3J_{1,2}=2.6\,\text{Hz}$, H-1); 4.15 (dd, 1H, $^3J_{5,OH}=7.5\,\text{Hz}$, $^3J_{4,5}=2.3\,\text{Hz}$, H-5); 3.95–3.85 (m, 2H, H-3,4); 3.75 (dt, 1H, $^3J_{2,3}=^3J_{2,OH}=5.5\,\text{Hz}$, $^3J_{1,2}=2.6\,\text{Hz}$, H-2); 3.65 (s, 3H, COO*Me*); 3.20 (s, 3H, O*Me*). ^{13}C NMR (125.8 MHz, DMSO-d_6): $\delta=172.9$ (*C*OOMe); 108.9 (C-1); 83.0 (C-4); 81.8 (C-2); 75.9 (C-3); 69.0 (C-5); 54.6 (O*Me*); 51.8 (COO*Me*).

Methyl (Methyl 2,3,5-Tri-*O*-Benzoyl-α,β-D-Galactofuranosid)uronate (4)

Compound **3** (400 mg, 1.8 mmol) was benzoylated conventionally with pyridine (15 mL) and benzoyl chloride (0.65 mL, 5.4 mmol). When the reaction was complete, the mixture was quenched with ice, diluted with CH_2Cl_2, and washed successively with 15% $KHSO_4$ solution, saturated $NaHCO_3$ solution, and water. The crude product (^{1}H NMR: α:β = 30:70) was chromatographed (15:1 toluene–EtOAc) to give **4α,β** (847 mg, 88%); TLC (R_f 0.42, 15:1 toluene–EtOAc); HRMS (ESI): calcd for $C_{29}H_{27}NaO_{10}$: 557.1418; found: 557.1428. Small amount of pure **4β** was obtained by preparative HPLC (15:1 toluene–EtOAc), which also gave a mixture enriched sufficiently in the α anomer, allowing complete spectrum assignment.

Methyl (Methyl 2,3,5-Tri-O-Benzoyl-α-D-Galactofuranosid)uronate (4α)

^{1}H NMR (500.13 MHz, $CDCl_3$): δ = 8.29 (m, 2H), 8.09 (m, 2H), 8.04 (m, 2H), (o-Ph); 7.45 (m, 4H), 7.32 (m, 2H), (m-Ph); 7.62–7.56 (m, 3H), (p-Ph); 6.08 (dd, 1H, $^3J_{2,3}$ = 7.5 Hz, $^3J_{3,4}$ = 6.0 Hz, H-3); 5.72 (d, 1H, $^3J_{4,5}$ = 3.5 Hz, H-5); 5.54 (dd, 1H, $^3J_{2,3}$ = 7.5 Hz, $^3J_{1,2}$ = 4.7 Hz, H-2); 5.38 (d, 1H, $^3J_{1,2}$ = 4.7 Hz, H-1); 4.75 (dd, 1H, $^3J_{3,4}$ = 6.0 Hz, $^3J_{4,5}$ = 3.5 Hz, H-4); 3.81 (s, 3H, COOMe); 3.44 (s, 3H, OMe). ^{13}C NMR (125.8 MHz, $CDCl_3$): δ = 167.7 (COOMe); 166.0, 165.9, 165.7, (3 C=O); 133.6, 133.5, 133.4, (3 p-Ph); 130.2, 130.0, 129.9, (3 o-Ph); 129.1, 129.0, 128.8, (3 i-Ph); 128.5, 128.5, 128.4, (3 m-Ph); 100.7 (C-1); 79.5 (C-4); 77.2 (C-2); 75.3 (C-3); 72.7 (C-5); 55.3 (OMe); 52.6 (COOMe).

Methyl (Methyl 2,3,5-Tri-O-Benzoyl-β-D-Galactofuranosid)uronate (4β)

Colorless syrup; $[\alpha]_D^{21}$ −13.4 (c 1.8, $CHCl_3$). ^{1}H NMR (500.13 MHz, $CDCl_3$): δ = 8.12 (m, 2H), 8.09 (m, 2H), 8.02 (m, 2H), (o-Ph); 7.60 (m, 2H), 7.53 (m, 1H), (p-Ph); 7.46 (m, 2H), 7.39 (m, 2H), 7.26 (m, 2H), (m-Ph); 5.94 (d, 1H, $^3J_{4,5}$ = 2.8 Hz, H-5); 5.57 (dd, 1H, $^3J_{3,4}$ = 5.4 Hz, $^3J_{2,3}$ = 1.2 Hz, H-3); 5.52 (d, 1H, $^3J_{2,3}$ = 1.2 Hz, H-2); 5.29 (s, 1H, H-1); 4.84 (dd, 1H, $^3J_{3,4}$ = 5.4 Hz, $^3J_{4,5}$ = 2.8 Hz, H-4); 3.82 (s, 3H, COOMe); 3.47 (s, 3H, OMe). ^{13}C NMR (125.8 MHz, $CDCl_3$): δ = 167.8 (COOMe); 165.9, 165.6, 165.6, (3 C=O); 133.6, 133.5, 133.4, (3 p-Ph); 130.1, 130.0, 129.9, (3 o-Ph); 129.1, 129.0, 128.8, (3 i-Ph); 128.5, 128.5, 128.4, (3 m-Ph); 106.7 (C-1); 82.4 (C-2); 81.9 (C-4); 77.8 (C-3); 71.4 (C-5); 54.9 (OMe); 52.8 (COOMe).

Methyl 1-O-Acetyl-2,3,5-Tri-O-Benzoyl-α,β-D-Galactofuranuronate (5)

A mixture of Ac_2O (0.3 mL), AcOH (0.4 mL), and H_2SO_4 (0.03 mL) was added with stirring at 0°C to a solution of **4** (300 mg, 0.56 mmol) in acetic acid (0.8 mL). The solution was kept at 0°C for 1 h and then allowed to attain room temperature. After 2.5 h, the reaction was quenched with ice, diluted with CH_2Cl_2, and washed successively with water, saturated $NaHCO_3$ solution, and water. The combined organic layer was dried (Na_2SO_4) and concentrated (^{1}H NMR, α:β = 25:75). Column chromatography (toluene:EtOAc 15:1) gave **5α,β** (237 mg, 75%); TLC (R_f 0.36, 15:1 toluene–EtOAc); HRMS (ESI): calcd for $C_{30}H_{26}NaO_{11}$: 585.1367; found: 585.1378.

Methyl 1-O-Acetyl-2,3,5-Tri-O-Benzoyl-α-D-Galactofuranuronate (5α)

^{1}H NMR (500.13 MHz, $CDCl_3$): δ = 8.26 (m, 2H), 8.05 (m, 4H), (o-Ph); 7.61–7.58 (m, 2H, p-Ph); 7.50–7.40 (m, 6H, m-Ph, 1H, p-Ph); 6.69 (d, 1H, $^3J_{1,2}$ = 5.0 Hz, H-1); 6.07 (dd, 1H, $^3J_{2,3}$ = 6.6 Hz, $^3J_{3,4}$ = 5.7 Hz, H-3); 5.82 (dd, 1H, $^3J_{2,3}$ = 6.6 Hz, $^3J_{1,2}$ = 5.0 Hz,

H-2); 5.76 (d, 1H, $^3J_{4,5}$=4.5 Hz, H-5); 4.84 (dd, 1H, $^3J_{3,4}$=5.7 Hz, $^3J_{4,5}$=4.5 Hz, H-4); 3.77 (s, 3H, OMe); 2.03 (s, 3H, Ac). ^{13}C NMR (125.8 MHz, CDCl$_3$): δ = 169.2 (MeCO); 167.1 (COOMe); 165.9, 165.4, 165.4, (3 C=O); 133.8, 133.7, 133.6, (3 p-Ph); 130.2, 130.0, 129.9, (3 o-Ph); 128.6, 128.4, 128.2, (3 m-Ph); 93.2 (C-1); 80.8 (C-4); 76.2 (C-2); 75.0 (C-3); 72.4 (C-5); 52.8 (COOMe); 21.1 (MeCO).

Methyl 1-*O*-Acetyl-2,3,5-Tri-*O*-Benzoyl-β-D-Galactofuranuronate (5β)

^{1}H NMR (500.13 MHz, CDCl$_3$): δ = 8.09 (m, 4H), 7.99 (m, 2H), (o-Ph); 7.65–7.57 (m, 2H), 7.51 (m, 1H), (p-Ph); 7.48 (m, 2H), 7.37 (m, 2H), 7.24 (m, 2H), (m-Ph); 6.57 (br, 1H, H-1); 5.94 (d, 1H, $^3J_{4,5}$=3.2 Hz, H-5); 5.64 (dd, 1H, $^3J_{2,3}$=1.0 Hz, $^3J_{1,2}$=0.6 Hz, H-2); 5.62 (d't', 1H, $^3J_{3,4}$=4.7 Hz, $^3J_{2,3}$=$^4J_{1,3}$=1.0 Hz, H-3); 4.99 (dd, 1H, $^3J_{3,4}$=4.7 Hz, $^3J_{4,5}$=3.2 Hz, H-4); 3.80 (s, 3H, OMe); 2.20 (s, 3H, Ac). ^{13}C NMR (125.8 MHz, CDCl$_3$): δ = 168.9 (MeCO); 167.5 (COOMe); 165.7, 165.6, 165.4, (3 C=O); 133.8, 133.7, 133.5, (3 p-Ph); 130.1, 130.0, 129.9, (3 o-Ph); 128.8, 128.7, 128.6, (3 i-Ph); 128.6, 128.6, 128.4, (3 m-Ph); 99.4 (C-1); 84.3 (C-4); 81.7 (C-2); 77.6 (C-3); 71.5 (C-5); 52.9 (COOMe); 21.1 (MeCO).

Methyl (Ethyl 2,3,5-Tri-*O*-Benzoyl-1-Thio-α,β-D-Galactofuranosid)uronate (6)

BF$_3$·Et$_2$O (0.14 mL, 1.11 mmol) was added at 0°C to a solution of **5** (200 mg, 0.36 mmol) and EtSH (60 μL, 0.75 mmol) in CH$_2$Cl$_2$ (5 mL). The mixture was stirred at 0°C for 2 h, diluted with CH$_2$Cl$_2$, and washed successively with saturated NaHCO$_3$ and water. The organic layer was concentrated (^{1}H NMR, α:β = 15:85) and chromatography (15:1 toluene–EtOAc) gave **6α,β** (120 mg, 60%); TLC (R_f 0.36, 15:1 toluene–EtOAc); HRMS (ESI): calcd for C$_{30}$H$_{28}$NaO$_9$S: 587.1346; found: 587.1357. Small amounts of pure **6α** and **6β** were obtained by preparative HPLC (15:1 toluene–EtOAc).

Methyl (Ethyl 2,3,5-Tri-*O*-Benzoyl-1-Thio-α-D-Galactofuranosid)uronate (6α)

Colorless syrup; $[\alpha]_D^{21}$+126.7 (c 0.4, CHCl$_3$). ^{1}H NMR (500.13 MHz, CDCl$_3$): δ = 8.22 (m, 2H), 8.10 (m, 2H), 8.04 (m, 2H), (o-Ph); 7.59 (m, 2H), 7.54 (m, 1H), (p-Ph); 7.45 (m, 4H), 7.33 (m, 2H), (m-Ph); 5.91 (dd, 1H, $^3J_{3,4}$=5.5 Hz, $^3J_{2,3}$=4.4 Hz, H-3); 5.87 (dd, 1H, $^3J_{1,2}$=5.4 Hz, $^3J_{2,3}$=4.4 Hz, H-2); 5.78 (d, 1H, $^3J_{4,5}$=4.4 Hz, H-5); 5.73 (d, 1H, $^3J_{1,2}$=5.4 Hz, H-1); 4.68 (dd, 1H, $^3J_{3,4}$=5.5 Hz, $^3J_{4,5}$=4.4 Hz, H-4); 3.78 (s, 3H, OMe); 2.75 (q, 2H, ^3J=7.4 Hz, SCH$_2$); 1.28 (t, 3H, ^3J=7.4 Hz, SCH$_2$CH$_3$). ^{13}C NMR (125.8 MHz, CDCl$_3$): δ = 167.7 (COOMe); 165.8, 165.5, 165.4, (3 C=O); 133.7, 133.6, 133.4, (3 p-Ph); 130.2, 130.1, 129.9, (3 o-Ph); 129.0, 129.0, 128.8, (3 i-Ph); 128.6, 128.5, 128.3, (3 m-Ph); 86.2 (C-1); 81.0 (C-4); 77.9 (C-2); 76.7 (C-3); 72.1 (C-5); 52.7 (COOMe); 25.4 (SCH$_2$); 14.9 (SCH$_2$CH$_3$).

Methyl (Ethyl 2,3,5-Tri-*O*-Benzoyl-1-Thio-β-D-Galactofuranosid)uronate (6β)

Mp. 136°C, colorless crystals from EtOAc-petroleum ether); $[\alpha]_D^{21}$ – 81.3 (c 1.0, CHCl$_3$), Ref. [3], $[\alpha]_D^{21}$ – 51.7 (c 2.35, CHCl$_3$). ^{1}H NMR (500.13 MHz, CDCl$_3$): δ = 8.13

(m, 2H), 8.10 (m, 2H), 8.03 (m, 2H), (*o*-Ph); 7.60 (m, 2H), 7.54 (m, 1H), (*p*-Ph); 7.48 (m, 2H), 7.40 (m, 2H), 7.27 (m, 2H), (*m*-Ph); 5.97 (d, 1H, $^3J_{4,5}$ = 2.9 Hz, H-5); 5.76 (br s, 1H, H-1); 5.61 (d't', 1H, $^3J_{3,4}$ = 5.3 Hz, $^3J_{2,3}$ = $^4J_{1,3}$ = 1.2 Hz, H-3); 5.55 (t', 1H, $^3J_{1,2}$ = $^3J_{2,3}$ = 1.2 Hz, H-2); 5.04 (ddd, 1H, $^3J_{3,4}$ = 5.3 Hz, $^3J_{4,5}$ = 2.9 Hz, $J_{1,4}$ = 0.7 Hz, H-4); 3.80 (s, 3H, OMe); 2.73 (m, 2H, SCH$_2$); 1.35 (t, 3H, ^3J = 7.4 Hz, SCH$_2$C*H*$_3$). ^{13}C NMR (125.8 MHz, CDCl$_3$): δ = 167.6 (COOMe); 165.7, 165.5 (2), (3 C=O); 133.7, 133.5, 133.4, (3 *p*-Ph); 130.0, 130.0, 129.9, (3 *o*-Ph); 129.0, 129.0, 128.8, (3 *i*-Ph); 128.5, 128.5, 128.4, (3 *m*-Ph); 88.3 (C-1); 83.0 (C-2); 81.6 (C-4); 78.0 (C-3); 71.6 (C-5); 52.7 (COOMe); 25.2 (SCH$_2$); 15.0 (SCH$_2$C*H*$_3$).

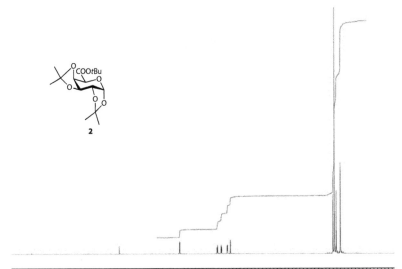

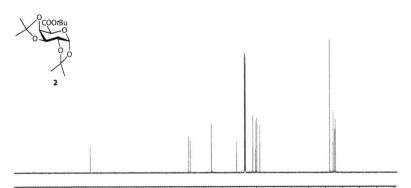

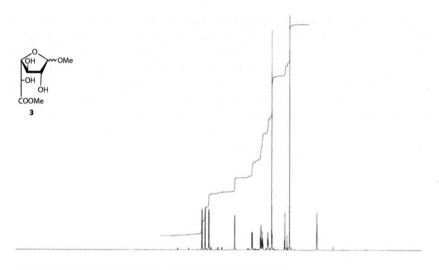

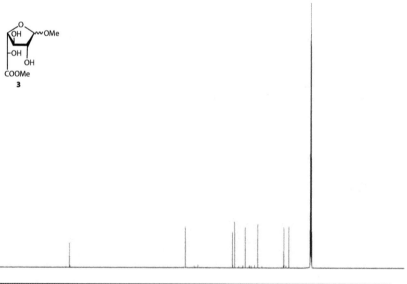

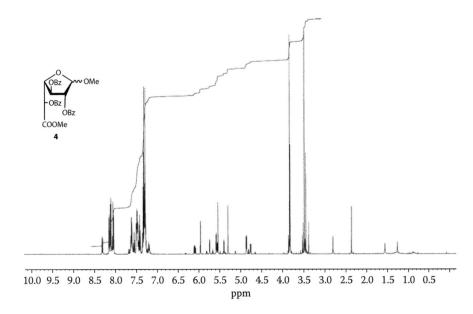

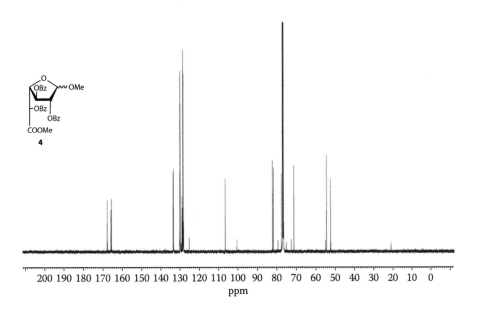

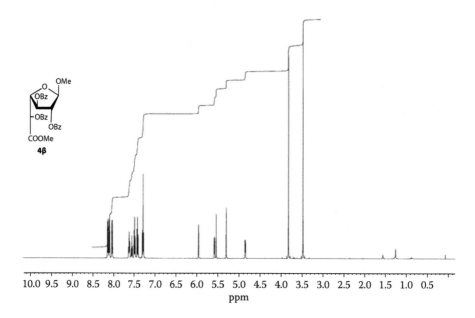

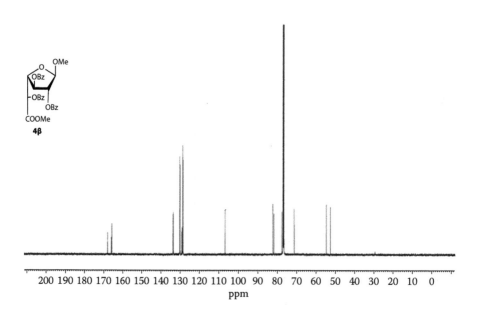

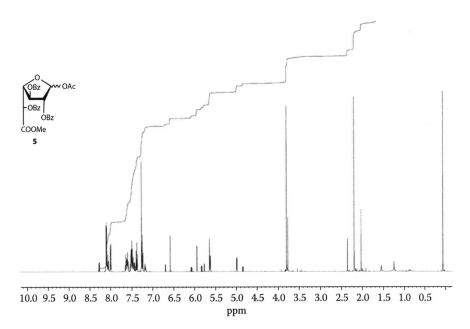

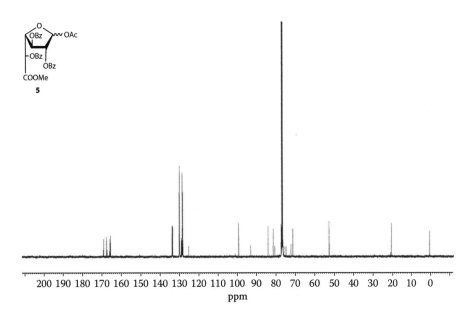

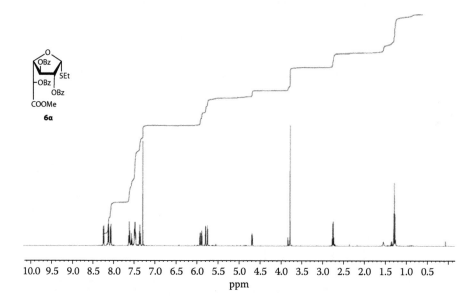

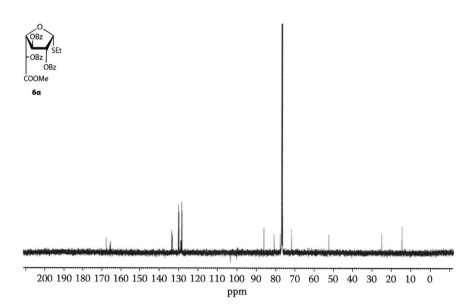

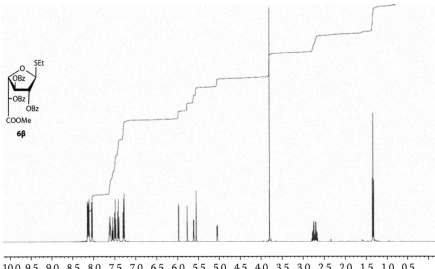

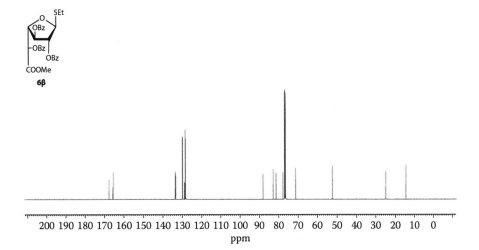

REFERENCES

1. Corey, E. J. and Samuelsson, B. *J. Org. Chem.* 1984, *49*, 4735–4735.
2. Tipson, R. S. *Methods Carbohydr. Chem.* 1963, *2*, 246–250.
3. Choudhury, A. K. and Roy, N. *Synlett* 1997, 105–106.
4. Matsuhiro, B.; Zanlungo, A. B.; and Dutton, G. G. S. *Carbohyd. Res.* 1981, *97*, 11–18; Schmidt, H. W. H. and Newkom, N. *Helv. Chem. Acta* 1966, *49*, 510–517.
5. Cimpoia, A. R.; Hunter, P. J.; Evans, C. A.; Jin, H.; Breining, T.; and Mansour, T. S. *J. Carbohyd. Chem.* 1994, *13*, 1115–1119.

38 p-Tolyl 2,3,5-Tri-O-Benzoyl-1-Thio-α-D-Arabinofuranoside: A Useful Thioglycoside Building Block in the Synthesis of Oligoarabinofuranosides

Maju Joe, Yu Bai, Lucía Gandolfi-Donadío,[†] and Todd L. Lowary*

CONTENTS

Experimental Methods 342
   General Methods 342
      p-Tolyl 2,3,5-Tri-O-Benzoyl-1-Thio-α-D-Arabinofuranoside 343
Waste Disposal Information 344
Acknowledgments 344
References 347

Furanose residues are important constituents of glycoconjugates of many bacterial,[1] parasitical,[2] fungal,[3] and plant species.[4] Although many different organisms produce furanose-containing glycans, arguably the most impressive examples of such compounds are found in mycobacteria.[1,5] This genus of bacteria contains a number of

---

* Corresponding author.

† Checker.

species, including the well-known human pathogens *Mycobacterium tuberculosis*, *Mycobacterium leprae*, and *Mycobacterium ulcerans*, the causes of tuberculosis, leprosy, and buruli ulcer, respectively. The cell wall of these organisms is composed, in large part, of two polysaccharides, arabinogalactan, and lipoarabinomannan; a major component of both these molecules is a D-arabinofuranan moiety.[5]

It has been known for several years that the clinically used antituberculosis agent, ethambutol, acts by inhibiting the action of at least one of the arabinofuranosyltransferases involved in mycobacterial arabinan biosynthesis.[6] This discovery, and the need for developing new antituberculosis agents due to the emergence of drug-resistant *M. tuberculosis* strains,[7] has led to heightened interest in the chemistry and biochemistry of arabinofuranose residues.[8] In particular, the identification of arabinofuranosyltransferase inhibitors has received increasing attention.[9] Given the xenobiotic nature of arabinofuranose-containing glycans in humans, the biosynthetic pathways leading to the formation of mycobacterial D-arabinan are believed to be attractive targets for drug action.[9,10] However, the processes by which these polysaccharides are assembled are not well understood, and much additional research in this area is needed before new potent inhibitors of these enzymes can be identified.[9,10] Such studies, in turn, require synthetic substrates that can be used for fundamental biochemical studies leading to the characterization of the appropriate biosynthetic enzymes.[11]

In previous investigations, arabinofuranose thioglycosides have been used to assemble oligoarabinofuranosides[11,12] and we describe here a 100 g scale synthesis of *p*-tolyl 2,3,5-tri-*O*-benzoyl-α-D-arabinofuranoside.[13] This species can be easily converted to a host of other differentially protected arabinofuranoside thioglycosides, which are of use in the preparation of mycobacterial arabinan fragments.[11,12] The procedure described provides a good yield of the product, requires no chromatography, and is suitable for further scale-up without any major modifications.

EXPERIMENTAL METHODS

GENERAL METHODS

Reactions were carried out in oven-dried glassware.* All reagents used were purchased from commercial sources and were used without further purification. The reaction was monitored by TLC on Silica Gel 60 F_{254} (0.25 mm, E. Merck). Spots were detected under UV light or by charring with acidified *p*-anisaldehyde solution in ethanol.† Melting points were determined with a Fisher-Johns apparatus and are uncorrected. Optical rotations were measured with a Perkin–Elmer 343 polarimeter at 25°C. The ^{1}H NMR spectrum was recorded at 500 MHz and chemical shifts were referenced to $CDCl_3$ at 7.26 ppm. The ^{1}H data are reported as though they are first order. The ^{13}C NMR (APT) spectrum was recorded at 125 MHz and ^{13}C chemical shifts were referenced to internal $CDCl_3$ (77.06, $CDCl_3$). Assignments of resonances in NMR spectra were done using ^{1}H–^{1}H COSY and HMQC experiments. Solutions in organic solvents were dried with Na_2SO_4‡ and

---

* The entire operation should be done in an efficient fume hood.
† Prepared by dissolving *p*-anisaldehyde (5 mL), glacial acetic acid (2 mL) and concentrated sulfuric acid (7 mL) in 95% ethanol (186 mL).
‡ Anhydrous Na_2SO_4 was purchased from Fischer Scientific and used as received.

concentrated under vacuum at <40°C on a rotary evaporator. Electrospray mass spectra were recorded on samples suspended in mixtures of THF with CH_3OH and added NaCl.

p-Tolyl 2,3,5-Tri-*O*-Benzoyl-1-Thio-α-ᴅ-Arabinofuranoside[13]

A 2 L, two-necked, round-bottom flask equipped with a rubber septum fitted with an argon inlet needle, a 200 mL pressure-equalizing addition funnel capped with a rubber septum, and a magnetic stirbar, was charged with methyl 2,3,5-tri-*O*-benzoyl-α-ᴅ-arabinofuranoside[14] (100 g, 0.21 mol) and *p*-thiocresol (29.0 g, 0.23 mol).*,† Dichloromethane (600 mL)‡ was added, followed by activated 4 Å molecular sieves (15 g, powdered) and the suspension was stirred for 30 min. The reaction mixture was then cooled to 2°C–3°C (bath, crushed ice) and boron trifluoride etherate (79 mL, 0.62 mol)*,§ was added dropwise over the course of 45 min. The cooling bath was removed after 3 h and the reaction mixture was warmed to rt over 2 h and then stirred for an additional 12 h.¶ The reaction mixture was diluted with dichloromethane (300 mL) and cooled again to 2°C–3°C (crushed ice), and triethylamine (88 mL, 0.63 mol)** was added dropwise with efficient stirring.†† The reaction mixture was then filtered to remove molecular sieves and the filtered solid was washed with dichloromethane (100 mL). The combined organic layers were successively washed with chilled water (1 × 1000 mL), chilled satd. aq. sodium bicarbonate solution (1 × 1000 mL),‡‡ and water (1 × 1000 mL). The organic layer was separated, dried, filtered, and concentrated. The thick syrup§§ obtained was triturated with methanol (500 mL)¶¶ and allowed to stand for 1 h, whereupon the compound solidified.***

---

* Boron trifluoride etherate and *p*-thiocresol were purchased from Aldrich Chemical Company, Inc. and were used without any further purification.

† Harmful if swallowed, inhaled, or absorbed through skin. Causes eye, skin, and respiratory tract irritation. Stench.

‡ Dichloromethane (VWR International, ACS grade) was used as received.

§ Causes eye and skin burns. Causes digestive and respiratory tract burns if swallowed or inhaled. Flammable liquid and vapor. Moisture sensitive.

¶ The progress of the reaction can be monitored by TLC: elution with 4:1 hexanes–EtOAc, R_f=0.36 (methyl glycoside), R_f=0.44 (thioglycoside). The compounds should be applied in dilution to get clear separations; if concentrated, poor separation will result.

   After 12 h, TLC showed complete conversion of the starting material to the desired thioglycoside (R_f = 0.44), and presence of a negligible amount of material, which cochromatographed with 2,3,5-tri-*O*-benzoyl-α,β-arabinofuranose.

** Triethylamine was purchased from Fischer Scientific and was used without any further purification. The addition should be done at 2°C–3°C (crushed ice), and the temperature should be maintained during the addition.

†† The reaction mixture can also be worked up by directly pouring the dichloromethane solution (after the initial dilution and filtration, to remove molecular sieves) into about 1 L of chilled sat. aq. sodium bicarbonate solution. In this case, care should be taken because there will be vigorous evolution of carbon dioxide. It is advised to add in small volumes to keep carbon dioxide generation under control.

‡‡ Sodium bicarbonate was purchased from EMD Chemicals Inc. (a division of Merck KGaA).

§§ Once most of the dichloromethane is evaporated as indicated by a thick syrupy appearance of the residue, the flask can be removed from the rotary evaporator. Do not allow the syrupy residue to become hard solid (if left longer on rotary evaporator).

¶¶ Methanol (Fischer Scientific, ACS grade) was used as received. For better results, make sure the solids are evenly dispersed in methanol before filtration.

*** Cooling to 2°C–5°C may be necessary to induce crystallization, when working on a small scale (e.g., ~1 g).

The solid product was collected by filtration and washed sequentially with methanol (200 mL) and hexane (300 mL), and the product dried under vacuum.[†††] Yield, 95.5 g (80%), mp 85°C–87°C (from MeOH, twice), Lit.[13] mp 82°C–83°C; $[\alpha]_D$ +85° (c 1.0, CHCl$_3$), Lit.[13] $[\alpha]_D$ +86°; ^{1}H NMR (500 MHz, CDCl$_3$, δ) 8.16–8.10 (m, 2H, Ar), 8.08–8.00 (m, 4H, Ar), 7.66–7.55 (m, 2H, Ar), 7.55–7.45 (m, 5H, Ar), 7.45–7.35 (m, 2H, Ar), 7.35–7.30 (m, 2H, Ar), 7.15–7.10 (m, 2H, Ar), 5.77 (br s, 1H, H-1), 5.72 (dd, 1H, $J_{2,3}$ 1.4, $J_{1,2}$ 1.3 Hz, H-2), 5.73 (br d, 1H, $J_{3,4}$ 4.8 Hz, H-3), 4.87 (ddd, 1H, $J_{3,4}$ 4.8, $J_{4,5}$ 3.7, $J_{4,5'}$ 5.1 Hz, H-4), 4.81 (dd, 1H, $J_{4,5}$ 3.7, $J_{5,5'}$ 11.9 Hz, H-5), 4.74 (dd, 1H, $J_{4,5'}$ 5.1, $J_{5,5'}$ 11.9 Hz, H-5′), 2.28 (s, 3H, ArCH$_3$); ^{13}C NMR (125 MHz, CDCl$_3$, δ) 166.1 (C=O), 165.6 (C=O), 165.3 (C=O), 138.2 (Ar), 133.6 (Ar), 133.5 (Ar), 133.0(6) (Ar), 133.0(1) (Ar), 130.0 (Ar), 129.9 (Ar), 129.8 (Ar), 129.7(7) (Ar), 129.7(2) (Ar), 129.5 (Ar), 129.0 (Ar), 128.9 (Ar), 128.5(6) (Ar), 128.5(3) (Ar), 128.3 (Ar), 91.7 (C-1), 82.5 (C-2), 81.0 (C-4), 78.1 (C-3), 63.5 (C-5), 21.1 (ArCH$_3$). HRMS: [M + Na]$^+$ calcd for C$_{33}$H$_{28}$O$_7$S, 591.1448. Found: 591.1445. Anal. calcd for C$_{33}$H$_{28}$O$_7$S: C, 69.70; H, 4.96. Found: C, 69.61; H, 5.06.

WASTE DISPOSAL INFORMATION

All toxic materials were disposed of in accordance with "Prudent Practices in the Laboratory"; National Academy Press; Washington, DC, 1995.

ACKNOWLEDGMENTS

This chapter was supported by the University of Alberta, The Natural Sciences and Engineering Research Council of Canada and the Alberta Ingenuity Centre for Carbohydrate Science. The authors thank C. S. Callam and R. R. Gadikota for initial synthetic work.[13]

[†††] The product obtained is pure enough for further synthetic manipulations such as glycosylations, debenzoylations, etc. If necessary, the product can be recrystallized from hot (62°C–64°C) methanol; 1.0 g of compound requires about 65–70 mL of methanol.

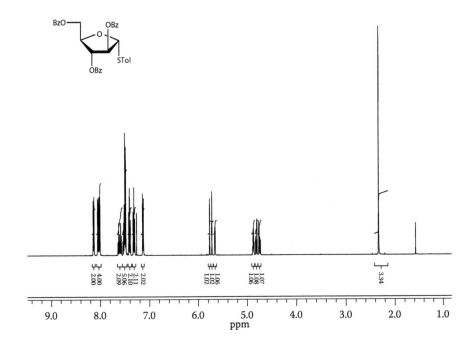

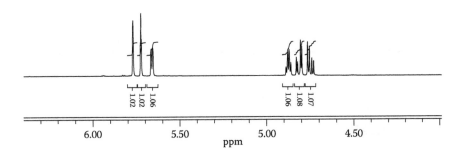

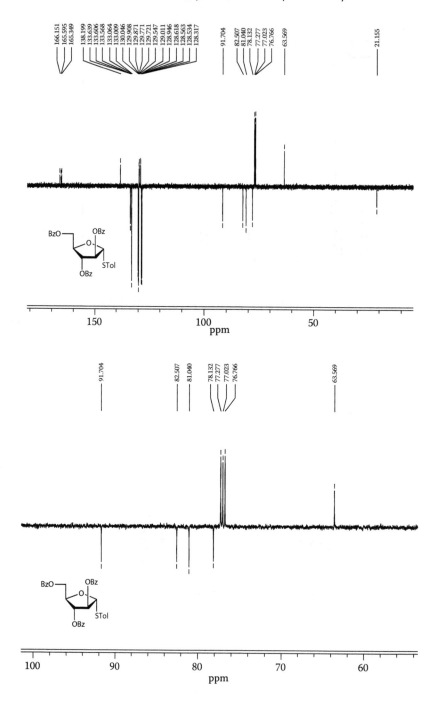

REFERENCES

1. Peltier, P.; Euzen, R.; Daniellou, R.; Nugier-Chauvin, C.; Ferrieres, V. *Carbohydr. Res.* 2008, *343*, 1897–1923.
2. (a) Gerold, P.; Eckert, V.; Schwarz, R.T. *Trends Glycosci. Glycotechnol.* 1996, *8*, 265–271. (b) de Lederkremer, R. M.; Colli, W. *Glycobiology* 1995, *5*, 547–552.
3. (a) Unkefer, C. J.; Gander, J. *J. Biol. Chem.* 1990, *265*, 685–689. (b) Mendonça-Previato, L.; Gorin, P. A. J.; Travassos, L. R. *Infect. Immun.* 1980, *29*, 934–939. (c). Groisman, J. F.; de Lederkremer, R. M. *Eur. J. Biochem.* 1987, *165*, 327–332. (d) Komatsu, K.; Shigemori, H.; Kobayashi, J. *J. Org. Chem.* 2001, *66*, 6189–6192.
4. Ryder, M. H.; Tate, M. E.; Jones, G. P. *J. Biol. Chem.* 1984, *259*, 9704–9710.
5. Brennan, P. J. *Tuberculosis* 2003, *83*, 91–97.
6. Belanger, A. E.; Besra, G. S.; Ford, M. E.; Mikusova, K.; Belisle, J. T.; Brennan, P. J.; Inamine, J. M. *Proc. Natl. Acad. Sci. USA* 1996, *93*, 11919–11924.
7. Nachega, J. B.; Chaisson, R. E. *Clin. Infect. Dis.* 2003, *36*, S24–S30.
8. Crick, D. C.; Mahapatra, S.; Brennan, P. J. *Glycobiology* 2001, *11*, 107R–118R.
9. (a) Lowary, T. L. *Mini-Rev. Med. Chem.* 2003, *3*, 694–707. (b) Brennan, P. J.; Crick, D. C. *Curr. Top. Med. Chem.* 2007, *7*, 475–488.
10. Berg, S.; Kaur, D.; Jackson, M.; Brennan, P. J. *Glycobiology* 2007, *17*, 35R–56R.
11. For some examples see: (a) Birch, H. J.; Alderwick, L. J.; Bhatt, A.; Rittmann, D.; Krumbach, K.; Singh, A.; Bai, Y.; Lowary, T. L.; Eggeling, L.; Besra, G. *Mol. Microbiol.* 2008, *69*, 1191–1206. (b) Khasnobis, S.; Zhang, J.; Angala, S. K.; Amin, A. G.; McNeil, M. R.; Crick, D. C.; Chatterjee, D. *Chem. Biol.* 2006, *13*, 787–795. (c) Zhang, J.; Khoo, K. H.; Wu, S. W.; Chatterjee, D. *J. Am. Chem. Soc.* 2007, *129*, 9650–9662. (d) Ayers, J. D.; Lowary, T. L.; Morehouse, C. B.; Besra, G. S. *Bioorg. Med. Chem. Lett.* 1998, *8*, 437–442. (e) Pathak, A. K.; Pathak, V.; Kulshrestha, M.; Kinnaird, D.; Suling, W. J.; Gurcha, S. S.; Besra, G. S.; Reynolds, R. C. *Tetrahedron* 2003, *59*, 10239–10248.
12. For some examples see: (a) Joe, M.; Bai, Y.; Nacario, R. C.; Lowary, T. L. *J. Am. Chem. Soc.* 2007, 129, 9885–9901. (b) Gadikota, R. R.; Callam, C. S.; Wagner, T.; Fraino, B. D.; Lowary, T. L. *J. Am. Chem. Soc.* 2003, 125, 4155–4165. (c) Zhu, X.; Kawatkar, S.; Rao, Y.; Boons, G.-J. *J. Am. Chem. Soc.* 2006, *128*, 11948–11957. (d) Ishiwata, A.; Akao, H.; Ito, Y. *Org. Lett.* 2006, *8*, 5525–5528. (e) Crich, D.; Pedersen, C. M.; Bowers, A. A.; Wink, D. J. *J. Org. Chem.* 2007, *72*, 1553–1565. (f) Yin, H.; D'Souza, F. W.; Lowary, T. L. *J. Org. Chem.* 2002, *67*, 892–903. (g) Marott, K.; Sanchez, S.; Bamhaoud, T.; Prandi. J. *Eur J. Org. Chem.* 2003, 3587–3598.
13. Callam, C. S.; Gadikota, R. R.; Lowary, T. L. *J. Org. Chem.* 2001, *66*, 4549–4558.
14. (a) Fletcher, H. G. Jr. *Methods Carbohydr. Chem.* 1963, *2*, 228–230. (b) Callam, C. S.; Lowary, T. L. *J. Chem. Educ.* 2001, *78*, 312–312.

39 Ethylene Dithioacetals of Common Hexoses

Rui C. Pinto, Marta M. Andrade, Cécile Ouairy,[†] and Maria Teresa Barros*

CONTENTS

Experimental Methods 350
  General Methods 350
    General Procedure 350
    D-Galactose Ethylene Dithioacetal (**1**) 350
    D-Glucose Ethylene Dithioacetal (**2**) 350
    D-Mannose Ethylene Dithioacetal (**3**) 351
References 354

Dithioacetals are 1,3-dithianes, where two sulfur atoms are attached to one carbon atom. The sulfurs act as electron withdrawing groups, making the proton attached to the central carbon slightly acidic. Thus, treatment of dithioacetals with base results in anion formation, which can act as a nucleophilic species in subsequent reactions.

Dithioacetal chemistry is used in a variety of ways in carbohydrate derivatization.[1] Among other things, it allows access to those hydroxyl groups of sugars, which are usually engaged in the formation of the pyranose/furanose ring. Most commonly, dialkyl (diethyl) dithioacetals are chosen for this purpose, which can be easily obtained by reaction of the sugar with ethanethiol in strong acidic medium.[2–5] The

---

* Corresponding author.
[†] Checker.

resulting acyclic structure of the sugar allows the employment of protecting group strategies different from those adopted for pyranose or furanose rings. Dithioacetals can be later hydrolyzed to regenerate the aldehyde and cyclize, if one free suitably positioned OH group is available.[1] A different option is the use of benzenethiol (thiophenol), but harsher conditions are needed (fuming HCl or trifluoroacetic acid[6]) to form diphenyl dithioacetals in satisfactory yields.[1]

A suitable alternative offer ethylene dithioacetals,[7,8] which can be obtained by reaction of aldoses with ethan-1,2-dithiol, the latter having the advantage of being less volatile, thus facilitating preparative procedures. Herein, we describe the synthesis of ethylene dithioacetals for three hexoses, but similar procedure can be applied to other common hexoses and pentoses.

EXPERIMENTAL METHODS

GENERAL METHODS

All reagents were purchased from Aldrich. All reactions must be performed in a well-ventilated fume hood. Melting points were determined with a capillary apparatus and are uncorrected. NMR spectra were recorded for solutions in DMSO-d_6 with a Bruker AMX-400 MHz instrument. IR spectra were measured in a PerkinElmer Spectrum BX. Elemental analyses were performed on Thermo Finnigan-CE Flash EA 1112 CHNS series analyzer.

General Procedure

1 g of hexose and 0.56 mL of ethan-1,2-dithiol (1.2 equiv.) were added to 2 mL of concentrated HCl, at 0°C (ice bath). After the time indicated for each case, cold MeOH (10 mL) was added, and the white solid formed after standing for 1–2 days in the freezer at −20°C was filtered off and recrystallized several times from methanol to give odorless and colorless crystals.

D-Galactose Ethylene Dithioacetal (1)

Reaction time: 10 min. Yield 0.90–0.97 g (63%–68%), mp 155°C–156°C (from methanol); $[\alpha]_D$ −6.4 (c 1, H$_2$O). ^{1}H NMR (DMSO-d6) δ 4.69 (d, 1H, J 7.9 Hz, OH), 4.54 (d, 1H, J 9.9 Hz, H-1), 4.44 (t, 1H, J 5.4 Hz, OH), 4.34 (d, 1H, J 8.0 Hz, OH), 4.12 (d, 1H, J 6.7 Hz, OH), 4.02 (d, 1H, J 7.6 Hz, OH), 3.67 (dd, 1H, J 12.7 Hz, J 6.2 Hz, H-5), 3.60–3.53 (q, 2H, J 9.6 Hz, J 9.3 Hz, H-2 and H-3), 3.36–3.35 (m, 3H, H-4 and H-6), 3.18–3.05 (m, 4H, (CH$_2$)$_2$S). ^{13}C NMR (DMSO-d6) δ 74.2 (C-2), 70.7 (C-3), 69.8 (C-5), 69.5 (C-4), 63.1 (C-6), 56.2 (C-1), 38.1, 37.3 (2 CH$_2$-S). IR (KBr) 3416, 3238, 2957, 2906, 1438, 1384, 1253, 1222, 1206, 1091, 1048, 1030, 1018, 862, 721, 668 cm^{-1}. HRMS (ESI) m/z calcd for C$_8$H$_{16}$NaO$_5$S$_2$: (M + Na)$^+$ 279.0337, found: 279.0345. Anal. calcd for C$_8$H$_{16}$O$_5$S$_2$: C, 37.48; H, 6.29; S, 25.02. Found: C, 37.50; H, 6.28; S, 24.83.

D-Glucose Ethylene Dithioacetal (2)

Reaction time: 30 min. Yield 0.60–0.67 g (42%–47%), mp 142°C–144°C (from methanol); $[\alpha]_D$ −15.4 (c 1, H$_2$O). ^{1}H NMR (DMSO-d6) δ 5.15 (d, 1H, J 5.7 Hz, OH), 4.58 (d, 1H, J 8.6 Hz, H-1), 4.53 (t, 2H, J 5.7 Hz, 2×OH), 4.34–4.32 (m, 2H, 2×OH),

3.83–3.81 (m, 1H, *H*-3), 3.58–3.53 (m, 1H, *H*-6a), 3.47–3.37 (m, 4H, *H*-2, *H*-4, *H*-5, *H*-6b), 3.16–3.05 (m, 4H, (CH$_2$)$_2$S). ^{13}C NMR (DMSO-d6) δ 77.8, 73.5, 71.2 (*C*-2, *C*-4, *C*-5), 69.6 (*C*-3), 63.1 (*C*-6), 55.6 (*C*-1), 37.9, 37.4 (2 CH$_2$-S). IR (KBr) 3497, 3404, 3281, 1403, 1295, 1271, 1231, 1204, 1120, 1085, 1053, 1024, 954, 852, 799, 779, 613 cm^{-1}. HRMS (ESI) *m/z* calcd for C$_8$H$_{16}$NaO$_5$S$_2$: (M + Na)$^+$ 279.0337; found: 279.0329. Anal. calcd for C$_8$H$_{16}$O$_5$S$_2$: C, 37.48; H, 6.29; S, 25.02. Found: C, 37.69; H, 6.43; S, 24.94.

D-Mannose Ethylene Dithioacetal (3)

Reaction time: 10 min. Yield 0.85 g (60%), mp 154°C–155°C (from methanol); [α]$_D$ 8.6 (*c* 1, H$_2$O). ^{1}H NMR (DMSO-d6) δ 4.86 (d, 1H, *J* 2.4 Hz, *H*-1), 4.76 (d, 1H, *J* 6.6 Hz, O*H*), 4.41 (t, 1H, *J* 5.4 Hz, O*H*), 4.35 (t, 1H, *J* 5.5 Hz, O*H*), 4.28 (d, 1H, *J* 7.8 Hz, O*H*), 4.17 (d, 1H, *J* 7.4 Hz, O*H*), 3.60–3.51 (m, 4H, *H*-2, *H*-3, *H*-4, *H*-6a), 3.46–3.27 (m, 3H, *H*-5, *H*-6b, 1 × (CH$_2$)$_2$S), 3.22–3.17 (m, 1H, 1 × (CH$_2$)$_2$S), 3.12–3.04 (m, 2H, 2 × (CH$_2$)$_2$S). ^{13}C NMR (DMSO-d6) δ 74.6, 71.6 (*C*-2, *C*-4), 71.1 (*C*-5), 69.5 (*C*-3), 63.8 (*C*-6), 55.9 (*C*-1), 38.2, 37.8 (2 CH$_2$-S). IR (KBr) 3386, 3281, 2918, 1417, 1312, 1204, 1088, 1021, 962, 884, 718, 604 cm^{-1}. HRMS (ESI) *m/z* calcd for C$_8$H$_{16}$NaO$_5$S$_2$: (M + Na)$^+$ 279.0337; found: 279.0336. Anal. calcd for C$_8$H$_{16}$O$_5$S$_2$: C, 37.48; H, 6.29; S, 25.02. Found: C, 37.74; H, 6.48; S, 25.16.

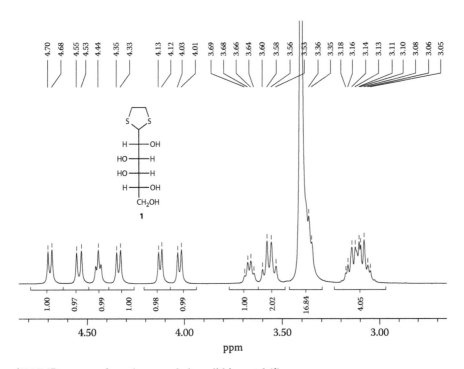

^{1}H NMR spectra of D-galactose ethylene dithioacetal (**1**).

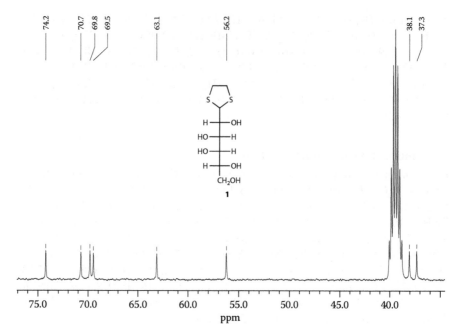

^{13}C NMR spectra of D-galactose ethylene dithioacetal (**1**).

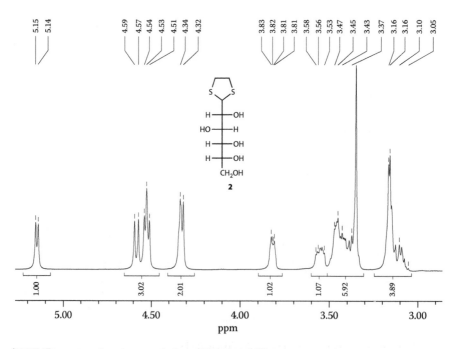

^{1}H NMR spectra of D-glucose ethylene dithioacetal (**2**).

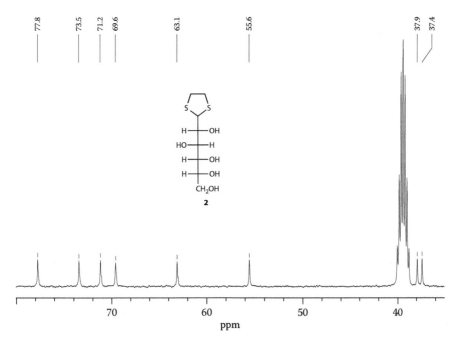

^{13}C NMR spectra of D-glucose ethylene dithioacetal (**2**).

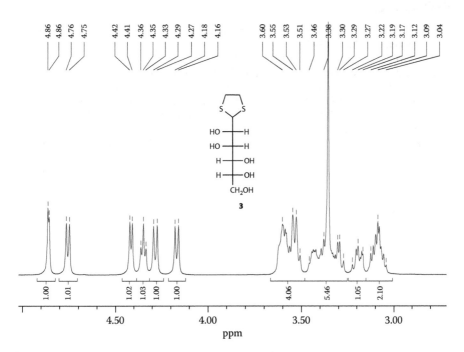

^{1}H NMR spectra of D-mannose ethylene dithioacetal (**3**).

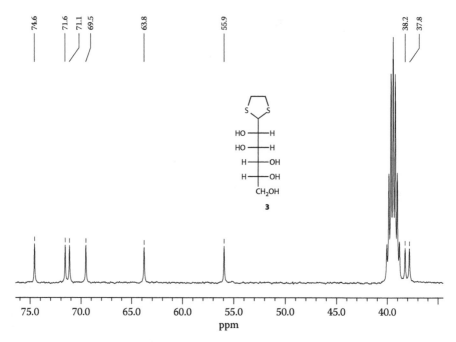

^{13}C NMR spectra of D-mannose ethylene dithioacetal (**3**).

REFERENCES

1. Norris, P.; Horton, D. *Preparative Carbohydrate Chemistry*; Eds. Hanessian, S.; Marcel Dekker: New York, 1997, pp. 35–52.
2. Bai, Y.; Lowary, T. L. *J. Org. Chem.* 2006, *71*, 9658–9671.
3. Maeda, T.; Nishimura, S.-I. *Chem. Eur. J.* 2008, *14*, 478–487.
4. Mahidhar, Y. V.; Rajesh, M.; Chaudhuri, A. *J. Med. Chem.* 2004, *47*, 3938–3948.
5. Pinilla, I. M.; Martínez, M. B.; Galbis, J. A. *Carbohydr. Res.* 2003, *338*, 549–555.
6. Funabashi, M.; Arai, S.; Shinohara, M. *J. Carbohydr. Chem.* 1999, *18*, 333–341.
7. DeJongh, D. C. *J. Org. Chem.* 1965, *30*, 1563–1570.
8. Zinner, H.; Bock, W.; Klöcking, H.-P. *Chem. Ber.* 1959, *92*, 1313–1319.

40 Preparation of 2,6-Anhydro-Aldose Tosylhydrazones

Marietta Tóth, László Somsák,* and David Goyard[†]

CONTENTS

Experimental Methods 357
   General Methods 357
   General Procedure 357
      2,6-Anhydro-3,4,5,7-Tetra-*O*-Benzoyl-D-*Glycero*-D-*Gulo*-Heptose
      Tosylhydrazone (**2a**) 358
      3,4,5,7-Tetra-*O*-Acetyl-2,6-Anhydro-D-*Glycero*-D-*Gulo*-Heptose
      Tosylhydrazone (**2b**) 358
      3,4,5,7-Tetra-*O*-Acetyl-2,6-Anhydro-D-*Glycero*-L-*Manno*-Heptose
      Tosylhydrazone (**2c**) 358
      4,5,7-Tri-*O*-Acetyl-2,6-Anhydro-3-Deoxy-3-Phthalimido-D-*Glycero*-D-
      Gulo-Heptose Tosylhydrazone (**2d**) 359
      3,4,5-Tri-*O*-Acetyl-2,6-Anhydro-D-*Manno*-Hexose Tosylhydrazone (**2e**) ... 359
Acknowledgments 359
References 365

---

* Corresponding author.
[†] Checker.

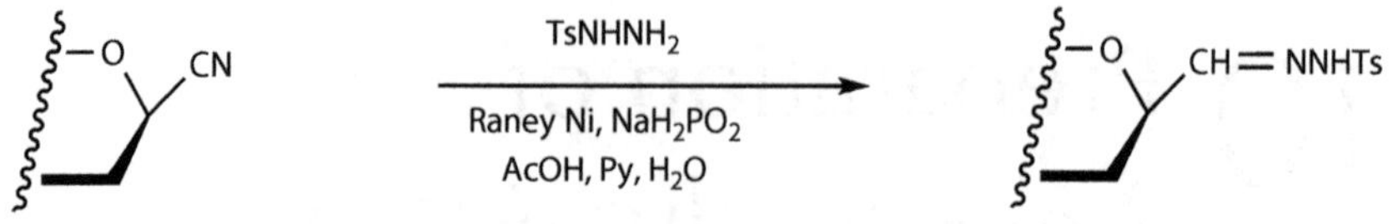

1a–e

TsNHNH$_2$

Raney Ni, NaH$_2$PO$_2$
AcOH, Py, H$_2$O

2a–e

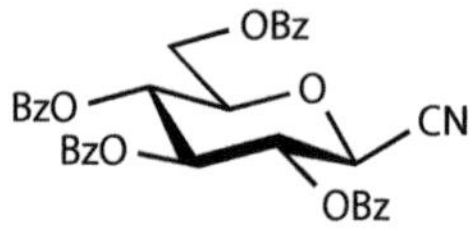

a

a (64%)

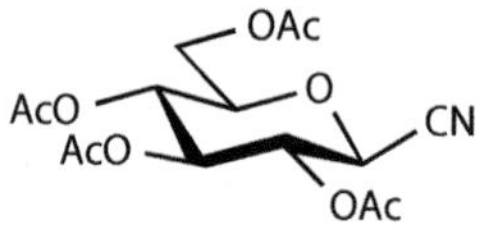

b

b (60%)

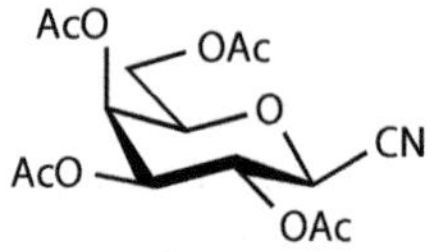

c

c (87%)

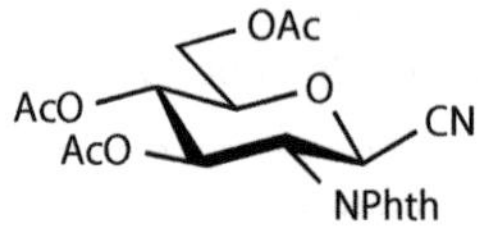

d

d (58%)

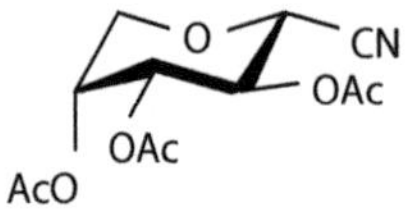

e

e (73%)

Hydrazones are readily available compounds, which can be transformed into a large variety of other structures, and have many industrial and biological applications.[1] Tosylhydrazones are a similarly valuable subclass of hydrazones whose most important synthetic uses are (a) nucleophilic addition to the C=N double bond, (b) electrophilic additions to hydrazone-derived azaenolates, (c) Bamford–Stevens and Shapiro reactions, and (d) reductions, just to mention a few.[2] The most widely applied general method to obtain hydrazone derivatives is the condensation of an aldehyde or ketone with an (un)substituted hydrazine in the presence of an acidic catalyst. With acid sensitive aldehydes, this condensation can be performed under neutral conditions as well.[1] Carboxylic acid derivatives such as imino esters and ortho esters are also converted to hydrazones.[1]

2,6-Anhydro-aldoses (C-glycopyranosyl aldehydes) are rather difficult to obtain.[3–7] On the other hand, 2,6-anhydro-aldononitriles (glycopyranosyl cyanides) are much more easily available,[8–11] and the direct transformation of nitriles to aldehyde tosylhydrazones[12] by using Raney-Ni and NaH_2PO_2 was also elaborated.[13] Herein, the direct synthesis of 2,6-anhydro-aldose tosylhydrazones from 2,6-anhydro-aldononitriles is described.[14]

EXPERIMENTAL METHODS

GENERAL METHODS

Melting points were measured in open capillary tubes or on a Kofler hot stage and are uncorrected. Optical rotations were determined with a Perkin-Elmer 241 polarimeter at rt. Nuclear magnetic resonance (NMR) spectra were recorded with Bruker 360 (360/90 MHz for $^1H/^{13}C$) or Bruker 400 (400/100 MHz for $^1H/^{13}C$) spectrometers. Chemical shifts are referenced to internal tetramethylsilane (^1H) or to the residual solvent signals (^{13}C). Proton chemical shifts and scalar coupling constants were extracted from the resolution enhanced 1D proton spectra. Microanalyses were performed on a Carlo-Erba analyzer Type 1106. Thin-layer chromatography (TLC) was performed on DC-Alurolle Kieselgel 60 F_{254} (Merck), and the plates were visualized under UV light and by gentle heating. For column chromatography, Kieselgel 60 (Merck, particle size 0.063–0.200 mm) was used. Solutions in organic solvents were dried over anhydrous $MgSO_4$ and concentrated under diminished pressure at 40–50°C (water bath). Raney nickel was purchased from Merck.

GENERAL PROCEDURE

Raney nickel* (1.5 g/1 mmol, from an aqueous suspension, Merck) was added at room temperature to a vigorously stirred solution of pyridine (5.7 mL/1 mmol), acetic acid (3.4 mL/1 mmol), and water (3.4 mL/1 mmol). Sodium hypophosphite[†] (0.74 g, 8.4 mmol), tosylhydrazine (0.20–0.32 g, 1.1–1.7 mmol), and the corresponding anhydro-aldononitrile **1** (1 mmol) were added to the mixture. The reaction mixture was stirred at room temperature (**1b–e**), while **1a** was transformed at 40°C. When the reaction was complete (TLC, 1:1 ethyl acetate–hexane), the insoluble materials were filtered off with suction and washed with dichloromethane (10 mL).[‡] The organic layer of the filtrate was separated, washed with water (3 mL), 10% aq. HCl (2 × 3 mL), cold, saturated aq. $NaHCO_3$ (2 × 3 mL), water (3 mL), dried, and concentrated. Traces

---

* The quality of the Raney nickel is essential; use of old Raney nickel results in incomplete conversion and lower yield.

† A round bottom flask three to five times larger than the final volume is recommended, since the addition of NaH_2PO_2 is accompanied by vigorous effervescence and foaming.

‡ Raney nickel is potentially highly flammable when dry. After filtration, the remaining Raney nickel was immediately collected and kept as a suspension in water before final disposal.

of pyridine were removed by repeated co-evaporations with toluene. Chromatography (gradient elution, eluent: 1:2–1:1 ethyl acetate–hexane) gave **2a–d**, while **2e** was obtained by crystallization from ethyl acetate–hexane.

2,6-Anhydro-3,4,5,7-Tetra-*O*-Benzoyl-D-*Glycero*-D-*Gulo*-Heptose Tosylhydrazone (2a)

Prepared from **1a** (0.50 g, 0.86 mmol) with 1.7 eq. tosylhydrazine. Yield, 0.42 g (64%) colorless syrup; R_f = 0.20 (3:7 ethyl acetate–petroleum ether); $[\alpha]_D$ +4 (*c* 1, CHCl$_3$); ^{1}H NMR (CDCl$_3$) δ 8.12 (brs, 1H, NH), 8.04–7.74 (m, 8H, OBz), 7.58 (d, 2H, *J* 7.9 Hz, Ts), 7.57–7.21 (m, 12H, OBz), 7.16 (d, 1H, $J_{1,2}$ 6.3 Hz, H-1), 6.90 (d, 2H, *J* 7.9 Hz, Ts), 5.93, 5.67, 5.41 (3 pseudo t, 3H, *J* 9.5 Hz, H-3, H-4, H-5), 4.58 (dd, 1H, $J_{7,7'}$ 12.1 Hz, H-7'), 4.43 (dd, 1H, H-7), 4.36 (dd, 1H, $J_{2,3}$ 9.5 Hz, H-2), 4.15 (ddd, 1H, $J_{6,7}$ 5.3 Hz, $J_{6,7'}$ 2.1 Hz, H-6), 2.19 (s, 3H, CH$_3$); ^{13}C NMR (CDCl$_3$) δ 166.3, 165.9, 165.6, 165.3 (C=O), 144.1 (C-1), 143.7, 135.2 (Ts quaterners), 133.6, 133.4, 133.2, 129.8, 129.6, 129.3, 128.4, 127.3 (Ts, OBz), 128.7, 128.6 (OBz quaterners), 78.1, 76.2, 73.7, 70.7, 69.3 (C-2, C-3, C-4, C-5, C-6), 63.2 (C-7), 21.6 (CH$_3$); IR (KBr) $\tilde{v}$ 3200, 1732, 1452, 1268, 1166, 1094, 710 cm^{-1}. Anal. Calcd for C$_{42}$H$_{36}$N$_2$O$_{11}$S: C, 64.94; H, 4.67; N, 3.61. Found: C, 64.82; H, 4.74; N, 3.72.

3,4,5,7-Tetra-*O*-Acetyl-2,6-Anhydro-D-*Glycero*-D-*Gulo*-Heptose Tosylhydrazone (2b)

Prepared from **1b** (0.35 g, 0.98 mmol) with 1.7 eq. tosylhydrazine. Yield, 0.29 g (60%) **2b** colorless syrup and 0.02 g **1b** (conversion: 94%); R_f=0.35 (1:1 ethyl acetate–hexane); $[\alpha]_D$ −8 (*c* 1.33, CHCl$_3$); ^{1}H NMR (CDCl$_3$) δ 9.16 (brs, 1H, NH), 7.80 (d, 2H, *J* 7.9 Hz, Ts), 7.34 (d, 2H, *J* 7.9 Hz, Ts), 7.00 (d, 1H, $J_{1,2}$ 6.3 Hz, H-1), 5.26, 5.05, 4.97 (3 pseudo t, 3H, *J* 9.5–10.0 Hz, H-3, H-4, H-5), 4.24 (dd, 1H, $J_{7,7'}$ 12.2 Hz, H-7), 4.07 (dd, 1H, H-7'), 3.99 (dd, 1H, $J_{2,3}$ 9.5 Hz, H-2), 3.72 (ddd, 1H, $J_{6,7}$ 5.3 Hz, $J_{6,7'}$ 1.8 Hz, H-6), 2.42 (s, 3H, CH$_3$-Ts), 2.07, 2.03, 2.01, 1.72 (4 s, 12H, 4×OAc); ^{13}C NMR (CDCl$_3$) δ 170.8, 170.6, 170.2, 169.6 (C=O), 144.3, 135.5 (Ts quaterners), 143.7 (C-1), 129.8, 128.0 (Ts), 77.8, 75.9, 73.1, 69.6, 68.3 (C-2, C-3, C-4, C-5, C-6), 62.1 (C-7), 21.6 (CH$_3$-Ts), 20.8, 20.7, 20.3 (CH$_3$); IR (KBr) $\tilde{v}$ 3186, 1754, 1368, 1226, 1166, 1036 cm^{-1}. Anal. Calcd for C$_{22}$H$_{28}$N$_2$O$_{11}$S: C, 50.00; H, 5.34; N, 5.30. Found: C, 50.15; H, 5.48; N, 5.21.

3,4,5,7-Tetra-*O*-Acetyl-2,6-Anhydro-D-*Glycero*-L-*Manno*-Heptose Tosylhydrazone (2c)

Prepared from **1c** (4.00 g, 11.2 mmol) with 1.1 eq. tosylhydrazine. Yield, 5.32 g (90%) crude product as a colorless syrup suitable for further transformation; an analytical sample was achieved by column chromatography; R_f=0.36 (1:1 ethyl acetate–petroleum ether); $[\alpha]_D$ +6 (*c* 0.97, CHCl$_3$); ^{1}H NMR (DMSO-d$_6$) δ 11.62 (brs, 1H, NH), 7.67 (d, 2H, *J* 7.9 Hz, Ts), 7.42 (d, 2H, *J* 7.9 Hz, Ts), 7.00 (d, 1H, $J_{1,2}$ 6.7 Hz, H-1), 5.29 (d, 1H, $J_{5,6}$ < 1 Hz, H-5), 5.22 (dd, 1H, $J_{4,5}$ 3.1 Hz, H-4), 4.95 (dd, 1H, $J_{3,4}$ 10.4 Hz, H-3), 4.24–4.20 (m, 1H, H-6), 4.14 (dd, 1H, $J_{2,3}$ 9.8 Hz, H-2), 4.00 (dd, 1H, $J_{6,7'}$ 4.9 Hz, $J_{7,7'}$ 11.6 Hz, H-7'), 3.93 (dd, 1H, $J_{6,7}$ 7.4 Hz, H-7), 2.37 (s, 3H, CH$_3$-Ts), 2.11, 1.98, 1.90, 1.66 (4 s, 12H, 4×OAc); ^{13}C NMR (CDCl$_3$) δ 170.6, 170.5, 170.2, 170.1 (C=O), 144.1 (C-1), 144.1, 135.5 (Ts quaterners), 129.6, 127.9 (Ts), 78.2, 74.3, 71.0, 67.6, 66.9

(C-2, C-3, C-4, C-5, C-6), 61.7 (C-7), 21.4 (CH$_3$-Ts), 20.6, 20.2 (CH$_3$); IR (KBr) $\tilde{\nu}$ 3208, 1752, 1372, 1228, 1166, 1054 cm^{-1}. Anal. Calcd for C$_{22}$H$_{28}$N$_2$O$_{11}$S: C, 50.00; H, 5.34; N, 5.30. Found: C, 49.91; H, 5.45; N, 5.42.

4,5,7-Tri-O-Acetyl-2,6-Anhydro-3-Deoxy-3-Phthalimido-D-*Glycero*-D-*Gulo*-Heptose Tosylhydrazone (2d)

Prepared from **1d** (0.50 g, 1.13 mmol) with 1.2 eq. tosylhydrazine.* Yield, 0.40 g (58%) white needles; mp 207°C dec. (from EtOAc–Hexane); R_f=0.24 (1:1 ethyl acetate–petroleum ether); [α]$_D$ +65 (c 1.01, CHCl$_3$); ^{1}H NMR (DMSO-d$_6$) δ 11.48 (brs, 1H, NH), 7.90–7.80 (m, 4H, Phth), 7.34 (d, 2H, J 7.9 Hz, Ts), 7.10 (d, 1H, J$_{1,2}$ 5.5 Hz, H-1), 7.07 (d, 2H, J 7.9 Hz, Ts), 5.62, 5.02, 4.30 (3 pseudo t, 3H, J 9.5–10.0 Hz, H-3, H-4, H-5), 4.87 (dd, 1H, J$_{2,3}$ 10.4 Hz, H-2), 4.16 (dd, 1H, J$_{6,7}$ 4.8 Hz, J$_{7,7'}$ 12.5 Hz, H-7), 4.07–4.03 (m, 2H, H-6, H-7'), 2.27 (s, 3H, CH$_3$-Ts), 2.02, 1.99, 1.76 (3 s, 9H, 3×OAc); ^{13}C NMR (CDCl$_3$) δ 170.8, 170.3, 169.7, 168.0, 167.5 (C=O), 144.0 (C-1), 144.2, 135.1 (Ts quaterners), 131.6, 131.5 (Phth quaterners), 134.4, 123.9 (Phth) 129.6, 127.8 (Ts), 76.1, 73.9, 71.3, 68.9 (C-2, C-4, C-5, C-6), 62.3 (C-7), 52.3 (C-3), 21.8 (CH$_3$-Ts), 20.9, 20.7, 20.6 (CH$_3$); IR (KBr) $\tilde{\nu}$ 3194, 1750, 1718, 1384, 1230, 1166, 1042 cm^{-1}. Anal. Calcd for C$_{28}$H$_{29}$N$_3$O$_{11}$S: C, 54.63; H, 4.75; N, 6.83. Found: C, 54.72; H, 4.92; N, 6.95.

3,4,5-Tri-O-Acetyl-2,6-Anhydro-D-*Manno*-Hexose Tosylhydrazone (2e)

Prepared from **1e** (1.00 g, 3.50 mmol) with 1.2 eq. tosylhydrazine. Yield, 1.16 g (73%) white needles; mp 83–86°C (from EtOAc:Hexane); R_f=0.41 (1:1 ethyl acetate–petroleum ether); [α]$_D$ −35 (c 1.01, CHCl$_3$); ^{1}H NMR (CDCl$_3$) δ 8.93 (brs, 1H, NH), 7.81 (d, 2H, J 7.9 Hz, Ts), 7.33 (d, 2H, J 7.9 Hz, Ts), 7.03 (d, 1H, J$_{1,2}$ 6.8 Hz, H-1), 5.33 (brs, 1H, H-5), 5.18 (dd, 1H, J$_{3,4}$ 10.0 Hz, H-3), 5.09 (dd, 1H, J$_{4,5}$ 3.1 Hz, H-4), 3.99 (d, 1H, J$_{5,6}$ < 1 Hz, J$_{6,6'}$ 13.1 Hz, H-6), 3.89 (dd, 1H, J$_{2,3}$ 9.5 Hz, H-2), 3.68 (d, 1H, J$_{5,6'}$ < 1 Hz, H-6'), 2.42 (CH$_3$-Ts), 2.15, 2.01, 1.75 (3 s, 9H, 3×OAc); ^{13}C NMR (CDCl$_3$) δ 170.6, 170.2, 170.0 (C=O), 144.3 (C-1), 144.0, 135.3 (Ts quaterners), 129.5, 127.9 (Ts), 78.5, 70.5, 68.4, 67.1 (C-2, C-3, C-4, C-5), 67.8 (C-6), 21.4 (CH$_3$-Ts), 20.8, 205, 20.2 (CH$_3$); IR (KBr) $\tilde{\nu}$ 3202, 1748, 1372, 1224, 1166, 1050 cm^{-1}. Anal. Calcd for C$_{19}$H$_{24}$N$_2$O$_9$S: C, 49.99; H, 5.30; N, 6.14. Found: C, 50.07; H, 5.39; N, 6.05.

ACKNOWLEDGMENTS

Financial support from the Hungarian Scientific Research Fund (Grant: OTKA CK77712) is gratefully acknowledged. The work was also supported by the TÁMOP 4.2.1/B-09/1/KONV-2010-0007 project co-financed by the European Union and the European Social Fund.

---

* Purification of **2d** could also be achieved by dropwise addition with stirring of a solution of the crude mixture in a minimum of CH$_2$Cl$_2$ into Et$_2$O, to give the title compound as a white powder.

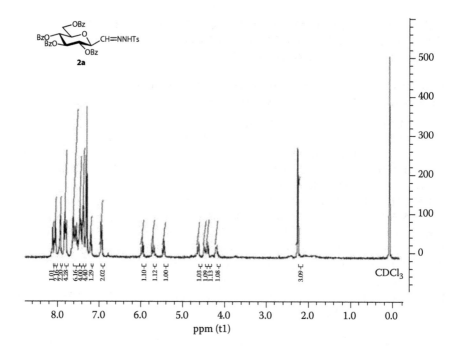

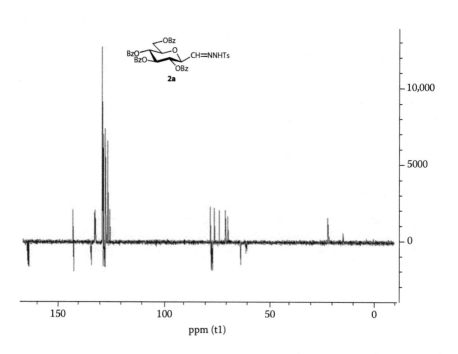

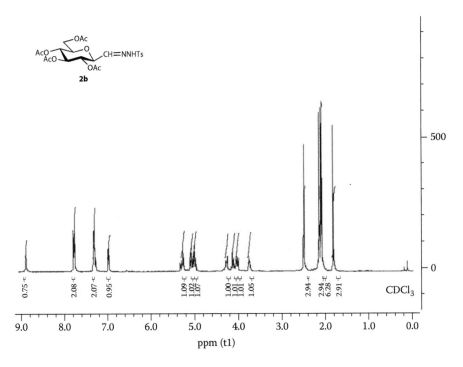

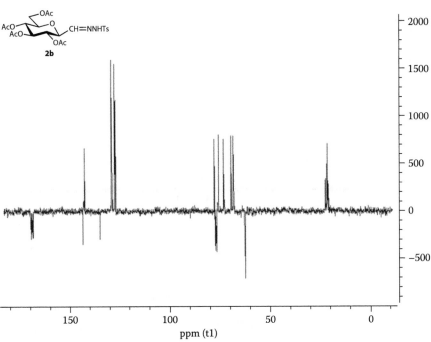

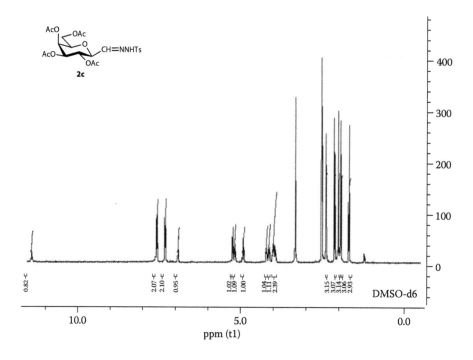

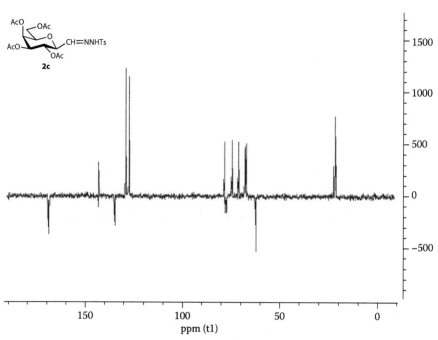

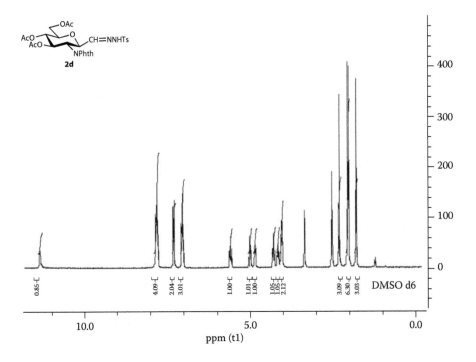

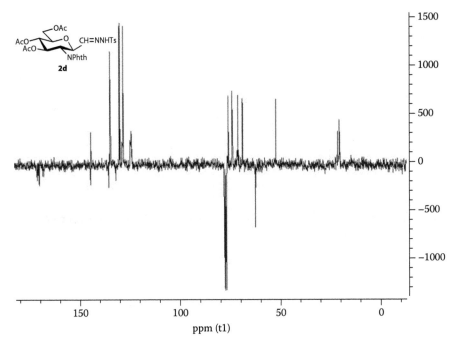

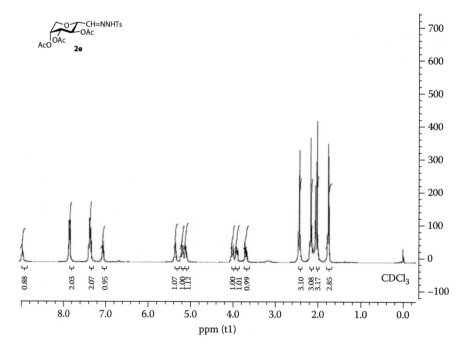

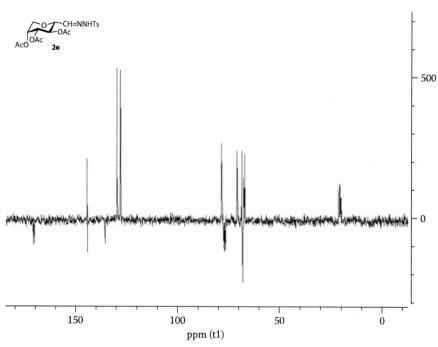

REFERENCES

1. Dumić, M.; Korunčev, D.; Kovačević, K.; Polak, L.; Kolbah, D. In *Methoden der Organischen Chemie (Houben-Weyl)*; Klamann, D.; Hagemann, H. (Eds.); Thieme: Stuttgart, 1990; pp. 434–631.
2. Chamberlin, A. R.; Sheppeck II, J. E. In *Encyclopedia of Reagents for Organic Synthesis;* Paquette, L. A. (Ed.); John Wiley & Sons: Chichester, U.K., 1995; pp. 4953–4958.
3. Dettinger, H.-M.; Kurz, G.; Lehmann, J. *Carbohydr. Res.* 1979, *74*, 301–307.
4. Kobertz, W. R.; Bertozzi, C.; Bednarski, M. D. *J. Org. Chem.* 1996, *61*, 1894–1897.
5. Dondoni, A.; Scherrmann, M.-C. *J. Org. Chem.* 1994, *59*, 6404–6412.
6. Dondoni, A.; Marra, A. *Tetrahedron Lett.* 2003, *44*, 13–16.
7. Norsikian, S.; Zeitouni, J.; Rat, S.; Gerard, S.; Lubineau, A. *Carbohydr. Res.* 2007, *342*, 2716–2728.
8. Myers, R. W.; Lee, Y. C. *Carbohydr. Res.* 1984, *132*, 61–85.
9. Myers, R. W.; Lee, Y. C. *Carbohydr. Res.* 1986, *154*, 145–163.
10. Köll, P.; Förtsch, A. *Carbohydr. Res.* 1987, *171*, 301–315.
11. Somsák, L.; Nagy, V. *Tetrahedron: Asymm.* 2000, *11*, 1719–1727. Corrigendum 2247.
12. Tóth, M.; Somsák, L. *Tetrahedron Lett.* 2001, *42*, 2723–2725.
13. Staskun, B.; van Es, T. *S. Afr. J. Chem.* 2008, *61*, 144–156.
14. Tóth, M.; Kövér, K. E.; Bényei, A.; Somsák, L. *Org. Biomol. Chem.* 2003, *1*, 4039–4046.

41 Preparation of Exo-Glycals from (C-Glycopyranosyl) formaldehyde Tosylhydrazones

Marietta Tóth, Sándor Kun,
László Somsák,* and David Goyard†

CONTENTS

Experimental Methods 369
    General Methods 369
    General Procedure 369
        2,6-Anhydro-3,4,5,7-Tetra-*O*-Benzoyl-1-Deoxy-D-*Gluco*-Hept-1-
        Enitol (**2a**) 370
        3,4,5,7-Tetra-*O*-Acetyl-2,6-Anhydro-1-Deoxy-D-*Galacto*-Hept-1-
        Enitol (**2b**) 370
        4,5,7-Tri-*O*-Acetyl-2,6-Anhydro-1,3-Dideoxy-3-Phthalimido-D-*Gluco*-
        Hept-1-Enitol (**2c**) 370
        3,4,5-Tri-*O*-Acetyl-2,6-Anhydro-1-Deoxy-D-*Arabino*-Hex-1-Enitol (**2d**) ... 370
Acknowledgments 371
References 375

---

* Corresponding author.
† Checker.

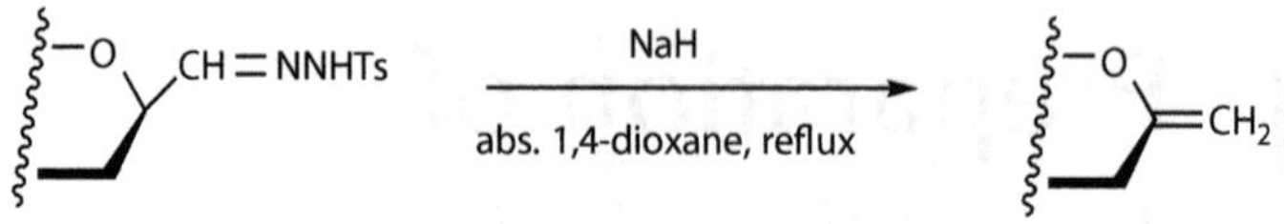

1a–d → NaH, abs. 1,4-dioxane, reflux → **2a–d**

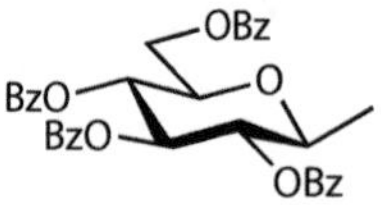

a (72%)

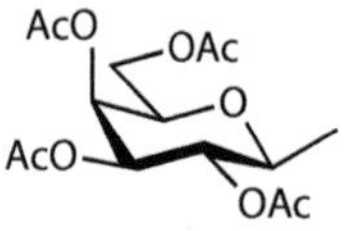

b (82%)

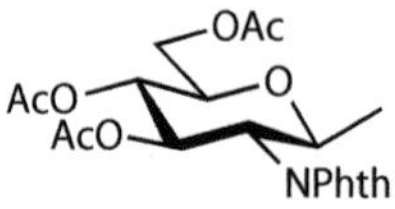

c (74%)

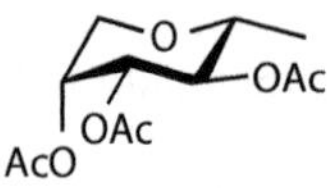

d (86%)

Unsaturated carbohydrates, especially glycals (1,4- or 1,5-anhydro-2-deoxy-hex- or hept-1-enitols) and *exo*-glycals (2,5- or 2,6-anhydro-1-deoxy-hex- or hept-1-enitols), play an important role in getting a better insight into the action of carbohydrate derivatives in living organisms. They themselves are glycomimetics and offer many synthetic possibilities for further transformations. The synthesis[1,2] and synthetic uses[3] of glycals and *exo*-glycals[4,5] are well documented and reviewed.[6] Exomethylene glycals are relatively easily available in the ether- or silyl-protected series.[4,7] Since such glycals are normally prepared at highly basic conditions and/or with the aid of organometallic reagents, *O*-acyl-protected derivatives are not so readily accessible due to the incompatibility of ester protecting groups at such reaction conditions. Herein, the direct synthesis of *O*-acyl-protected *exo*-glycals from (*C*-glycopyranosyl)formaldehyde tosylhydrazones is described.[8,9]

EXPERIMENTAL METHODS

GENERAL METHODS

Melting points were measured in open capillary tubes or on a Kofler hot stage and are uncorrected. Optical rotations were determined with a Perkin-Elmer 241 polarimeter at room temperature. Nuclear magnetic resonance (NMR) spectra were recorded with Bruker 360 (360/90 MHz for ^{1}H/^{13}C) or Bruker 400 (400/100 MHz for ^{1}H/^{13}C) spectrometers. Chemical shifts are referenced to internal TMS (^{1}H) or to the residual solvent signals (^{13}C). Proton chemical shifts and scalar coupling constants were extracted from the resolution-enhanced 1D proton spectra. Microanalyses were performed on a Carlo-Erba analyzer Type 1106. Thin-layer chromatography (TLC) was performed on DC-Alurolle Kieselgel 60 F_{254} (Merck), and the plates were visualized under UV light and/or by gentle heating. For column chromatography, Kieselgel 60 (Merck, particle size 0.063–0.200 mm) was used. Organic solutions were dried over anhydrous $MgSO_4$ and concentrated under diminished pressure at 40–50°C (water bath).

GENERAL PROCEDURE

In a flame-dried three-necked flask protected from atmospheric moisture (anhydrous $CaCl_2$-filled drying tube), sodium hydride* was added to dry 1,4-dioxane† (25 mL) containing powdered molecular sieves (3 Å). The suspension was heated to reflux and, with stirring, a solution of tosylhydrazone **1** (1 mmol) in dry 1,4-dioxane (25 mL) was added dropwise during 15–20 min from a dropping funnel protected from atmospheric moisture (anhydrous $CaCl_2$-filled drying tube). The mixture was refluxed for an additional hour, when TLC (1:1 ethyl acetate–hexane) showed the reaction to be complete. After cooled to rt, the insoluble material was filtered off and washed with a few mL of dry 1,4-dioxane. The combined filtrates were concentrated, and the residue was chromatographed (a solution of the residue in minimum of CH_2Cl_2 was applied on top of a column of silica gel [100 g/g of the crude product]).

---

* The amount of sodium hydride was 0.24 g (10 mmol) when a ~60% commercial suspension of NaH (Aldrich 45,291-2, S79600-249) was used. In these cases the oily suspension was taken up in hexane, the solvent was decanted from the slurry (3 times), and the rest of the solvent was removed by putting it onto an unglazed bisque plate. The necessary amount of NaH strongly depends on the quality of the chemical: sometimes as few as 1.5 equivalents proved sufficient.

    The amount of sodium hydride was 0.076 g (3 mmol) when a 95% NaH (Aldrich 223441, 59496AK) was used. In these cases the NaH was added was supplied.

† Best results were obtained when dioxane was dried as follows: a mixture of dioxane (1 L) and cc. HCl (100 mL) was refluxed for 3 h in N_2 atmosphere. After cooling, the lower (aqueous) phase was separated and dioxane was dried over solid KOH (150–200 g) overnight. After filtration, the pre-dried dioxane thus obtained was refluxed under N_2 over freshly cut sodium or sodium sand (for the preparation of sodium sand see Ref. [10]) in the presence of benzophenone until the solution became dark blue. Dioxane was then distilled and stored over molecular sieves.

    During checking, extra dry 1,4-dioxane from Acros Organics (cat. # 326890010) was used with similar efficiency.

2,6-Anhydro-3,4,5,7-Tetra-O-Benzoyl-1-Deoxy-D-*Gluco*-Hept-1-Enitol (2a)

Prepared from **1a** (0.20 g, 0.26 mmol) and purified by flash chromatography (1:4 ethyl acetate–hexane). Yield, 0.11 g (72%), colorless syrup; $[\alpha]_D$ +43 (c 0.98, CHCl$_3$); ^{1}H NMR (CDCl$_3$) δ 8.08–8.03 (m, 4H, OBz), 7.93–7.87 (m, 4H, OBz), 7.59–7.26 (m, 12H, Bz), 5.98–5.80 (m, 3H, H-3, H-4, H-5 strongly coupled), 4.96 (t, 1H, $J_{1,1'}$ 1.5 Hz, $J_{1,3}$ 1.5 Hz, H-1), 4.71 (t, 1H, $J_{1',3}$ 1.5 Hz, H-1′), 4.71 (dd, 1H, $J_{6,7}$ 3.1 Hz, $J_{7,7'}$ 12.1 Hz, H-7′), 4.53 (dd, 1H, $J_{6,7}$ 4.7 Hz, H-7), 4.32–4.27 (m, 1H, H-6); ^{13}C NMR (CDCl$_3$) δ 166.3, 165.7, 165.2, 165.1 (C=O), 153.3 (C-2), 133.7, 133.5, 133.3, 130.1, 129.9, 128.7, 128.6, 128.5 (OBz), 129.7, 129.1, 129.0, 128.9 (OBz quaterners), 97.3 (C-1), 77.0, 73.3, 69.9, 69.1 (C-3, C-4, C-5, C-6), 63.0 (C-7); IR (KBr) $\tilde{\nu}$ 1732, 1602, 1452, 1270, 1094, 708 cm^{-1}. Anal. Calcd for C$_{35}$H$_{28}$O$_9$: C, 70.94; H, 4.76. Found: C, 71.08; H, 4.89.

3,4,5,7-Tetra-O-Acetyl-2,6-Anhydro-1-Deoxy-D-*Galacto*-Hept-1-Enitol (2b)

Prepared from **1b** (0.40 g, 0.76 mmol) and purified by flash chromatography (1:3 ethyl acetate–hexane). Yield, 0.21 g (82%), colorless syrup; $[\alpha]_D$ +74 (c 1.45, CHCl$_3$); (Ref. [11]; $[\alpha]_D$ +70 (c 1.10, CHCl$_3$); ^{1}H NMR (CDCl$_3$) δ 5.69 (ddd, 1H, $J_{3,4}$ 10.5 Hz, H-3), 5.52 (dd, 1H, $J_{5,6}$ 1.5 Hz, H-5), 5.06 (dd, 1H, $J_{4,5}$ 3.1 Hz, H-4), 4.82 (dd, 1H, $J_{1,1'}$ 2.1 Hz, $J_{1,3}$ 1.5 Hz, H-1), 4.51 (dd, 1H, $J_{1',3}$ 1.6 Hz, H-1′), 4.21 (dd, 1H, $J_{7,7'}$ 11.5 Hz, H-7), 4.15 (dd, 1H, H-7′), 4.02 (ddd, 1H, $J_{6,7}$ 6.8 Hz, $J_{6,7'}$ 6.4 Hz, H-6), 2.17, 2.14, 2.07, 2.01 (4 s, 12H, 4 × OAc), data show good coincidence with lit.[12] values; ^{13}C NMR (CDCl$_3$) δ 170.5, 170.2, 170.0, 169.6 (C=O), 154.1 (C-2), 96.1 (C-1), 75.7, 71.3, 67.7, 67.0 (C-3, C-4, C-5, C-6), 61.7 (C-7), 20.8, 20.7, 20.6 (CH$_3$); IR (KBr) $\tilde{\nu}$ 2942, 1748, 1666, 1372, 1216, 1084 cm^{-1}. Anal. Calcd for C$_{15}$H$_{20}$O$_9$: C, 52.33; H, 5.85. Found: C, 52.39; H, 5.98.

4,5,7-Tri-O-Acetyl-2,6-Anhydro-1,3-Dideoxy-3-Phthalimido-D-*Gluco*-Hept-1-Enitol (2c)

Prepared from **1c** (0.06 g, 0.26 mmol) and purified by column chromatography (1:4 ethyl acetate–hexane; Kieselgel 60 was stirred with a 5% aq. solution of Na$_2$CO$_3$ for 1 day, then washed with water and dried in an oven under diminished pressure to get Kieselgel of pH 9–11). Yield, 0.08 g (74%), colorless syrup; $[\alpha]_D$ +29 (c 1.08, CHCl$_3$); ^{1}H NMR (CDCl$_3$) δ 7.88 (dd, 2H, Phth), 7.76 (dd, 2H, Phth), 5.92 (pseudo t, 1H, $J_{4,5}$ 9.7 Hz, H-4), 5.30 (pseudo t, 1H, $J_{5,6}$ 9.8 Hz, H-5), 5.07 (ddd, 1H, $J_{3,4}$ 9.8 Hz, H-3), 4.80 (pseudo t, 1H, $J_{1,1'}$ 1.8 Hz, $J_{1,3}$ 1.5 Hz, H-1), 4.42 (dd, 1H, $J_{7,7'}$ 12.3 Hz, H-7), 4.24 (pseudo t, 1H, $J_{1',3}$ 1.8 Hz, H-1′), 4.22 (dd, 1H, H-7′) 4.01 (ddd, 1H, $J_{6,7}$ 4.2 Hz, $J_{6,7'}$ 1.8 Hz, H-6), 2.06, 2.04, 1.87 (3 s, 9H, 3 × OAc); ^{13}C NMR (CDCl$_3$) δ 170.7, 170.0, 169.5, 167.0 (C=O), 151.9 (C-2), 131.4 (Phth quaterners), 134.6, 123.8 (Phth), 95.7 (C-1), 75.8, 70.8, 68.3 (C-4, C-5, C-6), 61.8 (C-7), 51.4 (C-3), 20.7, 20.6, 20.5 (CH$_3$); IR (KBr) $\tilde{\nu}$ 1748, 1732, 1380, 1222, 1048, 722 cm^{-1}. Anal. Calcd for C$_{21}$H$_{21}$NO$_9$: C, 58.47; H, 4.91; N, 3.25. Found: C, 58.32; H, 5.04; N, 3.12.

3,4,5-Tri-O-Acetyl-2,6-Anhydro-1-Deoxy-D-*Arabino*-Hex-1-Enitol (2d)

Prepared from **1d** (0.20 g, 0.70 mmol) and purified by flash chromatography (1:3 ethyl acetate–hexane). Yield, 0.10 g (86%) white needles; mp 98°C–100°C (from EtOAc–hexane); $[\alpha]_D$ −94 (c 0.99, CHCl$_3$); ^{1}H NMR (DMSO-d$_6$) δ 5.42 (d, 1H, $J_{3,4}$

10.0 Hz, H-3), 5.30 (ddd, 1H, $J_{5,6}$ 3.2 Hz, $J_{5,6'}$ 1.6 Hz, H-5), 5.10 (dd, 1H, $J_{4,5}$ 3.2 Hz, H-4), 4.69 (t, 1H, $J_{1,1'}$ 1.6 Hz, $J_{1,3}$ 1.6 Hz, H-1), 4.49 (t, 1H, $J_{1',3}$ 1.6 Hz, H-1'), 4.02 (dd, 1H, $J_{6,6'}$ 12.6 Hz, H-6), 3.92 (dd, 1H, H-6'), 2.12, 2.10, 1.99 (3 s, 9H, 3 × OAc); ^{13}C NMR (CDCl$_3$) δ 170.3, 170.0, 169.5 (C=O), 154.5 (C-2), 96.9 (C-1), 70.3, 67.8, 67.7 (C-3, C-4, C-5), 68.3 (C-6), 21.0, 20.9, 20.8 (CH$_3$); IR (KBr) $\tilde{v}$ 1748, 1662, 1372, 1218, 1070 cm^{-1}. Anal. Calcd for C$_{12}$H$_{16}$O$_7$: C, 53.01; H, 5.92. Found: C, 53.11; H, 5.84.

ACKNOWLEDGMENTS

Financial support from the Hungarian Scientific Research Fund (Grant: OTKA CK77712) is gratefully acknowledged. The work was also supported by the TÁMOP 4.2.1/B-09/1/KONV-2010-0007 project co-financed by the European Union and the European Social Fund.

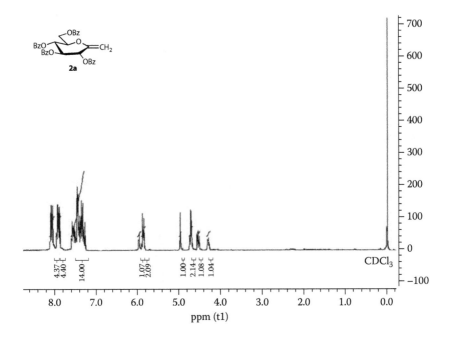

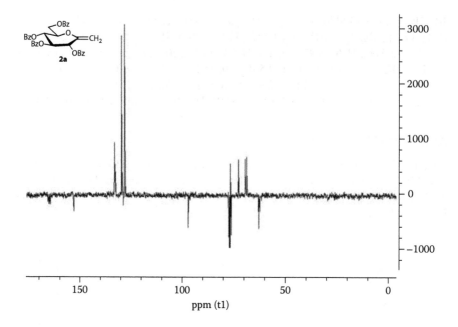

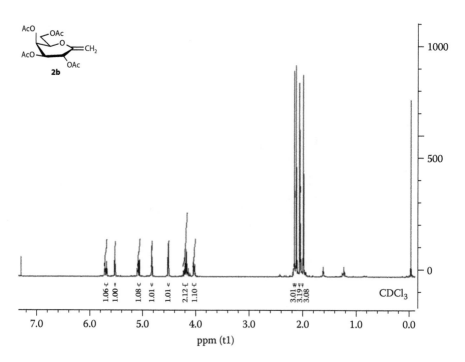

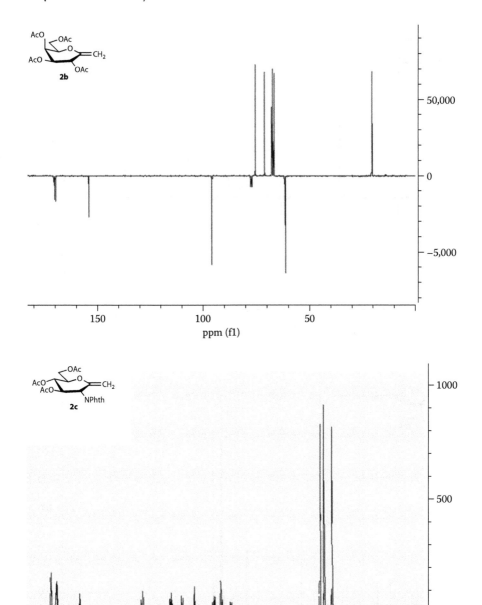

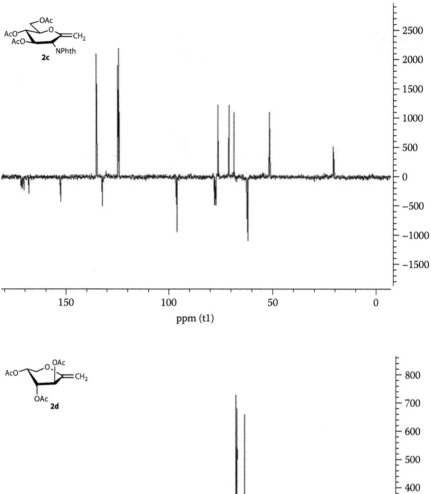

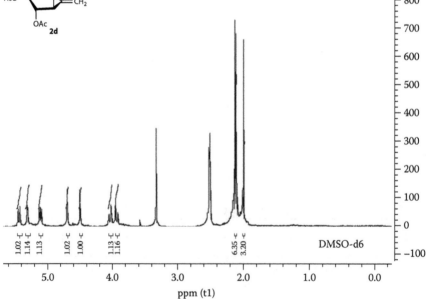

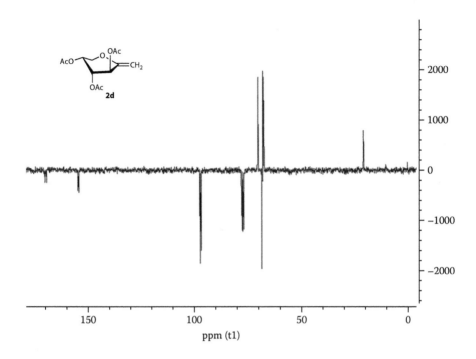

REFERENCES

1. Somsák, L. *Chem. Rev.* 2001, *101*, 81–135.
2. Priebe, W.; Grynkiewicz, G. In *Glycoscience: Chemistry and Chemical Biology*; Fraser-Reid, B.; Tatsuta, K.; Thiem, J. Eds.; Springer: Berlin, Heidelberg, Germany, 2001; pp. 749–784.
3. Tolstikov, A. G.; Tolstikov, G. A. *Usp. Khim.* 1993, *62*, 621–643.
4. Taillefumier, C.; Chapleur, Y. *Chem. Rev.* 2004, *104*, 263–292.
5. Lin, C.-H.; Lin, H.-C.; Yang, W.-B. *Curr. Top. Med. Chem.* 2005, *5*, 1431–1457.
6. Ferrier, R. J.; Hoberg, J. O. *Adv. Carbohydr. Chem. Biochem.* 2003, *58*, 55–119.
7. Gueyrard, D.; Haddoub, R.; Salem, A.; Bacar, N. S.; Goekjian, P. G. *Synlett* 2005, 520–522.
8. Tóth, M.; Somsák, L. *J. Chem. Soc. Perkin. Trans.* 2001, *1*, 942–943.
9. Tóth, M.; Kövér, K. E.; Bényei, A.; Somsák, L. *Org. Biomol. Chem.* 2003, *1*, 4039–4046.
10. Salaün, J.; Marguerite, J. *Org. Synth. Coll.* 1990, *7*, 131–135 (http://www.orgsyn.org/orgsyn/pdfs/CV7P0131.pdf).
11. Brockhaus, M.; Lehmann, J. *Carbohydr. Res.* 1977, *53*, 21–31.
12. Fritz, H.; Lehmann, J.; Schlesselmann, P. *Carbohydr. Res.* 1983, *113*, 71–92.

REFERENCES

42 Synthesis of O-(6-Deoxy-α- and β-L-Galactopyranosyl) Hydroxylamines (α- and β-L-Fucopyranosyl-hydroxylamines)

Isabelle Bossu, Barbara Richichi,[†]
Pascal Dumy, and Olivier Renaudet*

CONTENTS

Experimental Methods 378
   General Methods 378
      O-(2,3,4-Tri-*O*-Acetyl-6-Deoxy-α-ʟ-Galactopyranosyl)-*N*-
      Hydroxyphthalimide (**2**) and *O*-(2,3,4-Tri-*O*-Acetyl-6-Deoxy-β-ʟ-
      Galactopyranosyl)-*N*-Hydroxyphthalimide (**3**) 379
      O-(6-Deoxy-α-ʟ-Galactopyranosyl)Hydroxylamine
      (*O*-α-ʟ-Fucopyranosylhydroxylamine) (**4**) 380
      O-(6-Deoxy-β-ʟ-Galactopyranosyl)Hydroxylamine
      (*O*-β-ʟ-Fucopyranosylhydroxylamine) (**5**) 380
Acknowledgments 381
References 385

* Corresponding author.
† Checker.

Synthesis of O-(6-Deoxy-α- and β-L-Galactopyranosyl)Hydroxylamines(α- and β-L-Fucopyranosylhydroxylamines).

In the last decade, chemoselective oxime ligation has proved to be an attractive synthetic strategy in glycochemistry.[1] For example, many glycosylhydroxylamines have been efficiently conjugated through oxime linkage to aldehyde or ketone-containing biomolecules such as peptides[2] or oligonucleotides.[3] These key building blocks were also shown useful for the preparation of combinatorial libraries[4] and antitumoral synthetic vaccines,[5] for the immobilization of glycoclusters on surfaces,[6] for chemical engineering,[7] or for the construction of diverse other neoglycoconjugates.[8] Thus, a simple and efficient synthetic method that ensures direct incorporation of anomeric hydroxylamine functionality is essential to achieve that purpose.

Synthesis of glycosylhydroxylamines from glycosyl bromides using phase transfer catalysis in high yields and stereoselectivity has been previously described.[9] More recently, we have reported a complementary strategy that allows the formation of both alpha and beta glycosylhydroxylamine,[10] which is essential to assess the influence of anomeric configuration in biological processes. Because of the involvement of fucosylated glycoconjugates in a wide range of biological processes,[11] we exemplify herein the efficiency of this strategy with the synthesis of the title O-(6-deoxy-L-galactopyranosyl)hydroxylamines 4 and 5. It has to be noted that the glycosylation stereoselectivity may vary since it strongly depends on the anomeric ratio of the starting fluoride derivative (1).[10c]

EXPERIMENTAL METHODS

GENERAL METHODS

All chemical reagents and dry dichloromethane were purchased from Aldrich (Saint Quentin Fallavier, France) or Acros (Noisy-Le-Grand, France) and were used without further purification. Progress of reactions was monitored by thin-layer chromatography using silica gel $60\,F_{254}$ precoated plates (Merck). Spots were visualized by UV light and by charring with 10% H_2SO_4 in EtOH for protected derivatives or 1% ninhydrine in EtOH for hydroxylamine derivatives. Silica gel 60 (0.063–0.2 mm or 70–230 mesh, Merck) was used for column chromatography. Optical rotations were measured with a Perkin-Elmer 241 polarimeter. Melting points were measured on a Büchi melting point apparatus (model B545). ^{1}H- and ^{13}C-NMR spectra were recorded on Bruker AC300 spectrometers and chemical shifts (δ) were reported in parts per million (ppm). Spectra were referenced to the residual proton solvent peaks relative to the signal of $CDCl_3$ (δ 7.27 and 77.23 ppm for ^{1}H- and ^{13}C-NMR, respectively) or relative to the signal of D_2O (δ 4.79 ppm for ^{1}H-NMR). Proton and carbon assignments were done by GCOSY and GHMQC experiments. The anomeric configuration was established from $J_{1,2}$ coupling constants. High-resolution mass spectra (HRMS) were recorded at the University of Bern (Switzerland) by electron spray ionization (ESI) on an Applied Biosystems/Sciex QSTAR Pulsar in the positive mode.

O-(2,3,4-Tri-*O*-Acetyl-6-Deoxy-α-ʟ-Galactopyranosyl)-*N*-Hydroxyphthalimide (2) and *O*-(2,3,4-Tri-*O*-Acetyl-6-Deoxy-β-ʟ-Galactopyranosyl)-*N*-Hydroxyphthalimide (3)

2,3,4-tri-*O*-acetyl-6-deoxy-ʟ-galactopyranosyl fluoride (**1**, anomeric mixture, α/β, 1/4, 490 mg, 1.68 mmol), *N*-hydroxyphthalimide (273 mg, 1.68 mmol, 1 equiv.), and triethylamine (233 μL, 1.68 mmol, 1 equiv.) were added to a stirred suspension of 4 Å molecular sieves in dry CH_2Cl_2 (5 mL). After the addition of $BF_3 \cdot Et_2O$ (850 μL, 6.71 mmol, 4 equiv.), the solution was stirred at room temperature (rt) under argon gas. After 30 min, TLC indicated complete disappearance of the fluoride derivative (**1**). CH_2Cl_2 (10 mL) was added, and the organic layer was washed with 10% $NaHCO_3$ (3×30 mL), which made the aqueous phase colorless, and brine (2×30 mL). The organic phase was dried over $MgSO_4$, filtered and concentrated under reduced pressure. The resulting yellow oil, containing a mixture of **2** and **3**, was chromatographed (20% → 40% EtOAc–pentane).*

O-(2,3,4-Tri-*O*-acetyl-6-deoxy-α-ʟ-galactopyranosyl)-*N*-hydroxyphthalimide (**2**) was precipitated by dropping its solution in ether into stirred pentane to give a white, amorphous solid (253 mg, 35%, 0.58 mmol); R_f=0.46 (2:3 EtOAc–pentane)†; ^{1}H NMR ($CDCl_3$): δ 7.87–7.76 (m, 4H, H_{Pht}), 5.59 (dd, 1H, $J_{1,2}$ 3.9 Hz, H-1), 5.55 (dd, 1H, $J_{3,4}$ 3.3 Hz, $J_{2,3}$ 11.2 Hz, H-3), 5.45 (dd, 1H, $J_{4,5}$ 1.1 Hz, $J_{3,4}$ 3.3 Hz, H-4), 5.27(dd, 1H, $J_{1,2}$ 3.9 Hz, $J_{2,3}$ 11.2 Hz, H-2), 5.09 (bq, 1H, $J_{5,6}$ 6.3 Hz), 2.23 (s, 3H, $COCH_3$), 2.20 (s, 3H, $COCH_3$), 2.05 (s, 3H, $COCH_3$), 1.21 (d, 3H, $J_{5,6}$ 6.3 Hz, CH_3); ^{13}C NMR ($CDCl_3$): δ 171.2 ($C=O_{Ac}$), 170.8 ($C=O_{Ac}$), 170.2 ($C=O_{Ac}$), 163.5 ($C=O_{Pht}$), 135.1 (CH_{Pht}), 129.2 (C_{Pht}), 124.1 (CH_{Pht}), 102.5 (C-1), 71.3 (C-4), 67.6 (C-2 or C-3), 67.5

---

* Analytical RP-HPLC shows α/β=1/1.2 (column: Nucleosil 120 Å 3 μm C_{18} particles, 30×4.6 mm²; flow: 1.3 mL/min; UV monitoring: 214 and 250 nm; linear A–B gradient 5% → 100% B in 15 min, A: 0.09% CF_3CO_2H in water; B: 0.09% CF_3CO_2H in 90% acetonitrile). The α/β ratio, which may vary from preparation to preparation, can also be established by NMR spectroscopy.

† The $[\alpha]_D$ of the compound obtained from different preparations, varied between −204° and −211° (*c* ~ 1, $CHCl_3$).

(C-2 or C-3), 67.4 (C-5), 21.2 ($COCH_3$), 21.1 ($COCH_3$), 20.9 ($COCH_3$), 16.2 (CH_3); ESI⁺-HRMS: $[M+Na]^+$ calcd for $C_{20}H_{21}NO_{10}Na$: 458.1063; found: 458.1058. Anal. calcd for $C_{20}H_{21}NO_{10}$: C, 55.17; H, 4.86; N, 3.22. Found: C 55.0; H, 4.75; N, 3.14.

O-(2,3,4-Tri-O-acetyl-6-deoxy-β-L-galactopyranosyl)-N-hydroxyphthalimide (**3**) was precipitated by dropping its solution in CH_2Cl_2 into pentane (367 mg, 50%, 0.84 mmol); R_f=0.32 (2:3 EtOAc–pentane);* ¹H NMR ($CDCl_3$): δ 7.90–7.77 (m, 4H, H_{Pht}), 5.46 (dd, 1H, $J_{1,2}$ 8.3 Hz, $J_{2,3}$ 10.3 Hz, H-2) 5.29–5.27 (m, 1H, H-4), 5.12 (dd, 1H, $J_{3,4}$ 3.4 Hz, $J_{2,3}$ 10.3 Hz, H-3), 4.99 (d, 1H, $J_{1,2}$ 8.3 Hz, H-1), 3.84 (bq, 1H, $J_{5,6}$ 6.3 Hz), 2.24 (s, 3H, $COCH_3$), 2.23 (s, 3H, $COCH_3$), 2.03 (s, 3H, $COCH_3$), 1.27 (d, 3H, $J_{5,6}$ 6.3 Hz, CH_3); ¹³C NMR ($CDCl_3$): δ 171.2 (C=O_{Ac}), 170.5 (C=O_{Ac}), 170.3 (C=O_{Ac}), 163.1 (C=O_{Pht}), 135.1 (CH_{Pht}), 129.2 (C_{Pht}), 124.2 (CH_{Pht}), 106.8 (C-1), 71.4 (C-3), 70.6 (C-5), 70.1 (C-4), 67.5 (C-2), 21.2 ($COCH_3$), 21.1 ($COCH_3$), 20.9 ($COCH_3$), 16.4 (CH_3); ESI⁺-HRMS: $[M+Na]^+$ calcd for $C_{20}H_{21}NO_{10}Na$: 458.1063; found: 458.1079. Anal. calcd for $C_{20}H_{21}NO_{10}$: C, 55.17; H, 4.86; N, 3.22. Found: C 55.03; H, 4.59; N, 3.13.

O-(6-Deoxy-α-L-Galactopyranosyl)Hydroxylamine (O-α-L-Fucopyranosylhydroxylamine) (4)†

O-(2,3,6-Tri-O-acetyl-6-deoxy-α-L-galactopyranosyl)-N-hydroxyphthalimide (**2**) (520 mg, 1.20 mmol) was dissolved in EtOH (3 mL) containing methylhydrazine (3.1 mL, 60 mmol, 50 equiv.).‡ After stirring overnight at rt, the solvent was evaporated with a high vacuum pump, and the residue was stirred with absolute EtOH (2 mL) for 30–60 min at rt§ to give pure, amorphous O-(6-deoxy-α-L-galactopyranosyl)hydroxylamine (**4**), 55%–77%.¶ R_f=0.15 (3:7 EtOH–CH_2Cl_2); ¹H NMR (CD_3OD) δ: 4.86 (d, 1H, $J_{1,2}$=4.4 Hz, H-1), 3.99 (bq, 1H, $J_{5,6}$=6.4 Hz, H-5) 3.76 (dd, 1H, $J_{3,4}$=4.0 Hz, $J_{3,2}$=10.0 Hz, H-3), 3.67–3.63 (m, 2H, H-2, H-4), 1.21 (d, 1H, $J_{5,6}$=6.4 Hz, CH_3); ¹³C NMR (CD_3OD) δ: 104.9 (C-1), 74.5 (C-4), 72.4 (C-2), 70.5 (C-3), 68.5 (C-5), 17.4 (CH_3); ESI⁺-HRMS: $[M+H]^+$ calcd for $C_6H_{14}NO_5$, 180.0871; found: 180.0866. Anal. calcd for $C_6H_{13}NO_5$: C, 40.22; H, 7.31; N, 7.82. Found: C, 39.91; H, 7.69; N, 7.50.

O-(6-Deoxy-β-L-Galactopyranosyl)Hydroxylamine (O-β-L-Fucopyranosylhydroxylamine) (5)*

To a stirred solution of methylhydrazine (4.58 g, 5.23 mL, 99.48 mmol) in EtOH (5.0 mL), **3** (865 mg, 1.98 mmol) was added. After stirring overnight at rt, the solvent was evaporated under reduced pressure. The white solid obtained was suspended in absolute EtOH (10.0 mL) vigorously stirred for 30 min at rt, filtered and washed with

---

* The $[\alpha]_D$ of the compound obtained from different preparations, varied between +10° and +14° ($c \sim 1$, $CHCl_3$).

† Caution: Due to the high reactivity of hydroxylamine with aldehydes and ketones, acetone should not be used for labware washing.

‡ If methylhydrazine is not available, this reagent can be freshly prepared following published procedures [12].

§ A longer time may lead to crystallization of the 1,2-benzenedioic acid N-methylhydrazide (R_f=0.9, EtOH-CH_2Cl_2 3:7, UV detection).

¶ The yield varies depending of the amount of EtOH needed for washing the solid, to remove the UV positive material. The $[\alpha]_D$ of the compound obtained from different preparations varied between −177° and −204°; ($c \sim 1$, H_2O).

absolute EtOH (20.0 mL) to give pure O-(6-deoxy-β-L-galactopyranosyl)hydrox-
ylamine (**5**, 248 mg, 70%) as white solid*; R_f=0.15 (3:7 EtOH–CH$_2$Cl$_2$); ^{1}H NMR
(D$_2$O) δ 4.53 (d, 1H, $J_{1,2}$=8.1 Hz, H-1), 3.87 (bq, 1H, $J_{5,6}$=6.4 Hz, H-5), 3.81–3.79
(m, 1H, H-4), 3.71 (dd, 1H, $J_{3,4}$=3.3 Hz, $J_{2,3}$=9.6 Hz, H-3), 3.55 (dd, 1H, $J_{1,2}$=8.1 Hz,
$J_{2,3}$=9.6 Hz, H-2), 1.33 (d, 3H, $J_{5,6}$=6.4 Hz, CH$_3$); ^{13}C NMR (D$_2$O): δ 105.9 (C-1), 73.4
(C-3), 71.7 (C-4), 71.2 (C-5), 69.5 (C-2), 15.7 (CH$_3$); ESI$^+$-HRMS: [M+H]$^+$ calcd for
C$_6$H$_{14}$NO$_5$, 180.0871; found: 180.0875. Anal. calcd for C$_6$H$_{13}$NO$_5$: C, 40.22; H, 7.31;
N, 7.82. Found: C, 40.13; H, 6.91; N, 7.79.

ACKNOWLEDGMENTS

This chapter was supported by the Université Joseph Fourier, the Centre National de
la Recherche Scientifique (CNRS) and COST D-34. We are grateful to the NanoBio
program for access to the facilities of the Synthesis platform.

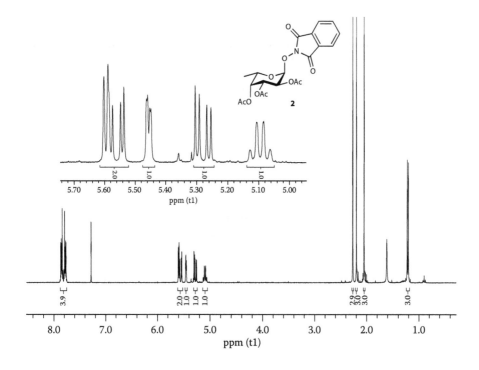

---

* The [α]$_D$ of the compound obtained from different preparations varied between +14° and −25° (c ~ 1).

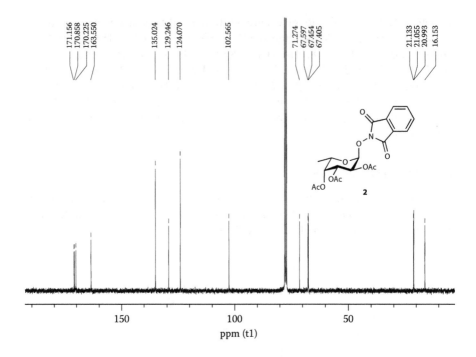

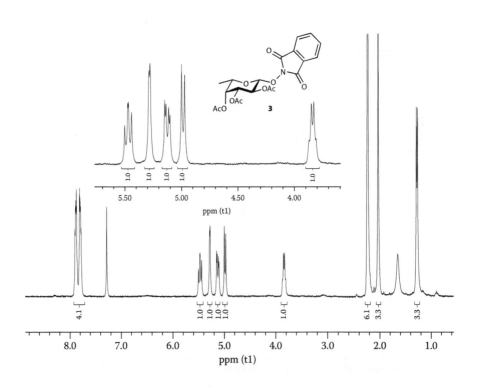

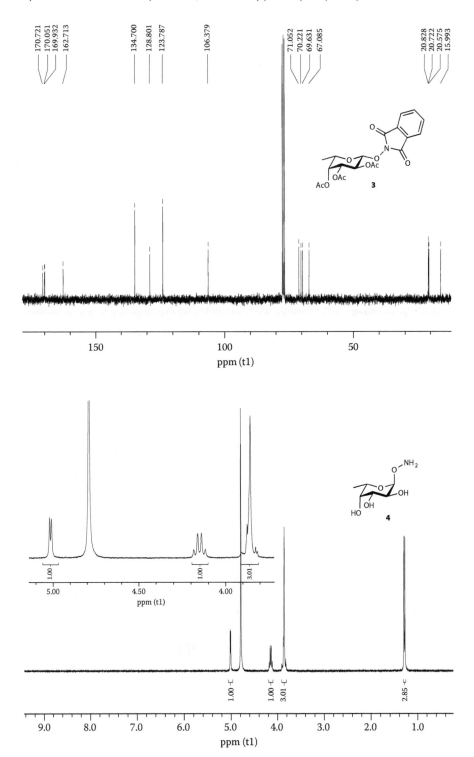

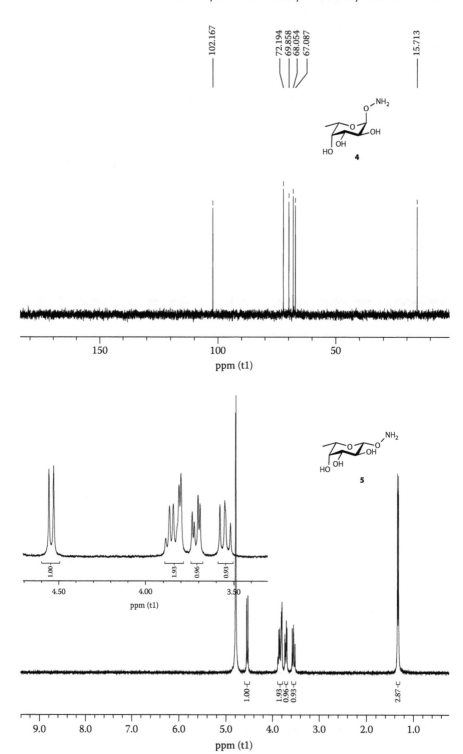

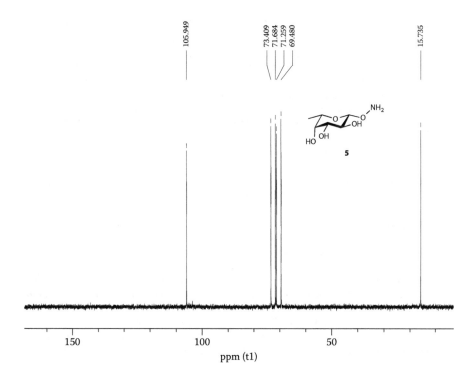

REFERENCES

1. (a) Roy, R. The chemistry of neoglycoconjugates. In *Carbohydrate Chemistry*, Boons, G.-J. (Ed.). Blackie Academic & Professional, London, U.K., 1998, pp. 243–321. (b) Hang, H.; Bertozzi, C. R. *Acc. Chem. Res.* 2001, *34*, 727–736. (c) Peri, F.; Nicotra, F. *Chem. Commun.* 2004, *6*, 623–627. (d) Langenhan, J. M.; Thorson, J. S. *Curr. Org. Synth.* 2005, *2*, 59–81. (e) Renaudet, O. *Mini-Rev. Org. Chem.* 2008, *5*, 274–286.

2. (a) Rodriguez, E. C.; Winans, K. A.; King, D. S.; Bertozzi, C. R. *J. Am. Chem. Soc.* 1997, *119*, 9905–9906. (b) Rodriguez, E. C.; Marcaurelle, L. A.; Bertozzi, C. R. *J. Org. Chem.* 1998, *63*, 7134–7135. (c) Marcaurelle, L. A.; Shin, Y.; Goon, S.; Bertozzi, C. R. *Org. Lett.* 2001, *3*, 3691–3694. (d) Lagnoux, D.; Darbre, T.; Lienhard Schmitz, M.; Reymond, J.-L. *Chem. Eur. J.* 2005, *11*, 3941–3950. (e) Renaudet O.; Dumy, P. *Org. Lett.* 2003, *5*, 243–245. (f) Renaudet O.; Dumy, P. *Bioorg. Med. Chem. Lett.* 2005, *15*, 3619–3622. (g) Singh, Y.; Renaudet, O.; Defrancq, E.; Dumy, P. *Org. Lett.* 2005, *7*, 1359–1362. (h) Garanger, E.; Boturyn, D.; Renaudet, O.; Defrancq, E.; Dumy, P. *J. Org. Chem.* 2006, *71*, 2402–2410. (i) Renaudet, O.; Boturyn, D.; Dumy, P. *Bioorg. Med. Chem. Lett.* 2009, *19*, 3880–3883.

3. (a) Forget, D.; Renaudet, O.; Defrancq, E.; Dumy, P. *Tetrahedron Lett.* 2001, *42*, 7829–7832. (b) Forget, D.; Renaudet, O.; Boturyn, D.; Defrancq, E.; Dumy, P. *Tetrahedron Lett.* 2001, *42*, 9171–9174. (c) Edupuganti, O. P.; Renaudet, O.; Defrancq, E.; Dumy, P. *Bioorg. Med. Chem. Lett.* 2004, *14*, 2839–2842.

4. (a) Renaudet, O.; Reymond, J.-L. *Org. Lett.* 2003, *5*, 4693–4696. (b) Duléry, V.; Renaudet, O.; Wilczewski, M.; Van der Heyden, A.; Labbé, P.; Dumy, P. *J. Comb. Chem.* 2008, *10*, 368–371. (c) Ruff, Y.; Lehn, J. M. *Biopolymers* 2008, *89*, 486–496.

5. (a) Grigalevicius, S.; Chierici, S.; Renaudet, O.; Lo-Man, R.; Dériaud, E.; Leclerc, C.; Dumy, P. *Bioconjugate Chem.* 2005, *5*, 1149–1159. (b) Renaudet, O.; BenMohamed, L.; Dasgupta, G.; Bettahi, I.; Dumy, P. *ChemMedChem* 2008, *3*, 737–741. (c) Bettahi, I.; Dasgupta, G.; Renaudet, O.; Chentoufi, A. A.; Zhang, X.; Carpenter, D.; Yoon, S.; Dumy, P.; BenMohamed, L. *Cancer Immunol. Immunother.* 2009, *58*, 187–200.

6. (a) Renaudet, O.; Dumy, P. *Org. Biomol. Chem.* 2006, *4*, 2628–2636. (b) Dubois, M. P.; Gondran, C.; Renaudet, O; Dumy, P.; Driguez, H.; Fort, S.; Cosnier, S. *Chem. Comm.* 2005, *34*, 4318–4320. (c) Wilczewski, M.; Van der Heyden, A.; Renaudet, O.; Dumy, P.; Coche-Guéerente, L.; Labbé, P. *Org. Biomol. Chem.* 2008, *6*, 1114–1122. (d) Dendane, N.; Hoang, A.; Renaudet, O.; Vinet, F.; Dumy, P.; Defrancq, E. *Lab Chip* 2008, *8*, 2161–2163.

7. (a) Chen, X.; Lee, G. S.; Zettl, A.; Bertozzi, C. R. *Angew. Chem. Int. Ed.* 2004, *43*, 6112–6116. (b) Yarema, K. J.; Mahal, L. K.; Bruehl, R. E.; Rodriguez, E. C.; Bertozzi, C. R. *J. Biol. Chem.* 1998, *273*, 31168–31179.

8. (a) Andreana, P. R.; Xie, W.; Cheng, H. N.; Qiao, L.; Murphy, D. J.; Gu, Q.-M.; Wang, P. G. *Org. Lett.* 2002, *4*, 1863–1866. (b) Tejler, J.; Leffler, H.; Nilsson, U. J. *Bioorg. Med. Chem. Lett.* 2005, *15*, 2343–2345. (c) Brunner, H.; Schönherr, M.; Zabel, M. *Tetrahedron: Asymmetry* 2003, *14*, 1115; (d) Mitchell, M. B.; Whitcombe, I. W. A. *Tetrahedron Lett.* 2000, *41*, 8829–8834. (e) Liu, H.; Wang, L.; Brock, A.; Wong, C.-H.; Schultz, P. G. *J. Am. Chem. Soc.* 2003, *125*, 1702–1703. (f) Renaudet, O.; Dumy, P. *Eur. J. Org. Chem.* 2008, 5383–5386.

9. Cao, S.; Tropper, F. D.; Roy, R. *Tetrahedron* 1995, *51*, 6679–6686.

10. (a) Renaudet O.; Dumy, P. *Tetrahedron Lett.* 2001, *42*, 7575–7578. (b) Renaudet O.; Dumy, P. *Tetrahedron Lett.* 2004, *45*, 65–68. (c) Duléry, V.; Renaudet, O.; Dumy, P. *Carbohydr. Res.* 2007, *342*, 894–900.

11. (a) Simanek, E. E.; McGarvey, G. J.; Jablonowski, J. A.; Wong, C.-H. *Chem. Rev.* 1998, *98*, 833–862. (b) Ilver, D.; Arnqvist, A.; Ogren, J.; Frick, I.-M.; Kersulyte, D.; Incecik, E. T.; Berg, D. E.; Covacci, A.; Engstrand, L.; Thomas Borén, T. *Science* 1998, *279*, 373–377. (c) Fukuda, M. *Cancer Res.* 1996, *56*, 2237–2244. (d) Mitchell, E.; Houles, C.; Sudakevitz, D.; Wimmerova, M.; Gautier, C.; Pérez, S.; Wu, A. M.; Gilboa-Garber N.; Imberty, A. *Nature Struct. Biol.* 2002, *9*, 918–921.

12. (a) Jain, R. S.; Mathur, M. A.; Sisler, H. H. *Inorg. Chem.* 1980, *19*, 2192–2195. (b) Horvitz, D. Preparation of methylhydrazine, 1963, US Patent 3113152. (c) Shiro, H.; Yoichi, H.; Takeo, H. Process for preparation of monomethylhydrazine, 1989, US Patent 4855501.

43 Functionalization of Terminal Positions of Sucrose—Part I: Synthesis of 2,3,3',4,4'-Penta-O-Benzylsucrose and Differentiation of the Terminal Positions (1,6,6')

Mateusz Mach, A. Zawisza,[†]
*B. Lewandowski, and S. Jarosz**

CONTENTS

Experimental Methods 389
   General Methods 389
      1',6,6'-Tri-O-Tritylsucrose (**2**) 390
      2,3,3',4,4'-Penta-O-Benzyl-1',6,6'-Tri-O-Tritylsucrose (**3**)........................ 391
      2,3,3',4,4'-Penta-O-Benzylsucrose (**4**).. 391
      2,3,3',4,4'-Penta-O-Benzyl-6,6'-Di-O-p-Nitrobenzoylsucrose (**5**) 392
      2,3,3',4,4'-Penta-O-Benzyl-1'-O-Benzyloxymethyl-6,6'-Di-O-p-
      Nitrobenzoylsucrose (**6**) 392
      2,3,3',4,4'-Penta-O-Benzyl-1'-O-Benzyloxymethylsucrose (**7**) 392
      2,3,3',4,4'-Penta-O-Benzyl-1'-O-Benzyloxymethyl-6'-O-Tert-
      Butyldiphenylsilylsucrose (**8**).. 393

* Corresponding author.
† Checker.

1'-*O*-Benzyloxymethyl-6,6'-Di-*O*-*Tert*-Butyldiphenylsilyl-2,3,3',4,4'-
Penta-*O*-Benzylsucrose (**9**)..393
2,3,3',4,4'-Penta-*O*-Benzyl-1'-*O*-Benzyloxymethyl-6-*O*-*Tert*-
Butyldiphenylsilylsucrose (**10**)..394
References..411

Sucrose is by far the cheapest and most common disaccharide, exploited mainly by the food industry. Its derivatives have also found application in other areas: surfactants, biodegradable polymers, biochemistry, and supramolecular chemistry.[1] Thus, sucrose has become a useful synthon for advanced materials in many research laboratories. There is, however, only a limited number of communications describing chemical transformations of sucrose in detail. This results mostly from insufficient knowledge of important factors (steric, electronic, etc.) that control selectivity and reactivity of individual functional groups of this disaccharide. Several examples of selective transformations of hydroxyl groups of sucrose were described in a recent review.[1] Most of the methodologies involve simple etherification, esterification, and oxidation reactions. Clearly, there is a need for synthetic procedures, which would provide sucrose derivatives with high added value. The following chapters provide such procedures, leading to sucrose derivatives modified at the terminal positions.

The synthetic efforts in our laboratory have been focused on functionalization of sucrose molecule that allows preparation of analogs modified at any terminal position (C6, C6', or C1'). This required protection of secondary hydroxyl groups that would be easily removable under other than acidic conditions (since the glycosidic bond of sucrose is very sensitive toward acid hydrolysis) and sufficiently stable during subsequent preparation of analogs. We have proposed a three-step procedure to prepare 2,3,3',4,4'-penta-*O*-benzylsucrose (**4**), having all terminal positions (C-6,1',6') unprotected.[2] Tritylation of the primary hydroxyl groups of sucrose with 3.5 eqv. of trityl chloride afforded the 6,1',6'-tri-*O*-tritylsucrose (**2**) in high yield.* Subsequent benzylation of **2** with benzyl bromide, followed by removal of the trityl groups under controlled conditions, allowed us to obtain compound **4**. The final step proved to be very demanding because of very high sensitivity of the glycosidic bond of sucrose toward hydrolysis. We have found that the desired product of detritylation could be obtained in *ca.* 60% yield when detritylation was effected with an acetic acid–toluene–water mixture (Scheme 43.1).

Compound **4** served as starting material for the preparation of a series of sucrose derivatives with different substitution pattern at the terminal positions (Scheme 43.2).[4] The Mitsunobu reaction performed on **4**, using 2.2 eqv. of *p*-nitrobenzoic acid afforded the diester **5** in 75% yield. Subsequent protection of the *O*-1' with (freshly prepared) benzyloxymethyl chloride followed by hydrolysis of the ester groups under the Zemplen conditions led to the diol **7**. The 6 and 6' positions in such derivative were differentiated using *tert*-butyldiphenylsilyl chloride. Reaction of **7** with 1.2 eqv. of the silylating agent led to compound **8** having the silyl group at the 6' position (65% yield). Formation of the monosubstituted regioisomer **10** with the 6-OH protection

---

* Protection of all primary hydroxyl groups can be achieved also with silyl chloride as reported by Khan, who prepared 6,1',6'-tri-*O*-silylatedsucrose in good yield [3].

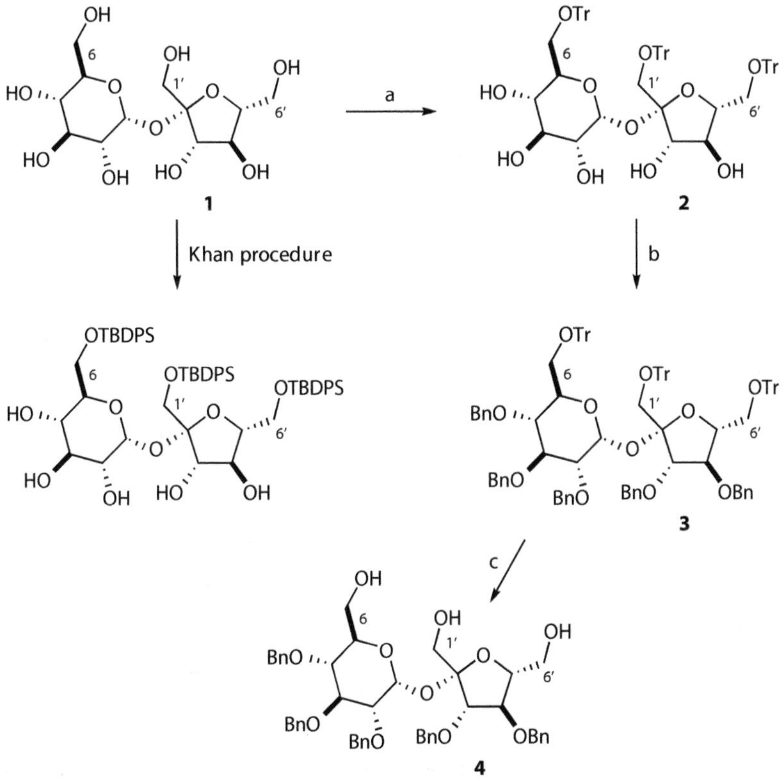

SCHEME 43.1 Preparation of 2,3,3′,4,4′-penta-*O*-benzylsucrose. a. TrCl (3.5 eqv.), DMAP, Py, 80%; b. BnBr, NaH, DMF, 98%; c. AcOH/H$_2$O, 60%.

was not observed. Reaction of the diol **7** with excess of silyl chloride (TBDPSCl) furnished the double protected derivative **9**. This compound was *selectively* deprotected at the 6′-position, giving the regioisomeric 2,3,3′,4,4′-penta-*O*-benzyl-1′-*O*-benzyloxymethyl-6-*O*-*tert*-butyldimethylsilylsucrose (**10**) in 85% yield over two steps.

EXPERIMENTAL METHODS

GENERAL METHODS

Nuclear magnetic resonance (NMR) spectra were recorded in CDCl$_3$ (internal Me$_4$Si) at 303 K with a Bruker Avance III 600 MHz spectrometer (operating at 600.262 and 150.936 MHz for ^{1}H and ^{13}C, respectively).

Mass spectra (ESI) were recorded with PE SCIEX API 365 or Mariner PerSeptive Biosystems apparatus. Optical rotations were measured at room temperature (rt) with a digital Jasco polarimeter DIP-360 for solutions in chloroform ($c = 1$). Column chromatography was performed on silica gel (Merck, 70–230 or 230–400 mesh). THF was distilled from potassium prior to use. Solutions in organic solvents were dried over anhydrous sodium or magnesium sulfate and concentrated at diminished pressure.

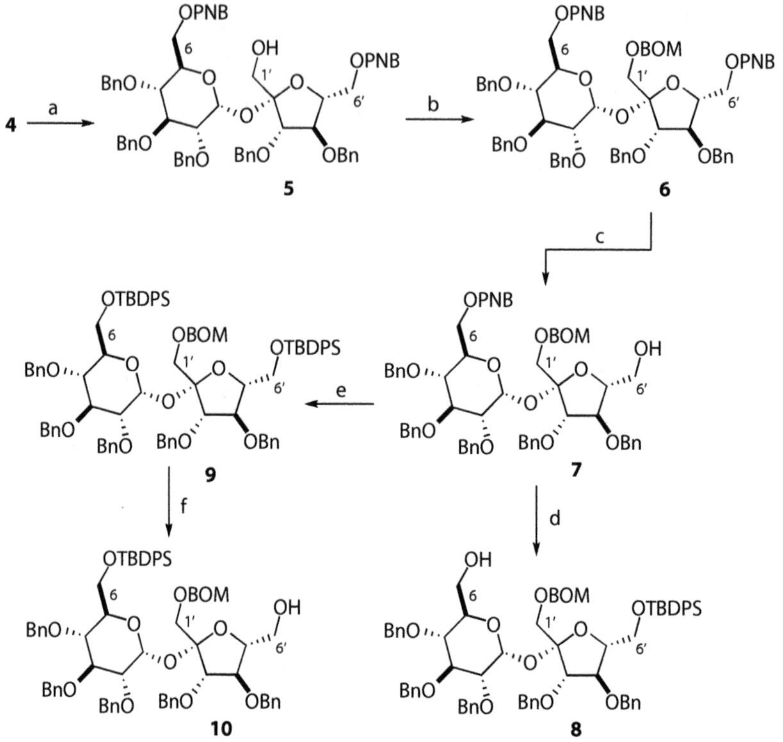

SCHEME 43.2 Functionalization of terminal positions of penta-O-benzylsucrose. a. p-nitrobenzoic acid, DEAD, Ph_3P, Py, 73%; b. BOMCI, py, 80%; c. MeONa, MeOH, 65%; d. TBDPSCI (1.2 eqv.), DMAP, DIPEA, CH_2Cl_2, 70%; e. TBDPSCI 3 eqv., DMAP, DIPEA, CH_2Cl_2, 95%; f. HF/PY (1 eqv.), MeOH/Et_2O, 68%.

Acetylation reactions were carried out in dry methylene chloride with acetic anhydride, in presence of pyridine or triethylamine.

1′,6,6′-Tri-O-Tritylsucrose (2)

Sucrose (**1**, 20 g, 0.0584 mol) was dissolved in boiling pyridine (120 mL). DMAP (1 g, 4.18 mmol) and trityl chloride were added (60 g, 0.2162 mol), and the mixture was stirred for 12 h at 60°C–70°C. Pyridine was evaporated and the residue was partitioned between EtOAc (500 mL) and water (200 mL). The organic layer was washed with water (2 × 100 mL) and brine (100 mL), dried, and concentrated, and the residue was chromatographed (2:1 → 1:1 hexane–EtOAc, containing 1% of methanol) to afford 1′,6,6′-tri-O-tritylsucrose (**2**) as white solid (47–50 g, 75%–80%), mp. 233°C–234°C. ESI-MS: 1091 [M($C_{69}H_{64}O_{11}$) +Na$^+$].

This compound was characterized as a pentaacetate*: [α]$_D$ +70.7. ^{1}H NMR δ: 5.83 (d, $J_{3',4'}$ = 5.4 Hz, 1H, H-3′), 5.36 (dd, 1H, $J_{3',4'}$ = 5.4 Hz, H-4′), 5.31 (d, $J_{1,2}$ = 4.2 Hz, 1H,

---

* In general, all sucrose derivatives containing the free hydroxyl groups were converted into acetate(s), since the resonances in the ^{1}H- NMR spectra of the acetates were better resolved than in the spectra of the parent alcohols.

H-1), 5.23 (dd, $J_{3,4}$=9.6 Hz, $J_{4,5}$=8.7 Hz, 1H, H-4), 5.19 (dd, $J_{2,3}$=9.6 Hz, $J_{3,4}$=9.6 Hz, 1H, H-3), 4.80 (dd, 1H, $J_{2,3}$=9.6 Hz, H-2), 4.12 (dd, $J_{4',5'}$=5.0 Hz, $J_{5',6'}$=6.0 Hz, 1H, H-5'), 3.97 (dd, $J_{4,5}$=9.6 Hz, $J_{5,6A}$=2.4 Hz, 1H, H-5), 3.37 and 3.27 (2H, $J_{1'A,1'B}$=10.6 Hz, H-1'), 3.32 and 3.29 (2H, $J_{6'A,6'B}$=10.8 Hz, H-6'), 3.17 and 2.76 (2H, $J_{5,6}$=1.8 and 3.0 Hz, $J_{6A,6B}$=10.2 Hz, H-6), 1.98, 1.96, 1.93, 1.91, 1.59 (5×s, 5×3H, 5×OAc).

^{13}C NMR δ: 170.2, 169.9, 169.5, 169.5, 168.8 (5×$\underline{C}$O), 105.4 (C-2'), 90.1 (C-1), 87.1, 86.9, 86.1 (C$_q$ trityl), 80.0, 76.2, 76.2, 70.8, 70.0, 69.2, 68.4 (C-2,3,3',4,4',5,5'), 63.9, 63.0, 60.6 (C-1',6,6'), 20.9, 20.8, 20.6, 20.5, 20.4 (5×OC(O)$\underline{C}$H$_3$).

Anal: Calcd for C$_{79}$H$_{74}$O$_{16}$: C, 74.16; H, 5.88. Found: C, 74.0; H, 5.9.

2,3,3',4,4'-Penta-O-Benzyl-1',6,6'-Tri-O-Tritylsucrose (3)

6,6'-Di-O-tritylsucrose (2, 62.5 g, 0.0585 mol) and imidazole (0.1 g, 1.5 mmol) were dissolved in DMF (200 mL) and cooled to 0°C–5°C (ice-water bath). Sodium hydride (60% dispersion in mineral oil, 23.4 g) was added in several portions with stirring. After 30 min, benzyl bromide (41.7 mL, 0.351 mol) was added dropwise (in such a rate to keep the temperature below 40°C), and the mixture was stirred at rt for 2 h. Excess of hydride was destroyed by careful addition of water and the mixture was partitioned between water (200 mL) and diethyl ether (300 mL). The layers were separated, the aqueous phase was extracted with diethyl ether (2×200 mL), the combined organic extracts were washed with water (3×200 mL) and brine (100 mL), dried, and concentrated. Column chromatography (20:1 → 9:1 hexane–EtOAc) of the residue provided 1',6,6'-tri-O-trityl-2,3,3',4,4'-penta-O-benzylsucrose in virtually theoretical yield, mp. 98°C–100°C (Et$_2$O–MeOH), [α]$_D$ +17.7. ^{1}H NMR δ: 6.36 (d, $J_{1,2}$=3.6 Hz, 1H, H-1). ^{13}C NMR δ: 104.2 (C-2'), 88.1 (C-1), 87.1, 86.7, 85.9 (C$_q$ trityl), 84.6, 82.0, 80.5, 79.4, 78.3, 77.6, 70.8 (C-2,3,3',4,4',5,5'), 75.8, 74.7, 73.1, 72.4, 71.9 (5×O$\underline{C}$H$_2$Ph), 67.1, 62.1, 61.8 (C-1',6,6'). ESI-MS: 1542 [M(C$_{104}$H$_{94}$O$_{11}$) +Na$^+$].

Anal: Calcd for C$_{104}$H$_{94}$O$_{11}$: C, 82.19; H, 6.23. Found: C, 82.2; H, 6.2.

2,3,3',4,4'-Penta-O-Benzylsucrose (4)

2,3,3',4,4'-Penta-O-benzyl-1',6,6'-tri-O-tritylsucrose (3, 2 g, 1.32 mmol) was placed in a round-bottomed flask containing glacial acetic acid (8 mL). The suspension was stirred and heated under reflux until the substrate dissolved. Water (0.5 mL) was added and the refluxing was continued until thin-layer chromatography (TLC) (4:1, hexane–EtOAc) indicated that all starting material was consumed (1–1.5 h). After concentration, the residue was partitioned between water (5 mL) and EtOAc (10 mL), and the pH of the aqueous phase was made neutral by addition of solid sodium hydroxide. The aqueous layer was extracted with EtOAc (2×10 mL), the combined organic extracts were washed successively with water (10 mL) and brine (10 mL), dried, and concentrated, and chromatography (4:1 → 2:1 → 1:2 hexane–EtOAc,) gave solid 4 (0.62 g, 68%), mp. 72°C–75°C (Et$_2$O–hexane), [α]$_D$ +18.8. ESI-MS: 815 [M(C$_{47}$H$_{52}$O$_{11}$) +Na$^+$].

This compound was characterized as a triacetate: [α]$_D$ +45.6.

^{1}H NMR δ: 5.65 (d, $J_{1,2}$=3.6 Hz, 1H, H-1), 2.00, 1.99, 1.98 (3×s, 3×3H, 3×OAc).

^{13}C NMR δ: 170.7, 170.6, 170.0 (3×$\underline{C}$O), 103.3 (C-2'), 90.0 (C-1), 83.5, 81.8, 79.4, 78.5, 77.2, 69.5, 69.3 (C-2,3,3',4,4',5,5'), 75.6, 75.0, 73.0 (double intensity), 72.7 (5×O$\underline{C}$H$_2$Ph), 64.9, 64.7, 63.1 (C-1',6,6'), 20.8, 20.78, 20.7 (3×OC(O)$\underline{C}$H$_3$).

Anal: Calcd for C$_{53}$H$_{58}$O$_{14}$: C, 69.27; H, 6.36. Found: C, 69.2; H, 6.5.

2,3,3′,4,4′-Penta-*O*-Benzyl-6,6′-Di-*O*-*p*-Nitrobenzoylsucrose (5)

Triphenylphosphane (1.68 g, 6.4 mmol) and *p*-nitrobenzoic acid (840 mg, 5.0 mmol) were added to a solution of 2,3,3′,4,4′-penta-*O*-benzylsucrose (4, 1.18 g, 1.5 mmol) in pyridine (20 mL), followed by diethyl azadicarboxylate (4.8 mL of a *ca.* 40% solution in toluene). The mixture was stirred at rt for 3 h, the solvent was evaporated, and the residue was chromatographed (4:1 → 3:2 hexane–EtOAc) to afford alcohol 5 as an oil (1.2–1.35 g, 73%–82%), $[\alpha]_D$ +27.0. ESI-MS: 1113 [M ($C_{61}H_{58}O_{17}N_2$) +Na$^+$].

This compound was characterized as an acetate, $[\alpha]_D$ +73.6. ^{1}H NMR (200 MHz) δ: 8.10 (m, 8H, two *p*-nitrobenzoyl groups), 5.80 (d, $J_{1,2}$ = 3.0 Hz, 1H, H-1), 2.03 (s, 3H OAc).

^{13}C NMR (50 MHz) δ: 169.9 (<u>C</u>OCH$_3$), 164.3, 164.2 (2×<u>C</u>O, *p*-nitrobenzoyl), 103.5 (C-2′), 89.8 (C-1), 83.6 (C-3′), 81.9 (C-3), 80.9 (C-4′), 79.4 (C-2), 77.9 (C-5′), 77.2 (C-4), 75.9, 74.9, 73.5, 73.0, 72.5 (5×O<u>C</u>H$_2$Ph), 69.5 (C-5), 65.4 (C-6′), 64.9 (C-1′), 64.5 (C-6), 20.8 (C(O)<u>C</u>H$_3$).

Anal: Calcd for $C_{63}H_{60}N_2O_{18}$: C, 66.78; H, 5.34; N, 2.47. Found: C, 66.4; H, 5.6; N, 2.9.

2,3,3′,4,4′-Penta-*O*-Benzyl-1′-*O*-Benzyloxymethyl-6,6′-Di-*O*-*p*-Nitrobenzoylsucrose (6)

Freshly prepared benzyloxymethyl chloride[5] (8.9 mL, 64 mmol) was added dropwise, under argon, to a stirred boiling solution of 2,3,3′,4,4′-penta-*O*-benzyl-6,6′-di-*O*-*p*-nitrobenzoylsucrose (5) (17.5 g, 16 mmol) in pyridine (50 mL) containing a catalytic amount of DMAP (0.1 g) and refluxing was continued for 2 h. Pyridine was evaporated, the residue was dissolved in diethyl ether, the solution was washed with water and brine, and dried. Column chromatography (6:1 → 3:1 hexane–EtOAc,) afforded compound 6 (15.5 g, 80%), $[\alpha]_D$ +50.7.

^{1}H NMR (200 MHz) δ: 5.70 (d, $J_{1,2}$ = 4.2 Hz, 1H, H-1).

^{13}C NMR (50 MHz) δ: 164.3, 164.2 (2×<u>C</u>O), 104.7 (C-2′), 94.8 (O<u>C</u>H$_2$O), 89.5 (C-1), 83.9 (C-3′), 82.0 (C-4′), 81.0 (C-5′), 79.5 (C-2), 77.8 (C-3), 77.1 (C-4), 75.8, 74.8, 73.5, 72.7, 72.3 (5×O<u>C</u>H$_2$Ph), 69.7 (C-5), 69.3 (O<u>C</u>H$_2$Ph, BOM), 69.3 (C-1′), 65.5 (C-6′), 64.1 (C-6).

Anal: Calcd for $C_{69}H_{66}N_2O_{16} \times H_2O$: C, 67.42; H, 5.58; N, 2.28. Found: C, 67.59; H, 5.30; N, 2.03.

2,3,3′,4,4′-Penta-*O*-Benzyl-1′-*O*-Benzyloxymethylsucrose (7)

A solution of 2,3,3′,4,4′-penta-*O*-benzyl-1′-*O*-benzyloxymethyl-6,6′-di-*O*-*p*-nitrobenzoylsucrose (6, 15.5 g, 12.8 mmol) in THF (15 mL) was added to methanol (60 mL) containing MeONa (2.3 g), and the reaction mixture was stirred for 1 h at rt. After concentration, the residue was extracted with EtOAc and water. The organic layer was concentrated and dried, and chromatography (hexane/EtOAc, 3:1–1:1) afforded title compound 7 (7.5–9.5 g, 64%–81%), $[\alpha]_D$ +25.7.

ESI-MS: 935 [M($C_{55}H_{60}O_{12}$) +Na$^+$].

The compound was characterized as a diacetate: $[\alpha]_D$ +43.2.

^{1}H NMR δ: 5.68 (d, $J_{1,2}$ = 3.0 Hz, 1H, H-1), 1.96 and 1.95 (2×s, 2×3H, 2×OAc).

^{13}C NMR δ: 170.6, 170.6 (2×$\underline{C}$O), 104.4 (C-2′), 94.7 (O$\underline{C}$H$_2$O), 89.7 (C-1), 83.8 (C-3′), 81.8 (C-4′), 81.6 (C-5′), 79.6 (C-2), 78.2 (C-3), 77.3 (C-4), 75.5, 74.8, 73.0, 72.7, 72.4 (5×O$\underline{C}$H$_2$Ph), 69.5, 69.1 (C-5, C-1′), 69.0 (O$\underline{C}$H$_2$Ph, BOM), 64.8 (C-6′), 63.0 (C-6), 20.7 and 20.6 (2×OAc).

Anal: Calcd for C$_{59}$H$_{64}$O$_{14}$: C, 71.07; H, 6.47. Found: C, 70.86; H, 6.70.

2,3,3′,4,4′-Penta-*O*-Benzyl-1′-*O*-Benzyloxymethyl-6′-*O*-*Tert*-Butyldiphenylsilylsucrose (8)

To a stirred solution of 2,3,3′,4,4′-penta-*O*-benzyl-1′-*O*-benzyloxymethylsucrose (**7**, 10.7 g, 11.7 mmol) in dry dichloromethane (100 mL) containing diisopropylethylamine (6 mL, 35.1 mmol) and DMAP (0.7 g, 0.6 mmol), *t*-butyldiphenylchlorosilane (3.6 mL, 14.1 mmol) was added at rt with a syringe pump (at a rate of 0.14 mL/h), and the stirring was continued for additional 12 h. EtOAc and water were added; the organic layer was separated, washed with water and brine, dried, and concentrated; and the residue was purified by column chromatography (9:1 → 1:2 hexane–EtOAc) to afford **8** as a pale yellow oil (9.31 g, 70%), [α]$_D$ +28.8.

ESI-MS: 1173 [M (C$_{71}$H$_{78}$O$_{12}$Si) +Na$^+$].

This compound was characterized as acetate, [α]$_D$ +32.5.

^{1}H NMR δ: 5.92 (d, $J_{1,2}$=3.6 Hz, 1H, H-1), 1.90 (s, 3H, OAc), 1.04 (s, 9H, *t*-Bu).

^{13}C NMR δ: 170.5 ($\underline{C}$O), 104.0 (C-2′), 94.8 (O$\underline{C}$H$_2$O), 89.0 (C-1), 84.1 (C-3′), 82.0 (C-3), 81.4 (C-5′), 80.9 (C-4′), 80.0 (C-2), 77.2 (C-4), 75.6, 74.7, 73.3, 72.7, 72.1 (5×O$\underline{C}$H$_2$Ph), 69.7 (C-1′), 69.5 (C-5), 68.9 (O$\underline{C}$H$_2$Ph, BOM), 64.3 (C-6′), 63.1 (C-6), 26.9 (C($\underline{C}$H$_3$)$_3$), 20.8 (OC(O)$\underline{C}$H$_3$), 19.2 ($\underline{C}$(CH$_3$)$_3$).

Anal: Calcd for C$_{73}$H$_{80}$O$_{13}$Si: C, 73.64; H, 6.76. Found: C, 73.34; H, 6.91.

1′-*O*-Benzyloxymethyl-6,6′-Di-*O*-*Tert*-Butyldiphenylsilyl-2,3,3′,4,4′-Penta-*O*-Benzylsucrose (9)

Sodium hydride (50% suspension in mineral oil, 0.5 g, 10.4 mmol) was added to a solution of 2,3,3′,4,4′-penta-*O*-benzyl-1′-*O*-benzyloxymethylsucrose (**7**, 2.0 g, 2.2 mmol) in dry THF (30 mL) containing a catalytic amount (~50 mg) of imidazole, and the mixture was stirred at rt for 0.5 h. *tert*-Butyldiphenylchlorosilane (1.4 mL, 5.5 mmol) was added and stirring was continued for 12 h. Excess of hydride was destroyed by careful addition of water, and the mixture was partitioned between diethyl ether and water. The organic layer was separated, washed with water, dried, and concentrated; and the product was isolated by column chromatography (9:1 → 6:1 hexane–EtOAc,) to afford product **9** (2.9 g, 95%), [α]$_D$ +27.7. ESI-MS: 1411 [M (C$_{87}$H$_{96}$O$_{12}$Si$_2$) +Na$^+$].

1H NMR δ: 6.13 (d, $J_{1,2}$=3.6 Hz, 1H, H-1), 1.173, 1.169 (2×s, 2×9H, 2×*t*-Bu).

1H NMR δ: 5.92 (d, $J_{1,2}$=4.2 Hz, 1H, H-1), 1.05, 1.04 (2×s, 2×9H, 2×*t*-Bu).

13C NMR δ: 104.2 (C-2′), 94.8 (O$\underline{C}$H$_2$O), 89.5 (C-1), 84.4 (C-3′), 82.3 (C-3), 81.9 (C-5′), 80.7 (C-4′), 80.5 (C-2), 77.2 (C-4), 75.8, 74.7, 73.3, 72.7, 72.1 (5×O$\underline{C}$H$_2$Ph), 71.6 (C-5), 69.9 (C-1′), 69.5 (O$\underline{C}$H$_2$Ph, BOM), 65.5 (C-6′), 64.5 (C-6), 27.0, 26.9 (2×C($\underline{C}$H$_3$)$_3$), 19.0, 18.4 (2×$\underline{C}$(CH$_3$)$_3$).

Anal: Calcd for C$_{87}$H$_{96}$O$_{12}$Si$_2$: C, 75.18; H, 6.96. Found: C, 74.99; H, 6.80.

2,3,3',4,4'-Penta-O-Benzyl-1'-O-Benzyloxymethyl-
6-O-*Tert*-Butyldiphenylsilylsucrose (10)

HF-Py complex (1 M in methanol, 80 mL) was added to a solution of 2,3,3',4,4'-penta-O-benzyl-1'-O-benzyloxymethyl-6,6'-di-O-*tert*-butyldiphenylsilylsucrose (**9**, 1.48 g, 1.06 mmol) in MeOH/Et$_2$O (70 mL, 4:1), and the mixture was stirred at rt for 10 h until TLC (3:1 hexane–EtOAc) showed that the reaction was almost complete. EtOAc and water were added; the organic layer was separated, washed with water and brine, dried, and concentrated; and the product was isolated by column chromatography (9:1 → 1:2 hexane–EtOAc,) to afford **10** (0.564 g, 68%), [α]$_D$ +24.6. ESI-MS: 1173 [M (C$_{71}$H$_{78}$O$_{12}$Si) +Na$^+$]. A small amount of the diol **7** was recovered.

Compound **10** was characterized as an acetate, [α]$_D$ +27.3.

^{1}H NMR δ: 6.00 (d, $J_{1,2}$=3.6 Hz, 1H, H-1), 1.72 (s, 3H, OAc), 1.18 (s, 9H, *t*-Bu).

^{13}C NMR δ: 170.6 (C̲O), 104.3 (C-2'), 94.8 (OC̲H$_2$O), 89.6 (C-1), 83.9 (C-3'), 82.1 (C-3), 81.6 (C-4'), 80.1 (C-2), 77.9 (C-5'), 77.3 (C-4), 75.8, 74.9, 73.0, 72.7, 72.4 (5×OC̲H$_2$Ph), 71.8 (C-5), 69.6 (C-1'), 69.6 (OC̲H$_2$Ph, BOM), 64.5 (C-6'), 62.3 (C-6), 26.8 (C(C̲H$_3$)$_3$), 20.7 (OC(O)C̲H$_3$), 19.3 (C̲(CH$_3$)$_3$).

Anal: Calcd for C$_{73}$H$_{80}$O$_{13}$Si: C, 73.64; H, 6.76. Found: C, 73.24; H, 6.69.

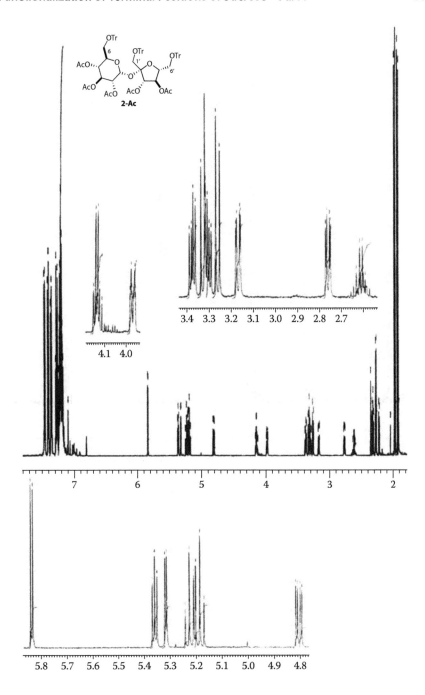

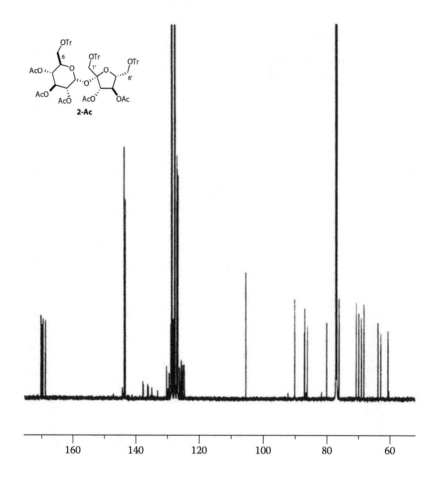

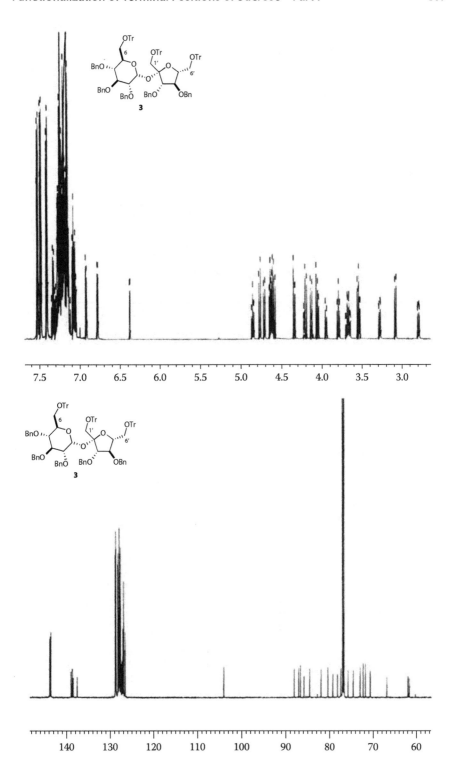

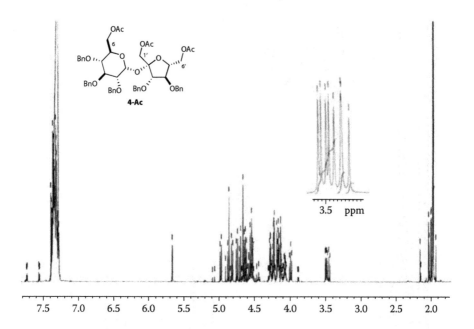

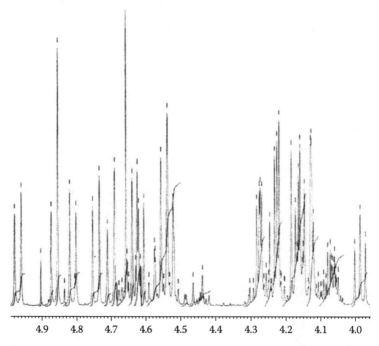

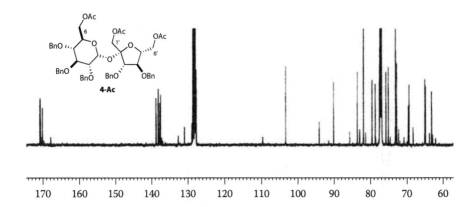

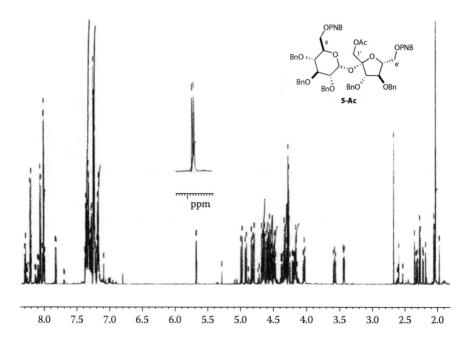

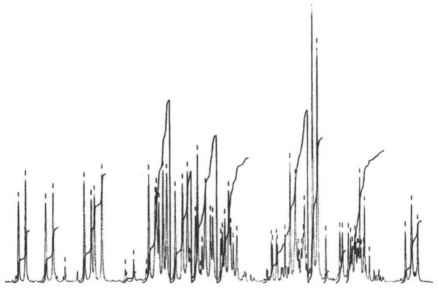

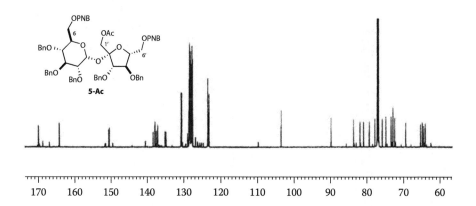

5-Ac

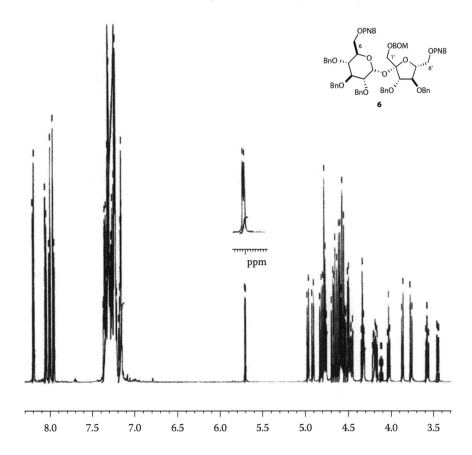

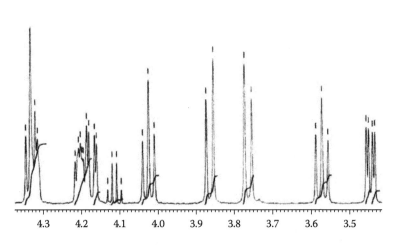

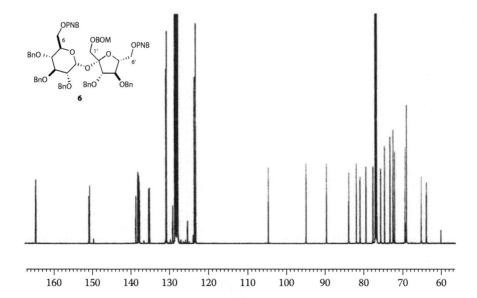

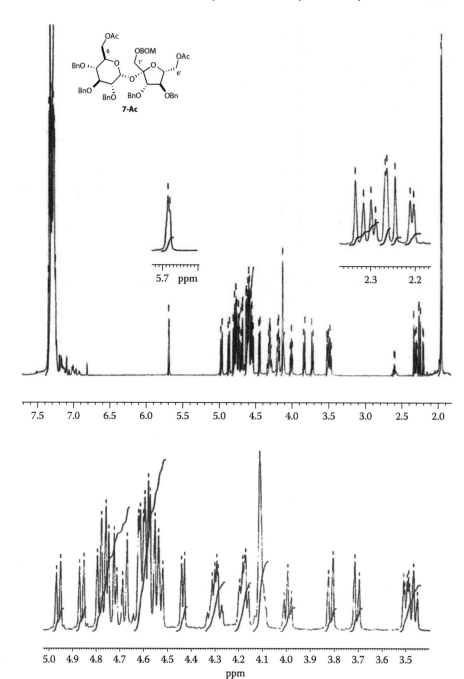

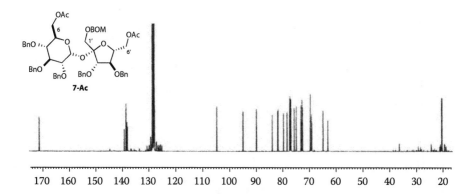

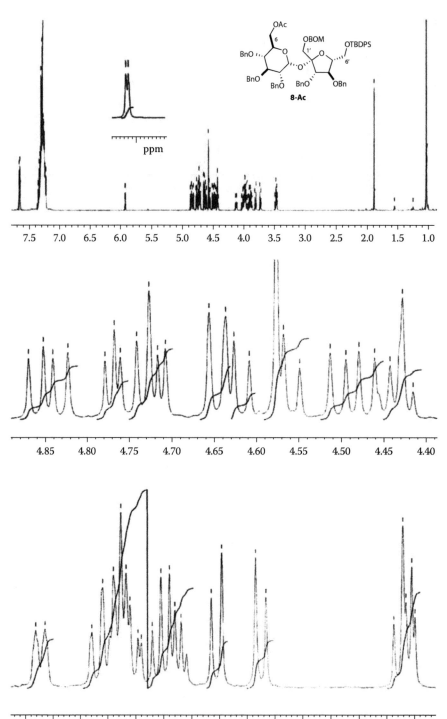

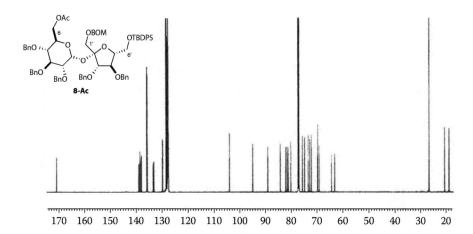

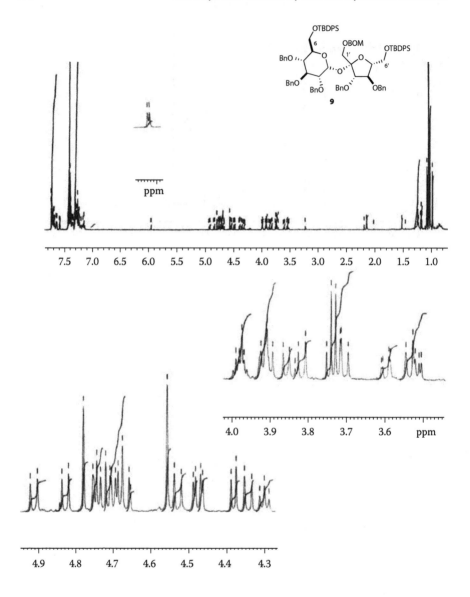

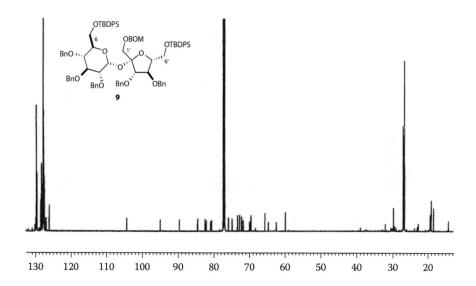

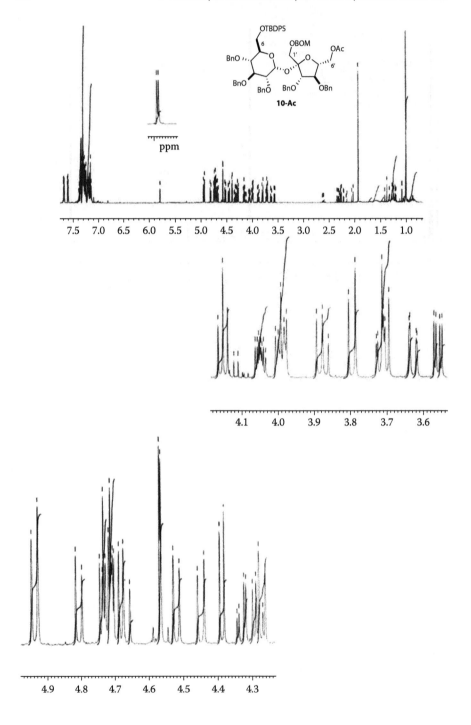

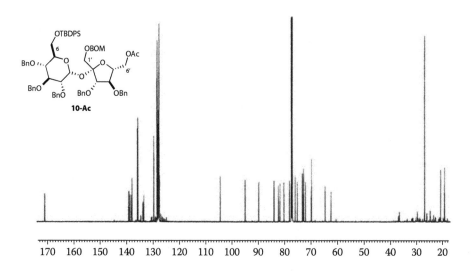

REFERENCES

1. Queneau, Y.; Jarosz, S.; Fittreman, J.; Lewandowski, B., *Adv. Carbohydr. Chem. Biochem.*, 2007, *61*, 217–292.
2. Jarosz, S.; Kościołowska, I., Patent, PL 177187 (1999); Jarosz, S.; Mach, M., *J. Carbohydr. Chem.*, 1997, *16*, 1111–1122.
3. Karl, H.; Lee, C. H.; Khan, R., *Carbohydr. Res.*, 1982, *101*, 31–38.
4. Jarosz, S.; Mach, M.; Frelek, J., *J. Carbohydr. Chem.*, 2000, *19*, 693–705.
5. Connor, D. S.; Klein, G. W.; Taylor, G. N.; Boeckman, Jr., R. K.; Medwick, J. B., *Org. Synth. Coll.*, 1988, *6*, 101–103.

REFERENCES

44 Functionalization of Terminal Positions of Sucrose—Part II[‡]: Preparation of 1',2,3,3',4,4'-Hexa-O-Benzylsucrose and 6,6'-*Bis*-O-(2-Hydroxyethyl)-1',2,3,3',4,4'-Hexa-O-Benzylsucrose

*B. Lewandowski, A. Listkowski,
K. Petrova,[†] and S. Jarosz**

CONTENTS

Experimental Methods 414
  General Methods 414
    6,6'-Di-O-Tritylsucrose (**1**) 416
    1',2,3,3',4,4'-Hexa-O-Acetyl-6,6'-Di-O-Tritylsucrose (**1A**) 417
    1',2,3,3',4,4'-Hexa-O-Benzyl-6,6'-Di-O-Tritylsucrose (**2**) 417
    1',2,3,3',4,4'-Hexa-O-Benzyl-6,6'-Dichloro-6,6'-Dideoxysucrose (**3A**) 418

[‡] For Part I, see Chapter 43.
* Corresponding author.
[†] Checker.

6,6'-Di-*O*-Acetyl-1',2,3,3',4,4'-Hexa-*O*-Benzylsucrose (**4**)........................ 418

1',2,3,3',4,4'-Hexa-*O*-Benzylsucrose (**5**).. 419

6,6'- Di-*O*-Allyl-1',2,3,3',4,4'-Hexa-*O*-Benzylsucrose (**6**) 419

1',2,3,3',4,4'-Hexa-*O*-Benzyl-6,6'-*Bis*-(*O-Tert-*

Butoxycarbonylmethylsucrose (**7**) 420

1',2,3,3',4,4'-Hexa-*O*-Benzyl-6,6'-*Bis*-(*O*-2-Hydroxyethyl) Sucrose (**8**)..... 420

References... 430

The strategy used for synthesis of 1',2,3,3',4,4'-hexa-*O*-benzylsucrose (**5**), having only *O*-6 and *O*-6' unprotected, was similar to the one described for the preparation of penta-*O*-benzylsucrose.[1] Accordingly, reaction of sucrose with 2.2 eqv. of trityl chloride provided the di-tritylated derivative **1** in 50% yield. Benzylation of the remaining hydroxyl groups followed by detritylation with iodine in dichloromethane/methanol[2] gave **5**. The latter compound was also prepared via an alternative route based on the known conversion of the free sucrose into 6,6'-dichloro-6,6'-dideoxysucrose (**3**),[3] followed by benzylation of the remaining six hydroxyl groups with potassium hydroxide as a base.* Subsequent reaction with tetrabutyl-ammonium acetate afforded the corresponding 6,6'-di-*O*-acetyl derivative **4**, which was followed by transesterification to give **5** (Scheme 44.1).[1]

1',2,3,3',4,4'-Hexa-*O*-benzylsucrose (**5**) was used as the starting material for the preparation of more complex derivatives. One of the synthetic routes described here led to the elongated diol **8** (with hydroxyethylene groups at positions *O*-6 and *O*-6').[4] This compound can be efficiently prepared through two different routes. The first one (***route a***) involved allylation of both hydroxyl groups in **5** with allyl bromide (→**6**), subsequent cleavage of both double bonds, followed by reduction of the aldehyde functions, which afforded the desired diol **8**. Alternatively (***route b***), diol **5** was alkylated with *tert*-butyl bromoacetate (under PTC conditions)[4] to the diester **7**, which, upon reduction with lithium aluminum hydride, afforded the target compound **8** (Scheme 44.2).

EXPERIMENTAL METHODS

GENERAL METHODS

Nuclear magnetic resonance (NMR) spectra were recorded at 400 MHz for solutions in $CDCl_3$ with a Bruker AMX-400 spectrometer. Chemical shift values (δ) are reported downfield from TMS. Most of the proton resonances were assigned by the $^1H-^1H$-COSY and the carbon resonances by the $^1H-^{13}C$-HMQC experiments. Mass spectra (ESI) were recorded with PE SCIEX API 365 or Mariner PerSeptive Biosystems apparatus. Optical rotations were measured at room temperature (rt) with a Digital Jasco polarimeter DIP-360 for solutions in chloroform (*c*, 1), except for compound **1**. Column chromatography was performed on silica gel (Merck, 70–230 or 230–400 mesh). THF was distilled from potassium prior to use. Solutions in organic solvents were dried over anhydrous sodium or magnesium sulfate.

---

* Typically, we use NaH as a base for benzylation of sucrose derivatives. However, in this case elimination of HCl was observed. Thus, sodium hydride was replaced with potassium hydroxide.

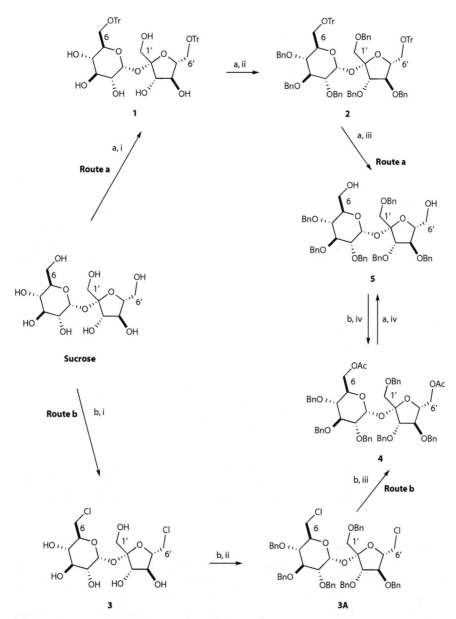

SCHEME 44.1 Preparation of 1',2,3,3',4,4'-hexa-O-benzylsucrose (**5**). (a,i) TrCl (2.2 eqv.), DMAP, Py, 50%; (a,ii) BnBr, NaH, DMF, 84%; (a,iii) I$_2$, CH$_2$Cl$_2$/MeOH, 58%; (a,iv) (CH$_3$CO)$_2$O, Py, 94%; (b,i) see Ref. [3]; (b,ii) BnBr, KOH, Bu$_4$NBr, DMF, 77%; (b,iii) Bu$_4$N$^+$OAc$^-$, DMF, 72%; (b,iv) MeONa, MeOH, 82%.

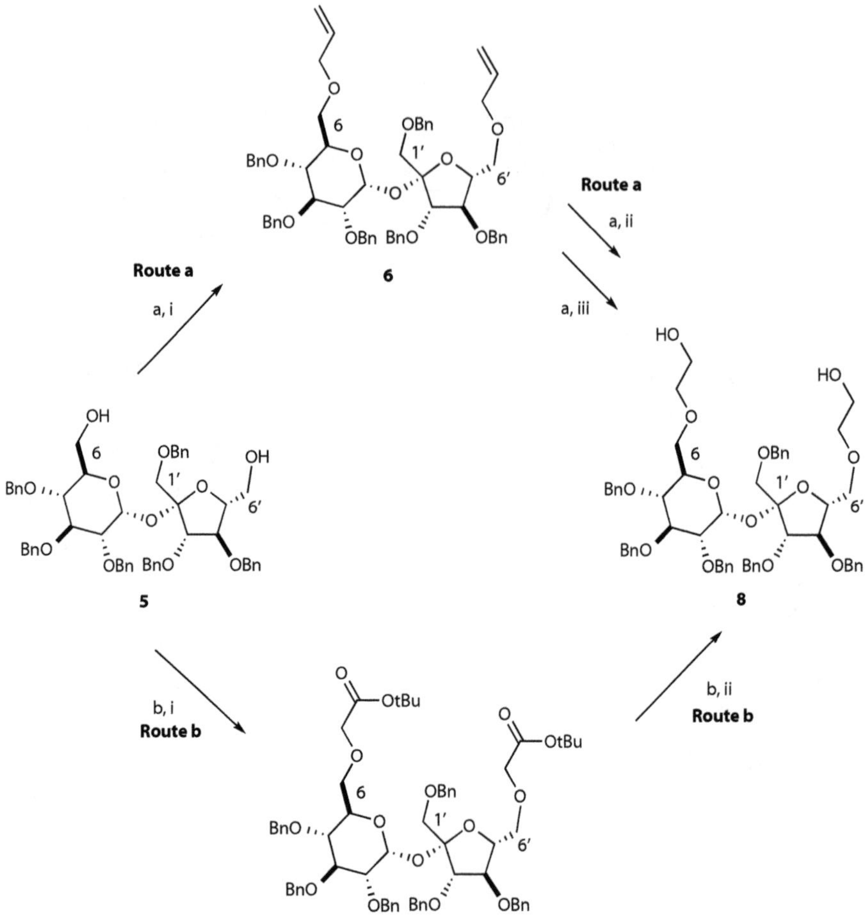

SCHEME 44.2   Synthesis of 6,6'-*bis*-*O*-(2-hydroxyethyl)-1',2,3,3',4,4'-hexa-*O*-benzylsucrose (**8**). (a,i) AllBr, NaH, DMF, 79%; (a,ii) NaIO$_4$, OsO$_4$, THF/H$_2$O; (a,iii) NaBH$_4$, CH$_2$Cl$_2$/MeOH, 47%; (b,i) BrCH$_2$CO$_2$tBu, Bu$_4$NBr, 50% aq. NaOH/PhMe, 83%; (b,ii) LiAlH$_4$, THF, 69%.

6,6'-Di-*O*-Tritylsucrose (1)

Sucrose (18 g, 0.053 mol) was dissolved in boiling pyridine (300 mL). Upon cooling to rt, DMAP (65 mg, 0.55 mmol) and trityl chloride were added (33 g, 0.12 mmol), and the mixture was stirred for 48 h at rt. The reaction was monitored by thin-layer chromatography (TLC), and it was terminated when formation of the tri-substituted derivative was observed. The solvent was evaporated at rt, and the residue was chromatographed (1:2 hexane-EtOAc, 100:5:2 EtOAc-methanol-water) to afford 6,6'-di-*O*-tritylsucrose (**1**) as a white solid* (21.7 g, 50%), mp. = 99°C–102°C, [α]$_D$ +38.7

---

* Tri-*O*-tritylated as well as several mono- and other di-tritylated derivatives were also formed (TLC).

(CH$_3$OH, 1.09). ^{1}H NMR (400 MHz) δ:7.21 (m, 30H, Ar-H), 5.80 (d, 1H, $J_{1,2}$=3.6 Hz, H-1), 4.34 (t, 1H, $J_{3',4',5'}$= 8.6 Hz, H-4'), 4.18 (d, 1H, $J_{3',4'}$=8.4 Hz, H-3'), 4.11 (d, 2H, $J_{5,6}$=7.1 Hz, H-6), 3.89 (m, 2H, H-5, H-5'), 3.53 (t, $J_{2,3,4}$=9.5 Hz 1H, H-3), 3.45 (d, 2H, $J_{5',6'}$=11.7 Hz, H-6'), 3.41 (s, 2H, H-1'), 3.27 (t, 1H, $J_{3,4,5}$=11.0 Hz, H-4), 3.09 (dd, 1H, $J_{1,2}$=3.8 Hz, $J_{2,3}$=9.3 Hz, H-2). ^{13}C NMR δ: 143.7, 143.6 (quat. C-Tr), 136.1, 128.8, 128.0, 127.5, 127.2, 123.8 (C$_{Ar}$), 104.8 (C-2'), 90.9 (C-1), 87.4, 87.1 (2×$\underline{C}$Ph$_3$), 79.2, 77.3, 74.7, 74.3, 71.6, 71.2, 70.9 (C-2,3,3',4,4',5,5'), 66.1, 64.4, 62.8 (C-1',6,6'). ESI-MS: 849 [M(C$_{50}$H$_{50}$O$_{11}$) +Na$^+$]. Anal: Calcd for C$_{50}$H$_{50}$O$_{11}$: C, 72.62; H, 6.09. Found: C, 72.70; H, 6.02.

1',2,3,3',4,4'-Hexa-O-Acetyl-6,6'-Di-O-Tritylsucrose (1A)

Compound **1** (0.1 g, 0.012 mmol) was dissolved in pyridine (10 mL), acetic anhydride (0.148 g, 0.14 mL) was added, and the mixture was stirred at rt overnight. After concentration, the residue was chromatographed (2:1 hexane-EtOAc) to afford the hexaacetate **1A** (0.13 g, 96%), mp. = 103°C–105°C, [α]$_D$ +69.5. ^{1}H NMR δ: 7.23 (m, 30H, Ar-H), 5.84 (d, 1H, $J_{1,2}$=3.9 Hz, H-1), 5.36 (t, 1H, $J_{3',4',5'}$=5.2 Hz, H-4'), 5.31 (d, 1H, $J_{3',4'}$=5.4 Hz, H-3'), 5.21 (m, 2H, $J_{3,4}$=9.3 Hz, H-3, H-4), 4.81 (dd, 1H, $J_{1,2}$=3.2 Hz, $J_{2,3}$=9.2 Hz, H-2), 4.14 (m, 1H, H-6A), 3.96 (d, 1H, $J_{6A,6B}$=8.9 Hz, H-6B), 3.33 (m, 4H, H-6'A, H-1'), 3.17 (d, 1H, $J_{5,6}$=9.8 Hz, H-5), 2.75 (dd, 1H, $J_{5',6'}$=8.0 Hz, H-5'), 2.16 (s, 6H, H-OAc), 1.98 (s, 3H, H-OAc), 1.96 (s, 3H, H-OAc), 1.93 (s, 3H, H-OAc), 1.92 (s, 3H, H-OAc). ^{13}C NMR δ: 170.2, 170.0, 169.5, 168.9 (6×$\underline{C}$O), 143.7, 143.3 (quat. C-Tr), 128.8, 128.6, 127.8, 127.7, 127.1, 127.0, 126.8 (C$_{Ar}$), 105.4 (C-2'), 90.1 (C-1), 87.1, 86.9 (2×$\underline{C}$Ph$_3$), 86.1, 80.1, 76.2, 70.8, 70.0, 69.2, 68.4 (C-2,3,3',4,4',5,5'), 63.9, 63.0, 60.6 (C-1',6,6'), 20.9, 20.8, 20.6, 20.5, 20.4 (6×OC(O)$\underline{C}$H$_3$). ESI-MS: 1101 [M(C$_{62}$H$_{62}$O$_{17}$) +Na$^+$]. Anal: Calcd for C$_{62}$H$_{62}$O$_{17}$: C, 69.00; H, 5.79. Found: C, 68.82; H, 5.63.

1',2,3,3',4,4'-Hexa-O-Benzyl-6,6'-Di-O-Tritylsucrose (2)

Sodium hydride (60% dispersion in mineral oil, 1.74 g, 0.044 mmol) was added in portions at 5°C–10°C to a stirred solution of 6,6'-di-O-tritylsucrose (**1**, 3.0 g, 3.63 mmol) and imidazole (0.007 g, 0.099 mmol) in DMF (30 mL), and the mixture was stirred at rt for 30 min. Benzyl bromide (5.58 g, 3.88 mL, 0.033 mol) was added dropwise at a rate to keep the temperature below 40°C. The cooling was removed, and when the starting material was consumed (4–5 h, TLC, 5:1 hexane-ethyl acetate), the reaction was quenched by dropwise addition of H$_2$O (with stirring, until effervescence ceased). The mixture was poured into cold H$_2$O (500 mL) and extracted with Et$_2$O (4 × 150 mL). The extracts were washed with H$_2$O (2 ×150 mL), the organic phase was dried with Na$_2$SO$_4$ and concentrated, and the residue was chromatographed (hexane, then gradient 12:1 → 17:3 hexane-EtOAc) to afford 1',2,3,3',4,4'-hexa-O-benzyl-6,6'-di-O-tritylsucrose (**2**) as a white, amorphous solid (4.2 g, 84%), [α]$_D$ +20.6. ^{1}H NMR δ: 7.20 (m, 60H, Ar-H), 6.40 (d, 1H, $J_{1,2}$=3.6 Hz, H-1), 4.87 (t, 1H, $J_{3',4',5'}$=8.9 Hz, H-4'), 4.66 (m, 7H, H-3', H-4, H-5, 2Ar-CH_2), 4.35 (dd, 2H, $J_{5,6}$=3.26, $J_{6A,6B}$=11.78, H-6), 4.12 (m, 6H, H-5', H-2, 2Ar-CH_2), 3.93 (d, 1H, J=9.8 Hz, Ar-CH_2), 3.79 (t, 1H, $J_{2,3,4}$=9.2 Hz, H-3), 3.67 (dd, 2H, $J_{5',6'}$=10.6 Hz, $J_{6'A,6'B}$=17.5 Hz, H-6'), 3.54 (t, 2H, $J_{1'A,1'B}$=8.2 Hz, H-1'), 3.28 (d, 1H, J=9.9 Hz, Ar-CH_2), 3.06 (d, 1H, J=9.8 Hz, Ar-CH_2), 2.78 (d, 1H, J=9.0 Hz, Ar-CH_2). ^{13}C NMR

δ: 143.9, 143.7 (quat. C-Tr), 139.0, 138.7, 138.5, 137.6 (C_q benzyl groups), 128.9, 128.8, 128.3, 128.2, 128.1, 127.9, 127.7, 127.4, 127.2, 127.0, 126.7 (C_{Ar}), 104.2 (C-2′), 88.1 (C-1), 87.1, 86.7 ($2 \times \underline{C}Ph_3$), 85.9, 84.6, 82.0, 80.5, 79.3, 78.3, 77.6, 75.9, 74.7, 73.1, 72.4, 71.9, 70.8 (C-2,3,3′,4,4′,5,5′, $6 \times O\underline{C}H_2Ph$), 67.1, 62.0, 61.7 (C-1′,6,6′).

Anal: Calcd for $C_{92}H_{86}O_{11}$: C, 80.79; H, 6.34. Found: C, 80.84; H, 6.39.

1′,2,3,3′,4,4′-Hexa-O-Benzyl-6,6′-Dichloro-6,6′-Dideoxysucrose (3A)

To a stirred solution of 6,6′-dichloro-6,6′-dideoxysucrose (3)[3] (0.68 g, 1.794 mmol) in DMF (40 mL), was added powdered KOH (0.90 g, 16.2 mmol), tetrabutylammonium bromide (0.06 g) and benzyl bromide (2.76 g, 1.92 mL, 16.2 mmol) and the mixture was stirred at rt overnight. The mixture was partitioned between water (80 mL) and ether (80 mL); the organic phase was separated, washed with water, dried, and concentrated; and the residue was chromatographed (8:1 → 7:1 hexane–EtOAc) to afford 1′,2,3,3′,4,4′-hexa-O-benzyl-6,6′-dichloro-6,6′-dideoxysucrose as a colorless oil (1.27 g, 77%), $[\alpha]_D$ +32. ^{1}H NMR δ: 7.29 (m, 30H, Ar-H), 5.69 (d, 1H, $J_{1,2} = 3.2$ Hz, H-1), 4.90 (dd, 2H, $J_{5,6} = 3.1$ Hz, $J_{6A,6B} = 10.8$ Hz, H-6), 4.74 (d, 1H, $J = 10.9$ Hz, Ar-CH_2), 4.53 (m, 10H, H-1′,2′,3′,4,4′, $2 \times$ Ar-CH_2), 4.19 (d, 1H, $J = 9.2$ Hz, Ar-CH_2), 4.10 (d, 2H, $J_{5′,6′} = 4.0$ Hz, H-6′), 3.96 (t, 1H, $J_{2,3,4} = 9.2$ Hz, H-3), 3.71 (m, 3H, H-5, Ar-CH_2), 3.57 (m, 5H, H-5′, $2 \times$ Ar-CH_2). ^{13}C NMR δ: 138.6, 138.2, 138.1, 137.9, 137.7 (C_q benzyl groups), 128.4, 127.9, 127.8, 127.6 (C_{Ar}), 105.2 (C-2′), 90.3 (C-1), 84.0, 83.3, 81.4, 80.5, 79.7, 78.1, and 70.1 (C-2,3,3′,4,4′,5,5′), 75.5, 75.1, 73.5, 73.1, 72.5, 72.4, 70.7 (C-1′ + 6 O$\underline{C}$H$_2$Ph), 45.0, 44.9 (C-6,6′). ESI-MS: 941 [M($C_{54}H_{56}O_9Cl_2$) +Na$^+$]. Anal: Calcd for $C_{54}H_{56}O_9Cl_2$: C, 70.50; H, 6.14; Cl, 7.71. Found: C, 70.42; H, 6.31; Cl, 7.57.

6,6′-Di-O-Acetyl-1′,2,3,3′,4,4′-Hexa-O-Benzylsucrose (4)

Tetrabutylammonium acetate (2.81 g, 9.33 mmol) was added to a solution of the foregoing 6,6′-dichloro-6,6′-dideoxy-1′,2,3,3′,4,4′-hexa-O-benzylsucrose (3A) (0.39 g, 0.424 mmol) in toluene (50 mL), the mixture was boiled under reflux for 2 h and then kept at rt overnight. After concentration, the residue was dissolved in CH$_2$Cl$_2$ (50 mL), the solution was washed with water (3×50 mL), and the aqueous phase was extracted with CH$_2$Cl$_2$ (2×). The organic phases were combined, dried, and concentrated; and chromatography (5:1 → 3:1 hexane/EtOAc) gave 4 as a colorless oil (0.29 g, 72%). $[\alpha]_D$ +50.6. ^{1}H NMR δ: 7.22 (m, 30H, Ar-H), 5.66 (d, 1H, $J_{1,2} = 3.3$ Hz, H-1), 4.95 (d, 1H, $J = 10.3$ Hz, Ar-CH_2), 4.84 (d, 1H, $J = 10.2$ Hz, Ar-CH_2), 4.77 (d, 1H, $J = 10.3$ Hz, Ar-CH_2), 4.57 (m, 8H, H-2′,3,4,4′,6A,6B, Ar-CH_2), 4.43 (s, 2H, Ar-CH_2), 4.28 (s, 1H, Ar-CH_2), 4.10 (m, 5H, H-1′,6″, Ar-CH_2), 3.98 (t, 1H, H-3), 3.69 (d, 1H, $J = 10.3$ Hz, Ar-CH_2), 3.50 (m, 3H, H-5, H-5′, Ar-CH_2), 1.97 (s, 6H, $2 \times$ OAc). ^{13}C NMR δ: 170.7 ($\underline{C}$O), 138.7, 138.1, 137.9, 137.8, 137.7 (C_q benzyl groups), 128.4, 128.0, 127.9, 127.8, 127.6 (C_{Ar}), 104.7 (C-2′), 89.8 (C-1), 83.7, 81.8, 81.7, 79.7, 78.2, 77.2, and 69.1 (C-2,3,3′,4,4′,5,5′), 75.6, 74.9, 73.4, 73.0, 72.7, 72.4, 71.1 (C-1′, 6×O$\underline{C}$H$_2$Ph), 64.8, 63.0 (C-6,6′), 20.8, 20.7 ($2 \times$ OC(O)$\underline{C}$H$_3$). ESI-MS: 989 [M($C_{58}H_{62}O_{13}$) +Na$^+$]. Anal: Calcd for $C_{58}H_{62}O_{13}$: C, 72.03; H, 6.46. Found: C, 72.24; H, 6.63.

1',2,3,3',4,4'-Hexa-*O*-Benzylsucrose (5)

Route a

6,6'-Di-*O*-trityl-1',2,3,3',4,4'-hexa-*O*-benzylsucrose (**2**, 3.0 g, 2.19 mmol) was dissolved in dichloromethane–methanol (1:3, 60 mL) to which iodine (0.557 g, 2.19 mmol) was added, and the mixture was boiled under reflux for 4–5 h (TLC, 1:1 hexane–EtOAc). Aq 10% sodium thiosulfate was added until the mixture became colorless (~200 mL), and the product was extracted with diethyl ether (4 × 100 mL). The combined organic extracts were washed with water and brine, dried, and concentrated. Chromatography (4:1 → 2:1 → 3:2 hexane–EtOAc) of the residue afforded 1',2,3,3',4,4'-hexa-*O*-benzylsucrose (**5**) as a colorless oil (1.12 g, 58%), [α]$_D$ +40.8. ^{1}H NMR δ: 7.26 (m, 30H, Ar-H), 5.49 (d, 1H, $J_{1,2}$=2.9 Hz, H-1), 4.86 (d, 2H, $J_{6A,6B}$ = 10.6 Hz, H-6), 4.66 (m, 7H, H-3,3',4,4', Ar-CH_2), 4.46 (3d, 3H, Ar-CH_2), 4.32 (m, 2H, Ar-CH_2), 4.14 (m, 1H, H-5), 3.98 (m, 2H, H-6'), 3.82 (m, 2H, H-1'), 3.60 (m, 3H, H-5', Ar-CH_2), 3.50 (dd, 1H, $J_{1,2}$=3.2 Hz, $J_{2,3}$=9.6 Hz, H-2), 3.43 (dd, 2H, J=10.2 Hz, Ar-CH_2). ^{13}C NMR δ: 138.6, 138.3, 138.1, 138.0, 137.7 (C$_q$ benzyl groups), 128.4, 127.9, 127.8, 127.7, 127.6 (C$_{Ar}$), 103.9 (C-2'), 90.7 (C-1), 83.5, 81.7, 81.0, 79.9, 79.5, 77.6, and 71.3 (C-2,3,3',4,4',5,5'), 75.6, 75.0, 73.4, 73.1, 73.0, 72.5 (C-1', 6×O$\underline{C}$H$_2$Ph), 61.9, 61.0 (C-6,6'). *m/z*: 905 [M(C$_{54}$H$_{58}$O$_{11}$) +Na$^+$]. Anal: Calcd for C$_{54}$H$_{58}$O$_{11}$: C, 73.45; H, 6.62. Found: C, 73.23; H, 6.84.

Conventional acetylation of **5** gave virtually theoretical yield of material, which was identical in all respect with the above described substance **4**.

Route b

Compound **4** (0.22 g, 0.227 mmol, obtained from **3** as described above) was dissolved in methanol (25 mL) containing catalytic amounts of sodium methoxide, and the mixture was stirred for 3 h. After concentration, the residue was chromatographed (1:1 hexane–EtOAc) to give colorless oil (0.16 g, 82%), which was identical in all respect to the above-described substance **5**.

6,6'- Di-*O*-Allyl-1',2,3,3',4,4'-Hexa-*O*-Benzylsucrose (6)

A solution of 1',2,3,3',4,4'-hexa-*O*-benzylsucrose (**5**, 0.58 g, 0.66 mmol) in DMF (6 mL) was added dropwise to a slurry of NaH (60% dispersion in mineral oil, 0.095 g, 1.98 mmol) in DMF (10 mL) containing a catalytic amount of imidazole (~10 mg). The mixture was cooled to 0°C in an ice bath and stirred with exclusion of moisture for 30 min, allyl bromide (0.383 g, 0.274 mL) was then added dropwise, and the mixture was stirred for 5 h at rt. Excess of hydride was destroyed by careful addition of water, the mixture was partitioned between water and ether (50 mL each); the organic phase was washed with water, dried, and concentrated; and the product **6** was isolated by column chromatography (4:1 hexane–EtOAc) as a colorless oil (0.50 g, 79%), [α]$_D$ +29.9. ^{1}H NMR δ: 7.32 (m, 30H, Ar-H), 5.93 (m, 3H, H-1, CH-allyl groups), 5.30 (dd, 4H, $J_{HA,HB}$=17.3 Hz, CH_2-allyl groups), 5.18 (t, 4H, $J_{3',4'}$=10.8 Hz, H-3', H-4', Ar-CH_2), 4.94 (t, 3H, $J_{3,4}$=11.1 Hz, H-4, Ar-CH_2), 4.82 (dd, 3H, $J_{6A,6B}$=10.9 Hz, H-6, Ar-CH_2), 4.72 (d, 1H, J=10.8 Hz, Ar-CH_2), 4.61 (d, 1H, J=10.8 Hz, Ar-CH_2), 4.44 (d, 4H, $J_{6'A,6'B}$=7.7 Hz, H-6', Ar-CH_2), 4.14 (dd,

1H, $J_{1,2} = 5.7\,Hz$, $J_{2,3} = 12.7\,Hz$, H-2), 4.03 (dd, 4H, $J_{CH_2,CH} = 5.4\,Hz$, $J_{CH_2A,B} = 11.2\,Hz$, OCH_2CH=CH$_2$), 3.70 (t, 1H, $J_{2,3,4} = 10.4\,Hz$, H-3), 3.61 (m, 5H, H-1', H-5 Ar-CH_2), 3.46 (m, 2H, H-5', Ar-CH_2). ^{13}C NMR δ: 138.6, 138.4, 138.2 (C_q benzyl groups), 134.7, 134.0 ($\underline{C}$H allyl groups), 128.3, 128.2, 127.9, 127.8, 127.7, 127.6, 127.5, 127.4 (C_{Ar}), 117.2, 117.0 ($\underline{C}H_2$, allyl groups), 108.2 (C-2'), 102.7 (C-1), 84.7, 82.3, 77.9, 77.3, 77.0, 76.7 (C-2,3,3',4,4',5,5'), 75.7, 75.0, 74.8, 72.5, 70.3, 68.9 (C-1',6,6', O$\underline{C}H_2$Ph, O$\underline{C}H_2$CH=CH$_2$). ESI-MS: 985 [M($C_{60}H_{66}O_{11}$) +Na$^+$].

1',2,3,3',4,4'-Hexa-O-Benzyl-6,6'-Bis-(O-Tert-Butoxycarbonylmethylsucrose (7)

1',2,3,3',4,4'-Hexa-O-benzylsucrose (**5**, 0.33 g, 0.377 mmol) was dissolved in toluene (15 mL), to which 50% aq. sodium hydroxide (15 mL) and tetrabutylammonium bromide (0.01 g, 0.03 mmol) were added. *tert*-Butyl bromoacetate (0.44 g, 0.33 mL, 2.26 mmol) was added dropwise and the mixture was stirred at rt for 4 h. Water (30 mL) and diethyl ether (30 mL) were added to the mixture; the organic layer was separated, washed with water, dried, and concentrated; and the product was chromatographed (7:1 hexane–EtOAc) to afford 6,6'-*bis*-1',2,3,3',4,4'-hexa-O-benzyl-(O-*tert*-butoxycarbonylmethyl) sucrose (**7**, 0.35 g, 83%) as a colorless oil, [α]$_D$ +30.7. 1H NMR δ: 7.33 (m, 30H, Ar-H), 5.67 (d, $J1,2 = 3.64\,Hz$, 1H, H-1), 4.91 (d, 1H, $J = 10.9\,Hz$, Ar-CH_2), 4.86 (d, 1H, $J = 10.9\,Hz$, Ar-CH_2), 4.77 (d, 2H, $J = 10.9\,Hz$, Ar-CH_2), 4.72 (d, 2H, $J = 10.9\,Hz$, Ar-CH_2), 4.65 (m, 2H, $J_{3',4'} = 11.5\,Hz$, H-3', Ar-CH_2), 4.58 (d, 3H, $JHA,HB = 7.2\,Hz$, CH_2CO, Ar-CH_2), 4.5 (d, 2H, $JHA,HB = 7.1\,Hz$, CH_2CO, Ar-CH_2), 4.41 (t, $J = 10.18\,Hz$, 2H, Ar-CH_2), 4.13 (s, 2H, H-6), 4.04 (d, $J = 14.7\,Hz$, 2H, H-6), 3.96 (d, $J = 14.8\,Hz$, 2H, H-6'), 3.87 (m, 2H, H-4, H-5'), 3.80 (m, 2H H-4', H-5), 3.72 (t, 1H, $J3,4 = 10.9\,Hz$, H-3), 3.65 (m, 2H, H-2, Ar-CH_2), 3.52 (m, 3H, Ar-CH_2) 1.44 (s, 18H, *tert*butyl). 13C NMR δ: 169.4, 169.2 (2×CO), 139.0, 138.8, 138.3, 138.0 (6×Cq benzyl), 128.3, 127.9, 127.7, 127.6, 127.5 (CAr), 104.6 (C-2'), 90.1 (C-1), 83.8, 82.4, 81.9, 81.4, 81.3 (C-2,3,3',4,4',5,5'), 79.7 (C(CH$_3$)$_3$), 75.4, 74.8, 73.4, 72.9, 72.7, 72.5, 72.3, 71.1, 70.5, 69.8, 69.0 (6×OCH_2Ph, 2×CH_2COO, C-1',6,6'), 28.1 (C(CH$_3$)$_3$). ESI-MS: 1133.4 [M($C_{66}H_{78}O_{15}$) +Na$^+$]. Anal: Calcd for $C_{66}H_{78}O_{15}×H_2O$: C, 70.21; H, 7.09. Found: C, 70.18; H, 7.13.

1',2,3,3',4,4'-Hexa-O-Benzyl-6,6'-Bis-(O-2-Hydroxyethyl) Sucrose (8)

Route a

6,6'-Di-O-allyl-1',2,3,3',4,4'-hexa-O-benzylsucrose (**6**) (0.39 g, 0.409 mmol) was dissolved in THF (6 mL) and a solution of NaIO$_4$ (0.526 g, 2.45 mmol) in H$_2$O (6 mL) was added, followed by OsO$_4$ (0.04 mL of a 2% solution in toluene). The resulting mixture was stirred at rt for 1.5 h and then partitioned between water (100 mL) and ether (80 mL). The organic phase was separated, dried, and concentrated. The residue was dissolved in 1:1 CH$_2$Cl$_2$–MeOH (10 mL) and cooled to −78°C. NaBH$_4$ (0.21 g, 5.54 mmol) was added in several portions, the mixture was stirred for 1 h at −78°C and then for 2 h at rt. Water (20 mL) was added, and the product was extracted with CH$_2$Cl$_2$ (25 mL). The organic layer was dried and concentrated, and the crude product was chromatographed (hexane/EtOAc, 1:1 then 2:3) to afford the title compound **8** as a pale yellow oil (0.185 g, 47%), [α]$_D$ +44.3. IR (film) ν: 2916, 2866, 1454, 1086, 1072, 736, 697 cm^{-1}; ^{1}H NMR δ: 7.30 (m, 30H, Ar-H), 6.13 (d, $J_{1,2} = 3.2\,Hz$,

1H, H-1), 4.96 (d, 1H, $J=10.9\,Hz$, Ar-CH_2), 4.79 (dd, 1H, $J_{1,2}=3.8\,Hz$, $J_{2,3}=11.2\,Hz$, H-2), 4.68 (m, 2H, Ar-CH_2), 4.63 (m, 6H, H-6,H-6', H-3, H-4), 4.48 (m, 5H, Ar-CH_2), 4.13 (m, 2H, H-5, Ar-CH_2), 3.90 (m, 3H, Ar-CH_2, H-5'), 3.64 (m, 4H, CH_2 from 2-hydroxyethyl), 3.57 (s, 1H, Ar-CH_2), 3.53 (m, 2H, CH_2 from 2-hydroxyethyl), 3.46 (m, 2H, CH_2 from 2-hydroxyethyl), 3.39 (t, 2H, $J=11.0\,Hz$), 3.30 (m, 4H, H-1',H-3', H-4').

^{13}C NMR δ: 139.2, 138.8, 138.2, 138.1, 137.9 ($6\times C_q$ benzyl), 128.3, 128.1, 127.9, 127.7 (C_{Ar}), 104.0 (C-2'), 87.7 (C-1), 83.3, 82.0, 79.0, 78.9, and 71.9 (C-2,3,3',4,4',5,5'), 75.2, 74.6, 73.4, 73.0, 72.9, 72.5, 72.3, 68.4, 61.7 (C-1',6,6', $6\times O\underline{C}H_2Ph$, $4\times CH_2$ from 2-hydroxyethyl). ESI-MS: 993.5 [M($C_{58}H_{66}O_{13}$) +Na$^+$]. Anal: Calcd for $C_{58}H_{66}O_{13}\times0.5$ H_2O: C, 71.07; H, 6.89. Found: C, 71.01; H, 7.12.

Route b

Compound **7** (0.150 g, 0.135 mmol) was dissolved in dry THF (12 mL), to which a suspension of LiAlH$_4$ (0.107 g, 2.804 mmol) in THF (4 mL) was added, and the mixture was stirred at rt for 3 h. EtOAc (10 mL) was added, followed by aqueous saturated sodium sulfate solution (2 mL) to destroy excess of the hydride. Inorganic salts were filtered off and washed with EtOAc. The solvents were removed in vacuum and chromatography of the residue (1:2 hexane–EtOAc) gave **8** (0.09 g, 69%), which was identical in all respects to the independently prepared material **8** described above.

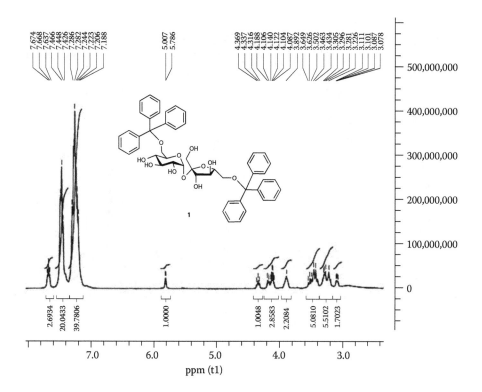

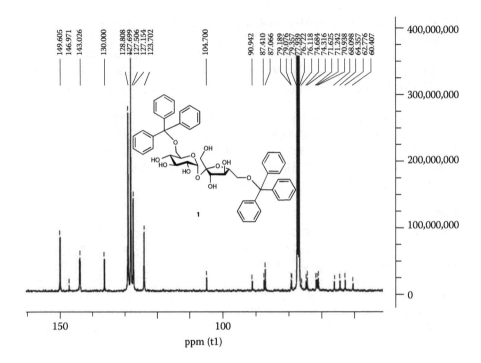

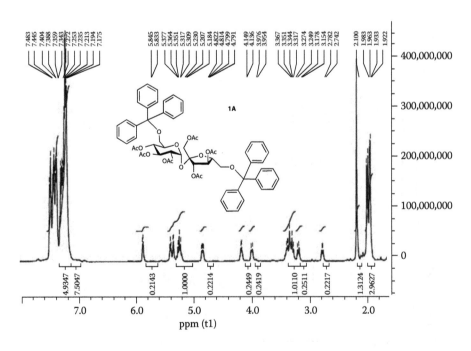

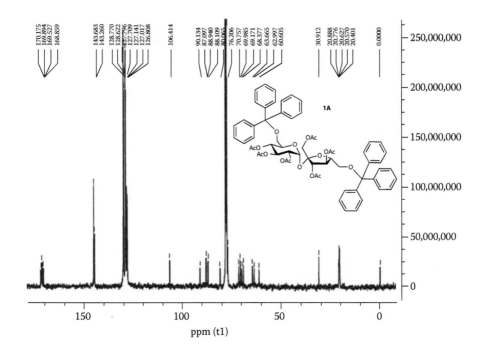

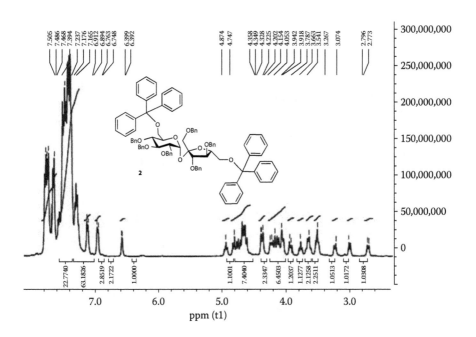

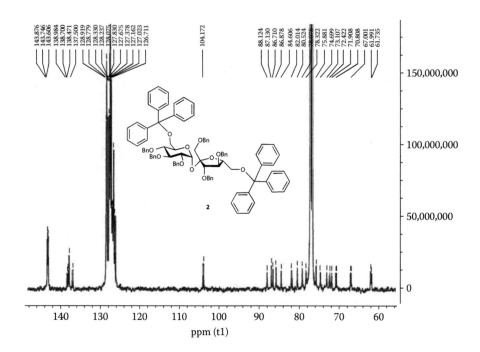

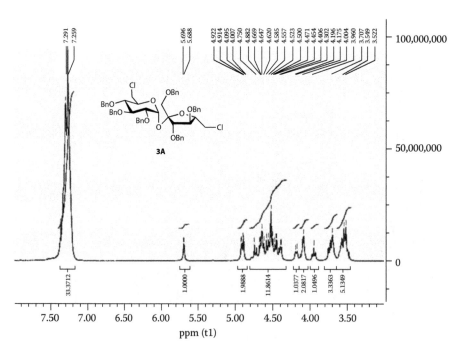

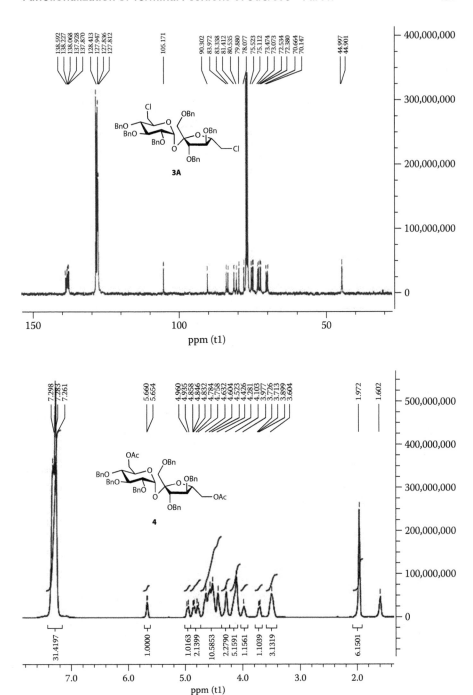

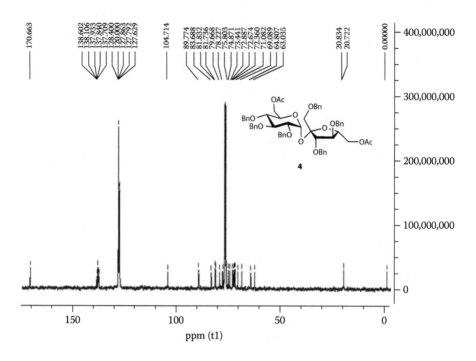

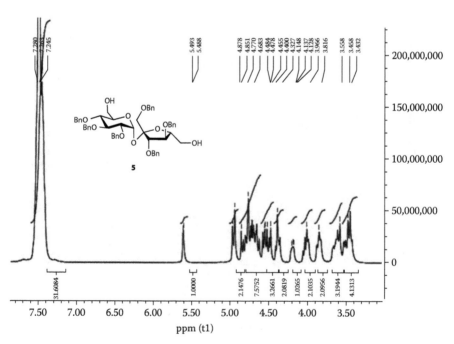

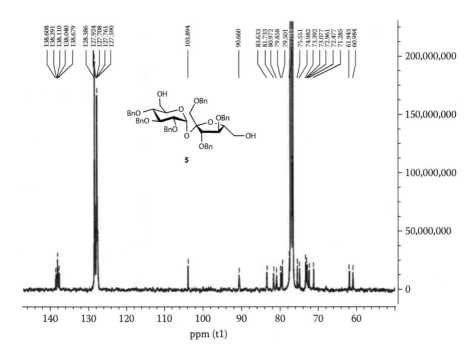

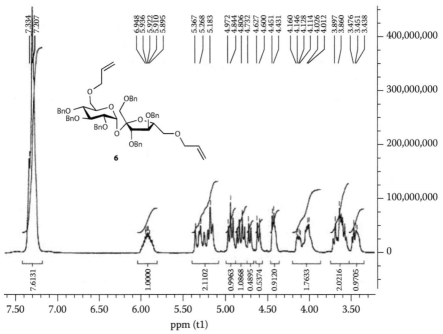

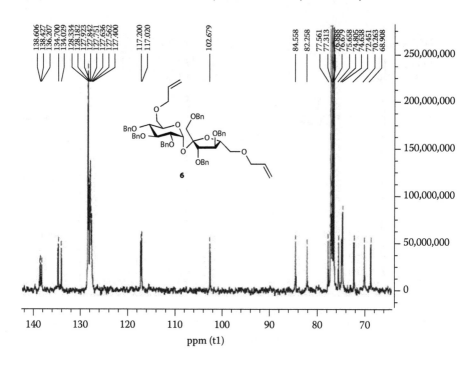

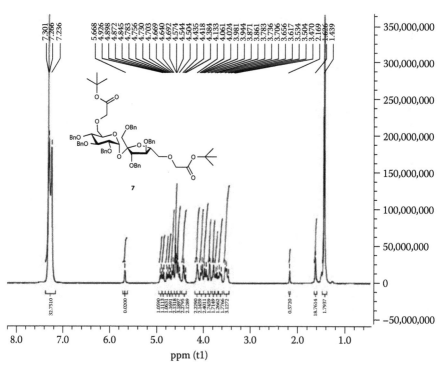

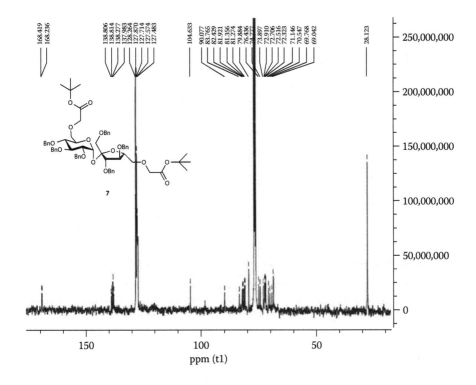

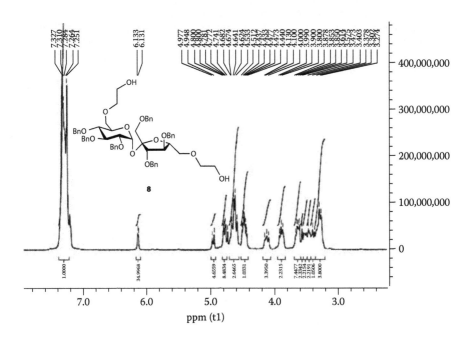

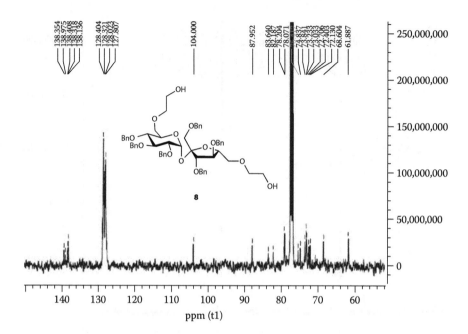

REFERENCES

1. Mach, M.; Jarosz, S.; Listkowski, A., *J. Carbohydr. Chem.*, 2001, *20(6)*, 485–493; Jarosz, S.; Listkowski, A., *J. Carbohydr. Chem.*, 2003, *22*, 753–763.
2. Szarek, W. A.; Zamojski, A.; Tiwari, K. N.; Ison, E.R., *Tetrahedron Lett.*, 1986, *27*, 3827; Ramasamy, K. S.; Bandaru, R.; Averett, D., *Synth. Comm.*, 1999, *29*, 2881–2894.
3. Whistler, R. L.; Anisuzzaman, A. K. M., *Methods Carbohydr. Chem.*, 1980, *8*, 227–231.
4. Jarosz, S.; Listkowski, A.; Lewandowski, B.; Ciunik, Z.; Brzuszkiewicz, A., *Tetrahedron*, 2005, *61*, 8485–8493.

Index

A

**2-Acetamido-4,6-*O*-benzylidene-
2-deoxy-D-glucopyranose**
preparation, 200
spot visualization, 200
Acetolysis
deoxysugars, of, 3
***N*-Acetylglucosamine**
benzylidenation of, 200
***N*-Acetylneuraminic acid**
acetylated glycal, preparation, 245
benzyl glycosides NMR data, 251, 255
chloride, NMR data, 246, 249
Arabinofuranose
1,2,3,5-tetra-*O*-benzoyl-α-D-, 234
1,2,3,5-tetra-*O*-benzoyl-α,β-D-, 234
Arabinopyranose
1,2,3,4-tetra-*O*-benzoyl-α-D-, 234
α-D-Arabinofuranoside
p-tolyl 2,3,5-tri-*O*-benzoyl-1-thio-
preparation, 343
Azido-functionalized carbohydrates
preparation, 177
Azobisisobutyronitrile (AIBN)
radical initiator, 55

B

BAIB/TEMPO oxidation, 99, 102
***S*-Benzoxazolyl (SBox) glycosides**, 188
Benzylidenation
N-acetylglucosamine, of, 200
[Bis(acetoxy)iodo]benzene (BAIB), 100
**Bis(trimethylsilyl)trifluoroacetamide
(BTSFA)**, 84
Butenolides, pyranose-fused, 137
**4-[(*tert*-Butyloxycarbonyl)glycylamido]
benzyl 5-acetamido-3,5-dideoxy-
D-*glycero*-D-*galacto*-non-2-
ulopyranosidonic acid**
preparation, 256
**BTSFA, *see* Bis(trimethylsilyl)
trifluoroacetamide**

C

CAN (ceric ammonium nitrate)
chemoselective removal of the *N*-benzyl
group with, 262

Cellobiose
benzyl 2,3,6,2′,3′6′-hexa-*O*-benzyl β
glycoside, 221
Cellobioside
benzyl 2,3,6,2′,3′6′-hexa-*O*-benzyl-β-, 224
benzyl 2,3,6,2′,3′4′-hexa-*O*-benzyl-β-, 224
benzyl 2,3,6,2′,3′-penta-*O*-benzyl-
4′,6′-*O*-benzylidene-β-, 223
benzyl 2,3,6,2′,3′-penta-*O*-benzyl-
4′,6′-*O*-benzylidene-α-, 223
"Click chemistry," 95
Copper (I)-catalyzed 1,3-cycloaddition, 96
Cross-coupling reactions, 91
Cross-metathesis, 285

D

Debenzylation
regioselective of *C*-glycosylpropene, 167
Dehydration
pyranosides, of, 15
Deoxygenation
using hypophosphorous acid, 56
1-Deoxynojirimycin
iminoxylitols related to, 259
Diazomethane
methyl ester preparation with, 308
Diazo transfer, 206
Diels–Alder reactions, cycloaddition, 296
Dimethyl sulfide
methylation, catalysis by, 27
**Diphenylsulfoxide-trifluoromethanesulfonic
(triflic) anhydride**
thioglycosides activator, 67
**Dithioacetals, *see* Ethylene dithioacetals
preparation**

E

Ethylene dithioacetals preparation
D-galactose ethylene dithioacetal, 350
D-glucose ethylene dithioacetal, 350–351
D-mannose ethylene dithioacetal, 351–354
***Exo*-glycals**, 367
2,6-anhydro-3,4,5,7-tetra-*O*-benzoyl-
1-deoxy-D-*gluco*-hept-1-enitol, 370
3,4,5,7-tetra-*O*-acetyl-2,6-anhydro-1-
deoxy-D-*galacto*-hept-1-enitol, 370
3,4,5-tri-*O*-acetyl-2,6-anhydro-1-
deoxy-D-*arabino*-hex-1-enitol, 370

4,5,7-tri-*O*-acetyl-2,6-anhydro-1,3-dideoxy-3-phthalimido-D-*gluco*-hept-1-enitol, 370
Exomethylene glycals, 368

F

Fucopyranosylhydroxylamines, 377
Fructopyranose
1,2:4,5-di-*O*-isopropylidene-3-*O*-[(methylsulfanyl)thiocarbonyl]-β-D-
deoxygenation of, 59
preparation, 58

G

Galactofuranose
1,6-anhydro-α-D-, 271
1,6-anhydro-2,3,5-tri-*O*-acetyl-α-D-, 271
1,6-anhydro-2,3,5-tri-*O*-benzoyl-α-D-, 271
1,2,3,5,6-penta-*O*-benzoyl-α,β-D-, 233
β-D-Galactofuranoside
methyl 2,3,5-tri-*O*-benzoyl-6-*O*-benzyl-, 270
Galactopyranose
1-*O*-acetyl-2,3,4,6-tetra-*O*-benzyl-β-D-, 216
6-*O*-benzyl-1,2:3,4-di-*O*-isopropylidene-α-D-, 270
2,3,4,6-tetra-*O*-acetylglycosyl bromide, 280
2,3,4,6-tetra-*O*-benzyl-D-, 216
2,3,6-tri-*O*-benzyl-preparation, 216
β-D-Galactopyranoside
1-azido-3,6-dioxaoct-8-yl 2,3,4,6-tetra-*O*-acetyl-, 177
methyl 3-*O*-benzyl-
methylation of, 30
methyl 3-*O*-benzyl-2,4,6-tri-*O*-methyl-
preparation of, 30
methyl 3-*O*-benzyl-2,6-di-*O*-methyl-
preparation, 31
methyl 2,3-di-*O*-methyl-6-*O*-trityl-
preparation, 32
methyl 2,3,4-tri-*O*-methyl-6-*O*-trityl-
preparation, 32
NMR data for, 32
methyl 6-*O*-trityl-
methylation of, 31
phenyl 4,6-*O*-benzylidene-2-deoxy-1-thio-2-(2,2,2-trichlorethoxycarbamido)-, 118
phenyl 2-amino-2-*N*-benzyl-4,6-*O*-benzylidene-2,3-*N,O*-carbonyl-2-deoxy-1-thio-β-D-, 119
α-D-Galactopyranosyl
chloride, 2,3,4,6-tetra-*O*-benzyl-
preparation, 77
3-*C*-(prop-1-ene), 85

β-D-Galactopyranosyl
acetylated *N*-hydroxysuccinimide, 29
hydroxylamine, preparation, 291
(2,3,4,6-tetra-*O*-acetyl)-3-prop-1-ene, 281
Galactose
acetobromo preparation, 280
ethylene dithioacetal preparation, 350
gem-Difluorocarba preparation via TIBAL-induced rearrangement, 132
Galacturonate, methyl
bromide, 308
methyl (allyl β-D-), 309
methyl (allyl 4-*O*-acetyl-β-D-), 309
methyl (allyl 4-*O*-acetyl-2,3-di-*O*-benzyl-β-D-), 310
methyl (allyl 4-*O*-benzoyl-β-D-), 310
methyl (allyl 4-*O*-benzoyl-2,3-di-*O*-benzyl-β-D-), 310
methyl (allyl 2,3-di-*O*-benzyl-β-D-)-, 311
methyl (allyl 2,3,4-tri-*O*-acetyl-β-D-), 308
1,2,3,4-tetra-*O*-acetyl-α-D-, 308
Galacturonic acid
methyl 1,2,3,4-tetra-*O*-acetyl-α-D-uronate, 307
Glucofuranose
1,2:5,6-di-*O*-isopropylidene-α-D-
deoxygenation of, 58
oxidation to 3-ulose, 141
Glucopyranose
2-acetamido-4,6-*O*-benzylidene-2-deoxy-D-
preparation, 200
1,6-anhydro-4-*O*-benzyl-2-methyl-β-D-
deoxygenation of, 56
1,6-anhydro 4-*O*-benzyl-2-deoxy-2-*C*-methyl-3-*O*-[(methylsulfanyl)thiocarbonyl]-β-D-
preparation, 59
deoxygenation of, 59
2-azido-4,6-*O*-benzylidene-2-deoxy-α,β-D-
preparation of, 208
1,3,4,6-tetra-*O*-acetyl-2-azido-2-deoxy-α,β-D-
preparation, 207
1,3,4,6-tetra-*O*-acetyl-2-*C*-(4,6-di-*O*-acetyl-2,3-dideoxy-α-D-*erythro*-hex-2-enopyranosyl)-2-deoxy-α/β-D-glucopyranose
preparation, 162
2,3,6-tri-*O*-benzyl-D-, 216
α-D-Glucopyranoside
methyl 6-*O*-trityl-
methylation of, 32
methyl 2,3,4-tri-*O*-methyl-6-*O*-trityl-
preparation, 32

methyl 2,3,4-tri-*O*-benzyl-6-*O*-(methyl
  4-*O*-acetyl-2,3-di-*O*-benzyl-β-D-
  mannopyranosyluronate)-, 69
β-D-Glucopyranoside
  1,3-benzoxazol-2-yl
    2,3,4,6-tetra-*O*-aceatyl-1-thio-
    preparation, 182
  benzyl 2,3,4,6-tetra-*O*-benzyl-β-D-
    galactopyranosyl-(1→4)-2,3,6-
    tri-*O*-benzyl-
    preparation, 215
  4,5-dihydro-1,3-thiazol-2-yl
    2,3,4,6-tetra-*O*-acetyl-1-thio-, 190
  ethyl 2,3,4,6-tetra-*O*-acetyl-1-thio-, 191
  methyl (phenyl 5-acetamido-4,7,8,9-
    tetra-*O*-acetyl-3,5-dideoxy-
  methyl 6-benzoyl-2,3-di-*O*-benzyl-
    4-*O*-methyl-
    preparation
  methyl 2,3-di-*O*-benzyl-6-*O*-benzoyl-
    methylation of, 33
    preparation, 29
    NMR data for, 29, 33
  methyl 2,3-di-*O*-benzyl-4,6-di-*O*-methyl-
    preparation, 35
  methyl (phenyl 3-*O*-benzoyl-2-deoxy-2-
    phthalimido-1-thio-)uronate, 102
  phenyl 3-*O*-benzoyl-2-deoxy-2-
    phtalimido-1-thio-
    NMR data for, 102
    preparation, 100
    TEMPO oxidation of, 102
  phenyl 2-amino-2-*N*-benzyl-4,6-*O*-
    benzylidene-2,3-*N,O*-carbonyl-
    2-deoxy-1-thio-, 117
  phenyl 2-amino-4,6-*O*-benzylidene-2,3-
    N,O-carbonyl-2-deoxy-2-*N*-(4-
    methoxybenzyl)-1-thio, 117
  phenyl 2-amino-4,6-*O*-benzylidene-
    2,3-*N,O*-carbonyl-2-deoxy-2-*N*-
    (4-nitrobenzyl)-1-thio-, 117
  phenyl 2-amino-4,6-*O*-benzylidene-
    2,3-*N,O*-carbonyl-2-deoxy-2-*N*-
    (prop-2-enyl)-1-thio-β-, 118
  phenyl 2-amino-4,6-*O*-benzylidene-
    2,3-*N,O*-carbonyl-2-deoxy-2-*N*-
    (prop-2-ynyl-1-thio-, 118
  phenyl 4,6-*O*-benzylidene-2-deoxy-1-thio-2-
    (2,2,2-trichlorethoxycarbamido)-, 116
  phenyl 2,3,4,6-tetra-*O*-acetyl-1-thio-, 189
  2-thio-D-*glycero*-α-D-*galacto*-non-2-
    ulopyranosid)onate
    preparation, 183
  p-tolyl 2,3,4,6-tetra-*O*-acetyl-1-thio-, 193
  2-trimethylsilylethyl 2-amino-2-*N*-
    benzyl-4,6-*O*-benzylidene-
    2,3-*N,O*-carbonyl-2-deoxy-, 116

2-trimethylsilylethyl 4,6-*O*-benzylidene-
  2-deoxy-2-(2,2,2-
  trichlorethoxycarbamido)-, 115
α-D-Glucopyranosyl chloride
  2,3,4,6-tetra-*O*-acetyl-
    preparation, 76
β-D-Glucopyranosyluronic Acid
  phenyl 3-*O*-benzoyl-2-deoxy-2-
    phthalimido-1-thio
    preparation, 102
Glucose
  ethylene dithioacetal
    preparation, 350
Glycal
  N-acetylneuraminic acid, of, 245
  dimerization, 159
  exo-, 367
  exomethylene, 368
**4-(Glycylamido)benzyl 5-acetamido-3,5-
  dideoxy-D-*glycero*-D-*galacto*-
  non-2-ulopyranosidonic acid**
    preparation, 256
Glycosides
  conversion (acetolysis) into 1-*O*-acetates, 4, 5
C-Glycosylation
  from unprotected *O*-glycosides, 83
O-Glycosylation
  chemoselective, by preactivation, 43
  Koenigs–Knorr, 176
  SnCl₄-catalyzed, 177
Glycosyl chlorides
  glycopyranoses/glycofuranoses,
    preparation of, 73
C-Glycosylpropene
  regioselective debenzylation, 167
Grubbs' second-generation catalyst, 286

H

Hanessian's stain, 261
Hept-1-enitol
  2,6-anhydro-3,4,5,7-tetra-*O*-benzoyl-
    1-deoxy-D-*gluco*-, 370
  3,4,5,7-tetra-*O*-acetyl-2,6-anhydro-
    1-deoxy-D-*galacto*-, 370
  4,5,7-tri-*O*-acetyl-2,6-anhydro-1,3-
    dideoxy-3-phthalimido-D-*gluco*-, 370
Hex-1-enitol
  3,4,5-tri-*O*-acetyl-2,6-anhydro-1-
    deoxy-D-*arabino*-, 370
**Hex-2-and hex-3-enopyranoside
  enol ethers**, 11
  preparation, 16
Hydrazinolysis, 291
Hydroxylamine
  6-deoxy-α-L-galactopyranosyl, 380
  6-deoxy-β-L-galactopyranosyl, 380

O-α-L-fucopyranosyl, 380
O-β-L-fucopyranosyl, 380
O-β-D-galactopyranosyl, 291
Hypophosphorous acid
　use in deoxygenation, 53

I

Iminosugars, 259
1,5-Iminoxylitol
　1,5-di-(1-/2-benzotriazolyl)-N-benzyl-
　　1,5-dideoxy-, 261
　rac-(1R,5R)-2,3,4-tri-O-acetyl-1,5-di-C-
　　allyl-1,5-dideoxy-, 262
　2,3,4-tri-O-acetyl-1,5-di-C-allyl-N-
　　benzyl-1,5-dideoxy-, 262
Iodocyclization, 84, 168, 169
Iodoethers, bicyclic, 85
p-Iodophenyl-α-D-mannopyranoside
　use in Sonogashira cross-coupling
　　reactions, 91
**1,2:5,6-di-O-isopropylidene-α-D-ribo-
　hexofuranosid-3-ulose**
　preparation, 141

K

Knochel's procedure, 260
Koenigs–Knorr glycosylation, 176

L

Lactose
　benzyl per-O-benzyl-β-glycoside, 215
　benzylation, 215
β-Lactoside
　1-azido-3,6-dioxaoct-8-yl
　　2,3,6,2′,3′,4′,6′-hepta-O-acetyl-, 178
Levoglucosenone
　analogue preparation, 295
LiBr
　as solubilizer for N-acetyl-D-
　　glucosamine, 200
Linker (spacer) for glycoconjugates
　introduction into sugars, 177

M

Madsen and Lauritsen benzylation, 306
Methanolic HCl
　preparation, 309
α-D-Mannofuranosyl chloride
　2,3:5,6-di-O-isopropylidene-
　　preparation, 77
　2,3,4,6-tetra-O-acetyl-
　　preparation, 77

α-D-Mannopyranoside
　p-iodophenyl 2,3,4,6-tetra-O-acetyl-
　　in palladium-catalyzed
　　　Sonogashira coupling, 92
　methyl 2,3-O-isopropylidene-4-O-
　　(methylthio)thiocarbonyl-
　　prop-2-ynyl 2,3,4,6-tetra-O-acetyl-, 275
　　"click chemistry" with, 96
　6-O-triphenylmethyl-
　　deoxygenation of, 57
　　preparation, 57
　propargyl 2,3,4,6-tetra-O-acetyl-
　　preparation, 275
Mannose
　ethylene dithioacetal
　　preparation, 351
Me₂S, 27
Methylation
　Purdie, enhanced rate of, 27
　selective, of uronic acids, 102
**Methyl (2R)-2-acetamido-3-(α-D-
　galactopyranosylpropylthio)
　propanoate**
　preparation by non-photochemical
　　reaction, 86
　preparation by photochemical reaction, 85
**Methyl (5-acetamido-4,7,8,9-tetra-O-
　acetyl-3,5-dideoxy-2,6-anhydro-
　D-glycero-D-galacto-non-2-
　enopyranos)onate**
　preparation, 249
**Methyl (5-acetamido-4,7,8,9-tetra-
　O-acetyl-3,5-dideoxy-β-D-
　glycero-D-galacto-non-2-
　ulopyranosyl)onate chloride**
　preparation, 246
Methyl glycuronates
　preparation of, 100
**Methyl (5-acetamido-4,7,8,9-tetra-
　O-acetyl-3,5-dideoxy-2,6-
　anhydro-D-glycero-D-galacto-
　non-2-enopyranos)onate**
　large scale preparation, 249
　small scale preparation, 249
**Methyl (5-acetamido-4,7,8,9-tetra-
　O-acetyl-3,5-dideoxy-β-D-
　glycero-D-galacto-non-2-
　ulopyranosyl)onate chloride
　preparation**
　large scale preparation, 247
　small scale preparation, 246
Methyl sulfide/dimethyl sulfide
　methylation, catalysis by, 27
**(E)-Methyl 4-(2,3,4,6-tetra-O-acetyl-
　β-D-galactopyranosyl)
　but-2-enoate**
　preparation, 286

Methyl thiosialoside, 182
**Methyl 2-{[4-(2,3,4,6-tetra-*O*-acetyl-α-D-
   mannopyranosyloxy)methyl]-1*H*-
   1,2,3-triazol-1-yl}acetate**
   preparation, 96
Mitsunobu reaction, 392

N

**4-[(4-Nitrophenoxy)adipoylglycylamido]
   benzyl 5-acetamido-3,5-dideoxy-
   D-*glycero*-D-*galacto*-non-2-
   ulopyranosidonic acid**
   preparation, 257
Nucleotides
   by prosphoramidate approach, 107

P

Prop-1-ene
   3-*C*-(3,4,6-tri-*O*-benzyl-α-D-
      glucopyranosyl), 169
   3-*C*-(3,4,6-tri-*O*-benzyl-α-D-
      fructofuranosyl), 170
Purdie methylation
   enhanced rate by dimethyl sulfide, 28
Pyridinium dichromate
   in oxidation of carbohydrates, 141
Pyridinium perchlorate
   catalyst for benzylidenation, 200

Q

**Quantitative structure activity
   relationship (QSAR)**, 92

R

α-L-Rhamnopyranose
   1,3-di-*O*-acetyl-2,4-di-*O*-benzyl-, 7
   1-*O*-acetyl-2,3,4-tri-*O*-benzyl-, 6
   2,3,4-tri-*O*-acetyl-α-L-rhamnopyranosyl-
      (1→3)-α-*O*-acetyl-2,4-di-*O*-benzyl-, 6
α-L-Rhamnopyranoside
   3-azidopropyl 2-acetamido-3,6-di-*O*-
      benzyl-2,4-dideoxy-β-D-*threo*-
      hex-3-enopyranosyl-(1→4)-2,3,6-
      tri-*O*-benzyl-β-D-glucopyranosyl-
      (1→2)-3,4-di-*O*-benzyl-, 17

S

Samarium iodide
   C-sialylation mediator, 239, 240
***C*-Sialylation**, 240
**Sonogashira coupling cross-coupling
   reactions**, 91

Sucrose
   1′-*O*-benzyloxymethyl-6,6′-di-*O-tert*-
      butyldiphenylsilyl-
      2,3,3′,4,4′-penta-*O*-benzyl, 402
   1′-*O*-acetyl-2,3,3′,4,4′-penta-*O*-benzyl-
      6,6′-di-*O-p*-nitrobenzoyl-, 392
   6,6′-di-*O*-acetyl-2,3,3′,4,4′-penta-*O*-
      benzyl-1′-*O*-benzyloxymethyl-, 392
   1′,6,6′-tri-*O*-acetyl-2,3,3′,4,4′-penta-
      O-benzyl-, 391
   2,3,3′,4,4′-penta-*O*-benzyl-1′-*O*-
      benzyloxymethyl-6′-*O-t*-
      butyldiphenylsilyl-, 393
   2,3,3′,4,4′-penta-*O*-benzyl-1′-*O*-
      benzyloxymethyl-6,6′-di-*O-t*-
      butyldiphenylsilyl-, 393
   2,3,3′,4,4′-penta-*O*-benzyl-1′-*O*-
      benzyloxymethyl-, 392
   2,3,3′,4,4′-penta-*O*-benzyl-1′-*O*-
      benzyloxymethyl-6,6′-di-*O-p*-
      nitrobenzoyl-, 392
   2,3,3′,4,4′-penta-*O*-benzyl-,
      1′-*O*-benzyloxymethyl-, 392
   1′,2,3,3′,4,4′-hexa-*O*-benzyl-, 419
   6,6′-*bis*-*O*-(2-hydroxyethyl)-
      1′,2,3,3′,4,4′-hexa-*O*-benzyl, 418
   6,6′-di-*O*-acetyl-1′,2,3,3′,4,4′-hexa-*O*-
      benzyl, 418
   6,6′-di-*O*-allyl-1′,2,3,3′,4,4′-hexa-
      O-benzyl, 419
   6,6′-di-*O*-trityl, 416
   1′,2,3,3′,4,4′-hexa-*O*-acetyl-6,6′-di-*O*-trityl, 417
   1′,2,3,3′,4,4′-hexa-*O*-benzyl-6,6′-*bis*-
      (*O-tert*-butoxycarbonylmethyl), 420
   1′,2,3,3′,4,4′-hexa-*O*-benzyl-6,6′-*bis*-
      (*O*-2-hydroxyethyl), 420
   1′,2,3,3′,4,4′-hexa-*O*-benzyl-6,6′-
      dichloro-6,6′-dideoxy, 418
   1′,2,3,3′,4,4′-hexa-*O*-benzyl-6,6′-di-
      O-trityl, 417
   1′,2,3,3′,4,4′-hexa-*O*-benzyl, 419
   1′,6,6′-tri-*O*-trityl, 389
   2,3,3′,4,4′-penta-*O*-acetyl-1′,6,6′-tri-
      O-trityl-, 390
   2,3,3′,4,4′-penta-*O*-benzyl-1′,6,6′-tri-
      O-trityl-, 391
   2,3,3′,4,4′-penta-*O*-benzyl, 391
   2,3,3′,4,4′-penta-*O*-benzyl-6,6′-di-*O-p*-
      nitrobenzoyl-, 392
   2,3,3′,4,4′-penta-*O*-benzyl-6,6′-di-*O-p*-
      nitrobenzoyl, 392
   2,3,3′,4,4′-penta-*O*-benzyl-1′-*O*-
      benzyloxymethyl-
      6,6′-di-*O-p*-nitrobenzoyl, 392
   2,3,3′,4,4′-penta-*O*-benzyl-1′-*O*-
      benzyloxymethyl-
      6-*O-tert*-butyldiphenylsilyl, 404

2,3,3',4,4'-penta-*O*-benzyl-1'-*O*-
  benzyloxymethyl, 392
2,3,3',4,4'-penta-*O*-benzyl, 391
2,3,3',4,4'-penta-*O*-benzyl-1',6,6'-
  tri-*O*-trityl, 391
1',6,6'-tri-*O*-trityl, 390
N,N'-Sulfuryldiimidazole
  in preparation of enol ethers, 11

T

TCT/DMF chlorination
  mechanism, 74
    glycosyl chlorides, preparation with, 76
TEMPO/BAIB oxidation, 99, 102
Thioglycosides
  activation with Ph$_2$SO and Tf$_2$O, 67
  preparation from glycosyl halides, 181
  preparation from peracetates, 187
  remote activation, 188
Thioimidates
  preparation from glycosyl halides, 181
  preparation from peracetates, 187
TIBAL-induced rearrangement, 132
***p*-Toluenesulfenyl chloride**
  preparation, 46
  use in chemoselective *O*-glycosylation, 46, 47
Tosylhydrazone of
  3,4,5,7-tetra-*O*-acetyl-2,6-anhydro-
    D-*glycero*-D-*gulo*-heptose, 358
  3,4,5,7-tetra-*O*-acetyl-2,6-anhydro-
    D-*glycero*-L-manno-heptose, 358
  3,4,5,7-tetra-*O*-benzoyl-D-glycero-
    D-gulo-heptose, 358
  4,5,7-tri-*O*-acetyl-2,6-anhydro-3-
    deoxy-3-phthalimido-D-*glycero*-
    D-*gulo*-heptose, 359
  3,4,5-tri-*O*-acetyl-2,6-anhydro-
    D-manno-hexose, 359
**N-2,2,2-Trichloroethoxycarbonyl (Troc)-
  protected 2-aminoglycosides**
  conversion into *N*-alkylated 2,3-*N,O*-
    carbonyl-protected glycosides, 113
Trifluoromethanesulfonyl azide (TfN$_3$)
  preparation, 207

U

Uridine
  5'-(2-acetamido-2-deoxy-α-D-glucopyranosyl
    diphosphate) disodium salt, 109

Uronate
  bromide, 308
  methanolysis of, 328
  methyl l,2,3,4-tetra-*O*-acetyl-α-D-
    galactopyran, 308
  methyl 1-*O*-acetyl-2,3,5-tri-*O*-
    benzoyl-α-D-galactofuran, 331
  methyl 1-*O*-acetyl-2,3,5-tri-*O*-
    benzoyl-α,β-D-galactofuran, 331
  methyl 1-*O*-acetyl-2,3,5-tri-*O*-
    benzoyl-β-D-galactofuran, 332
  methyl (4-*O*-acetyl-2,3-di-*O*-
    benzyl-β-D-mannopyranosyl)-
    (1→6)-(methyl
    2,3,4-tri-*O*-benzyl-α-D-
    glucopyranosid), 69
  methyl (allyl β-D-galactopyranosid), 309
  methyl (allyl 2,3,4-tri-*O*-acetyl-β-D-
    galactopyranosid), 308
  methyl (allyl 4-*O*-acetyl-β-D-
    galactopyranosid), 309
  methyl (allyl 4-*O*-acetyl-2,3-di-
    O-benzyl-β-D-galactopyranosid), 310
  methyl (allyl 4-*O*-benzoyl-β-D-
    galactopyranosid), 310
  methyl (allyl 4-*O*-benzoyl-2,3-di-
    O-benzyl-β-D-galactopyranosid), 310
  methyl (allyl 2,3-di-*O*-benzyl-β-D-
    galactopyranosid), 311
  methyl (ethyl 2,3,5-tri-*O*-benzoyl-1-
    thio-α,β-D-galactofuranosid), 327, 332
  methyl (ethyl 2,3,5-tri-*O*-benzoyl-1-
    thio-β-D-galactofuranosid), 332
  methyl (methyl α-D-galactofuranosid), 330
  methyl (methyl α,β-D-galactofuranosid), 330
  methyl (methyl β-D-galactofuranosid), 330
  methyl (methyl 2,3,5-tri-*O*-
    benzoyl-α-D-galactofuranosid), 331
  methyl (methyl 2,3,5-tri-*O*-benzoyl-
    α,β-D-galactofuranosid), 330
  methyl (methyl 2,3,5-tri-*O*-benzoyl-
    β-D-galactofuranosid), 331
  tert-butyl 1,2:3,4-di-*O*-isopropylidene-
    α-D-galactopyran, 330

V

Vilsmeier-Haack (V-H) electrophile, 74

W

Wittig olefination, 139–141

Milton Keynes UK
Ingram Content Group UK Ltd.
UKHW021900071024
449327UK00021B/1595